Pediatric Kidney Disease

A CASE-BASED APPROACH

Pediatric Kidney Disease

A CASE-BASED APPROACH

Farahnak Assadi, MD
Distinguished Emeritus Professor and Chief
Department of Pediatrics
Division of Nephrology
Rush University Medical College
Chicago, Illinois

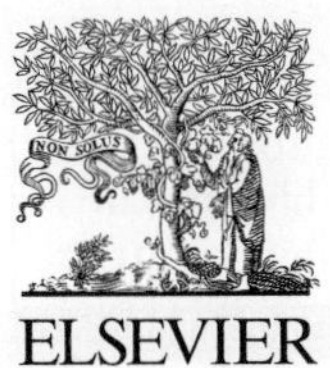

ELSEVIER

Elsevier
1600 John F. Kennedy Blvd.
Ste 1800
Philadelphia, PA 19103-2899

PEDIATRIC KIDNEY DISEASE: A CASE-BASED APPROACH ISBN: 978-0-44328-337-6

Executive Content Strategist: Nancy Anastasi Duffy
Senior Content Development Specialist: Ambika Kapoor
Publishing Services Manager: Deepthi Unni
Project Manager: Gayathri S
Design Direction: Renee Duenow

Printed in India

Last digit is the print number: 9 8 7 6 5 4 3 2 1

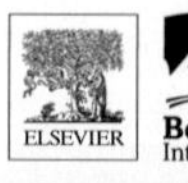

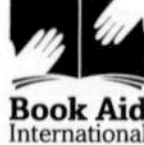

I dedicate this book to my family for their constant support, encouragement, patience, and love. Thank you as well to my mentors, teachers, and colleagues for shaping my medical education and making me the physician and educator I am today. This book is also dedicated to my trainees—medical students, residents, and fellows—with the hope of igniting the flame of patient safety and physician accountability as nonnegotiable core responsibilities for the next generation of physicians to come. Most of all, I dedicate this book to my patients and patients' families who have entrusted me with their care and taught me so much by listening to them, understanding their stories, see through their eyes, and feel through their souls, with unconditional empathy, compassion, and love, whose participation has enriched my clinical experience immensely.

PREFACE

The primary purpose of writing *Pediatric Kidney Disease: A Case-Based Approach* is to provide complete state-of-the-art reviews and assessments of kidney diseases in children that are frequently encountered in real-world routine daily clinical practice.

More than 400 cases are divided into nine chapters consisting of acute and chronic kidney failures, congenital anomalies of the kidney and urinary tract, fluid, electrolytes and acid-base disorders, genetic disorders, glomerulonephritis, hypertension, tubulointerstitial diseases, and urinary tract infections. Each chapter contains extensive discussions of clinical characteristics, differential diagnosis, and treatments of relevant kidney disease.

Each case report begins with a succinct summary of the patient's history, signs and symptoms, examinations, and initial investigations followed by questions and answers. The answers and comments provide a detailed discussion on each topic, with further case references where appropriate.

The format of case reports will illuminate the basic principles and pathophysiology of diseases of the kidney and define diagnosis and treatment. The selected case reports focus on the essential aspects of the patient's presentation findings and management needed to assist in the differential diagnosis. They develop a process of logical questioning from the presentation of the signs and symptoms and laboratory data, and they are presented in the way in which our patients come to us with their signs and symptoms or are referred to us by our colleagues. Each question is followed by a detailed discussion that reviews recent publications and translates emerging areas of science into data that is useful at the bedside. The content is an evidence-based medicine approach, resulting in improved quality, safety, and cost-effectiveness of patient care. An updated bibliography concludes each set of clinical presentations. This format will help readers stay abreast of developing areas of clinical nephrology. These true-to-life cases will help readers recognize important clinical symptoms and signs and develop the diagnostic and management skills needed for the cases they will encounter in their routine daily clinical practice.

The book is ideal for residents and fellows rotating on nephrology services. The material is also useful as a first-line resource for other practicing physicians who need quick access to current scientific and clinical information on managing pediatric kidney disease.

Farahnak Assadi, MD
Distinguished Emeritus Professor and Chief
Department of Pediatrics
Division of Nephrology
Rush University Medical College
Chicago, Illinois

ACKNOWLEDGMENTS

Many of the individuals to whom I am most indebted are only indirect contributors to this book. They are the people who saw some glimmer of hope in the author early in his career and nurtured him in what has been the most rewarding life in pediatrics and nephrology. From my residency years, Professor Robert Kay and Professor Arthur Hervada were great teachers and always highly supportive when my knowledge had profound limitations. During my fellowship training at the University of Pennsylvania, the Children's Hospital of Philadelphia, Professor David Cornfield and Professor Michael Norman established the groundwork for my subsequent work in nephrology. They provided an intellectual environment, and I have always been grateful for their efforts on my behalf.

In the beginning of my career at the University of Illinois, one could hardly have had better mentors than Professor Ira Rosenthal and Professor George Honig. After moving to Thomas Jefferson University, I received extraordinary help from Professor Robert Brent and Professor Michael Norman. They supported my efforts to establish the core of an outstanding nephrology program at Dupont Hospital for Children. Leading the Division of Nephrology at Rush University Medical Center has been one of the greatest fortunes of my life. Professor Samuel Gotoff and Professor Kenneth Boyer have made it enjoyable to come to work each and every day for more than 15 years.

CONTENTS

1 Acute Kidney Injury 1
2 Congenital Anomalies of Kidney and Urinary Tract 47
3 Chronic Kidney Disease 89
4 Fluid, Electrolytes, and Acid-Base Disorders 125
5 Genetic Disorders 183
6 Glomerulonephritis 219
7 Hypertension 291
8 Tubulointerstitial Disease 325
9 Urinary Tract Infection 375
Index 407

CHAPTER 1

Acute Kidney Injury

Clinical Presentation 1

An otherwise healthy 4-year-old girl is brought to the emergency department because of fever and progressive lethargy. According to the child's mother, her daughter has been vomiting after each meal for the past 3 days and has had five episodes of nonbloody, liquid diarrhea today. The mother also states that the girl drank only 200 mL of juice and water yesterday and only drank half as much today. The girl has urinated only once today. She looks toxic on arrival with a delayed capillary refill, a glazed stare, tachypnea (28 breaths/min), and tachycardia (145 beats/min). Her temperature is 39°C and blood pressure (BP) is 80/30 mm Hg. She has diffused abdominal tenderness and no rash. The diagnosis of septic shock was made and antibiotics therapy including gentamicin, vancomycin, and amoxicillin was initiated after the initial fluid resuscitation. The urine dipstick showed a pH of 7.0, specific gravity 1.010, blood 1+, and no protein. You are now concerned about acute kidney injury (AKI) secondary to circulatory collapse.

Which ONE of the following tests is the most sensitive urinary biomarker for the early detection of acute kidney injury (select all that apply)?

A. Serum creatinine.
B. Estimated glomerular filtration rate (eGFR).
C. Kidney injury molecule (KIM-1).
D. Neutrophil gelatinase-associated lipocalin (ANGAL).

The correct answer is A

Comment: A recent prospective cross-sectional study examined a panel of three most promising AKI biomarkers, including IL-28, NGAL, and KIM-2, in 86 children between 7 months and 24 years of age with circulatory collapse. The study results concluded that of a panel of three promising biomarkers, KIM-1 demonstrated the best performance in predicting AKI before a change in serum creatinine or eGFR becomes apparent.[1]

Clinical Presentation 2

A 2-year-old boy was admitted with hypoglycemia. His blood pressure was 105/68 mm Hg, heart rate 98 beats/min, and respiration 29 breaths/min. He was afebrile. His growth and development were normal. He had no clinical evidence of dehydration. Admission serum electrolytes (mEq/L) were sodium 142, potassium 5.6, chloride (Cl) 98, CO_2 12 mEq/L, glucose 58 mg/dL, blood urea nitrogen (BUN) 19 mg/dL, and creatinine 1.2 mg/dL. Arterial blood gas pH was 7.24, and PCO_2 was 15 mm Hg. Serum ketone measured by ketosis strip showed a 3+ reaction. Urinalysis revealed pH 5.0, specific gravity 2.018, and no blood or protein. The patient responded well to fluid therapy. Following the correction of electrolyte abnormalities, his serum creatinine fell to 0.4 mg/dL, blood pH rose to 7.40, blood glucose was 105 mg/dL, and serum was free of ketones.

What is the best explanation for the concurrent fall in the serum creatinine and serum ketone levels following correction of hypoglycemia (select all that apply)?

A. Prerenal azotemia.
B. AKI.
C. Falsely high serum creatinine.
D. Laboratory error.

The correct answer is C

Comment: Falsely high creatinine values have been previously reported when the Jaffe reaction is used for creatinine determination (option C).[1] The false elevation of serum creatinine concentration is not seen with lactic acidosis in the absence of ketosis. Therefore, when increased anion gap metabolic acidosis is present with an elevation of ketosis, the high serum creatinine levels, when measured by the Jaffe method, should be interpreted with caution and should not be considered definitive of renal dysfunction.

Clinical Presentation 3

Which one of the following statements regarding the validity of urinary beta-2 excretion is true in newborn infants (select all that may apply)?

A. Fractional excretion of beta-2 macroglobulin is a useful predictor of fetal hydronephrosis.
B. Glomerular-tubular balance for beta-2 macroglobulin is not influenced by urine flow rate.
C. Beta-2 macroglobulin is not a reliable predictor of renal tubular maturation and might be influenced by other factors than conceptional age.
D. The glomerular-tubular balance is established by conceptional age 35 weeks and can be used as a marker to assess the renal tubular toxicity caused by nephrotoxic drugs.

The correct answer is D

Comment: In the neonatal period, the proximal tubular transporting capacity is more vulnerable than the glomerular filtration rate in the states of hypoxia and nephrotoxic drugs.[1,2]

Fractional excretion of beta-2 is a reliable index to assess renal tubular maturation in newborns.[1] The test is helpful to identify high-risk newborns in whom AKI results from poor renal perfusion secondary to asphyxia days and nephrotoxic medications days or weeks before a rise in serum creatinine level is observed (option A).[2,3]

Clinical Presentation 4

An 18-year-old man receiving treatment for HIV infection presents with severe myalgias. His serum creatinine is 2.1 mg/dL, with a creatinine phosphokinase of 7400 U/L. His urinalysis is strongly positive for blood on dipstick, but he has only 2 to 4 red blood cells per high-power field.

Which ONE of the following medications is MOST likely to be associated with his acute renal failure (ARF)?

A. Acyclovir.
B. Adefovir.
C. Cidofovir.
D. Foscarnet.
E. Zidovudine.

The correct answer is E

Comment: Rhabdomyolysis is seen with increased frequency in association with HIV infection. Several factors contribute to this, including a high rate of alcohol and substance abuse in this population, muscle involvement, and direct drug toxicity. Although myopathy is a common complication of HIV infection, it usually does not produce severe enough muscle injury to cause myoglobinuric ARF. The antiretroviral drug zidovudine has been associated with severe myopathy and rhabdomyolysis as a result of mitochondrial DNA duplication in myocytes. None of the other listed agents is associated with rhabdomyolysis.[1]

Clinical Presentation 5

A 7-year-old boy develops multisystem organ failure with ARF in the setting of *Klebsiella pneumoniae* and sepsis. His BP is 87/50 mm Hg, with a heart rate of 96 beats/min with 6 g/kg/min continuous infusion of dopamine. He is mechanically ventilated and has a PO_2 of 74 torr while receiving 60% inspired oxygen. His pulmonary capillary occlusion pressure is 22 mm Hg. His urine output is <5 mL/h. Laboratory data include a creatinine of 4.3 mg/dL, BUN of 92 mg/dL, potassium of 5.3 mEq/L, and a bicarbonate of 19 mEq/L. You decide to begin renal replacement therapy (RRT).

Which ONE of the following statements comparing modalities of RRT is correct?

A. Continuous arteriovenous hemodiafiltration is associated with improved survival compared with intermittent hemodialysis.
B. Continuous venous hemodialysis (CVVHD) provides better solute control than continuous venous hemofiltration.
C. Sustained low-efficiency dialysis (SLED) and extended daily dialysis (EDD) are associated with improved survival compared with intermittent hemodialysis.
D. Continuous venovenous hemofiltration (CVVH) is associated with improved survival compared with peritoneal dialysis.
E. Sustained SLED and EDD are associated with improved survival compared with CVVH.

Correct answer is D

Comment: In a recent study in patients with infection-associated ARF, the mortality rate in patients treated with peritoneal dialysis was 47% compared with a mortality rate of 15% in patients treated with CVVH.[1] In studies comparing chronic RRT (CRRT) with intermittent hemodialysis, no consistent survival benefit has been observed for CRRT. In the largest randomized controlled trial, CRRT was associated with higher mortality, although the study was flawed by unbalanced randomization that resulted in a higher acuity of illness in the CRRT group.[2] There are no data to compare outcomes of SLED or EDD to outcomes with intermittent hemodialysis, or any from CRRT.[3] Although the mechanism of solute removal differs between CVVH (predominantly convective clearance) and CVVHD (predominantly diffusive clearance), similar degrees of solute control for urea and other low-molecular-weight solutes can be achieved with either modality.

Clinical Presentation 6

Which ONE of the following statements regarding treatment with loop diuretics in AKI is true?

A. It increases urine output and decreases the need for dialysis.
B. It decreases AKI mortality rate.

C. It shortens the duration of AKI.
D. It may cause severe hypokalemia.
E. The benefits of loop diuretics are augmented by concurrent use of dopamine.

The correct answer is D

Comment: Loop diuretics are frequently used in the management of patients with AKI. Because no oliguric ARF has a better prognosis than oliguric AKI, it has been suggested that converting a patient from an oliguric to no oliguric state improves outcomes. Increasing urine flow may wash out obstructing intraluminal cellular debris and casts, thereby reversing one of the mechanisms of renal dysfunction. In addition, by decreasing active transport in the thick ascending loop of Henle, loop diuretics may decrease energy requirements and protect cells in a region of compromised perfusion. Clinical studies, however, have not supported these arguments. In randomized controlled trials, diuretic therapy was not associated with any improvement in mortality, decrease in the duration of AKI, or alteration in the need for dialysis therapy. There is no evidence of augmentation of benefit with concomitant administration of dopamine. Diuretic therapy may, however, result in kaliuresis and hypokalemia.[1]

Clinical Presentation 7

A 6-year-old boy develops multisystem organ failure and ARF after a motor vehicle accident, in which he sustains severe trauma. His BP is 80/47 mm Hg with 0.07 g/kg per minute of norepinephrine. He is intubated and mechanically ventilated and has an oxygen saturation of 98% and an FIO_2 of 0.40%. His urine output is 15 mL/h. Laboratory studies demonstrate a serum creatinine of 2.9 mg/dL, BUN of 49 mg/dL, potassium of 4.8 mEq/L, and bicarbonate of 22 mEq/L. The critical care attending physician asks if you should initiate RRT.

Which ONE of the following statements regarding the timing of RRT initiation?

A. Early RRT initiation is associated with a 25% reduction in mortality.
B. Early initiation of RRT resulted in no change in mortality.
C. Early initiation of RRT reduced mortality by 15%.
D. Early initiation of RRT reduced mortality by about 40%.

The correct answer is D

Comment: There are very limited data regarding the timing of renal therapy initiation in ARF. In a single retrospective analysis, the survival in patients initiated on RRT with a BUN <60 mg/dL was 39% compared with a survival of only 20% in patients in whom RRT was not initiated until BUN was >60 mg/dL.[1] No randomized controlled trials have been conducted to evaluate this question.

Clinical Presentation 8

Which ONE of the following statements is true regarding the use of low-dose dopamine (<2 µg/kg/min) in the treatment of ischemic acute tubular necrosis (ATN)?

A. Decreases the ATN mortality rate.
B. Decreases the percentage of patients who are oliguric.
C. Decrease the likelihood of needing dialysis.
D. Decreases the duration of ATN.
E. None of the above.

The correct answer is E

Comment: When infused at low doses (0.5–2 μg/kg/min), dopamine increases plasma flow, glomerular filtration rate, and renal sodium excretion through activation of dopaminergic receptors.[1] At higher doses, dopamine binds to adrenergic receptors, resulting in vasoconstriction and inotropic effects. Infusions of low-dose dopamine have been used, and still are widely used, to increase urine output and to prevent or treat ATN among oliguric, critically ill patients. The ability of dopamine to achieve these goals is largely anecdotal, however, and has not been supported in rigorous clinical trials. In both a large, randomized trial of low-dose dopamine in critically ill patients with early evidence of ATN, and in a meta-analysis of 17 earlier studies, low-dose dopamine was not associated with any benefit with regard to the development of oliguria, duration of ATN, need for RRT, or mortality.[2]

Clinical Presentation 9

A 19-year-old woman with HIV infection, treated with active antiretroviral therapy, presents with nausea, vomiting, and abdominal and flank pain. Her serum creatinine is 2.8 mg/dL (baseline value was 0.7 mg/dL 2 weeks previously). Urine microscopy is remarkable for rectangular plate-like and needle-shaped crystals.

Which ONE of the following medications is most likely to have caused her AKI?

A. Adefovir.
B. Indinavir.
C. Nevirapine.
D. Ritonavir.
E. Zidovudine.

The correct answer is B

Comment: This patient presents with crystal-related AKI with indinavir. Indinavir sulfate forms needle-shaped crystals that may aggregate to form rectangular plates or rosettes. The actual renal failure may develop as a result of intratubular deposition with tubulointerstitial nephritis or with nephrolithiasis.[1,2] None of the other drugs listed is associated with crystal-induced AKI.

Clinical Presentation 10

A 17-year-old boy with a history of intravenous drug abuse is admitted with a 2-week history of fever and malaise. Blood cultures on admission are positive for coagulase-negative *Staphylococcus*, and an echocardiogram demonstrates vegetation on his aortic valve. His serum creatinine is 1.1 mg/dL. He is started on antibiotic therapy with vancomycin and gentamycin, his blood cultures resolve, and he is discharged to home to complete a 4-week course of intravenous antibiotics. He is readmitted 2 weeks later with recurrent fevers, having been noncompliant with his outpatient antibiotic regimen. Blood cultures are again positive for coagulase-negative *Staphylococcus*. His serum creatinine is now 2.4 mg/dL. Urinalysis reveals hematuria with some dysmorphic red blood cells but without any casts noted. Serum complement levels are slightly reduced below the lower limits of normal.

Which ONE of the following choices provides the MOST appropriate management of AKI?

A. Continue current antibiotic therapies.
B. Discontinue aminoglycoside therapy.

C. Discontinue vancomycin.
D. Discontinue both vancomycin and aminoglycoside antibiotic therapies.
E. Begin intravenous methylprednisolone.

The correct answer is A

Comment: This patient presents with a syndrome most consistent with endocarditis-associated glomerulonephritis. Although red blood cell cats were not seen on urinalysis, there is hematuria with dysmorphic red blood cells, suggesting glomerular bleeding. The low serum complement levels are suggestive of an immune complex disease.[1] The treatment of endocarditis-associated glomerulonephritis is treatment of the underlying infection. The use of combination therapy with vancomycin and gentamicin to achieve more rapid sterilization of blood cultures is appropriate. Steroid therapy is not indicated, especially in the setting of active infection.

Clinical Presentation 11

A 5-year-old girl with a history of mitral valve prolapse and no history of renal disease develops *Streptococcus viridians* endocarditis. She is placed on intravenous ampicillin and gentamicin. Two weeks into her course of therapy, she develops worsening shortness of breath and lower extremity edema. On examination, she has an erythematous maculopapular rash across her legs and lower abdomen. Laboratory studies demonstrate a serum creatinine of 1.6 mg/dL. The leukocyte count is 9800/mm^3, with 4% eosinophils. Urinalysis demonstrates microscopic hematuria and pyuria. The urine stain for eosinophils is negative.

Which ONE of the following treatment options would be most appropriate in this patient?

A. Discontinue gentamicin, continue ampicillin.
B. Discontinue ampicillin and gentamicin and begin vancomycin.
C. Continue current antibiotics without any changes.
D. Continue current antibiotics and begin intravenous methylprednisolone.

The correct answer is B

Comment: The most likely diagnosis for this patient's AKI is allergic interstitial nephritis (AIN), with ampicillin being the most likely offending agent. The characteristic features of AIN that are present include the erythematous maculopapular rash, microscopic hematuria, and pyuria. Although eosinophilia is frequently associated with AIN, and her percentage of eosinophils is slightly elevated, her absolute eosinophil count is not elevated (<400/mm^3). Although eosinophilia has been suggested as a key diagnostic feature in AIN, its true diagnostic value is that it is present in only two-thirds of patients with AIN.[1] Aminoglycoside nephrotoxicity is a less likely diagnosis; it is not associated with cutaneous manifestations and would be expected to be associated with many tubular epithelial cells and granular casts in urine microscopy. The urine sediment does not suggest endocarditis-associated glomerulonephritis (GN). The primary treatment of AIN is discontinuation of the offending agent. Thus, choices A, D, and E are incorrect.[1]

There is no convincing evidence for the treatment of AIN with steroids, and they are relatively contraindicated in the presence of acute infection. Choice C is therefore inappropriate. The optimal therapy is therefore to discontinue the ampicillin and begin an alternative antibiotic agent to treat endocarditis (choice B).

Clinical Presentation 12

An 18-year-old man with a history of congenital AIDS is admitted with a 4-day history of progressive fatigue, weakness, confusion, myalgia, and oliguria. Medications before hospital admissions included indinavir, didanosine, stavudine, tenofovir, zidovudine, trimethoprim-sulfamethoxazole, and atorvastatin. On admission, his BP was 90/50 mm Hg, and he was in acute respiratory distress. On review of arterial blood gases, his pH was 6.93 with an HCO_3- of 5 mEq/L. His BUN was 78 mg/dL, serum creatinine 7.6 mg/dL, and creatinine kinase 124 U/L. Urine microscopy revealed no crystalluria. His plasma lactate level was 5.4 mmol/L, rising to 16.7 mmol/L on the third hospital day despite therapy with continuous venous hemofiltration using bicarbonate buffered fluids. Blood and urine cultures, bronchoscopy, and abdominal and pelvic computed tomography scans were all negative.

Which ONE of the following medications is the most likely cause of his ARF?

A. Indinavir.
B. Tenofovir.
C. Zidovudine.
D. Atorvastatin.
E. Trimethoprim-sulfamethoxazole.

The correct answer is B

Comment: Several recent case reports have described ATN in association with severe lactic acidosis in patients treated with tenofovir.[1,2] The other four drugs listed have also been associated with ARF; however, their patterns of renal failure are not consistent with this patient's presentation. Indinavir causes ARF through deposition of insoluble drug crystals in the kidneys or obstructive uropathy from indinavir stones. The absence of crystalluria makes indinavir toxicity unlikely. In addition, indinavir toxicity is not associated with lactic acidosis. Zidovudine has been associated with lactic acidosis; however, zidovudine-associated ARF is due to rhabdomyolysis, which can be excluded by the normal serum creatinine kinase. Atorvastatin is also associated with rhabdomyolysis and myoglobinuric ARF, which is not present in this patient. Trimethoprim-sulfamethoxazole may cause acute interstitial nephritis but is not associated with the severe lactic acidosis seen in this patient.

Clinical Presentation 13

A 16-year-old boy with end-stage liver disease, secondary to chronic hepatitis C infection, undergoes an orthotropic liver transplant. Preoperatively, his serum creatinine is 1.1 mg/dL and his bilirubin is 28 mg/dL. His intraoperative course is unremarkable, with a lowest recorded BP of 95/60 mm Hg. On the third postoperative day, he has tense ascites, and his bilirubin, which had fallen to 11 mg/dL, is 21 mg/dL. His BP is 110/72 mm Hg on no vasopressors. His central venous pressure is 16 mm Hg and pulmonary capillary occlusion pressure is 19 mm Hg. His urine output is 130 mL over 24 hours. After irrigating his Foley catheter, his intravesical pressure is reported as 37 cm H_2O. His serum creatinine is 2.6 mg/dL. His urine sodium 12 is <10 mEq/L. Urine microscopy demonstrates occasional bile-stained casts. A tacrolimus level is reported as 8 ng/dL.

Which ONE of the following options would be the MOST appropriate next step?

A. Infusion of 1500 mL 0.9% saline.
B. Infusion of 1599 mL 0.45% saline.

C. Infusion of selepressin.
D. Abdominal decomposition by paracentesis.
E. Initiation of continuous renal replacement therapy.

The correct answer is D

Comment: The abdominal compartment syndrome is characterized by increased intra-abdominal pressure resulting in decreased renal perfusion. It is most commonly seen in trauma patients who have received massive volume resuscitation but may be seen in a variety of other settings, including tight abdominal surgical closure or as a result of scarring after burn injuries, both of which result in mechanical limitation of the abdominal wall and in association with bowel obstruction and pancreatitis in which intra-abdominal fluid sequestration leads to increased intra-abdominal pressure. Previous reports have described this syndrome after liver transplantation. The diagnosis of abdominal compartment syndrome should be considered in patients developing ARF in the setting of tense distention of the abdomen.[1,2] The diagnosis is commonly made by measurement of intravesical pressure, which correlates with intra-abdominal pressure. This diagnosis can be excluded when the intravesical pressure is <10 mm Hg (<14 cm H_2O) and is virtually always present if the pressure is >25 mm Hg (34 cm H_2O), as in this case. The treatment consists of abdominal decompression, which may be achieved acutely by paracentesis, although the majority of patients ultimately require surgical decompression. Renal function usually recovers promptly following normalization of intra-abdominal pressure. Volume resuscitation with either crystalloid or colloid is not indicated because volume-responsive prerenal azotemia is unlikely given the elevated central venous and pulmonary artery pressures. Selepressin has been suggested as potentially beneficial for the treatment of hepatorenal syndrome (HRS). Although this diagnosis is also associated with a low urine sodium concentration, a diagnosis of HRS must be deferred until all other etiologist of ARF are excluded. This patient has no clinical parameters suggesting an urgent need for renal replacement therapy. Because his renal function may recover following abdominal decompression, initiation of CRRT is not appropriate.

Clinical Presentation 14

An 11-year-old boy develops ARF following operative repair of a 5.6-cm bowel perforation. He is oliguric, with urine output averaging 5 mL/h, and volume-overloaded, with a central venous pressure of 26 mm Hg. His BP is 110/65 mm Hg, his heart rate is 102 beats/min, and he has a transcutaneous oxygen saturation of 88% on a fractional inspired oxygen of 0.80 on volume-cycled mechanical ventilation. His preoperative serum creatinine was 0.6 mg/dL and has increased to 2.2 mg/dL on the first postoperative day. Following intravenous administration of 80 mg of furosemide, his urine output increases to 10 mL/h for 4 hours.

Which ONE of the following therapeutic interventions is most appropriate at this time?

A. Begin infusion of furosemide 5 mg/h.
B. Intravenous chlorothiazide 500 mg followed by 5 mg bumetanide.
C. Begin infusion of dopamine 1.5 μg/h.
D. Initial RRT.

The correct answer is D

Comment: The case describes a patient with oliguric renal failure resulting from ischemic ATN, complicated by severe volume overload with respiratory compromise. He has not responded to a bolus infusion of high-dose furosemide. The most appropriate intervention at this time would be the initiation of RRT for management of volume overload.[1] Clinical studies do not support the use of further diuretic therapy after an initial failure to respond. There is no role for the use of low-dose dopamine in the management of oliguric ARF. Dobutamine is an inotrope with vasodilatory properties. Although potentially beneficial in the management of prerenal azotemia resulting from heart failure, it has no role in the management of ischemic ATN.

Clinical Presentation 15

Which ONE of the statements regarding modality selection for RRT in acute renal failure (ARF) is MOST correct?

A. CRRT is associated with improved survival compared with intermittent hemodialysis after adjusting for comorbidity and acuity of illness.
B. Intermittent hemodialysis is associated with increased recovery of renal function compared with CRRT.
C. Sustained low-efficiency dialysis is associated with decreased mortality compared with intermittent hemodialysis.
D. There is no relationship between dose of therapy and outcome in either intermittent hemodialysis or CRRT.
E. Peritoneal dialysis is associated with decreased mortality compared with CRRT.

The correct answer is E

Comment: In contrast to peritoneal dialysis, CRRT is associated with intermittent hemodialysis, although there is some suggestion that CRRT may be with a significantly improved survival. After adjusting for comorbidities and acuity of illness, however, no survival benefit has been consistently observed when CRRT is compared with a higher rate of recovery of renal function. No studies comparing outcomes with sustained low-efficiency dialysis or other forms of slow hemodialysis and conventional intermittent hemodialysis have been reported. There are clear data that there is a relationship between increased doses of therapy and survival in ARF.[1]

Clinical Presentation 16

Which ONE of the following strategies will provide the greatest benefit in preventing acute contrast nephropathy in a 5-year-old child with a serum creatinine of 1.2 mg/dL?

A. Volume expansion with 0.9% saline (1 mL/kg/h for 4 hours before and 6 hours after procedure), and pretreatment with fenoldopam.
B. Volume expansion with 0.9% saline (1 mL/kg/h for 12 hours before and 12 hours after procedure), and pretreatment with N-acetylcysteine.
C. Volume expansion with 0.9% saline (1 mL/kg/h for 12 hours before and 12 hours after procedure), and pretreatment with acetazolamide.
D. Volume expansion with isotonic sodium bicarbonate (1 mL/kg/h for 4 hours before and 6 hours after procedure).

The correct answer is C

Comment: Volume expansion with saline is the mainstay of prevention of radiocontrast nephropathy. The optimal rate of infusion is 1 mL/kg/h for 12 hours before and 12 hours after radiocontrast administration. The data regarding the use of N-acetylcysteine and sodium bicarbonate are conflicting. A recent controlled study in children with compromised kidney function has shown that the treatment with 0.9% saline combined with acetazolamide before, during, and after the contest media exposure provides more protection against the contrast-induced nephropathy than the use of isotonic saline alone.[1]

Clinical Presentation 17

A 6-year-old girl is admitted with increasing ascites. Her serum creatinine on admission is 1.4 mg/dL. Following a large-volume paracentesis, her urine output precipitously decreases to <100 mL/d and her serum creatinine increases to 2.7 mg/dL. Ascitic fluid culture is sterile. Her urine sodium is 8 mEq/L. Following infusion of 1500 mL of 0.9% saline, she has no increase in her urine output.

Which ONE of the following medications will most likely provide the best balance between improved renal function and adverse effects?

A. Octreotide.
B. Dopamine.
C. Selepressin.
D. Omnipresent.
E. Spironolactone.

The correct answer is C

Comment: This patient has HRS. The only effective pharmacologic therapy currently available for the management of HRS is the administration of vasoconstrictors. Two classes of drugs have been used vasopressin analogues and adrenergic agonists with most given in combination with intravenous albumin to further treat arterial underfilling. The best success has been observed with the vasopressin v1-receptor agonist selepressin.[1] Ischemia from arterial vasoconstriction is the major complication associated with selepressin therapy, with ischemic side effects necessitating discontinuation of therapy in 5% to 10% of patients. Ornipressin is another vasopressin v1-receptor agonist. The incidence of ischemic complications in patients treated with ornipressin is 30% to 40%. Octreotide is a somatostatin analogue that causes splanchnic vasoconstriction. It is not effective at improving renal function in HRS when used as a single agent but has some benefits in combination with midodrine. Dopamine is not effective in the treatment of HRS. Spironolactone an aldosterone receptor antagonist is a highly effective diuretic in patients with advanced liver disease but has no impact on renal function in patients with HRS.

Clinical Presentation 18

Which ONE of the following statements regarding the use of low-dose dopamine (<2 μg/kg/min) in the treatment of ischemic ATN is correct?

A. It reduces postoperative mortality.
B. It increases the risk of postoperative arterial fibrillation.
C. It improves responsiveness to loop diuretics.
D. It decreases the need for dialysis therapy.

The correct answer is B

Comment: Two clinical studies in cardiac surgery patients have associated low-dose dopamine therapy with increased incidence of arterial arrhythmias, presumably mediated by adrenergic stimulation, which is present even at putative dopaminergic doses.[1] Low-dose dopamine has not been found to have any of these benefits in adequate prospective, comparative studies. Dopamine has been reported to cause hypothyroidism, not hyperthyroidism.[1,2]

Clinical Presentation 19

An 18-year-old woman with advanced liver disease secondary to sclerosing cholangitis is admitted with increasing ascites. Her serum creatinine 1 month ago was 1.2 mg/dL. On admission, her serum creatinine is 1.7 mg/dL. Her physical examination is remarkable for a BP of 110/70 mm Hg, massive ascites, and minimal peripheral edema. A paracentesis is performed with drainage of 9.2 L of fluid, accompanied by the administration of 75 g of hyperoncotic (25%) albumin. Two days later, her serum creatinine was 2.6 mg/dL, rising to 3.2 mg/dL despite the administration of 1.5 L of isotonic saline.

Which ONE of the following interventions is MOST appropriate currently?

A. Administration of octreotide.
B. Administration of octreotide and dopamine.
C. Administration of octreotide and midodrine.
D. Emergent splenorenal shunt.
E. Removal from liver transplant waiting list.

The correct answer is C

Comment: The patient described has AKI resulting from HRS. Prerenal azotemia has been effectively excluded based on the failure to respond to administration of isotonic saline. In a case series, pharmacologic therapy with vasoconstrictors such as the vasopressin analogue selepressin or the somatostatin analogue octreotide in combination with the adrenergic midodrine, has been associated with sustained improvement in renal function. The use of octreotide alone is not effective (choice A is incorrect) and the combination of octreotide and dopamine has not been evaluated (choice B is incorrect). There is no indication for emergent splenorenal shunt this surgery is performed to decompress the portal circulation in patients with intractable gastrointestinal bleeding from portal hypertension and is not associated with improvement in renal function (choice D is incorrect). The development of HRS does not contraindicate liver transplantation. Patients who respond to vasoconstrictor therapy have similar outcomes as patients who do not have HRS (choice E is incorrect).[1]

Clinical Presentation 20

A 14-year-old girl is admitted with severe community-acquired pneumonia and sepsis. On admission to the intensive care unit, she becomes acutely confused and hypoxic, and she is intubated after a respiratory arrest. After intubation, her BP decreases from 130/70 mm Hg to 100/55 mm Hg on a dopamine infusion of 8 g/kg/min, with a central venous pressure of 8 mm Hg. Ventilation settings are tidal volume 6 mL/kg, respiratory rate 35/min, positive end-expiratory pressure (PEEP) of 15 cm H_2O, and oxygen saturation 90% on 70% inspired oxygen. Plateau pressure (static airway pressure measured during an inspiratory pause) is 35 cm H_2O. Her chest x-ray shows bilateral pulmonary infiltrates with good central venous catheter and endotracheal tube placement. Her arterial gases are pH 7.19, PCO_2 65 mm Hg, pO_2 60 mm Hg, and bicarbonate 24 mEq/L. Central venous oxygen saturation is 51%. Urine output is 10 mL/h and serum creatinine has increased from 0.8 mg/dL on admission to 1.5 mg/dL. Her hemoglobin is 7.0 g/dL.

Which ONE of the following is the BEST management plan for her AKI?

A. Increase PEEP.
B. Transfuse 1 to 2 units of packed red blood cells.
C. Start a loop diuretic.
D. Start norepinephrine infusion and wean dopamine.

The correct answer is B

Comment: This patient should receive early goal-directed therapy for septic shock. Ventral venous pressure is within the 8- to 12-mm Hg range recommended for early goal-directed therapy of septic shock, but central venous oxygen saturation is low. Transfusion of packed red blood cells to achieve a hemoglobin of 10 g/dL is recommended to increase central venous oxygen saturation to ≥70%.[1,2] Dobutamine would be added to normalize central venous oxygen saturation if transfusion to a hemoglobin of 10 g/dL failed to achieve this goal. Furosemide infusion (choice C is incorrect) or increased PEEP (choice A) would exacerbate hypovolemic response (the impact of positive pressure ventilation with decreased venous return has caused hypovolemia in this patient, masked in part by positive intrathoracic pressure elevating the central venous pressure, and by dopamine-induced venoconstriction) and norepinephrine would continue to mask it (choice D is incorrect). Although increasing respiratory rate would improve hypercapnia and pH (choice E), any improvement in renal blood flow by this mechanism would be less substantial than the effects of volume expansion and would risk significantly increasing auto PEEP air trapping.[2] Finally, raising central venous oxygen saturation will also improve arterial oxygenation and might permit use of a lower fraction of inspired oxygen and perhaps less PEEP, further improving management. This is the best approach to improving systemic and renal perfusion for this patient.

Clinical Presentation 21

A 7-year-old girl with no history of kidney disease undergoes aortic valve replacement bypass surgery. In the initial postoperative period, she has a low cardiac index and requires hemodynamic support with an intra-aortic balloon pump and a continuous infusion of epinephrine. By the third postoperative day, however, she is hemodynamically stable with a mean arterial BP of 54 mm Hg of off-pressor support. She remains intubated, mechanically ventilated, and is sedated with continuous infusions of propofol and fentanyl. Despite net positive fluid balance, she has developed progressive oliguria, her BUN is 84 mg/dL, and her serum creatinine is 4.3 mg/dL. You are consulted by a cardiothoracic surgeon to initiate dialysis.

Which ONE of the following statements regarding the modality of RRT in this clinical setting is evidence based?

A. CRRT would be associated with a greater probability of survival compared with intermittent hemodialysis.
B. Intermittent hemodialysis would be associated with an increased risk of combined death and irreversible renal function.
C. SLED would provide more rapid correction of metabolic acidosis than CRRT.
D. CRRT would be associated with a greater probability of achieving negative net fluid balance than SLED.

The correct answer is C

Comment: There are no data establishing better survival or recovery of renal function with CRRT, intermittent hemodialysis, or SLED (choices A and B are not correct). CRRT has been demonstrated to be associated with a greater probability of achieving negative fluid balance without exacerbating hemodynamic instability, in comparison to intermittent hemodialysis[1]; however, hemodynamic stability during SLED is similar to that observed during CRRT (choice D is incorrect). Similarly, SLED requires a lower total anticoagulant dose than CRRT because of the shorter duration of treatment (choice E is incorrect). SLED has, however, been shown to provide more rapid correction of metabolic acidosis than CRRT (choice C is incorrect).[1]

Clinical Presentation 22

You are asked to see a 13-year-old boy, a trauma victim who sustained closed head trauma resulting in cerebral edema. He is intubated and mechanically ventilated. His BP is 90/60 mm Hg on no pressor agent, and his urine output is 40 mL/h. Laboratory testing reveals serum creatinine 8 mg/dL, potassium 5.9 mEq/L, bicarbonate 12 mEq/L, and serum creatinine phosphokinase 100,000 U/L. Bilateral infiltrates are present on his chest x-ray.

Which ONE of the following interventions is MOST appropriate at this time?

A. Begin infusion of mannitol, bicarbonate, and saline.
B. Administer intravenous calcium.
C. Initiate continuous venovenous hemofiltration (CVVH).
D. Administer high-dose (200 mg) furosemide.

The correct answer is C

Comment: This patient has severe acute renal failure in association with acute brain injury, cerebral edema, and elevated intracranial pressure. He also has significant rhabdomyolysis, with hyperphosphatemia and hypocalcemia. Mannitol or any intravenous fluids will exacerbate pulmonary edema, and diuretic therapy will not improve renal function or control hyperphosphatemia/hypocalcemia in this setting (choices A and B are incorrect). Furosemide therapy (choice D) might also precipitate tetany by lowering systemic ionized calcium. Calcium infusion is contraindicated in this severely hyperphosphatemia patient (choice B is incorrect). CVVH will provide better control of hyperphosphatemia and hypocalcemia, and correct azotemia and acidosis without raising intracranial pressure (a proven adverse effect of intermittent dialysis in the presence of cerebral edema) (choice C is correct).[1]

Clinical Presentation 23

A 7-year-old girl is to begin chemotherapy for a poorly differentiated non-Hodgkin lymphoma.

Which ONE of the following is NOT effective at reducing her risk of developing AKI as a result of induction chemotherapy?

A. Furosemide.
B. Rasburicase.
C. Allopurinol.
D. Isotonic saline.
E. Sodium bicarbonate.

The correct answer is A

Comment: The major risk for AKI in this patient is tumor lysis syndrome. A variety of therapies may be of benefit in preventing AKI in tumor lysis syndrome, including volume expansion with isotonic saline, inhibiting uric acid generation using the xanthine oxidase inhibitor allopurinol and using rasburicase (recombinant uricase) to convert uric acid to allantoin. Urinary alkalinization using sodium bicarbonate has also been recommended as a prophylactic measure to increase the urinary solubility of uric acid; however, urinary alkalinization may increase the risk of calcium phosphate precipitation in patients with concomitant hyperphosphatemia. There is, however, no role for loop-acting diuretics such as furosemide for the prevention of AKI in the tumor lysis syndrome.[1]

Clinical Presentation 24

A 5-year-old boy with a history of congenital heart disease, congestive heart failure, and chronic kidney disease undergoes cardiopulmonary bypass surgery. He receives furosemide at 5 mg/h and dopamine at 3 g/kg/min perioperatively. He is uneventfully extubated postoperatively, but then develops atrial fibrillation with a rate of 140 beats/min, fails therapy with adenosine, becomes hypotensive, and is reintubated. He is now oliguric, with an irregular heart rate of 120 beats/min, BP of 60/50 mm Hg, and central venous pressure of 4 mm Hg. The dopamine infusion is increased to 6 g/kg/min for treatment of hypotension. His serum creatinine is now 2.5 mg/dL, sodium 135 mEq/L, potassium 3.4 mEq/L, chloride 105 mEq/L, bicarbonate 20 mEq/L, BUN 70 mg/dL, and glucose 110 mg/dL. His urinalysis is unremarkable.

In addition to potassium repletion and discontinuation of his furosemide infusion, which ONE of the following interventions is MOST appropriate?

A. Add a beta-blocker to achieve rate control.
B. Give vasopressin and rapidly wean off dopamine.
C. Administer a bolus of normal saline and rapidly wean off dopamine.
D. Switch dopamine to phenylephrine.
E. Switch dopamine to dobutamine.

The correct answer is C

Comment: This patient has acute renal failure with a preexisting chronic kidney disease with pre-renal azotemia caused by furosemide-induced hypovolemia, masked by the use of dopamine and aggravated by development of uncontrolled atrial fibrillation. In addition to dopaminergic receptors, dopamine stimulates beta-adrenergic and alpha-adrenergic arterial receptors, which may be pro-arrhythmic (beta-adrenergic effect) and mask hypovolemia (by alpha-adrenergic arterial and venous constriction, and beta-adrenergic inotropic effect). Potassium repletion, discontinuation of furosemide infusion, and active volume expansion are required for this patient. Saline boluses to raise central venous pressure to 8 to 12 mm Hg should permit rapid weaning off pro-arrhythmic dopamine, and correction of hypovolemia will also remove a second mechanism of catecholamine-driven tachycardia.[1] If rate control is still inadequate and perfusion impaired, rate control with a blocker, and (if necessary) use of a pressor or cardioversion could be considered. If a pressor is required for this patient, phenylephrine would be preferred to norepinephrine to avoid beta-adrenergic stimulation. Dobutamine should be avoided for the same reason.

Clinical Presentation 25

A 17-year-old boy with a history of liver disease secondary to hepatitis C viral infection is admitted to the hospital with increasing abdominal girth. He has had a prior episode of gastrointestinal bleeding from esophageal varices and has been treated with endoscopic variceal banding. He has had poor intake of food and fluids for the past 3 days but denies any episodes of vomiting or hematemesis. On physical examination, his BP is 105/64 mm Hg with a heart rate of 69 beats/min, and a temperature of 37°C. His skin is grossly jaundiced. His neck veins are not visible when his head is elevated at a 30-degree angle. He has decreased breath sounds at the lung bases bilaterally, without rales. His abdomen is grossly distended and there is trace peripheral edema. His BUN is 26 mg/dL, serum creatinine 2.6 mg/dL, sodium 128 mEq/L, and bilirubin 8.4 mg/dL. His urine sodium concentration is $<$10 mEq/L. Urinalysis reveals many bile-stained epithelial cells and casts with no proteinuria. A diagnostic paracentesis reveals 110 white blood cells/mL with 45% neutrophils.

Which ONE of the following is the most effective therapy at reducing risk of developing AKI?

A. Administration of at least 1.5 L of isotonic saline.
B. Administration of 75 g of 25% albumin.

C. Initiation of octreotide.
D. Therapy with a combination of octreotide and midodrine.

The correct answer is A

Comment: The differential diagnosis of AKI in a patient with advanced liver disease includes prerenal azotemia, acute tubular necrosis, hepatorenal syndrome, and glomerular disease. In this patient, the primary differentiation is between prerenal azotemia and hepatorenal syndrome. Glomerular disease is unlikely given the absence of proteinuria and hematuria. Acute tubular necrosis is unlikely given the very low urine sodium concentration. Hepatorenal syndrome is differentiated from a prerenal state based on an assessment of effective intravascular volume and/or the response to a volume challenge. The appropriate intervention should therefore be intravascular volume expansion as both a diagnostic and therapeutic trial.[1] There is no evidence to support the administration of hypertonic albumin or other colloid solutions in the routine management of renal dysfunction in patients with advanced liver disease (choice B is incorrect). The combination of octreotide and midodrine is of potential benefit in patients with hepatorenal syndrome; however, this diagnosis has not yet been established in this patient (choice D is incorrect). Placement of a transjugular intrahepatic portosystemic shunt may be of benefit in some patients with hepatorenal syndrome, particularly if they have responded to vasoconstrictor therapy, but should not be used before establishment of the diagnosis and should probably be withheld until after a trial of vasoconstrictors (choice E is incorrect).

Clinical Presentation 26

A 4-year-old girl undergoes cardiac surgery for congenital heart disease with pulmonary hypertension and severe right heart failure, which is associated with chronic renal insufficiency (baseline serum creatinine, 1.5 mg/dL). After 4 hours of cardiopulmonary bypass, it is difficult to wean her from bypass. She returns to the ICU intubated and anuric on furosemide 15 mg/h. Her BP is 70/30 mm Hg on vasopressin, dopamine, and norepinephrine infusions. She is mechanically ventilated and has oxygen saturation of 90% on an inspired oxygen of 1.0 L with 15 cm H_2O PEEP and inhaled nitric oxide therapy. Central venous pressure is 35 mm Hg and venous oxygen saturation is 50%. Her weight has increased 2.5 kg from her postoperative weight, and the sternal wound has not been closed because of massive edema. Her chest x-ray demonstrates bilateral pulmonary edema. Her serum creatinine is 2.8 mg/dL, sodium 135 mEq/L, potassium 4.5 mEq/L, chloride 100 mEq/L, bicarbonate 12 mEq/L, BUN 70 mg/dL, and glucose 80 mg/dL. Urinalysis is not available. The surgical team plans to transfuse 5 units of fresh frozen plasma in preparation for a return to the operating room for placement of a right ventricular assist device and sternal closure. You are asked to initiate emergent RRT.

Which of the following RRTs would be most effective in this patient?

A. CVVH.
B. Peritoneal dialysis (PD).
C. CVVHD.
D. Intermittent hemodialysis.

The correct answer is A

Comment: The CVVH method uses hydrostatic pressure across a semipermeable membrane for ultrafiltration using convection to filter solutes.[1] Higher- and lower-molecular-weight solutes are transported with equal efficiency until the molecular radius of the solute exceeds the membrane pore size. A solute replacement fluid is required to allow sufficient solute clearance. The replacement fluid can be administered either before or after filtration. CVVH is the simplest and most efficient techniques of CRRT for removing fluids in critically ill patients with edema compared with PD, intermittent hemodialysis, and CAVVHD.[1,2]

Clinical Presentation 27

A 2-year-old boy develops oliguric acute renal failure in the setting of multiple organ failure after a motor vehicle accident. He is mechanically ventilated and requires pressor therapy with 0.15 g/kg/min of norepinephrine to maintain a mean arterial BP of 60 mm Hg.

Which ONE of the following statements regarding RRT in this setting is evidenced based?

A. Intermittent hemodialysis is associated with increased mortality compared with CRRT.
B. Survival with sustained low-efficiency hemodialysis is comparable to survival with CRRT.
C. Intermittent hemodialysis should be prescribed to deliver a single-pool Kt/V of 1.2 on a 3-times-per-week schedule.
D. CRRT should be prescribed to deliver an effluent flow rate of 25 mL/kg/h.
E. CRRT will provide greater volume removal with less hemodynamic instability than intermittent hemodialysis.

The correct answer is D

Comment: It has been shown that CRRT is able to provide greater net volume removal than intermittent hemodialysis, despite producing less hemodynamic instability. Despite this benefit, CRRT has not been demonstrated to provide a survival benefit compared with intermittent hemodialysis (choice A is incorrect). Choice B is incorrect because the optimal dose of intermittent hemodialysis when delivered on a 3-times-per-week basis in patients with acute renal injury is not known. There have been no studies comparing outcomes with sustained low-efficiency hemodialysis to outcomes with either conventional intermittent hemodialysis or any of the continuous therapies (choice E is incorrect). Large, single-center, randomized, controlled trials have demonstrated improved survival in CVVH when prescribed to deliver ultrafiltration rates of 35 mL/kg/h and 45 mL/kg/h compared with 20 mL/kg/h (choice C is incorrect). CVVH is the modality of choice in terms of fluid and solute removal in critically ill and hemodynamically unstable patients.[1,2]

Clinical Presentation 28

A 12-month-old boy sustains a cerebral hemorrhage with subsequent hydrocephalus requiring ventriculostomy after catheter-directed thrombosis of a sinus thrombosis. He is maintained on mechanical ventilation. Atracurium is administered for neuromuscular blockade, and fentanyl are administered for sedation and pain control. Hypertonic saline and mannitol are administered to reduce cerebral edema. A phenylephrine infusion is initiated to increase the mean arterial BP to maintain adequate cerebral perfusion pressure. His baseline serum creatinine was 0.3 mg/dL, rising to 1.2 mg/dL on hospital day 3 and 2.5 mg/dL on hospital day 5. On day 5, his creatinine phosphokinase is 8750 U/L. His troponin is 20 ng/mL, and the electrocardiogram shows a right bundle branch block with diffuse ST- and T-wave changes.

Which of the following medications was MOST likely to be responsible for AKI in this patient?

A. Atracurium.
B. Fentanyl.
C. Mannitol.

D. Phenylephrine.
E. Propofol.

The correct answer is E

Comment: The patient described in this case has the manifestations of propofol infusion syndrome, characterized by cardiac dysfunction, metabolic acidosis, and rhabdomyolysis with AKI.[1] Risk factors for this complication of sedation include prolonged therapy with high doses of propofol, and concomitant administration of catecholamines and/or corticosteroids in the setting of acute neurologic injury or acute inflammatory disease complicated by severe infection or sepsis. None of the other listed drugs is associated with this presentation.[1]

Clinical Presentation 29

A 4-year-old boy has his legs pinned under a pile of rubble in an earthquake event. He is extricated after 5 hours. On arrival in the emergency room, he is found to have a creatinine phosphokinase of 23,000 U/L and a serum creatinine of 1.9 mg/dL.

Which ONE of the following treatments would be associated with a decreased risk of AKI in this patient?

A. Intravenous saline 2–3 mL/kg/h before arriving to the emergency department.
B. Intravenous mannitol infusion 2–3 mL/kg/h.
C. Dopamine infusion 2 μg/kg/h.
D. Oral N-acetylcysteine plus 0.45% saline 2–3 mL/kg/h.

The correct answer is A

Comment: Several strategies have been proposed to prevent or attenuate the development of ARF in rhabdomyolysis. The most important is aggressive volume replacement. In patients with traumatic rhabdomyolysis, fluid restriction should be initiated in the field, even before the crushed extremity is released.[1] Urinary alkalinization has been advocated as a means to increase the solubility of heme proteins within the tubule. It has also been suggested that alkalinization may decrease the cycling of myoglobin, thereby reducing the generation of reactive oxygen species. The use of mannitol has also been advocated; however, it has not been shown to have greater efficacy than volume expansion with saline alone. No benefit has been demonstrated for dopamine, furosemide, or N-acetylcysteine in this setting.

Clinical Presentation 30

A previously healthy 16-year-old boy presented with a 4-day history of dark urine, reduced urine output, and bilateral flank pain. There was a history of a severe sore throat infection 2 weeks previous. A throat swab culture was sterile and his serum creatinine level was 0.7 mg/dL. His medical history otherwise was unremarkable and he was on no medications.

On examination, he was alert, interactive, and well perfused without any evidence of peripheral edema. His weight was 64.9 kg and height 172 cm. His body temperature was measured at 36.8°C, respiratory rate 18 breaths/min, heart rate 68 beats/min, normal jugular venous pressure, and blood pressure of 110/71 mm Hg. There was no associated lymphadenopathy or organomegaly. The remainder of the examination was unremarkable except for the presence of mild bilateral flank tenderness.

Laboratory investigation showed the following: Urine dipstick was positive for blood (4+) and protein (2+) and microscopy confirmed abundant red blood cells (>500 10^6/HPF) with nonsignificant white cells or casts. Urine culture was negative for any evidence of infection. Urine protein creatinine ratio was 31 mg/mmol. The results of blood tests confirmed ARF with plasma creatinine of 823 7.6 mg/L and urea of 287 mg/L. Plasma albumin was normal at 40 g/L, hemoglobin 14 g/dL, platelet 201 × 10^9/L, and normal clotting. His throat swab was negative and ASO titer was 190 IU/mL with anti-DNAse B 98 IU/mL. Serum complement levels were normal with C3 1.5 g/L and C4 0.31 g/L, and anti-nuclear antibody titer was negative. A renal ultrasound study demonstrated prominent kidneys with bipolar lengths of 11.4 cm and 12.0 cm. Both were hyperechoic, but with no evidence of any pelvicalyceal dilation or any other signs suggestive of obstruction.

His renal function continued to deteriorate with peak plasma creatinine of 11.0 mg/dL and urea 4121 mg/L. Hemodialysis was initiated. A diagnostic percutaneous renal biopsy was performed under local anesthesia.

What is the most likely cause of acute renal failure (select all that apply)?

A. Focal segmental glomerulonephritis.
B. Membranoproliferative glomerulonephritis.
C. Membranous glomerulonephritis.
D. ATN.
E. Immunoglobulin A (IgA) nephritis.

The correct answers are D and E

Comment: ARF is a rare but well-known complication of massive gross hematuria and has been reported in IgA nephropathy and paroxysmal nocturnal hemoglobinuria.[1] Renal biopsy in these patients usually shows extensive acute tubular necrosis with flattening of the epithelial cells, cytoplasmic vacuolation, blebbing, and the presence of red cell casts.[2]

ATN, possibly secondary to tubular obstruction because of the presence of large numbers of red blood cell (RBC) casts in the tubular lumen, is likely to be a major factor in the development of acute renal failure.[1–3] Free hemoglobin is thought to be directly toxic to renal tubules and can cause proximal tubular epithelium necrosis.[3]

Clinical Presentation 31

A previously healthy 11-year-old boy presented to the emergency department with fever, myalgias, and muscular weakness 2 days earlier. His urine had turned a dark-brown color. The patient also had diarrhea and occasional vomiting for 2 days.

On admission, the patient's blood pressure was 112/72 mm Hg, and his heart rate was 113/min. Axillary temperature was 39.0°C. Physical examination showed muscular weakness in both legs and flank tenderness. The findings of the respiratory, cardiac, and neurological examinations were normal.

The test results on admission were as follows: rapid testing for influenza A was positive; urine dipstick was positive for bilirubin (3+), blood (3+), and protein (3+). Laboratory tests showed a creatine kinase level of 318,000 U/L, urea nitrogen 18 mmol/L, creatinine 214 μmol/L, bicarbonate 16 mmol/L, and potassium 5 mEq/L. A diagnosis of massive rhabdomyolysis with AKI was made.

Rhabdomyolysis progressed with a peak creatine kinase level of 358,000 U/L, lactate dehydrogenase 134,000 U/L, serum myoglobin 44,873 μg/L, aspartate aminotransferase 8122 IU/L, alanine aminotransferase 1562 IU/L, metabolic acidosis, hyperkalemia of 5.4 mEq/L, hypocalcemia of 8.2 mg/dL, and hyperphosphoremia of 6.2 mg/dL. Ultrasound imaging showed enlarged kidneys with a loss of corticomedullar differentiation. Despite aggressive intravenous hydration with normal saline and urine alkalinization with sodium bicarbonate, urinary output decreased, and the patient developed anuric renal failure on day 2 with a creatinine level of 8.2 mg/dL and urea nitrogen level of 130 mg/dL. Hemodialysis was initiated on day 2.

Postdialysis laboratory investigations revealed that the levels of plasma amino acids and plasma carnitine fell within the control range, as did the urine organic acid profile. The free carnitine level was 41 μmol/L (control range, 30–50 μmol/L), and the total carnitine level was 46 μmol/L (control range, 43–65 μmol/L). The plasma acylcarnitine profile revealed a marked increase of long-chain acylcarnitines, with C12, C14, C16, and C18:1 concentrations of 0.4, 1.1, 0.7, and 0.8 μmol/L, respectively. (Control levels for all of these metabolites were <0.1–0.3 μmol/L.) The patient was discharged without any treatment at day 21.

Why did this patient develop rhabdomyolysis?

A. Carnitine palmitoyltransferase II (CPT II) deficiency-related rhabdomyolysis.
B. Infection-related rhabdomyolysis.

The correct answer is A

Comment: Our patient presented with classical clinical and biological symptoms of AKI resulting from rhabdomyolysis. The electrolyte abnormalities that occurred include hyperkalemia, metabolic acidosis, hyperphosphatemia, and hypocalcemia. The patient then had a transient episode of hypercalcemia (13 mg/dL), with the recovery of renal function resulting from the mobilization of calcium, normalization of serum phosphate, and increase in calcitriol.

The primary cause of AKI in this patient is rhabdomyolysis. Rhabdomyolysis may not be the only cause of AKI. Diagnosis of CPT II deficiency was suspected clinically by the occurrence of severe and recurrent rhabdomyolysis based on the acylcarnitine profile. The diagnosis was confirmed by measurement of CPT II enzyme activity, which showed a low CPT II activity of approximately 10% of control values. Molecular analysis in our patient identified compound heterozygosity for the p.Ser113Leu and p.Pro50His mutations in the *CPT2* gene.[1,2]

The management regimen includes the treatment of rhabdomyolysis-induced AKI and the prevention of further rhabdomyolysis episodes. Alkalinization of urine by sodium bicarbonate administration has been recommended by some authors. Hemodialysis is required in severe rhabdomyolysis with refractory hyperkalemia or prolonged oligo-anuric renal failure.

The prevention of CPT II deficiency-related rhabdomyolysis is mainly based on measures to limit energy depletion. For example, the following activities should be avoided: extended fasting; strenuous exercise, especially in the cold; increased body metabolism with fever; or treatment with anesthesia. Infusions of glucose during intercurrent infections and adequate hydration during episodes of diarrhea or vomiting are necessary to prevent catabolism. A high-carbohydrate and low-fat diet before and during prolonged exercise may also be prescribed. A beneficial effect of bezafibrate in the treatment of the mild form of CPT II deficiency has been shown.[1,2]

In summary, patients with recurrent episodes of rhabdomyolysis should be evaluated for CPT II deficiency. Screening may also be appropriate in patients with a single episode and no evidence of traumatic or toxic causes of rhabdomyolysis. Early recognition of the disease is crucial to initiating early treatment and preventing further recurrences of rhabdomyolysis.

Clinical Presentation 32

A 14-year-old boy presented with respiratory distress, an inability to walk, and widespread muscle pain after playing football. History revealed that the patient occasionally had weakness after exercise and infections and was hospitalized for widespread muscle pain and difficulty in breathing 3 years previously. In addition, his parents were second-degree relatives.

On physical examination, the patient's general well-being was moderate, he was conscious, but restless and looked pale. His blood pressure was 163/90 mm Hg. Urine output was 1.4 mL/kg/h and its color was dark brown. The urine examination by dipstick showed 3+ blood in the urine, but microscopic examination did not show erythrocytes. Whole blood count showed hemoglobin 9.0 g/dL, white blood cell 22,300/mm^3, and platelet count 280,000/mm^3. Blood chemistry results were as follows: blood glucose 88 mg/dL, BUN 19 mg/dL, creatinine 1.2 mg/dL, creatinine phosphokinase 2460 U/L (normal range, 10–145 U/L), AST 901 U/L, ALT 181 U/L, lactate dehydrogenase 2590 U/L, uric acid 9.8 mg/dL, Na 139 mg/dL, K 4.9 mg/dL, Cl 103 mg/dL, phosphate 4.1 mg/dL, and calcium 8.9 mg/dL. He had mild metabolic acidosis (pH: 7.34 and HCO_3; 18 BE: −5.0). Thyroid function tests were normal (free T4, free T3, thyroid-stimulating hormone). Electrocardiography and echocardiography were normal. There was increased echogenicity in the parenchyma of both kidneys on renal ultrasonography. Repeat laboratory analysis the following day showed deterioration: BUN 85 mg/dL, creatinine 4.8 mg/dL, uric acid 9.6 mg/dL, and urinary output 0.3 mL/kg/h.

What diagnostic tests would you order now?

A. CPT II analysis.
B. Lactate dehydrogenase.
C. Adenosine monophosphate deaminase analysis.
D. Glycogen phosphorylase kinase analysis.

The correct answer is A

Comment: Our patient initially presented with respiratory distress and widespread muscle pain following exercise, after which dark urine symptoms developed. During follow-up periods, clinical and laboratory findings showed acute kidney injury and rhabdomyolysis. Laboratory analyses ruled out hypothyroidism, hyperthyroidism, diabetic ketoacidosis, and severe electrolyte disturbances (hyponatremia, hypernatremia, hypokalemia, hypophosphatemia), which are part of the etiological spectrum of rhabdomyolysis. Therefore, a decision was made to analyze CPT II enzyme activity in leukocytes, which showed 0.03 nmol/min protein (normal range, 0.2–1 nmol/min protein), consistent with CPT II deficiency.

Long-chain fatty acids (LCFAs) are the main source of energy for muscles during prolonged exercise. LCFAs cannot diffuse into mitochondria passively. Instead, they are activated by LCFA-CoA synthase in the outer membrane of mitochondria and are transmitted into mitochondria through the carnitine palmitoyltransferase pathway, which contains two enzymes: carnitine palmitoyltransferase I in the outer membrane and CPT II in the inner membrane.[1]

CPT II deficiency, which has an autosomal recessive pattern of inheritance, is the most common LCFA disorder.[2] It may appear in the neonatal period, in the infantile period, or in adulthood. When it appears in adulthood, rhabdomyolysis attacks develop because of increased fatty acid and catecholamine metabolism resulting from prolonged exercise, cold weather, infections, hunger, emotional stress, general anesthesia, and administration of some drugs such as ibuprofen, diazepam, and valproate. Our patient had rhabdomyolysis and myoglobinuria, which led to an accumulation of iron in the proximal tubules.

The differential diagnosis includes metabolic conditions presenting with rhabdomyolysis and myoglobinuria attacks, such as adenosine monophosphate deaminase deficiency, muscle glycogen phosphorylase deficiency (McArdle disease: glycogen storage disease type V), muscle glycogen phosphorylase kinase deficiency (glycogen storage disease type VIII), muscle glycolytic disorders, and lactate dehydrogenase deficiency. In McArdle disease, exercise-induced increased creatinine kinase levels are pathognomonic, which is an important differentiation from CPT II deficiency. Besides these primary muscle diseases, drugs (valproic acid, propofol, isoniazid [INH], zidovudine, etc.), infections (influenza A and B), ischemia, vigorous exercise, polymyositis, snake poison, hyperthyroidism, hypothyroidism, toxins (cocaine, heroin, ethanol, fungi), pheochromocytoma, and trauma should also be considered in the differential diagnosis.[3]

Clinical Presentation 33

A 16-year-old otherwise healthy adolescent boy was admitted to our hospital with complaints of nausea, vomiting, headache, and fever lasting 4 days. His first complaints started 6 days before admission when he began to suffer from generalized myalgia and abdominal and back pain. He lived in a rural area. His and his family histories were unremarkable. On presentation, he looked acutely ill, and physical examination revealed conjunctival hemorrhage, pharyngeal injection together with facial flushing, diffuse abdominal tenderness, and excoriate lesions on his feet and soles. His heart rate was 110/min, BP 83/61 mm Hg, respiratory rate 33/min, and temperature was 39°C. Initial laboratory values were as follows: hemoglobin 11 g/dL, white blood cell 9100/mm^3, platelets 10,500/mm^3, C-reactive protein 230 mg/L, erythrocyte sedimentation rate 63 mm/h, serum creatinine level 4.6 mg/dL, and BUN 88 mg/dL. There was no hemolysis on blood smear examination. Prothrombin, partial thromboplastin time, and fibrinogen levels were normal. Aspartate aminotransferase (70 U/L), alanine aminotransferase (68 U/L), and lactic acid dehydrogenase (470 U/L) were elevated. Urinalysis showed microscopic hematuria, pyuria, hyposthenuria, and mild proteinuria. The initial chest radiograph was normal. There was increased echogenicity in the parenchyma of both kidneys on renal ultrasonography.

In the follow-up, his fever subsided and then he developed epistaxis and petechiae on his soft palate and entire body, as well as hypotension (64/41 mm Hg), bradycardia, and clinical shock. Urine output decreased to <0.5 mL/kg/h. Leukocytosis with a left shift (28,000/mm^3, 90% neutrophil), hypoalbuminemia (2.4 g/dL), striking elevations in BUN and serum creatinine levels (108/6.6 mg/dL, respectively), hyponatremia, hyperkalemia, and metabolic acidosis developed. He was treated with supportive care (fluid and inotropic agents) and CVVH with dialysis. On the fourth day of admission to the pediatric intensive care unit, his general condition was good, blood pressure returned to normal, urine output increased to 5 mL/kg/h, serum creatinine improved to 0.6 mg/dL, and platelet count increased to 360,000/mm^3. The patient was discharged from the pediatric intensive care unit after 7 days.

What is your diagnosis and what additional diagnostic tests would you perform?

A. Hemolytic uremic syndrome.
B. Hemolytic thrombocytopenic purpura.
C. Disseminated intravascular coagulation.
D. Hemorrhagic fever with renal syndrome.

The correct answer is D

Comment: This patient presented with fever, nausea, vomiting, headache, abdominal pain, and generalized myalgia. His clinical course progressed through clinical shock with hypotension, followed by oliguric, polyuric, and recovery phases. Laboratory examination showed thrombocytopenia, a left shift in leukocyte differential count, elevated levels of hepatic transaminases and lactate dehydrogenase, hypoalbuminemia, microscopic hematuria, pyuria, hyposthenuria, and mild proteinuria. He was living in a rural and endemic area for hantavirus infection, and the history was retaken regarding possible rodent exposure; his family stated that he walked barefoot in the forested area infested with rodent feces and he had excoriated lesions on his feet and soles. These findings led to the consideration of hemorrhagic fever with renal syndrome, and during hospitalization, hantavirus infection was proven serologically. Due to the presence of fever, thrombocytopenia and renal failure without laboratory findings of any bacterial or viral infection can be ruled out in the differential diagnosis.

Hantaviruses, which are members of the Bunyaviridae family, are the etiologic agents of a diverse group of rodent-borne hemorrhagic fevers and are responsible for considerable morbidity and mortality worldwide. Hantaviruses can lead to two different types of infection in humans, namely, hantavirus pulmonary syndrome and hemorrhagic fever with renal syndrome (HFRS). HFRS is the most common type of hantavirus infection in Europe and Asia (China, Korea, and the eastern part of Russia), and the most common virus types are Puumala, Dobrova, Hantaan, and Seoul. Because of the predominantly rural nature of the disease and its prevalence in developing regions of the Eurasian land mass, accurate case reporting and statistical data for HFRS are limited.[1] The presence of the virus in Turkey is not surprising because it circulates in neighboring countries. Although the exact incidence is not known in Turkey, 5.2% seroprevalence was found among the healthy but at-risk population of one of the affected provinces.[2]

Clinical Presentation 34

An 11-year-old boy was referred with the complaint of vomiting 6 times in a day. History was marked by premature birth at the 28th gestational week, birth asphyxia, cerebral palsy, motor intellectual disability, and epilepsy. He had been treated chronically with baclofen, diazepam, and L-dopa and had been hospitalized for chronic constipation and rectal bleeding twice. Evaluation for metabolic diseases was reported to be normal. His parents were not relatives, and he had two healthy siblings. Physical examination was characterized by normal vital signs, impaired anthropometric development including head circumference, severe mental-motor retardation, and spasticity in all extremities. Laboratory tests revealed low hemoglobin (10.8 g/dL), low mean corpuscular volume (74 fL), and normal kidney and liver function tests and electrolytes. Urinalysis showed microscopic hematuria; urine culture was sterile.

Persistent and bloody vomiting necessitated stopping enteral feeding and placement of a nasogastric tube. Abdominal ultrasonography could not be interpreted because of the presence of widespread intestinal air. The patient was transferred to the intensive care unit on the fourth day of follow-up because of deterioration of his general status and development of abdominal distension. Repeated ultrasonography showed free fluid in the abdomen. Abdominal computed tomography verified the presence of widespread fluid in the abdomen. In addition, computed tomography showed contracted urinary bladder with irregularly thickened wall and massive dilatation of the rectum resulting from fecal impaction. The patient had impaired renal function (BUN 26 mg/dL, creatinine 2.14 mg/dL, creatinine clearance 30 mL/min/1.73 m^2) and oliguria concurrently. Placement of a bladder catheter caused regression of abdominal distension.

What is the underlying etiology of ascites and acute kidney injury in our patient?

A. Rupture of the bladder from trauma.
B. Iatrogenic rupture of bladder.
C. Spontaneous rupture of the bladder from fecal impaction.
D. Rapture of the bladder because of diverticula.

The correct answer is C

Comment: The causes of ascites in children include trauma, infection, hepatocellular, pancreatic, and gastrointestinal abnormalities, and malignancies. Paracentesis and analysis of the fluid are often necessary for a specific diagnosis.[1]

Our patient had no history of hepatic, renal, pancreatic, or gastrointestinal disease other than chronic constipation. The diagnosis of bladder rupture in our patient was suspected by his inability to void, abdominal distension, and azotemia. The diagnosis was confirmed by tomography that showed intraperitoneal fluid, overdistended rectum from fecal impaction, contracted and laterally displaced bladder; and confirmed by exploratory laparoscopy. Diagnosis was further supported by clinical improvement and return of renal function to normal following the insertion of a Foley catheter suggested the diagnosis of spontaneous urinary ascites from chronic constipation and fecal impaction.

Clinical Presentation 35

A 2-year-old boy was admitted to a pediatric hematology department because of a 2-day history of fever of 39°C, vomiting, diarrhea, jaundice, and general malaise.

On admission, the patient was in overall good clinical condition, without fever or symptoms of a respiratory tract infection. Physical examination revealed slight yellowing of the skin and sclerae, and mild hepatomegaly (1 cm below the costal arch). Laboratory testing showed anemia with a hemoglobin level of 6.1 g/dL, platelet count of 218,000/mm^3 (normal reference range, 250,000–400,000/mm^3), biochemical features of hemolysis, including relative reticulocyte count of 32.5%, increased levels of lactate dehydrogenase at 5926 U/L (normal reference range, up to 920 U/L), iron at 234 µg/dL (normal reference range, up to 145 µg/dL), ferritin at 1309.98 ng/mL (normal reference range, up to 140 ng/mL), and total bilirubin at 4.4 mg/dL, as well as elevated inflammation markers, including a C-reactive protein level of 5.4 mg/dL (normal reference range, up to 1 mg/dL) and leukocyte 15,000/mm^3. The blood film showed anisocytosis, myelocytes, and spherocytes but no schistocytes. The direct antiglobulin test, routinely performed with immunoglobulin (Ig) G antibodies, was negative.

Additional testing showed acute kidney injury, with a creatinine level of 1.3 mg/dL, a glomerular filtration rate estimated using the Schwartz formula of 64 mL/min/1.73 m^2 and a urea level of 191 mg/dL. Serum sodium and potassium levels, as well as arterial blood gases, were normal. Urinalysis showed proteinuria of 135 mg/dL, with 3 to 4 erythrocytes per field of view and numerous hemoglobin deposits. Abdominal ultrasonography revealed enlarged kidneys (length, 70–77 mm) with increased echogenicity.

Based on the overall clinical picture and laboratory findings, autoimmune hemolytic anemia was suspected. Paroxysmal nocturnal hemoglobinuria was excluded based on normal CD59 and CD66b expression on granulocytes and CD55 and CD59 expression on erythrocytes.

The repeated antiglobulin test was positive and showed the presence of complement C3 fragments on RBCs, and biphasic hemolysins were detected in the serum. Parvovirus B19 infection was excluded (based on negative results of anti-PV B19 IgG and anti-PV B19 IgM testing), as were Epstein-Barr virus and cytomegalovirus infections.

The management included transfusion of filtered and irradiated packed RBCs (on three occasions) and protecting the patient from cold.

Further laboratory testing performed during the hospitalization period showed increases in creatinine and urea levels to 1.7 and 199 mg/dL, respectively, on the second day of hospital stay, along with platelet count reduction to 139,000/mm^3. Parameters of renal function normalized on the 10th day of treatment. Two weeks after discharge, all of the blood count and renal function parameters were normal, with no anemia noted. At that time, the hemoglobin level was 12.7 g/dL, and direct antiglobulin test results continued to be positive.

What is the likely diagnosis?

A. Hemolytic anemia.
B. Acquired aplastic anemia.
C. Paroxysmal cold hemoglobinuria (PCH).
D. Glucose-6-phosphate dehydrogenase deficiency.

The correct answer is C

Comment: AKI in paroxysmal cold hemoglobinuria results from a toxic effect of the released hemoglobin on renal tubules, mediated by tubular lumen occlusion caused by complexes formed of heme and Tamm-Horsfall protein.[1] A molecular mechanism for a toxic effect of heme has also been reported that results from a deficiency of heme oxygenase, which in turn is responsible for heme degradation. This process leads to increased levels of free iron and subsequent renal failure.

Intravascular hemolysis results from the activation of the complement cascade by cold-reactive, biphasic IgG antibodies. The direct antiglobulin test becomes positive with the use of anti-C3 serum. Protection from cold and symptomatic treatment are of paramount importance in the management of this condition. Glucocorticosteroids are of limited use in paroxysmal cold hemoglobinuria as their therapeutic effects are modest.

Clinical Presentation 36

A 15-day-old firstborn baby of nonconsanguineous parents presented to our hospital with poor feeding and an 18% weight loss on day 8 of life. He was born at 42 weeks' gestation by emergency cesarean section because of failure of progress with a birth weight of 4.078 kg. His antenatal history was uneventful with normal anomaly scans. He was noted to be a poor feeder but otherwise normal on physical examination. His parents were advised to top-up his feeds at home. His weight improved initially but he became progressively lethargic and floppy on day 17 of life. There was no history of fever, diarrhea, or vomiting.

On admission, he was clinically dehydrated with reduced skin turgor and a sunken fontanelle. His weight was 3.54 kg (weight loss of 13% compared with birth weight). He had otherwise no dysmorphic facial features. His respiratory, cardiovascular, and abdominal examinations were unremarkable. He had normal external genitalia with bilateral descended testes. Blood tests revealed his sodium to be 110 mmol/L, potassium of 8.1 mmol/L, urea of 65 mg/dL, plasma creatinine of 4.2 mg/dL, and uric acid 8.3 mg/dL. He was acidotic with a pH of 7.26, bicarbonate of 14.8 mmol/L, and base excess was −15.1. His liver function tests and albumin were normal. His hemoglobin was 176 (normal, 125–205) g/L, total white cell count was raised with neutrophil predominance at 21.3×10^9/L (normal, 6–18 $\times 10^9$/L). His urine dipstick showed 1+ protein, 1+ blood, and 3+ leukocytes. He was given boluses of normal saline, followed by intravenous bicarbonate and replacement intravenous fluid. Blood samples were sent for endocrine investigations to rule out congenital adrenal hyperplasia, all of which were normal.

On reassessment, he still appeared to be dehydrated with dry mucous membranes. His capillary refill was 3 seconds. He was given a further 20-mL/kg bolus of normal saline and then maintenance intravenous fluids with nasogastric feed. His total amount of fluid intake was up to 200 mL/kg/day. He had good urine output of 2 to 4 mL/kg/h. He also required two further corrections with sodium bicarbonate for his metabolic acidosis. With rehydration, his plasma creatinine gradually came down to 212 μmol/L 4 days after admission, although he remained hyponatremic with sodium requirement as high as 15 mmol/kg/day. He also had persistent acidosis despite rehydration and correction with sodium bicarbonate. Two days after admission, he was noted to have a swollen left index finger at the proximal interphalangeal joint. X-ray of the left hand showed soft-tissue swelling at the proximal interphalangeal joint of the index finger.

He was able to maintain good urine output all along and his urine was sent for tubulopathy screen. He had elevated urine albumin to creatinine ratio of 35 (normal, 1.7–12.2) mg/mmol, elevated urate to creatinine ratio of 5.31 (normal, 0.42–1.53) mg/mmol, elevated oxalate to creatinine ratio of 173 (normal, 4–98) μmol/mmol, and a normal urine calcium to creatinine ratio of 0.47 (normal, 0.06–0.74) mmol/mmol. Over the next few days, his plasma creatinine continued to improve to 115 μmol/L. Renal ultrasound showed that both kidneys were echogenic with multiple shadowing flecks within the medullary pyramids.

What is the likely diagnosis?

A. Lesch-Nyhan syndrome.
B. Lang disease.
C. Tourette syndrome.
D. Familial dysautonomia.

The correct answer is A

Comment: Hyperuricemia and AKI are essential features of Lesch-Nyhan syndrome. Hypoxanthine-guanine-phosphoribosyl-transferase (HPRT) test. HPRT enzyme is vital for the normal purine salvage pathway function. Varying degrees of residual HPRT activities are associated with the different phenotypes. The causes of AKI in Lesch-Nyhan syndrome are the precipitation and deposition of uric acid crystals that obstruct urine flow, particularly at the distal nephron of the kidneys. Dehydration and extracellular volume depletion may further aggravate the situation by increasing the concentration of uric acid in the tubular fluid and urine. Therefore, primary management consisted of cautious rehydration of the patient. The drug of choice to manage hyperuricemia associated with HRPT deficiency is allopurinol.

Lesch-Nyhan syndrome is a rare X-linked recessive disorder caused by a mutation of the gene encoding the enzyme HPRT.[1] It is characterized by the progressive development of hyperuricemia and neurological dysfunction, including spasticity and neurobehavioral symptoms, with possible subsequent self-mutilation behavior. Varying levels of residual HRPT activity co-relate with the overlapping phenotypes with different clinical pictures.[2] The classical Lesch-Nyhan syndrome patients with the most severe disease have a residual enzyme level of <1.5%; Lesch-Nyhan disease variants with 1.5% to 8% of residual HPRT activity present with hyperuricemia and neurological disability. Patients with at least 8% of residual HPRT activity (Kelly-Seemiller syndrome) present with hyperuricemia but have apparently normal neurological development.[3]

Clinical Presentation 37

A 2-year-old boy was admitted to pediatric intensive care with persistent fever and AKI. At the time of his initial visit to a general practitioner, he presented with high fever, respiratory symptoms (coughing, rhinitis), vomiting, abdominal pain, and cervical lymphadenopathy; he was prescribed oral amoxicillin and ibuprofen for a suspected upper respiratory tract infection. However, 3 days later, he had to be admitted to the local hospital because of persistent fever. Bacterial sepsis was suspected, and his antibiotic treatment was switched to intravenous amoxicillin-clavulanate, but without improvement. He had no history of any major illnesses or kidney disease and had no previous history of medication use. His condition worsened, and high spiking fever (temperatures ≥104°F) persisted, but repeated cultures (blood, urine) remained negative. Elevated serum creatinine and BUN levels were also noted, and he developed metabolic acidosis for which sodium bicarbonate was given. These symptoms led to a suspicion of a tubulointerstitial nephritis secondary to sepsis. He was admitted on the fifth day of illness because of increasing serum creatinine and BUN levels with a potential need for dialysis.

At presentation, the child had an ill-looking appearance and was tachycardic, with a normal BP, normal oxygen saturation, and a capillary refill of ≤2 seconds. Bilateral conjunctivitis, periorbital edema, a hyperemic pharynx, dry cracked lips with blood crusts, and cervical lymphadenopathy were also noted. Several petechiae were clearly visible on his shoulders and axillary areas, but no exanthema was present. Mild respiratory distress with wheezing on lung auscultation was noted in addition to a tender abdomen with normal peristalsis.

The results of the laboratory tests were: hemoglobin, 10.0 g/dL, leukocytes, 27,300/mm^3; platelets, 157,000/mm^3; activated partial thromboplastin time, 49 (reference, 28–38) seconds; prothrombin time, 64.7% (reference, 70%–120%); fibrinogen, 699 (reference, 200–400) mg/dL; C-reactive protein, 282 (reference, <5) mg/L; sodium, 134 mmol/L; potassium, 4.4 mmol/L; calcium, 9.8 mg/dL, phosphate, 6.1 mg/dL, BUN, 103 mg/dL; serum creatinine, 2.0 mg/dL; albumin, 3.3 g/dL, aspartate aminotransferase, 82 (reference, 11–50) U/L; alanine aminotransferase, 42 (reference, 7–40) U/L; and lactate dehydrogenase, 264 (reference, 160–370) U/L. Complement, creatine kinase, and uric acid levels were normal, whereas Ig levels (IgA, IgG, IgM) were all slightly elevated.

The urinalysis showed 2+ blood, 2+, mild proteinuria (protein-creatinine index/ratio 3.57 g/g creatinine). Blood and urine cultures were negative, but the polymerase chain reaction (PCR) assay of the nasopharyngeal smear was positive for human metapneumovirus, rhinovirus, and parainfluenza viruses. The chest x-ray did not show any abnormalities.

A Doppler renal ultrasound showed normal perfusion and increased corticomedullary differentiation and increased size of the kidneys (left kidney, 11.4 cm; right kidney, 10.4 cm; normal range, 5–7 cm). A moderate amount of ascites was noticed on the ultrasound image, but no additional abnormalities were detected. The patient was started on broad-spectrum intravenous antibiotics therapy and oxygen supplementation, but fever persisted. His condition deteriorated, and he became oliguric, subsequently developed progressive fluid overload with peripheral edema, hepatomegaly, and increasing ascites. Fluid restriction and administration of a loop diuretic were initiated.

What is the likely diagnosis?

A. Sepsis-induced AKI.
B. Ibuprofen-induced AKI.
C. Kawasaki disease (KD).
D. IgA nephritis.
E. Hemolytic uremic syndrome (HUS).

The correct answer is C

Comment: Establishing the correct diagnosis was challenging. Sepsis and associated AKI could have explained the clinical picture, including the coagulopathy, but repeated cultures of blood and urine were negative, and no improvement was noted with the administration of antibiotics. IgA nephropathy has been associated with several infections and might present as nephritis with increased corticomedullar differentiation. However, episodes of IgA nephropathy are often mild and rarely result in AKI, except in severe cases with nephrotic range proteinuria.[1] Tubulointerstitial nephritis or reduced renal perfusion secondary to ibuprofen (a nonsteroidal antiinflammatory drug) use could have explained AKI but was less likely given this patient's clinical presentation. HUS could explain the anemia and thrombocytopenia, but lactate dehydrogenase and complement levels were normal and there was no history of bloody diarrhea. Lupus nephritis was also a possible explanation, but autoimmune tests eventually came back negative, and a high C-reactive protein level is not a common presenting feature unless concurrent bacterial infection is present. Acute pyelonephritis was unlikely since repeated urine cultures were negative.

In light of the clinical course and renal ultrasound image, KD was suspected, and intravenous immunoglobulin (IVIG; 2 g/kg body weight) was administered on the sixth day of illness. Because fever persisted, the treatment with IVIG was repeated 48 hours later. The fever tapered, and the patient's temperature normalized shortly thereafter, whereas urinary output increased. The maximum levels of serum creatinine and BUN were 2.12 and 103 mg/dL, respectively, but dialysis was not needed. Renal function improved gradually, with a lowering of the serum creatinine and BUN levels from the ninth day of illness, but the hematuria, proteinuria, and leukocyturia persisted. The patient's anemia worsened, and iron supplementation was started after an erythropoietin infusion. The patient developed thrombocytosis (maximum, 1,000,000/mm^3), and the leukocyte count normalized. With this improved clinical status, he was transferred to the general pediatric ward after 5 days on the pediatric intensive care unit. On the 13th day of illness, he also developed peeling of the fingertips of both hands, which fulfilled the criteria for the complete form of KD. He was discharged soon after in good clinical condition. Renal function completely recovered, and no coronary abnormalities were detected during follow-up.

KD is a frequent cause of vasculitis in children younger than 5 years of age. The criteria for KD according to the American Heart Association the presence of at least four of the following six principal features[2]:

1. Fever persisting for at least 5 days
2. Erythema and edema of hands and feet; membranous desquamation of fingertips
3. Polymorphous exanthema
4. Bilateral, painless bulbar conjunctival injection without exudate
5. Changes in lips and oral cavity: erythema and cracking of lips, strawberry tongue, diffuse injection of oral and pharyngeal mucosa
6. Cervical lymphadenopathy (diameter ≥1.5 cm), usually unilateral.

Without treatment, 20% to 25% of these patients develop coronary abnormalities in comparison to <5% when timely treatment is administered.[3] In addition to cardiac involvement, several other organs and organ systems can be affected, including the gastrointestinal tract, joints, hematopoietic system, respiratory tract, and the neurological and urogenital tracts. AKI is rarely a presenting feature, in contrast to sterile pyuria, which is often seen.[4] However, renal complications ranging from nephrotic syndrome to full-blown renal failure requiring dialysis have been described.[4,5]

Clinical Presentation 38

A 10-year-old boy presented with symptoms of persistent vomiting during the preceding 3 days and anuria in the previous 24 hours. Vomiting was nonbilious and occurring up to 10 times per day. He was also quite thirsty and complained of leg cramps. There was no fever or diarrhea and no signs of a respiratory infection. No symptoms of abdominal pain or dysuria were present and he regularly passed stool (once a day). His medical history had been uneventful until the age of 7 years, when he started having episodes of vomiting. Screening for conditions such as *Helicobacter pylori* infection and celiac disease had been negative; psychogenic vomiting was suspected because these episodes seemed to coincide with periods of stress. He did not take any medication and his family history was negative for gastrointestinal and renal disease.

At physical examination, the boy was cooperative and alert and had a dry mouth and tongue. Heart rate was 105 beats/min, BP 118/75 mm Hg, and oxygen saturation 100%. Auscultation of the heart and lungs was normal. No abdominal distension was noticed and the rest of the examination did not reveal any abnormalities. He was 142.7 cm (standard deviation −1.5) in height and weighed 30.2 kg (standard deviation −1.5).

His laboratory results were as follows: hemoglobin 16.4; leukocytes 10.2 × 10^3/µL; thrombocytes 350,000/mm^3; sodium 131 mmol/L; potassium 3.7 mmol/L; chloride 77 mmol/L; calcium 9.8 mg/L; phosphate 10.2 mg/dL; magnesium 2.1 mg/dL; bicarbonate 36 mmol/L; BUN 51 mg/dL; serum creatinine 1.7 mg/dL; uric acid 8.1 mg/dL; C-reactive protein 0.9 mg/dL (reference, 0–0.5); aspartate aminotransferase 35 U/L (reference, 0–37); alanine aminotransferase 13 U/L (reference, 7–40); lactate dehydrogenase, 443 U/L (reference, 110–293); lipase 18 U/L (reference, 15–110); and parathyroid hormone 168 ng/L (15–65).

A renal ultrasound showed large kidneys (left, 10.2 cm; right, 10.3 cm), with increased cortical echogenicity and corticomedullary differentiation. The patient's serum creatinine and BUN had decreased to 1.5 and 43 mg/dL, respectively, within 24 hours. His urinalysis showed no proteinuria, but 2+ hematuria. After intravenous rehydration, he recovered well clinically with normalization of diuresis and an ability to take foods without vomiting the next day.

What is the diagnosis and how would you proceed?

A. Primary hyperoxaluria.
B. ATN.
C. Chronic glomerulopathy.
D. Prerenal azotemia.

The correct answer is A

Comment: In prerenal AKI with or without ATN, there should not be any abnormalities on renal ultrasound because no structural damage has taken place. That after rehydration, urinary output was immediately restored indicates a prerenal component of the renal dysfunction but does not explain the ultrasound abnormalities. He was not discharged and an additional workup was planned.

Hyperphosphatemia and hyperparathyroidism together typically point more toward chronic kidney disease (CKD)[1,2] than AKI, and this was the initial indication that there might have been a preexisting renal problem. The ultrasound image is unusual for ATN because, in that case, we expected a globally increased echogenicity.[3] In addition, there is usually a delay in the normalization of urinary output after rehydration.[4] In ATN, urinalysis typically shows epithelial cell casts and free renal tubular epithelial cells,[4] which were absent in this case. The ultrasound image thus indicated a different underlying condition than ATN and we decided to perform a renal biopsy to exclude underlying conditions such as glomerulonephritis, tubulointerstitial nephritis, and CKD. Autoimmune antibody testing (antinuclear antibodies, antistreptolysin O antibodies) and complement screening both came back negative. A biopsy showed normal glomeruli and no signs of tubulointerstitial nephritis. However, the tubules were filled with amorphous material consistent with the presentation of hyperoxaluria, which was later confirmed by biochemical testing.

The patient was suspected to have primary hyperoxaluria and treatment was commenced consisting of pyridoxine (vitamin B6), hyperhydration, and magnesium supplementation. Twenty-four-hour urine screening (performed before the start of therapy) showed hyperoxaluria. Genetic testing for primary hyperoxaluria (*AGXT*/*GRHPR* genes) also came back positive.

Hyperoxaluria is a condition characterized by the accumulation of oxalate in the body, with increased oxalate excretion in the urine and deposition of calcium oxalate in the kidneys and urinary tract, leading to nephrocalcinosis and urolithiasis. It is traditionally divided into primary, dietary, idiopathic, and enteric hyperoxaluria.[4] Primary hyperoxaluria is the most common form caused by genetic mutations and divided into type 1 (*AGXT* gene) and type 2 (*GRHPR* gene). These mutations lead to defective liver enzyme function (respectively, alanine-glyoxylate aminotransferase and glyoxylate reductase/hydroxypyruvate reductase) and subsequent overproduction of oxalate by the liver.[5] Extrarenal calcium oxalate depositions usually occur when the glomerular filtration rate decreases below 30 to 50 mL/min, and reduced oxalate excretion by the kidneys leads to a critical saturation point, inducing oxalate precipitation in several organs such as the skeleton, joints, nerves, and heart.[5] In dietary hyperoxaluria, an excessive oxalate intake (e.g., increased intake of coffee, chocolate, spinach, animal protein, and fruit juice) is the underlying cause,[5] whereas in the idiopathic form no specific cause has yet been determined. Enteric hyperoxaluria accounts for 5% of cases of hyperoxaluria and is often seen secondary to (fat) malabsorption related to intestinal surgery, intestinal bacterial overgrowth syndromes, or inflammatory bowel disease.[5] Under normal circumstances, most of the ingested oxalate is bound by free calcium in the gut and not absorbed. Malabsorption causes unabsorbed bile acids (normally absorbed in the proximal intestine) to bind calcium and magnesium salts in the intestine-forming complexes. This prevents the normal calcium-oxalate binding, leaving excess free oxalate to be absorbed in the colon, with subsequent oxalosis and hyperoxaluria. This explains the course in our patient.

Clinical Presentation 39

A 17-year-old girl presented to a local hospital emergency department with productive cough and shortness of breath as well as intermittent vomiting and diarrhea. Initial vital signs showed a heart rate of 101/min and blood pressure of 121/69 mm Hg. She weighed 89.3 kg on admission. Physical examination on presentation was significant for diminished breath sounds throughout and end-expiratory wheezing.

She was diagnosed with hypogammaglobulinemia and natural killer cell deficiency, with a low absolute number and decreased function of natural killer cells. She had an improvement in the frequency of her infections after starting therapy with intravenous immunoglobulin. At 16 years of age, she presented with cervical lymphadenopathy. A lymph node biopsy showed effacement of nodal architecture by a diffuse proliferation of atypical cells and areas of expansile, closely packed follicles lacking polarization. She was diagnosed with stage III follicular lymphoma and underwent six cycles of chemotherapy with rituximab, cyclophosphamide, doxorubicin, and prednisone that was completed about 2.5 years before presentation. During her chemotherapy, she was noted to have a normal serum creatinine of 0.5 to 0.6 mg/dL. She was seen 17 months before the current admission for recurrence of left-sided lymphadenopathy. A lymph node biopsy showed plasmacytosis with a mixed lymphocyte population, without diagnostic features of follicular lymphoma and no clonal B-cell population. At that time, she was noted to have a serum creatinine at her baseline of 0.6 mg/dL. Subsequently, she became pregnant and had a miscarriage. Since then, she had been lost to follow-up for about 10 months before the current admission.

On this admission, she was noted to have systolic BP in the 130 to 140 mm Hg range and mild pitting edema in her lower extremities. Her urine output was reported to be decreased but without gross hematuria or microscopic hematuria. She was treated with ceftriaxone and azithromycin for pneumonia and had an improvement in her cough and dyspnea. A urinalysis was performed and showed specific gravity 1.010, 2+ proteinuria, 1+ leukocyte esterase, and trace blood without red cells or red cell casts. Her spot urine protein to creatinine ratio was 1.95. An abdominal ultrasound was performed and showed a small amount of pelvic free fluid but was otherwise normal, with normal renal size and architecture and no hydronephrosis. Laboratory tests showed a serum creatinine level of 4.9 mg/dL, BUN of 36 mg/dL, serum albumin of 1.9 g/dL, C-reactive protein of 76 mg/L, and erythrocyte sedimentation rate >140 mm/h. Complete blood count showed a hemoglobin of 8.4 g/dL, white cell 15,500/mm^3 with 52% neutrophils and 37% lymphocytes, and platelet count 239 × 10^3/mm^3. Immunologic evaluation showed a mildly low IgG level of 662 mg/dL, with normal IgA and IgM. Complement C3 (130 mg/dL) and C4 (13 mg/dL) levels were normal. Anti–double-stranded DNA antibodies, antinuclear antibodies (ANA), antiextractable nuclear antigen antibodies, and antineutrophil cytoplasmic antibodies (ANCA) were negative. Lymphocyte subpopulation evaluation was significant for high absolute CD3, CD4, and CD8 counts (5389 cells/mm^3, 606 cells/mm^3, and 1244 cells/mm^3, respectively), low absolute CD19 count (4 cells/mm^3), and absent CD15+CD56 cells. A chest computed tomography scan showed multifocal right-sided pneumonia. Polymerase chain reaction testing of nasopharyngeal secretions was positive for *Mycoplasma pneumoniae* and rhinovirus/enterovirus.

An infectious workup showed positive cytomegalovirus DNA below quantifiable levels, nonreactive HIV p24-antigen levels, nonreactive rapid plasma reagin test, and negative hepatitis panel. Blood and urine cultures were obtained and remained negative. Hematologic workup showed a reticulocyte count of 2.07%, normal uric acid level at 6.4 mg/dL, and lactate dehydrogenase of 359 U/L. Indirect and direct Coombs were negative.

Given her elevated creatinine and proteinuria, a renal biopsy was performed. The biopsy showed numerous fractured tubular casts that were periodic acid-Schiff and silver-stain negative and fuchsinophilic on trichrome stain, with associated giant cells, tubulitis, acute tubular injury, and tubular rupture. The tubular casts had 3+ staining for lambda light chains and 0–1+ staining for kappa light chains.

What is the likely diagnosis for the proteinuria and acute kidney injury in this patient?

A. Thrombotic microangiopathy.
B. Focal segmental glomerulosclerosis.
C. Membranous nephropathy.

D. Drug-induced tubulointerstitial disease.
E. Light chain cast nephropathy (LCCN).

The correct answer D

Comment: The patient had light chain cast nephropathy as confirmed by renal biopsy. The biopsy findings of tubulitis, acute tubular injury with normal glomeruli appearance with no crescent formation, endocapillary proliferation, or segmental necrosis are pathognomonic of LCCN. Serum free light chains, serum immunofixation, urine protein electrophoresis, and urine immunofixation studies supported the renal biopsy diagnosis of LCCN.[1–3]

Monoclonal gammopathy is a biomarker of the clonal proliferation of cells producing monoclonal immunoglobulin.[4] Monoclonal gammopathies of renal significance are extremely rare in the pediatric population with limited pediatric case reports and limited literature available on pediatric LCCN.[5]

The likely cause of her LCCN was the new diagnosis of a B-cell lymphoma. Other risk factors include her history of hypogammaglobulinemia, natural killer cell deficiency, community-acquired pneumonia, and prior follicular lymphoma. She had a gradual improvement in her renal function after treatment of initiation of chemotherapy. Lymphoma-associated renal involvement occurs by a variety of mechanisms, which are summarized elsewhere.[1,2] Rare cases of LCCN have been described in association with lymphoma.[1,3]

Clinical Presentation 40

A 17-year-old boy with no relevant medical history or active medication presented with gross hematuria and hypogastric pain. Kidney ultrasound revealed medullary hyperechogenicity, suggestive of nephrocalcinosis, and bilateral cysts. A month later, he developed acute renal colic secondary to an obstructive 14-mm stone located in the right ureteropelvic junction, requiring the placement of a double J stent. The stone was removed by ureteroscopy. Infrared spectroscopy showed the stone to be of mixed type: carbapatite, brushite, and calcium oxalate mono- and dihydrate. Family history was negative for nephrolithiasis or cysts and the parents were not consanguineous. Kidney magnetic resonance imaging showed normal-sized kidneys, multiple renal cysts bilaterally, and the absence of liver cysts.

Serum creatinine was 2.3 mg/dL, calcium 12.1 mg/dL, ionized calcium 5.7 mg/dL, phosphorous 6.2 mg/dL, intact PTH <1.3 pg/mL. Total hydroxyvitamin D was 41 ng/mL, and 1,25-hydroxyvitamin D3 was elevated at 185 pg/mL. A 24-hour urine volume was 1500 mL, pH 6.2, creatinine 1500 mg, calcium 202 mg, oxalate 38 mg, and sodium 90 mEq/L.

Chest imaging was normal. Measurement of serum levels of angiotensin-converting enzyme and eye examination were also normal.

What is the differential diagnosis for this patient's hypercalcemia, suppressed PTH, and nephrolithiasis?

A. Squamous cell carcinoma.
B. Sarcoidosis.
C. CYP24A1 deficiency.
D. Lymphoma.

The correct answer is C

Comment: The diagnosis of CYP24A1 deficiency should be suspected in patients with bilateral kidney cysts, high levels of 1,25-dihydroxvitamin D3, nephrocalcinosis, and kidney stones composed of carbapatite, brushite, and/or oxalate calcium dihydrate, which are typically associated with hypercalciuria.

Diagnosis of sarcoidosis was unlikely in the absence of lung pathology and normal level of serum calcium and angiotensin-converting enzyme. Neoplasia was excluded in the absence of skin lesion or lymphadenopathy.

Genetic testing using a next-generation sequencing targeted gene panel revealed a homozygous variant in the CYP24A1 gene predicted to lead to a substitution of tryptophan for arginine at amino acid 396 (p.Arg396Trp); this variant has been previously reported to result in complete loss of function.[2] The patient's parents were both heterozygous for the variant.

This patient has non-parathyroid-related hypercalcemia, of which the most common cause is neoplasia. Both solid tumors and hematologic malignancies may increase bone resorption by various mechanisms: induction of osteolysis by bone metastases, release of osteoclast activating factor in multiple myeloma, secretion of PTH-related protein by some solid tumors (especially squamous cell carcinomas), or production of 1,25-dihydroxyvitamin D (usually by lymphomas).[1]

Nontumor etiologies of non-parathyroid-related hypercalcemia include excessive intake of vitamin D supplements or 1,25-dihydroxyvitamin D3 and increased endogenous production of 1,25-hydroxyvitamin D3 in patients with granulomatous disorders (especially sarcoidosis).

Other rare causes of hypercalcemia include lithium therapy, thiazide diuretics, hypervitaminosis A, thyrotoxicosis, pheochromocytoma, adrenal insufficiency, milk-alkali syndrome, and prolonged immobilization.

A rare additional cause of high vitamin D levels is a monogenic disorder caused by biallelic (or occasionally monoallelic) pathogenic variants in the gene encoding 25-hydroxyvitamin D3 24-hydroxylase. This enzyme, also known as CYP24A1, catalyzes the conversion of 1,25-dihydroxvitamin D3 and 25-hydroxyvitamin D3 into inactive 24-hydroxylated products that are excreted. CYP24A1 deficiency leads to persistently high levels of 1,25-dihydroxvitamin D3. Loss-of-function variants in CYP24A1 may lead to infantile hypercalcemia type 1 (OMIM 143880), also called hypersensitivity to vitamin D3. This hypersensitivity to vitamin D3 can be severe and potentially fatal in infants after prophylactic vitamin D3 supplementation for the prevention of rickets.[2] Adolescent and adult patients may present with recurrent calcium kidney stones, with or without nephrocalcinosis. Recently, medullary and/or corticomedullary junction cysts (a mean of 5.3 cysts per patient) were reported in 16 patients with CYP24A1 deficiency (half of whom had nephrolithiasis as the presenting symptom).[3] The mechanisms of cystogenesis remain unknown, but sustained hypercalciuria and/or exposure to increased calcitriol levels could contribute to kidney cyst development.

The diagnosis of CYP24A1 deficiency should be suspected in patients with bilateral kidney cysts, high levels of 1,25-dihydroxvitamin D3, nephrocalcinosis, and kidney stones composed of carbapatite, brushite, and/or oxalate calcium dihydrate, which are typically associated with hypercalciuria.

The management of CYP24A1 deficiency remains challenging. The patient received dietary counseling on the need to increase water intake; reduce intake of salt, protein, and oxalate; and maintain a diet moderately rich in calcium to enhance bone formation. The patient was also counseled to avoid vitamin D supplements and sun exposure. Thiazide diuretics must be used with caution when treating hypercalciuria, as they may worsen or cause hypercalcemia.

Clinical Presentation 41

A 10-year-old boy was referred and admitted for AKI. He had no significant past medical events and no family history of kidney disease. Before his admission, he had experienced vomiting and diarrhea for 4 days, leading to oliguria. Because these symptoms were shared with his parents and grandparents, acute viral gastroenteritis was clinically suspected and symptomatic treatment was started. Despite this symptomatic treatment, vomiting and diarrhea persisted.

At the time of admission, his physical examination was normal. He had no fever or edema, and his blood pressure was 142/72 mm Hg. Urinary tests showed microscopic hematuria and proteinuria <1 g/L. His laboratory results were as follows: serum creatinine 12.9 mg/dL; sodium 123 mmol/L; potassium 9.1 mmol/L; and bicarbonate 13 mmol/L. His electrocardiogram showed signs of hyperkalemia and he was transferred to the pediatric intensive care unit.

The father and grandfather demonstrated the same gastrointestinal symptoms. Their serum creatinine levels were 9.8 and 13.5 mg/dL, respectively. The mother had less severe AKI (serum creatinine, 1.7 mg/ dL). A renal biopsy was performed in the child, father, and grandfather (at day 6, 9, and 8 after their hospital admission, respectively), and histological analysis showed acute tubulointerstitial nephritis (TIN). Atrophic and necrotic lesions of the tubular epithelium were present in varying degrees in all three patients. Glomeruli and vessels were normal. Immunofluorescence analysis demonstrated the absence of immunoglobulin or complement deposits.

What is the most likely diagnosis of these four AKI family cases?

A. Sepsis.
B. Severe dehydration secondary to acute gastroenteritis.
C. Food poisoning.
D. None of the above.

The correct answer is C

Comment: In this report, four family members developed AKI within a few days following gastroenteritis. Their renal biopsies showed acute TIN. A toxic etiology was therefore suspected.[1] There was no history of nephrotoxic drug exposure. However, all patients ate wild mushrooms during the previous 2 weeks. Taken together, histological findings and analysis of symptoms supported the hypothesis of an orellanus syndrome secondary to ingestion of poisonous mushrooms from the *Cortinarius* genus.[2]

In cases of mushroom poisoning, the mycological identification is often uncertain and is not sufficient to confirm which mushroom was responsible for the toxicity. Therefore, identification of *Cortinarius* poisoning is classically performed by detecting the fungal toxin called orellanine in the biological fluids or in renal tissues.[3,4] The toxin has been detected by high-performance liquid chromatography in renal biopsy samples.[4,5] However, this analytical method is not generally available in clinical practice.

Treatment of orellanus syndrome is generally symptomatic, based on gastric washing and activated charcoal administration in the early phase and on renal replacement therapy in AKI phase.

Cortinarius poisoning is a rare syndrome that is responsible for a delayed toxic tubulointerstitial nephritis that can induce severe acute or chronic renal failure in children and adults.[2]

Our four family patients demonstrated typical orellanus syndrome characterized by a prerenal phase, with nonspecific digestive disorders occurring within 3 days (12 hours to 14 days) after ingestion of the mushrooms. Moreover, a flu-like syndrome was observed in one of our patients.[6] Liver injury has also been described but was not observed in our patients. Sometimes, because of the large duration of the asymptomatic phase, mushroom consumption is repeated in several meals, as in patients in this family. The renal phase was delayed (4–15 days, with a median of 8.5 days after the first mushroom meal).

In our report, all individuals presented with AKI, with variable degrees of severity. When the renal function is normal, a latent TIN may not be suspected in the absence of microscopic hematuria and leukocyturia. The tubular epithelium is the toxin's target, with a direct dose-dependent toxicity that explains the severity of tubulointerstitial injury in the case of the child in our report. The prognosis of *Cortinarius* poisoning is poor, and about 50% of patients present with acute renal failure that evolves into chronic renal failure.[2] In children, a very poor outcome had been described in previous published cases, indicating that all of the five reported cases rapidly developed acute renal failure requiring renal replacement therapy and kidney transplantation in one of them.

Clinical Presentation 42

A previously healthy 11-year-old boy presented to the pediatric emergency department with fever, myalgias, and muscular weakness since the previous day. His urine had turned a dark-brown color. The patient also had diarrhea and occasional vomiting for 2 days. The parents explained that a total dose of 2.1 g of ibuprofen (i.e., 60 mg/kg) had been administered as self-medication the day before.

On admission, the patient's blood pressure was 113/78 mm Hg, and his heart rate was 123/min. Axillary temperature was 39.5°C. Physical examination showed muscular weakness in both legs and flank tenderness. The findings of the respiratory, cardiac, and neurological examinations were normal.

The test results on admission were as follows: rapid testing for influenza A was positive; urine dipstick was positive for bilirubin (3+), blood (3+), and protein (3+). Laboratory tests showed a creatine kinase level of 318,000 U/L, urea nitrogen 45 mg/dL, creatinine 2.5 m/dL, bicarbonate 16 mmol/L, and potassium 5 mmol/L. A diagnosis of massive rhabdomyolysis with AKI was made.

Rhabdomyolysis progressed with a peak creatine kinase level of 348,000 U/L, lactate dehydrogenase 124,000 U/L, serum myoglobin 42,873 µg/L, aspartate aminotransferase 7122 IU/L, alanine aminotransferase 1462 IU/L, metabolic acidosis, hyperkalemia of 5.2 mmol/L, hypocalcemia of 6.5 mg/dL, and hyperphosphatemia of 7 mg/dL. Ultrasound imaging showed enlarged kidneys with a loss of corticomedullar differentiation. Despite aggressive intravenous hydration with normal saline and urine alkalinization with sodium bicarbonate, urinary output decreased, and the patient developed anuric renal failure on day 2 with a creatinine level of 663 µmol/L and urea nitrogen level of 35 mmol/L.

Hemodialysis was initiated on day 2. Nine hemodialysis sessions were necessary until day 16. The patient had no cardiac complication. His condition improved, with diuresis recovery on day 13. Creatine kinase levels and renal function normalized within 1 month.

Three months later, he presented with a second episode of myalgias and brown urine, with an elevated level of creatine kinase of 2801 U/L. The anamnesis revealed that this episode was also preceded by fever. The patient had remained entirely asymptomatic between the two episodes. The outcome was favorable with high fluid intake advice within 24 hours.

A medical history taken to determine etiology indicated that no trauma had occurred, and the boy had not used any illicit drug or toxic substance. Laboratory investigations revealed that the levels of plasma amino acids (ion exchange chromatography) and plasma carnitine fell within the control range, as did the urine organic acid profile. The free carnitine level was 41 µmol/L (control range, 30–50 µmol/L), and total carnitine level was 46 µmol/L (control range, 43–65 µmol/L). The plasma acylcarnitine profile revealed a marked increase of long-chain acylcarnitines, with C12, C14, C16, and C18:1 concentrations of 0.4, 1.1, 0.7, and 0.8 µmol/L, respectively; control level for all of these metabolites was <0.1–0.3 µmol/L). The patient was discharged without any treatment at day 21.

What is the diagnosis?

A. Influenza A infection.
B. High-intensity exercise.
C. Severe dehydration.
D. Rhabdomyolysis from CPT II deficiency.

The correct answer is D

Comment: Our patient presented with classical clinical and biological symptoms of AKI resulting from rhabdomyolysis. The electrolyte abnormalities that occurred include hyperkalemia, metabolic acidosis, hyperphosphatemia, and hypocalcemia. Hypocalcemia might be due to calcium entering the ischemic muscle cells and the precipitation of calcium-phosphate complexes in necrotic muscle.[1] The patient then had a transient episode of hypercalcemia (3 mmol/L), with the recovery of renal function resulting from the mobilization of calcium, normalization of serum phosphate, and increase in calcitriol. The urine and plasma organic acid profile, rise in lactic acid, plasma carnitine levels, and acylcarnitine levels suggested a CPT II deficiency in our patient.[2]

Diagnosis of CPT II deficiency was suspected clinically by the occurrence of severe and recurrent rhabdomyolysis and based on the acylcarnitine profile. The diagnosis was confirmed by the measurement of CPT II enzyme activity and subsequent molecular analysis.

Molecular analysis in our patient identified compound heterozygosity for the p.Ser113Leu and p.Pro50His mutations in the *CPT2* gene. There is a correlation between genotype and phenotype; both of these mutations are considered to be common mutations in patients with the mild form of CPT II deficiency,[3] and inheritance of these mutations is not associated with the more severe infantile or neonatal forms of the disease.[4]

Rhabdomyolysis is facilitated by the fact that mild myopathic CPT II deficiency is characterized by a thermolabile mutant enzyme protein. As such, these patients show susceptibility to high temperature, therefore explaining how myopathic episodes can be triggered by febrile illness. Some drugs, such as valproic acid, diazepam, or ibuprofen, may also trigger attacks of rhabdomyolysis in CPT II-deficient patients.[3] Our patient carefully followed the instructions and did not show any recurrence of rhabdomyolysis at 18 months after the acute episode.

In conclusion, patients with recurrent episodes of rhabdomyolysis should be evaluated for CPT II deficiency. Screening may also be appropriate in patients with a single episode and no evidence of traumatic or toxic causes of rhabdomyolysis. The biochemical diagnosis relies on the plasma (or blood spotted onto filter paper) acylcarnitine profile, which has to be performed during rhabdomyolysis or, at some interval between these episodes, in the fasting state.[5] Early recognition of the disease is crucial to initiating early treatment and preventing further recurrences of rhabdomyolysis.

The primary cause of AKI in this patient is the rhabdomyolysis. Rhabdomyolysis may not be the only cause of AKI. Indeed, our patient also presented with diarrhea and occasional vomiting and was probably dehydrated. Finally, a cumulative dose of 60 mg/kg body weight of ibuprofen was given as self-medication 1 day before admission. All of these elements may have contributed to a deterioration of the renal function resulting from hypoperfusion and/or vasoconstriction.

The management regimen includes the treatment of rhabdomyolysis-induced AKI and the prevention of further rhabdomyolysis episodes. Supportive treatment of rhabdomyolysis consists of the early and aggressive repletion of fluids. Alkalinization of urine by sodium bicarbonate administration has been recommended by some authors, but evidence supporting its clinical benefit is weak.[1] Hemodialysis is required in severe rhabdomyolysis with refractory hyperkalemia or prolonged oligo-anuric renal failure. The prevention of CPT II deficiency-related rhabdomyolysis is mainly based on measures to limit energy depletion. For example, the following activities should be avoided: extended fasting, strenuous exercise, especially in the cold, increased body metabolism with fever, or treatment with anesthesia. Infusions of glucose during intercurrent infections and adequate hydration during episodes of diarrhea or vomiting are necessary to prevent catabolism. A high-carbohydrate and low-fat diet before and during prolonged exercise may also be prescribed. A beneficial effect of bezafibrate in the treatment of the mild form of CPT II deficiency has been shown.[3]

Clinical Presentation 43

A previously healthy 3-year-old girl presented to the emergency department of a general hospital with high-grade fever, nausea, vomiting, diarrhea, and coughing. A week before presentation, she had a low-grade fever, a sore throat, a red tongue, and bilateral purulent conjunctivitis. Between these two episodes was a relatively symptom-free interval. There were no explicit environmental exposures, such as contact with rodents. She did not take any medication, especially no antibiotics or nonsteroidal antiinflammatory drugs. At the emergency department, she showed signs of shock with a decreased level of consciousness, confusion, tachypnea (44–48 breaths/min), tachycardia (151–162 beats/min), and low blood pressure (62/46 mm Hg). On physical examination, she displayed generalized exanthema with desquamation of the skin and lips, a red tongue, enlarged (almost kissing) tonsils, conjunctivitis, and cervical lymphadenopathy. Auscultation of the heart and lungs was unremarkable. Abdominal examination revealed bilateral flank pain. Fluid boluses were administered to stabilize the shock. There was no need for inotropic or vasopressor support. Antipyretics (acetaminophen) were given to lower the fever and, after the collection of blood cultures, broad-spectrum intravenous cephalosporin antibiotics (ceftriaxone) were started. This resulted in an improvement in her mental state and hemodynamic parameters. The next day, despite extensive fluid therapy, she was still oliguric and developed generalized edema. Laboratory tests showed AKI. Serum creatinine was 3.8 mg/dL and eGFR was 14 mL/min/1.73 m^2, BUN 46 mg/dL, albumin 2.4 g/dL, white blood cell 43 × 10^9/L, hemoglobin 9.1 g/dL, and platelets 402 × 10^9/L. Urinalysis revealed large blood, 2+ protein. She was transferred to the pediatric nephrology department.

On admission, she was clinically stable and normotensive. Further laboratory studies included normal serum complement C3, C4, and CH50, negative ANA, dsDNA, and ANCA. Echocardiogram and ophthalmology examination were normal.

A renal ultrasound was done, which showed both kidneys to be enlarged with a normal corticomedullary differentiation, normal flow in the renal artery and vein, and no dilation or signs of urolithiasis. A rapidly progressive glomerulonephritis seemed likely considering the hematuria, proteinuria, edema, reduced renal function, and enlarged kidneys seen on ultrasound.

A renal biopsy was performed and our patient was started on methylprednisolone pulse therapy for 3 consecutive days, followed by oral prednisone. The biopsy specimen was processed for light and immunofluorescence microscopy using standard techniques. Light microscopic sections showed on average 20 glomeruli, all unremarkable. There were no abnormalities of the arteries and arterioles. A distinct interstitial infiltrate was seen, most prominent in the medullary areas of the biopsy, consisting of both mononuclear cells and neutrophils. Furthermore, the interstitium was markedly hemorrhagic with relatively mild tubulitis. A few intraluminal pus collections were noted. Viral inclusions and viral cytopathic changes were not detected. Immunofluorescence studies showed no staining for IgG, IgA, IgM, C1q, C3, or light chains. The biopsy was consistent with a diffuse hemorrhagic interstitial nephritis. The blood culture revealed a group A beta-hemolytic streptococcus (*Streptococcus pyogenes*), for which antibiotic therapy could be narrowed down to intravenous penicillin. Fever disappeared, skin and eyes improved, and C-reactive protein and blood leukocytes declined. Following a regimen of fluid and dietary restrictions combined with methylprednisolone pulse therapy and subsequent oral prednisone, diuresis, and overall clinical condition improved, renal function recovered, and hematuria and proteinuria subsided. A short period of moderate polyuria occurred during recovery. After 11 days, our patient was discharged with normal renal function, minimal residual proteinuria, and normal blood pressure.

What is the cause of AKI?

A. Hemorrhagic interstitial nephritis.
B. Autoimmune disease.
C. Tubulointerstitial nephritis and uveitis (TINU) syndrome.
D. Acute post-streptococcal glomerulonephritis (APSGN).

The correct answer is D

Comment: The parents of our patient denied any medication use. Blood and biopsy analysis did not reveal eosinophilia. Thus, drug-induced AIN was highly unlikely in this young girl. Neither the clinical presentation nor the radiographic, laboratory, or histological findings supported a diagnosis of autoimmune disease. Tubulointerstitial nephritis and uveitis syndrome were excluded because the ophthalmic examination showed no signs of uveitis. Normal results for complement and immunoglobulin studies refuted other rate etiologies.[1–7]

Our patient had a low-grade fever, a sore throat, a red tongue, and bilateral purulent conjunctivitis a week before presentation, likely as a result of streptococcal infection. There are three mechanisms by which streptococcal infection can conduce to AKI.[8] First, APSGN may result from scarlet fever or group A streptococcal skin infections. Inasmuch as the glomerular structure appeared to be unaffected in the renal biopsy specimen, hypertension was absent and serum complement levels were normal, APSGN was not the cause of AKI in this young girl. Second, fulminant streptococcal sepsis is commonly associated with ischemic ATN because of poor renal perfusion. Although this may have contributed to the deterioration of renal function in our patient, it was probably not the main cause because tubular epithelial cell shedding was not found in the renal biopsy specimen. Third, and more rarely, AKI may be the consequence of group A *Streptococcus*-related AIN,[8–10] as was the case in our patient. Distinguishing among these three entities is important because they have different course, treatment, and prognosis.

Patients with AIN are usually normotensive. AIN is biochemically characterized by a varying degree of AKI, (tubular) proteinuria, hematuria, leukocyturia, hyposthenuria, tubular dysfunction, ranging from isolated glucosuria to Fanconi syndrome, (non-) hemolytic anemia, and eosinophilia/eosinophiluria. This latter finding is commonly associated with an allergic reaction underlying drug-induced AIN. Renal ultrasound may show normal-sized or enlarged kidneys with hyperechogenicity. The histological hallmarks of AIN are interstitial inflammation with a predominant mononuclear cell and eosinophil infiltrate, interstitial edema with or without fibrosis, tubulitis, minimal or absent glomerular alterations, and normal renal vessels.[9–12] Given the nonspecific nature of clinical signs and symptoms, a kidney biopsy is required for a definitive diagnosis of AIN.[10–12]

Treatment mainly consists of the removal of the offending agent and supportive care with dialysis if needed. The role of corticosteroids in the treatment of AIN is controversial,[10–12] except for cases with underlying autoimmune disease, with small retrospective studies showing therapeutic benefits. However, evidence from randomized controlled trials is lacking. Nevertheless, many clinicians opt for steroid treatment when confronted with severe renal failure and use a regimen similar to the one used in our case, namely, methyl-prednisolone pulses on 3 consecutive days, followed by oral prednisone tapered over several weeks.[12] With appropriate management, AIN has an excellent prognosis in the majority of children, with complete convalescence of renal function and normalization of the urinary sediment within several weeks to months.[10–12] Clinical and/or histopathological parameters consistently predicting renal outcome in AIN have not yet been established. Consequently, life-long follow-up is recommended for all AIN patients.[10,12]

Although the literature on AIN secondary to streptococcal infection is relatively scarce, several reports have documented this association, both in adults[8,9] and children.[10] In fact, AIN was first described as a clinical entity in patients with scarlet fever.[8,12] We feel confident that our patient represents a further case of group A *Streptococcus*-associated AIN because she presented with scarlet fever and her blood culture was positive for *Streptococcus pyogenes*. Additional support for the causative role of streptococci in the genesis of AIN can usually not be derived from the histopathological (i.e., light microscopic) findings because clues for a specific etiology are generally lacking in renal biopsy specimens.[10] With immunofluorescence staining, the renal interstitium can be assessed for deposition of complement and immunoglobulins. Immunofluorescence studies were negative in our patient.

Hemorrhagic interstitial nephritis can be caused by (hyper)acute humoral rejection, renal infarction, invasive procedures (e.g., needle biopsy), and various infections, among which are leptospirosis, rickettsiosis, hantavirus-associated HFRS and other hemorrhagic fever viruses (Marburg,

Ebola, and Flaviviridae).[1] With the noteworthy exception of hantavirus, all of these infectious agents seemed unlikely in the present case. Hantavirus was first considered to be the culprit in our patient for the following reasons: (1) HFRS is a well-known and relatively frequent cause of acute hemorrhagic interstitial nephritis[2]; (2) all five phases of HFRS were discernible in our patient, with a period of polyuria before full recovery[1–5]; (3) anti-hantavirus IgM antibodies were initially (weakly) positive; and (4) the young girl lives in a region of The Netherlands where hantavirus-infected rodents occur,[4,6] and direct contact with these animals is not a prerequisite for human infection because transmission of disease takes place via inhalation of aerosols contaminated by virus-infected rodent excreta.[3,6] However, HFRS was eventually discarded as a diagnosis because certain clinical manifestations (e.g., thrombocytopenia) were absent, and, more importantly, IgG for hantavirus remained negative.[1,3–5] Whereas specific serum antibodies may incidentally be lacking in hantavirus-infected patients,[7] an attempt to detect hantaviral antigen in the renal biopsy specimen was undertaken using reverse transcription PCR. Negative results were also obtained with this test. Streptococci are not listed among the causes of hemorrhagic interstitial nephritis.

Clinical Presentation 44

A 2-year-old White boy was transferred with persistent fever and AKI. At the time of his initial visit to the general practitioner, he presented with high fever, respiratory symptoms (coughing, rhinitis), vomiting, abdominal pain, and cervical lymphadenopathy; he was prescribed oral amoxicillin and ibuprofen for a suspected upper respiratory tract infection. However, 3 days later, he had to be admitted to the local hospital because of persistent fever. Bacterial sepsis was suspected, and his antibiotic treatment was switched to intravenous amoxicillin-clavulanate, but without improvement. He had no history of any major illnesses or kidney disease and had no history of medication use. His condition worsened, and high spiking fever (temperatures ≥104°F) persisted, but repeated cultures (blood, urine) remained negative. Elevated serum creatinine and BUN levels were also noted, and he developed metabolic acidosis for which sodium bicarbonate was given. These symptoms led to a suspicion of a tubulointerstitial nephritis secondary to sepsis.

He was transferred to our hospital on the fifth day of illness because of increasing serum creatinine and BUN levels with a potential need for dialysis. At presentation, the child had an ill-looking appearance and was tachycardic, with a normal BP, normal oxygen saturation, and a capillary refill of ≤2 seconds. Bilateral conjunctivitis, periorbital edema, a hyperemic pharynx, dry cracked lips with blood crusts, and cervical lymphadenopathy were also noted. Several petechiae were clearly visible on his shoulders and axillary areas, but no exanthema was present. Mild respiratory distress with wheezing on lung auscultation was noted in addition to a tender abdomen with normal peristalsis. The results of the laboratory tests were: hemoglobin, 10.0 g/dL (reference, 11–14); mean cell volume, 71.0 fL (reference, 73–85); leukocytes, 27,300/mm3; platelets, 157,000/mm^3; activated partial thromboplastin time, 49 seconds (reference, 28–38); prothrombin time, 64.7% (reference, 70%–120%); fibrinogen, 699 mg/dL (reference, 200–400); C-reactive protein, 282 mg/dL (reference <5); sodium, 134 mmol/L (reference, 135–144); potassium, 4.4 mmol/L (reference, 3.6–4.8); calcium, 2.23 mmol/L (reference, 2.15–2.65); phosphate, 1.57 mmol/L (reference, 1.0–1.9); BUN, 103 mg/dL (reference, 12–48); serum creatinine, 2.0 mg/dL (reference, 0.17–0.41); albumin, 33 g/L (reference, 34–48 g/L); aspartate aminotransferase, 82 U/L (reference, 11–50); alanine aminotransferase, 42 U/L (reference, 7–40); and lactate dehydrogenase, 264 U/L (reference, 160–370). Complement, creatine kinase, and uric acid levels were normal, whereas Ig levels (IgA, IgG, IgM) were all slightly elevated. Additional tests included autoimmune antibody testing, the results of which were negative for antinuclear antibodies and anticytoplasmic neutrophilic antibodies, and an echocardiogram, which revealed a structurally normal heart with normal coronaries.

The urinalysis showed mild proteinuria (protein/creatinine index/ratio 3.57 g/g creatinine; reference, <0.2 g/g creatinine), leukocyturia, and hematuria (3+). Blood and urine cultures remained negative, but the PCR assay of the nasopharyngeal smear was positive for human metapneumovirus, rhinovirus, and parainfluenza viruses. The chest x-ray did not show any abnormalities. A kidney ultrasonography was performed, with a Doppler of the renal vessels showing normal perfusion but with clearly increased corticomedullary differentiation and increased size of the kidneys (left kidney, 11.4 cm; right kidney, 10.4 cm; normal range, 5–7 cm). A moderate amount of ascites was noticed on the ultrasound image, but no additional abnormalities were detected. The patient was started on broad-spectrum intravenous antibiotic therapy and oxygen supplementation, but fever persisted. His condition deteriorated, and he became oliguric, subsequently developing progressive fluid retention with peripheral edema, hepatomegaly, and increasing ascites for which intravenous bumetanide (loop diuretic) was prescribed in addition to fluid restriction.

What is your diagnosis?

A. Sepsis with AKI.
B. Kawasaki disease (KD).
C. Ibuprofen-induced AKI (interstitial nephritis and/or decreased renal perfusion).
D. HUS.

The correct answer B

Comment: In light of the clinical course and renal ultrasound image, KD was suspected, and IVIG (2 g/kg body weight) was administered on the sixth day of illness. Since the fever persisted, the treatment with IVIG was repeated 48 hours later. The fever tapered, and the patient's temperature normalized shortly thereafter, whereas urinary output increased. The maximum levels of serum creatinine and BUN were 2.12 and 103 mg/dL, respectively, but dialysis was not needed. Renal function improved gradually, with a lowering of the serum creatinine and BUN levels from the ninth day of illness, but the hematuria, proteinuria, and leukocyturia persisted. The patient's anemia worsened, and iron supplementation was started after an erythropoietin infusion. The patient developed thrombocytosis (maximum 1,000,000/μL), and the leukocyte count normalized.

KD is a frequent cause of vasculitis in children younger than 5 years of age. The criteria for KD according to the American Heart Association[1] are (1) fever persisting at least 5 days and the presence of at least four of the following five principal features; (2) changes in extremities: erythema and edema of hands and feet; membranous desquamation of fingertips; (3) polymorphous exanthema; (4) bilateral, painless bulbar conjunctival injection without exudate; (5) changes in lips and oral cavity: erythema and cracking of lips, strawberry tongue, and diffuse injection of oral and pharyngeal mucosae; and (6) cervical lymphadenopathy (diameter ≥1.5 cm), usually unilateral.

KD occurs in all ethnic groups, with the highest incidence is found in Asian countries, particularly Japan (137.7 cases per 100,000 children aged <5 years),[2] and a lower incidence in White children.[3] It is slightly more common in boys, with a male to female ratio of 1.3:1.[4] The etiology of KD is still uncertain, although infectious and autoimmune causes have been suggested.[5] The most frequent and feared cardiac complications involve coronary aneurysms,[6] which in turn are associated with myocardial infarction and sudden death. KD has been recognized as the leading cause of acquired heart disease in children in the United States and Japan.[7] Treatment within 10 days of disease onset with IVIG is associated with a significant reduction of mortality because of cardiac complications.[8,9]

Without treatment, 20% to 25% of these patients develop coronary abnormalities in comparison to <5% when timely treatment is administered.[10] In addition to cardiac involvement, several other organs and organ systems can be affected, including the gastrointestinal tract, joints, hematopoietic system, respiratory tract, and the neurological and urogenital tracts. AKI is rarely a presenting feature, in contrast to sterile pyuria, which is often seen.[11] However, renal complications ranging from nephrotic syndrome to full-blown renal failure requiring dialysis have been described.[11,12]

Establishing the correct diagnosis in this case proved to be quite challenging. Sepsis and associated AKI could have explained the clinical picture, including the coagulopathy, but repeated cultures of blood and urine were negative, and no improvement was noted with the administration of antibiotics. IgA nephropathy has been associated with several infections and might present as nephritis with increased corticomedullar differentiation. However, episodes of IgA nephropathy are often mild and rarely result in AKI, except in severe cases with nephrotic range proteinuria.[13] Tubulointerstitial nephritis or reduced renal perfusion secondary to ibuprofen (a nonsteroidal antiinflammatory drug) use could have explained AKI but was less likely given this patient's clinical presentation. HUS could explain the anemia and thrombocytopenia, but lactate dehydrogenase and complement levels were normal and there was no history of bloody diarrhea. Lupus nephritis was also a possible explanation, but autoimmune tests eventually came back negative, and a high C-reactive protein level is not a common presenting feature unless concurrent bacterial infection is present. Because repeated urine cultures remained negative, it was believed that acute pyelonephritis was unlikely. Patients with tumors of the hematopoietic and lymphoid tissues can present with high fever and AKI secondary to tumor lysis syndrome or leukemic infiltration of the kidneys. However, because uric acid levels were normal and the results of ultrasound imaging were indicative of renal vasculitis, we considered that acute leukemia/lymphoma was not likely to be the underlying condition. Traditional renal ultrasonography, performed to exclude obstructive causes in AKI, provided an important clue in this case. The ultrasound image showed significantly enlarged kidneys with increased corticomedullary differentiation. This increased corticomedullary differentiation is caused by hyperechogenicity of the cortex in combination with a hypoechogenic medulla and is typically associated with renal vasculitis.[11,14–16] Renal ultrasound images in septic AKI are highly variable, ranging from kidneys with a normal appearance to those showing global parenchymal hyperechogenicity with a loss of corticomedullary differentiation.[17,18]

Our young patient also had high urinary α1-microglobulin levels (maximum, 64 mg/L), which suggested tubular injury. He eventually developed severe pyuria (9600 leukocytes/μL), but repeated urine cultures remained negative. Watanabe et al. studied sterile pyuria in patients with KD but were unable to determine whether the pyuria represented sterile urethritis or whether it originated from the kidney.[19] Respiratory symptoms can accompany KD, often caused by a concurrent upper respiratory tract infection. An association between viral infections and KD has previously been reported,[20] but no causal relationship has yet been established. Coagulopathies secondary to increased consumption of clotting factors have been described in KD and are associated with a complicated course of the disease.[21] We did not perform a biopsy in light of this coagulopathy and that, in our opinion, this would not have provided sufficient benefit to the patient to justify the procedure.

Treatment for KD usually consists of a combination of IVIG and high-dose aspirin. We chose not to administer aspirin because of the potential deleterious effect on the already compromised renal function and the coagulopathy. IVIG was administered even though at the time the patient did not yet completely fulfill the criteria for KD (fever ≥5 days and four principal features) because the risk of coronary artery lesions in incomplete KD is at least as high as in patients with complete KD.[10]

At the time of treatment initiation, the diagnosis was far from being clear-cut but the decision to administer IVIG proved to be the right one. This case highlights the need for timely treatment when there is a suspicion of KD, with treatment strongly recommended before the 10-day window of treatment efficacy closes since late treatment (≥10 days after illness onset) has proven to be ineffective in preventing coronary artery lesions.[22]

Clinical Presentation 45

A 7-year-old boy presented with rashes all over his body, joint pain, and pain in the abdomen for the past 11 days. He was admitted to a primary care hospital where he was diagnosed with renal dysfunction and decreased urine output and was referred. His history, surgical history, and family history were insignificant. There was no history of known allergies or consumption of nephrotoxic drugs. On physical examination, he had palpable purpuric rashes over his shins, lower limbs, and buttocks. His blood pressure was 124/90 mm Hg, and he had no edema. His systemic examination was unremarkable. He was anuric at presentation.

Laboratory parameters at admission were as follows: hemoglobin 11.3 g/dL, platelet count 532,000/mm^3, peripheral smear, no evidence of hemolysis, urea 110 mg/dL, creatinine 10 mg/dL, sodium 145 mEq/L, potassium 4.5 mEq/L, bicarbonate 22 mEq/L, calcium 9.1 mg/dL, phosphate 3.8 mg/dL, albumin 5.0 g/dL, cholesterol 154 mg/dL, normal C3, C4, negative ANA immunofluorescence, ANCA immunofluorescence. Urine examination showed 2+ protein, RBCs 2 to 4/hpf, white blood cells 60 to 80/hpf, and urine sediment showed no casts. Urine culture was sterile.

Renal ultrasound revealed mild left hydronephrosis, dilated left ureter with a diameter of 4.5 cm near the vesicoureteric junction, and dilated left lower ureter with a diameter of 4.5 mm. Urinary bladder showed floating echogenic foci.

In view of suspected IgA vasculitis and anuria, the child was planned for a kidney biopsy the next day; a single dose of methylprednisolone 20 mg/kg was administered and an urgent ultrasound abdomen was done.

He drastically improved after the dose of intravenous methylprednisolone. His urine output became 20 mL/kg/h, and he passed almost 750 to 1000 mL/h overnight. The next day, his serum creatinine had improved to 0.5 mg/dL, and he completely recovered.

The child completely normalized within 24 hours, with postobstructive diuresis. A kidney biopsy was withheld in view of complete normalization and bilateral hydronephrosis with left ureteric dilatation. The skin biopsy later showed evidence of leukocytoclastic vasculitis with IgA deposition.

What is your diagnosis (select all that apply)?

A. IgA vasculitis with crescentic glomerulonephritis.
B. Bilateral ureteritis.
C. Vesicoureteral reflux.
D. Acute tubular necrosis.

The correct answer is B

Comment: Ureteritis is a rare complication of Henoch-Schönlein purpura. It typically presents with severe symptoms. It results from ureteral vasculitis. As demonstrated in our cases, there was marked edema at a vesicoureteric junction on the left side, which resolved with corticosteroids. Only about 16 cases have been reported in the medical literature. It is important to remember that pain in the abdomen in Henoch-Schönlein purpura may also be due to ureteritis causing inflammation, spasm, or obstruction secondary to clot formation.[1]

There is a variable response, from self-remitting ureteritis, good response to surgical management,[2] and even progression to end-stage renal disease.[1] There is also a report of ureteritis progressing to diffuse immune complex glomerulonephritis on follow-up.[2]

References

Clinical Presentation 1

1. Assadi F, Sharbaf FG. Urine KIM-1 as a potential target biomarker of acute kidney injury after circulatory collapse in children. *Pediatr Emerg Care.* 2016;35:104–107.

Clinical Presentation 2

1. Assadi FK, John EG, Furnell L, Rosenthal IM. Falsely elevated serum creatinine concentration in ketoacidosis. *J Paediatr.* 1985;107:562–564.

Clinical Presentation 3

1. Assadi FK, John EG, Justice P, Furnell L. Beta 2-microglobulin clearance in neonates: index of tubular maturation. *Kidney Int.* 1985;28:153–157.
2. Assadi FK, Chow-Tung E. Renal handling of beta-2-microglobulin in neonates treated with gentamicin. *Nephron.* 1988;49:114–118.
3. Pacifica GM. Clinical pharmacology of gentamicin in neonates: regimen, toxicology and pharmacokinetics. *Med Exp.* 2015;2:M150501.

Clinical Presentation 4

1. Perazella MA. Acute renal failure in HIV-infected patients: a brief review of cases. *Am J Med Sci.* 2000;319:385–391.

Clinical Presentation 5

1. Kellum JA, Angus DC, Johnson JP, et al. Continuous venous intermittent renal replacement therapy: a meta-analysis. Intensive Care Med. 2092;28:29–37.
2. Mehta R, McDonald B, Gabbai F, et al. A randomized clinic trail of continuous versus intermittent dialysis for acute renal failure. *Kidney Int.* 2001;60:1151–1163.
3. Pho NH, Hien TT, Mai NTH, et al. Hemofiltration and peritoneal dialysis in infection- associated acute renal failure in Vietnam. *N Engl J Med.* 2002;347 895–890.

Clinical Presentation 6

1. Kellum JA. Use of diuretics in the acute care setting. *Kidney Int.* 1998;66:S67–S70.

Clinical Presentation 7

1. Kaarsou SA, Jaber BL, Pereira GJG. Impact of intermittent hemodialysis variables on clinical outcomes in acute renal failure. *Am J Kidney Dis.* 2000;35:980–991.

Clinical Presentation 8

1. Kellum JA, Decker JM. Use of dopamine in acute renal failure: a meta-analysis. *Crit Care Med.* 2001;29:1526–1531.
2. Australian and New Zealand Intensive Care Society Clinical Trials Group. Low-dose dopamine in patients with early renal dysfunction: a placebo-controlled randomized trial. *Lancet.* 2000;356:2139–2143.

Clinical Presentation 9

1. Perazella MA, Kashgarian M, Cooney E. Indinavir nephropathy in an AIDS patient with renal insufficiency and pyuria. *Clin Nephrol.* 1988;50:194–196.
2. Gagnon RF, Tsoukas CM, Walters AK. Light microscopy of indinavir urinary crystals. *Ann Intern Med.* 1998;138 421–323.

Clinical Presentation 10

1. Majumdar A, Chowdhary S, Ferreira MA, et al. Renal pathological findings in infective endocarditis. *Nehru Dial Transplant.* 2000;15:1782–1787.

Clinical Presentation 11

1. Roseert J. Drug-induced interstitial nephritis. Kidney Int. 2091;60:804–817.

Clinical Presentation 12

1. Peraxella MA. Acute renal failure in HIV-infected patients: a brief review of common causes. *Am J Med Sci.* 2000;319:385–391.
2. Schaaf B, Aries SP, Kramme E, et al. Acute renal failure associated with tenofovir treatment in a patient with acquired immunodeficiency syndrome. Clin Inf Dis. 2093;37:41–43.

Clinical Presentation 13

1. Baily J, Shapiro MJ. Abdominal compartment syndrome. *Crit Care.* 2000;4:23–29.
2. Biancofiore G, Bindi ML, Romanelli AM, et al. Intra-abdominal pressure monitoring in liver transplant recipients: a prospective study. *Intensive Care Med.* 2003;29:30–36.

Clinical Presentation 14

1. Mehta RL, Pascual MT, Soroko S, et al. Diuretics, mortality, and no recovery of renal function in acute renal failure. *JAMA.* 2002;288:2547–2553.

Clinical Presentation 15

1. Phi NH, Hien TT, Mai NTH, et al. Hemofiltration and peritoneal dialysis in infection- associated acute renal failure in Vietnam. *N Engl J Med.* 2002;347:895–902.

Clinical Presentation 16

1. Assadi F. Acetazolamide for prevention of contrast-induced nephropathy: a new use for an old drug. *Pediatr Cardiol.* 2006;27:238–242.

Clinical Presentation 17

1. Gines P, Guevara A, Arroyo V, et al. Hepatorenal syndrome. Lancet. 2093;362:1819–1827.

Clinical Presentation 18

1. Argalious M, Motta P, Khandwala F, et al. "Renal dose" dopamine is associated with the risk of new-onset arterial fibrillation after cardiac surgery. *Crit Care Med.* 2005;33:1327–1332.
2. Chiolero R, Borgeat A, Fisher A. Postoperative arrhythmias and risk factors after open heart surgery. *Thorac Cardiovasc Surg.* 1991;39:81–84.

Clinical Presentation 19

1. Gines P, Guevara M, Arroyo V, et al. Hepatorenal syndrome. Lancet. 2093;362:1819–1827.
2. Gines P, Cardenas A, Arroyo V, et al. Management of cirrhosis and ascites. *N Engl J Med.* 2004;350: 1646–1654.

Clinical Presentation 20

1. Kuiper JW, Groeneveld AB, Slutsky AS, et al. Mechanical ventilation and acute renal failure. *Cri Care Med.* 2005;33:1460–1461.
2. Rivers E, Nguyen B, Havstad S, et al. Early goal-directed therapy in the treatment of severe sepsis and septic shock. *N Engl J Med.* 2001;345:1368–1377.

Clinical Presentation 21

1. Augustine JJ, Sandy D, Seifert TH, et al. A randomized controlled trial comparing intermittent with continuous dialysis in patients with ARF. *Am J Kidney Dis.* 2004;44:1000–1007.

Clinical Presentation 22

1. Davenport A. Renal replacement therapy in the patient with acute brain injury. *Am J Kidney Dis.* 2001;37:457–466.

Clinical Presentation 23

1. Humphreys BD, Soiffer RJ, Mage CC. Renal failure associated with cancer and its treatment: an update. *J Am Soc Nephrol.* 2005;26:151–161.

Clinical Presentation 24

1. Murray PT. Use of dopaminergic agents for renoprotection in the ICU. *Yearbook of Intensive Care and Emergency Medicine.* New York: Springer-Verlag; 2003:637–764.

Clinical Presentation 25

1. Gines P, Guevara M, Arroyo V, et al. Hepatorenal syndrome. Lancet. 2093;362:1819–1827.

Clinical Presentation 26

1. Bent P, Tan HK, Bellomo R, et al. Early and intensive continuous hemofiltration for severe renal failure after cardiac surgery. *Ann Thorac Surg.* 2001;71:832–837.
2. Demirkilic U, Kuralay E, Yenicesu M, et al. Timing of replacement therapy for acute renal failure after cardiac surgery. *J Card Surg.* 2004;19:17–20.

Clinical Presentation 27

1. Augustine JJ, Sandy D, Seifert TH. A randomized controlled trial comparing intermittent with continuous dialysis in patients with acute renal failure. *Am J Kidney Dis.* 2004;44:1000–1007.
2. Tolwani A. Renal replacement therapies for acute renal failure: does dose matter? *Am J Kidney Dis.* 2005;45:1139–1143.

Clinical Presentation 28

1. Casserly B, O'Mahony E, Timm EG, et al. Propofol infusion syndrome: an unusual cause of renal failure. *Am J Kidney Dis*. 2004;44:e98–e101.

Clinical Presentation 29

1. Abassi ZA, Hoffman A, Better OS. Acute renal failure complicating crush injury. *Semin Nephrol*. 1998;18:558–565.

Clinical Presentation 30

1. Chow KM, Lai FM, Wang AY, et al. Reversible renal failure in paroxysmal nocturnal hemoglobinuria. *Am J Kidney Dis*. 2001;37:E172.
2. Zager RA, Gamelin LM. Pathogenetic mechanisms in experimental hemoglobinuric acute renal failure. *Am J Physiol*. 1989;256:F446–F4553.
3. Chan WL, Tang NL, Yim CC, et al. New features of renal lesion induced by stroma free hemoglobin. *Toxicol Pathol*. 2000;28:635–642.

Clinical Presentation 31

1. Mannix R, Tan ML, Wright R, Baskin M. Acute pediatric rhabdomyolysis: causes and rates of renal failure. *Pediatrics*. 2006;118:2119–2125.
2. Kelly KJ, Garland JS, Tang TT, Shug AL, Chusid MJ. Fatal rhabdomyolysis following influenza infection in a girl with familial carnitine palmityl transferase deficiency. *Pediatrics*. 1989;84:312–316.

Clinical Presentation 32

1. Al-Ismaili Z, Piccioni M, Zappitelli M. Rhabdomyolysis: pathogenesis of renal injury and management. *Pediatr Nephrol*. 2011;26:1781–1788.
2. Isackson PJ, Bennett MJ, Lichter-Konecki U. CPT2 gene mutations resulting in lethal neonatal or severe infantile carnitine palmitoyl-transferase II deficiency. *Mol Genet Metab*. 2008;94:422–4273.
3. van Adel BA, Tarnopolsky MA. Metabolic myopathies: update. *J Clin Neuromuscul Dis*. 2009;10:97–121.

Clinical Presentation 33

1. Tkachenko EA, Lee HW. Etiology and epidemiology of hemorrhagic fever with renal syndrome. *Kidney Int*. 1991;40:54.
2. Ertek M, Buzgan T. Refik Saydam National Public Health Agency; Ministry of Health, Ankara, Turkey. An outbreak caused by hantavirus in the Black Sea region of Turkey, January–May 2009. *Euro Surveill*. 2009;14:1–2.

Clinical Presentation 34

1. Bodner DR, Selzman AA, Spirnak JP. Evaluation and treatment of bladder rupture. *Semin Urol*. 1995;13:62–65.

Clinical Presentation 35

1. Hothi DK, Bass P, Morgan M, et al. Acute renal failure in a patient with paroxysmal cold hemoglobinuria. *Pediatr Nephrol*. 2007;22:593–596.

Clinical Presentation 36

1. Jinnah HA. Lesch-Nyhan disease: from mechanism to model and back again. *Dis Model Mech*. 2009;2:116–121.
2. Pela I, Donati MA, Procopio E, et al. Lesch–Nyhan syndrome presenting with acute renal failure in a 3-day-old newborn. *Pediatr Nephrol*. 2008;23:155–158.
3. Cherian S, Crompton CH. Partial hypoxanthine-guanine phosphoribosyltransferase deficiency presenting as acute renal failure. *Pediatr Nephrol*. 2005;20:1811–1813.

Clinical Presentation 37

1. Bu R, Li Q, Duan ZY, et al. Clinicopathologic features of IgA-dominant infection-associated glomerulonephritis: a pooled analysis of 78 cases. *Am J Nephrol*. 2015;41:98–106.
2. Council on Cardiovascular Disease in the Young; Committee on Rheumatic Fever, Endocarditis, Kawasaki Disease; American Heart Association. Diagnostic guidelines for Kawasaki Disease. *Circulation*. 2001;103:335–336.
3. Freeman A, Shulman S. Kawasaki disease: summary of the American Heart Association guidelines. *Am Fam Physician*. 2006;74:1141–1148.
4. Watanabe T. Kidney and urinary tract involvement in Kawasaki disease. *Int J Pediatr*. 2013;2013:831834.
5. Lande MB, Gleeson JG, Sundel RP. Kawasaki disease and acute renal failure. *Pediatr Nephrol*. 1993;7:593.

Clinical Presentation 38

1. Ozmen S, Danis R, Akin D, et al. Parathyroid hormone as a marker for the differential diagnosis of acute and chronic renal failure. *Ren Fail.* 2007;29:509–512.
2. Saliba W, El-Haddad B. Secondary hyperparathyroidism: pathophysiology and treatment. *J Am Board Fam Med.* 2009;22:574–581.
3. Daneman A, Navarro OM, Somers GR, et al. Renal pyramids: focused sonography of normal and pathologic processes. *Radiographics.* 2010;30:1287–1307.
4. Cochat P, Fargue S, Harambat J. Primary hyperoxaluria. In: Avner ED, Harmon PN, Niaudet P, Yoshikawa N, eds. *Pediatric nephrology.* 6th ed. Berlin Heidelberg: Springer; 2009:1065–1079.
5. Khan SR, Glenton PA, Byer KJ. Dietary oxalate and calcium oxalate nephrolithiasis. *J Urol.* 2007;178:2191–2196.

Clinical Presentation 39

1. Pérez NS, Garcia-Herrera A, Rosiñol L, et al. Lymphoplasmacytic lymphoma causing light chain cast nephropathy. *Nephrol Dial Transplant.* 2012;27:450–453.
2. Cohen LJ, Rennke HG, Laubach JP, et al. The spectrum of kidney involvement in lymphoma: a case report and review of the literature. *Am J Kidney Dis.* 2010;56:1191–1196.
3. Sethi S, Fervenza FC, Rajkumar SV. Spectrum of manifestations of monoclonal gammopathy-associated renal lesions. *Curr Opin Nephrol Hypertens.* 2016;25:127–137.
4. Rosner MH, Edeani A, Yanagita M, et al. Paraprotein–related kidney disease: diagnosing and treating monoclonal gammopathy of renal significance. *Clin J Am Soc Nephrol.* 2016;11:2280–2287.
5. Karafin MS, Humphrey RL, Detrick B. Evaluation of monoclonal and oligoclonal gammopathies in a pediatric population in a major urban center. *Am J Clin Pathol.* 2014;141:482–487.

Clinical Presentation 40

1. Guise TA, Wysolmerski JJ. Cancer-associated hypercalcemia. *N Engl J Med.* 2022;386:1443–1448.
2. Schingmann KP, Kaufmann M, Weber S, et al. Mutations in CYP24A1 and infantile hypercalcemia. *N Engl J Med.* 2021;365:401–421.
3. Hanna C, Potretze TA, Cogal AG, et al. High prevalence of kidney cysts in patients with CYP24A1 deficiency. *Kidney Int Rep.* 2021;6:1895–1903.

Clinical Presentation 41

1. Baker RJ, Pusey CD. The changing profile of acute tubulointerstitial nephritis. *Nephrol Dial Transplant.* 2004;19:8–11.
2. Saviuc P, Garon D, Danel V, et al. Cortinarius poisoning. Analysis of cases in the literature. *Néphrologie.* 2001;22:167–173.
3. Andary C, Rapior S, Delpech N, et al. Laboratory confirmation of Cortinarius poisoning. *Lancet.* 1989;1:213.
4. Rohrmoser M, Kirchmair M, Feifel E, et al. Orellanine poisoning: rapid detection of the fungal toxin in renal biopsy material. *J Toxicol Clin Toxicol.* 1977;35:63–66.
5. Nieminen L, Pyy K. Individual variation in mushroom poisoning induced in the male rat by Cortinarius speciosissimus. *Med Biol.* 1976;54:156–158.
6. Schumacher T, Hoiland K. Mushroom poisoning caused by species of the genus Cortinarius (Fries). *Arch Toxicol.* 1983;53:87–106.

Clinical Presentation 42

1. Bosch X, Poch E, Grau JM. Rhabdomyolysis and acute kidney injury. *N Engl J Med.* 2009;361:62–72.
2. Elsayed EF, Reilly RF. Rhabdomyolysis: a review, with emphasis on the pediatric population. *Pediatr Nephrol.* 2010;25:7–18.
3. Bonnefont JP, Djouadi F, Prip-Buus C, et al. Carnitine palmitoyltransferases 1 and 2: biochemical, molecular and medical aspects. *Mol Aspects Med.* 2004;25:495–520.
4. Thuillier L, Rostane H, Droin V, et al. between genotype, metabolic data, and clinical presentation in carnitine palmitoyltransferase 2 (CPT2) deficiency. *Hum Mutat.* 2003;21:493–501.
5. Laforêt P, Vianey-Saban C, Vissing J, et al. 162nd ENMC International Workshop: disorders of muscle lipid metabolism in adults 28–30 November 2008, Bussum, The Netherlands. *Neuromuscul Disord.* 2009;19:324–329.

Clinical Presentation 43

1. Lordemann A, Hjelle B, Theegarten D, et al. Young man with kidney failure and hemorrhagic interstitial nephritis. *Am J Kidney Dis*. 2009;54:1162–1166.
2. Ferluga D, Vizjak A. Hantavirus nephropathy. *J Am Soc Nephrol*. 2008;19:1653–1658.
3. Manigold T, Vial P. Human hantavirus infections: epidemiology, clinical features, pathogenesis and immunology. *Swiss Med Wkly*. 2014;144:w13937.
4. De Weerd EC, Douma CE, Wattel-Louis HW, et al. Acute kidney injury caused by hantavirus in the Netherlands. *Ned Tijdschr Geneeskd*. 2015;159:A8273.
5. Krautkrämer E, Zeier M, Plyusnin A. Hantavirus infection: an emerging infectious disease causing acute renal failure. *Kidney Int*. 2012;83:23–27.
6. Verner-Carlsson J, Lõhmus M, Sundström K, et al. First evidence of Seoul hantavirus in the wild rat population in the Netherlands. *Infect Ecol Epidemiol*. 2015;5:27215.
7. Groen J, Bruijn JA, Gerding MN, et al. Hantavirus antigen detection in kidney biopsies from patients with nephropathia epidemica. *Clin Nephrol*. 1996;46:379–383.
8. Chang JF, Peng YS, Tsai CC, et al. A possible rare cause of renal failure in streptococcal infection. *Nephrol Dial Transplant*. 2011;26:368–371.
9. Dharmarajan TS, Yoo J, Russell RO, et al. Acute post streptococcal interstitial nephritis in an adult and review of the literature. *Int Urol Nephrol*. 1999;31:145–148.
10. Ellis D, Fried WA, Yunis EJ, et al. Acute interstitial nephritis in children: a report of 13 cases and review of the literature. *Pediatrics*. 1981;67:862–870.
11. Papachristou F, Printza N, Farmaki E, et al. Antibiotics-induced acute interstitial nephritis in 6 children. *Urol Int*. 2006;76:348–352.
12. Ulinski T, Sellier-Leclerc AL, Tudorache E, et al. Acute tubulointerstitial nephritis. *Pediatr Nephrol*. 2012;27:1051–1057.

Clinical Presentation 44

1. Council on Cardiovascular Disease in the Young; Committee on Rheumatic Fever, Endocarditis, Kawasaki Disease; American Heart Association. Diagnostic guidelines for Kawasaki disease. *Circulation*. 2001;103:335–336.
2. Yanagawa H, Nakamura Y, Yashiro M, et al. Incidence of Kawasaki disease in Japan: the nationwide surveys of 1999–2002. *Pediatr Int*. 2006;48:356–361.
3. Gedalia A. Kawasaki disease: 40 years after the original report. *Curr Rheumatol Rep*. 2007;9:336–341.
4. Sonobe T. A summary of epidemiologic surveys conducted about Kawasaki disease over thirty years. *JMAJ*. 2005;48:30–33.
5. Scuccimarri R. Kawasaki disease. *Pediatr Clin North Am*. 2012;59:425–445.
6. Baer AZ, Rubin LG, Shapiro CA, et al. Prevalence of coronary artery lesions on the initial echocardiogram in Kawasaki syndrome. *Lancet*. 1984;2:1055–1058.
7. Rowley AH, Shulman S. *Nelson textbook of pediatrics*. (Kliegman RM ed.). 18th ed. Philadelphia: Saunders; 2007:1036–1042.
8. Newburger JW, Takahashi M, Burns JC, et al. The treatment of Kawasaki syndrome with intravenous gamma globulin. *N Engl J Med*. 1986;315:341–347.
9. Furusho K, Nakano H, Shinomiya K, et al. High-dose intravenous gammaglobulin for Kawasaki disease. *Lancet*. 1984;2:1055–1058.
10. Freeman A, Shulman S. Kawasaki disease: summary of the American Heart Association guidelines. *Am Fam Physician*. 2006;74:1141–1148.
11. Watanabe T. Kidney and urinary tract involvement in Kawasaki disease. *Int J Pediat*. 2013;2013:831834.
12. Lande MB, Gleeson JG, Sundel RP. Kawasaki disease and acute renal failure. *Pediatr Nephrol*. 1993;7:593.
13. Bu R, Li Q, Duan ZY, et al. Clinicopathologic features of IgA-dominant infection-associated glomerulonephritis: a pooled analysis of 78 cases. *Am J Nephrol*. 2015;41:98–106.
14. Nardi PM, Haller JO, Friedman AP, et al. Renal manifestation of Kawasaki's disease. *Pediatr Radiol*. 1985;15:116–118.
15. Riccabona M. Renal failure in neonates, infants, and children: the role of ultrasound. *Ultrasound Clin*. 2006;1:457–469.
16. Wang JN, Chiou YY, Chiu NT, et al. Renal scarring sequelae in childhood Kawasaki disease. *Pediatr Nephrol*. 2007;22:684–689.

17. Kamaya A, Wong-You-Cheong J. *Diagnostic Ultrasound: Abdomen and Pelvis*. Philadelphia: Elsevier; 2016:948–960.
18. Faubel S, Patel N, Lockhart ME, et al. Renal relevant radiology: use of ultrasonography in patients with AKI. *Clin J Am Soc Nephrol.* 2014;9:382–394.
19. Watanabe T, Abe Y, Sato S, et al. Sterile pyuria in patients with Kawasaki disease originates from both the urethra and the kidney. *Pediatr Nephrol.* 2007;22:987–991.
20. Chang LY, Lu CY, Shao PL, et al. Viral infections associated with Kawasaki disease. *J Formos Med Assoc.* 2014;113:148–151.
21. Kanegaye JT, Wilder MS, Molkara D, et al. Recognition of a Kawasaki disease shock syndrome. *Pediatrics.* 2009;123:e783–e789.
22. Muta H, Ishii M, Yashiro M, et al. Late intravenous immunoglobulin treatment in patients with Kawasaki disease. *Pediatrics.* 2012;129:291–297.

Clinical Presentation 45

1. Corbett ST, Lennington JN, Chua AN, et al. Stenosing ureteritis in a 7-year-old boy with Henoch-Schönlein purpura nephritis: a case report and review of the literature. *J Pediatr Urol.* 2010;6:538–542.
2. Kasahara K, Uemura O, Nagai T, et al. Stenosing ureteritis in Henoch-Schönlein purpura: report of two cases. *Pediatr Int.* 2015;57:317–320.

CHAPTER 2

Congenital Anomalies of Kidney and Urinary Tract

Clinical Presentation 1

A 2-day-old premature neonate was born with respiratory distress with an Apgar score of 7. His birth weight was 800 g. He was the third live birth child to a closely related family, with no history of any abnormalities in the other two siblings.

Examination revealed a dysgenic neonate with retraction of all intercostal respiratory muscles. He also showed features of Pierre Robin syndrome. His abdominal skin was redundant and wrinkled and the scrotum was empty. There were no other significant external abnormal findings. Blood electrolytes including blood urea nitrogen (BUN) and creatinine concentrations were normal. Abdominal ultrasound showed an absence of the right kidney.

What is the likely diagnosis?

A. Megacystis and megaureter
B. Megacystitis
C. Intestinal hypoperistalsis syndrome
D. Posterior ureteral valves
E. Prune belly syndrome

The correct answer is E

What other organs of the body can be affected in this condition?

A. Brain
B. Heart
C. Kidney and urinary tract
D. Liver

The correct answer is C

What is the prognosis of the patient with this disease?

A. Good after surgical repair of abnormalities.
B. Grave; usually dies within days after birth.

The correct answer is B
Comment: Prune belly syndrome, also known as Eagle-Barrett syndrome, is a rare disorder characterized by partial or complete absence of the abdominal muscles, failure of both testes to descend into the scrotum (bilateral cryptorchidism), and/or urinary tract malformations.[1]

The urinary malformations may include hydroureteronephrosis and vesicoureteral reflux.

Complications associated with prune belly syndrome may include underdevelopment of the lungs (pulmonary hypoplasia) and/or chronic renal failure. The exact cause of prune belly syndrome is not known.[1]

There is no cure for prune belly syndrome, though treatment options and our understanding of the condition are constantly growing. The prognosis for newborns with this condition varies and depends on the severity of symptoms and kidney function.[2]

Although the cause of prune belly syndrome is unknown, some cases have been reported in siblings, suggesting there may be a genetic component. It is known the prune belly syndrome develops as the fetus is growing before birth. Analysis of these cases suggests that urethral obstruction is an important factor contributing to the development of this syndrome.

Some babies who have prune belly syndrome may die in the uterus at 20 weeks of pregnancy or later (stillborn). Some babies with this condition die a few months after birth.

Clinical Presentation 2

A 2-month-old female infant was admitted to our hospital because of FTT associated with diarrhea and abdominal distension. She was the first child of nonconsanguineous healthy parents. Pregnancy was complicated by maternal hypertension and intrauterine growth restriction. Birth was by vaginal delivery at 38 weeks' gestation, with Apgar scores of 9 at 1 minute and 10 at 5 and 10 minutes. Her birth weight 2070 g, length 44 cm, and head circumference 31 cm. Jaundice on the first day of life led to phototherapy for 48 hours. There was a good weight gain up to the first month of life, with regular growth below the third percentile. After the second month of life, hypotonia and poor weight gain prompted hospitalization.

On admission, the infant was severely undernourished (weighing 2940 g), with abdominal distension, intermittent stridor, and axial hypotonia. Dysmorphic features included a large anterior fontanelle and dehiscence of the interparietal space extending to the posterior fontanelle, broad nasal bridge with orbital hypertelorism, epicanthus, high-arched palate, short neck, rhizomatic shortening of proximal extremities, low-set thumb, and overlapping toes.

Transfontanel and abdominal ultrasounds were normal. The skeletal radiograph did not show any calcific stippling of epiphyses. A chest computed tomography (CT) scan with angiography revealed two supra-aortic trunks with preserved permeability (proximal stem yielding to the right brachycephalic trunk and left carotid artery and distal stem corresponding to the left subclavian artery) and no apparent decrease in the diameter of the trachea, revealing a variant of normal cardiovascular structure. On further investigation, karyotype analysis was normal (46, XX), as were carbohydrate-deficient transferrin, phytanic, and pristanic acids, and the erythrocyte plasmalogens. Brain proton magnetic resonance (MR) spectroscopy revealed localized peaks at 0.9 and 1.3 ppm, possibly reflecting the presence of macromolecules and lipids/lactate, without other relevant changes in neuroimaging.

Laboratory investigations revealed increased plasma levels of very long-chain fatty acids and precursor of bile acids and deficient activity of dihydroxyacetonephosphate acyltransferase in fibroblasts. Two mutations in the *PEX1* gene were found in heterozygosity (c.2528G>A (p.G843D)/c.760dupT (p.S254fs*5)), confirmed by the patient's genetic study.

What is the likely diagnosis?

A. Zellweger syndrome (ZS)
B. Lowe syndrome
C. Potter syndrome.
D. Meckel-Joubert syndrome

The correct answer is A

Comment: This case has particular features that are consistent with a diagnosis of ZS, based on clinical phenotype and specific laboratory and genetic abnormalities.[1]

Zellweger spectrum disorders (ZSD) are a group of rare, genetic, multisystem disorders that were once thought to be separate entities. These disorders are now classified as different expressions (variants) of one disease process because of their shared biochemical basis. Collectively, they form a spectrum or continuum of disease. The most severe form of these disorders was previously referred to as ZS, the intermediate form was referred to as neonatal adrenoleukodystrophy, and the milder forms were referred to as infantile Refsum disease or Heimler syndrome, depending on the clinical presentation. ZSD can affect most organs of the body. Neurological deficits, loss of muscle tone (hypotonia), hearing loss, vision problems, liver dysfunction, and kidney abnormalities are common findings. ZSD often result in severe, life-threatening complications early during infancy. Some individuals with milder forms have lived into adulthood. ZSD are inherited in an autosomal recessive pattern.

ZSD are the result of a mutation in any of the 12 *PEX* genes, whereas most cases of ZSD are due to a mutation in the *PEX1* gene. These genes control peroxisomes, which are needed for normal cell function. Peroxisomes break down toxins and fats. They play an important role in the development of the bones, brain, eyes, nervous and cardiovascular systems, and kidneys.

Symptoms of ZS usually appear soon after birth. Facial abnormalities common in ZS include broad nose bridge, epicanthal folds (skin folds at the inner corners of the eyes), flattened face, high forehead, underdeveloped eyebrow ridges, and wide-set eyes.

Other symptoms include difficulty swallowing, hepatosplenomegaly, gastrointestinal bleeding, hearing and vision problems, jaundice, seizures, underdeveloped muscles, and movement problems.[2]

There is no cure for ZS. Some therapies may ease symptoms, but there are not any treatments that address the cause of ZSD. For example, a baby with difficulty eating may benefit from a feeding tube but will not be able to eat normally on his or her own in the future.

Clinical Presentation 3

Which of the following is incorrect in a newborn with unilateral renal agenesis?

A. Underdeveloped lungs
B. Undescended testis
C. Oligohydramnios
D. Low-set ears
E. None of the above

The correct answer is E

Comment: The kidneys develop between the fifth and 12th weeks of fetal life, and by the 13th week they are normally producing urine. When the embryonic kidney cells fail to develop, it leads to renal agenesis. Renal agenesis is often detected on fetal ultrasound because there will be a lack of amniotic fluid or oligohydramnios.[1]

When both kidneys are absent, this condition is not compatible with life. Approximately 40% of newborns with bilateral renal agenesis will be stillborn, and if born alive, will live only a few hours.

Neonates with bilateral renal agenesis will have several unique characteristics: dry loose skin, wide-set eyes, prominent folds at the inner corner of each eye, sharp nose, and large low-set ears with lack of ear cartilage. They will typically have underdeveloped lungs, absent urinary bladder, anal atresia, esophageal atresia, and unusual genitals. The lack of amniotic fluid causes some of the problems (undeveloped lungs, sharp nose, clubbed feet); other problems occur because the kidneys and those affected structures are formed at the same time of fetal life (such as the ears, genitals, and esophagus).

Newborns with unilateral renal agenesis may have no other symptoms at all. Unilateral renal agenesis is more common with intrauterine growth retardation (poor growth during pregnancy) and often results in premature birth. It is also more common when a mother is carrying multiple children, such as twins or triplets). Children with unilateral renal agenesis will generally live normal lives with no developmental effects. In fact, many times the solitary kidney is only detected incidentally when x-rays are done for other purposes. The remaining kidney will enlarge to carry out the function normally done by two kidneys.[1,2]

Clinical Presentation 4

Which of the following is associated with bilateral duplication of ureter?

A. Vesicoureteral reflux
B. Ectopic ureterocele
C. Ureteropelvic junction (UPJ) obstruction
D. Simple ectopic ureter
E. All of the above

The correct answer is E

Comment: Congenital ureter anomalies such as double ureters are uncommon developmental anomalies of the renal system. An abnormal branching pattern of the ureteric bud results in the formation of a double ureter.

Duplication of the ureters is frequently encountered by radiologists. Duplication may be either complete or incomplete and is often accompanied by various complications.[1,2] Incomplete duplication is most often associated with UPJ obstruction (UPJO) of the lower pole of the kidney. Complete duplication is most often associated with vesicoureteral reflux, ectopic ureterocele, or ectopic ureteral insertion, all of which are more common in girls than in boys. Vesicoureteral reflux affects the lower pole and can be outgrown, as in nonduplicated systems. Ectopic ureterocele and ectopic ureteral insertion affect the upper pole. The ectopic ureterocele produces a filling defect of variable size in the bladder; it can be identified with contrast material studies or ultrasound. Ectopic ureters may function poorly, be difficult to detect, and cause enuresis in girls. A fourth complication, UPJO, occurs only in the lower pole and is seen in more boys than girls. Anatomic variants or anomalies as well as suboptimal imaging techniques can either simulate or obscure duplication, making diagnosis difficult. However, familiarity with the embryology of duplication and an awareness of the potential pitfalls of excretory urography and voiding cystourethrography will foster an understanding of the varied appearances and associated complications of both incomplete and complete duplication.

Clinical Presentation 5

Surgical complications of UPJO include all the following EXCEPT?

A. Bleeding
B. Recurrent UPJO
C. Urinary extravasation and leakage
D. Pyelonephritis
E. Trauma to surrounding tissues
F. Fanconi syndrome

The correct answer is F

Comment: UPJO is one of the most common causes of hydronephrosis in children. If left untreated, it might cause loss of the affected kidney.[1,2]

During fetal life, the kidneys develop from the metanephric mesoderm up to the distal tubules. The collecting duct, major and minor calyces, renal pelvis, and ureters arise from the ureteric bud that originates from the mesonephric duct during the fifth week of the intrauterine phase. This explains why the UPJ is wholly made by the ureteric bud rather than the fusion of two different mesenchymal tissues.

UPJO results in impaired urine flow from the renal pelvis into the ureter, and if not detected and treated properly, can result in complete loss of the affected kidney.

Hydronephrosis can be detected as an incidental finding on antenatal ultrasound, which might reflect underlying UPJO.

Common symptoms in older children include periodic abdominal pain (loin pain), usually after diuresis, vomiting, fever, recurrent urinary tract infections, or hematuria secondary to infection.

All patients who have symptoms of UPJO should have a full set of blood tests, including complete blood count, kidney function tests, including creatinine, glomerular filtration rate (GFR), and BUN. A urine sample should be sent for analysis and culture because recurrent urinary tract infections are commonly seen in these patients.

In neonates who were found to have mild to moderate hydronephrosis on an antenatal scan, a follow-up scan should be done after 48 hours to avoid the transient neonatal dehydration period; however, in severe cases, a scan should be performed within the first 48 hours because urgent intervention might be needed.

The Society for Fetal Urology grading system is used to evaluate the severity of hydronephrosis as follows:

Grade 0: No hydronephrosis, intact central renal complex seen on ultrasound

Grade 1: Only renal pelvis visualized, dilated pelvis on ultrasound, no caliectasis

Grade 2: Moderately dilated renal pelvis and a few calyces

Grade 3: Hydronephrosis with nearly all calyces seen, large renal pelvis without parenchymal thinning

Grade 4: Severe dilatation of renal pelvis and calyces with accompanying parenchymal atrophy or thinness

UPJO is mainly a congenital condition that can be detected by antenatal ultrasound during the second trimester.[1,2]

Pediatric UPJO might be associated with other congenital anomalies such as an imperforated anus, multicystic kidney, and ipsilateral ureterovesical reflux. In similar patients, UPJO should be treated first because distal ureteric diseases are commonly not severe.

In cases of a duplex renal system, the lower moiety is more commonly affected; in this case, ureterovesical reflux is likely to be found and can be diagnosed using voiding cystourethrogram (VCUG).

Diuretic renography is one of the most important studies used to determine the split function of each kidney and identify any renal evidence of obstruction and is the gold standard for the evaluation of the severity of UJPO. The most commonly used agent in renogram studies is technetium 99m mercaptoacetyltriglycine, especially in the pediatric population. The agent is usually secreted by proximal renal tubules in a small amount that should be filtered by renal glomeruli. The kidney is considered to be significantly damaged if the split function in one of the kidneys is less than 40% of the total kidney function; this should be in correlation to the half-life of the agent. In the adult population, other agents can be used, such as diethylenetriamine pentaacetate.

VCUG should be used to rule out the ureterovesical reflux role to hydronephrosis if diuretic demography does not detect UPJO.

In patients with a split renal function of more than 40%, the diuretic renogram should be repeated at 3-, 6-, and 12-month intervals. Surgery is to be performed if function has deteriorated.

The indications for surgical treatment include:

1. UPJO with less than 40% in the split function of the affected kidney on the diuretic renogram.
2. Renal parenchymal atrophy from severe bilateral UPJO.
3. Recurrent infections despite using prophylactic antibiotics.
4. Symptomatic obstructive UPJO or that associated with an abdominal mass.

Dismembered pyeloplasty is the gold standard technique used by surgeons. The main advantage of this procedure is to save the crossing vessel if present.[1,2]

Nondismembered pyeloplasty is used in case of high insertion of the ureter and no crossing vessel. It is inferior to dismembered pyeloplasty.

Surgical complications of UPJO include:

1. Pyelonephritis
2. Urinary extravasation and leakage
3. Recurrent UPJO
4. Bleeding
5. Trauma to surrounding organs

Clinical Presentation 6

Which *one* of the following anomalies has not been reported in Meckel-Gruber syndrome?

A. Polycystic kidney disease
B. Polydactyly
C. Central nervous malformations
D. Pulmonary hypoplasia
E. Horseshoe kidney

The correct answer is E

Comment: Meckel-Gruber syndrome is a lethal, rare, autosomal recessive condition characterized by the triad of occipital encephalocele, large polycystic kidneys, and postaxial polydactyly. Associated abnormalities include oral cleft, genital anomalies, central nervous system malformations, including Dandy-Walker and Arnold-Chiari malformation, and liver fibrosis.[1,2] Pulmonary hypoplasia is the leading cause of death. Improvements in ultrasonography have enabled prenatal diagnosis as early as 10 weeks' gestation.

This syndrome was first described by Johann Friedrich Meckel the Younger in 1822. He described two sibling neonates, a boy and a girl who had the combination of microcephaly with occipital encephalocele, cleft palate, polydactyly, and large cystic kidneys. In the boy, the testes were near the lower pole of the kidneys and the external genitalia were more female-like. Meckel mentioned that he suspected that the infants were an example of heredity because he had seen other instances of anomalies within given families. More than a century after, Gruber reported similar cases he had encountered and added a few more from the literature for a total of 16 cases. Gruber named the disease dysencephalia splanchnocystica and mentioned that it was genetic because many of the abnormalities were among siblings.[3] Meckel syndrome is usually lethal in early infancy because of the severity of renal and central nervous system malformations.

Clinical Presentation 7

Constellation of kidney dysphasia associated with hypoplasia of cerebellar vermis, nystagmus, retinal dysplasia, ocular coloboma, mid-brain "molar sign" on a magnetic resonance imaging (MRI) scan and congenital hepatic fibrosis are characteristics of which of the following abnormalities?

A. Joubert syndrome
B. Meckle-Gruber syndrome
C. Short rib syndrome
D. VACTER-L syndrome

The correct answer is A

Comment: Joubert syndrome is an uncommon autosomal recessive condition characterized by hypoplasia of the cerebellar vermis (demonstrated by MRI as the "molar tooth sign"), intellectual disability, retinal dystrophy, ocular coloboma, rotatory nystagmus, polydactyly, cystic renal dysplasia, and congenital hepatic fibrosis. Its neurologic manifestations usually come to medical attention in infancy. The syndrome was initially described in a French-Canadian family with four affected siblings by pediatric neurologists in Montreal more than 40 years ago.[1] One of the original children had an occipital meningoencephalocele that was removed at birth.

The two different forms of renal disease that have been described in Joubert syndrome are cystic renal dysplasia and nephronophthisis (tubulointerstitial nephritis and cysts at the corticomedullary junction). Clinically, these children present with polydipsia, polyuria, anemia, growth failure, elevated creatinine, and later develop renal failure.

Recently, it has become known that Joubert syndrome is due to ciliary disorders and there is some overlap in clinical presentations with Meckel and Bardet-Biedl syndromes (e.g., occipital meningoencephalocele, congenital hepatic fibrosis, obesity, ambiguous genitalia). So far, the molecular genetics of Joubert syndrome includes eight mutations in the ciliary/basal body genes: *INPPFE*, *AH11*, *NPHP1*, *CEP290*, *TMEM67/MKS3*, *RPGR1P1L*, *ARL13B*, and *CC2D2A*.[2] At a molecular level, it has been demonstrated that Joubert and Meckel syndromes share at least one gene mutation (*TMEM67/MKS3*) and it seems logical to infer that in the future more common mutations will be found.

Some individuals may have a mild form of the disorder with minimal motor (movement) disability and good mental development or may have severe motor disability with moderate impaired mental development and multiorgan impairments.

Current treatment options are symptomatic and supportive. Infant stimulation and physical, occupational, and speech therapy may benefit some children, in addition to regularly monitoring symptoms. Routine screening for progressive eye, liver, and kidney complications associated with Joubert syndrome–related disorders is highly recommended.

Clinical Presentation 8

What is the most common renal lesion in VACTER-L anomaly?

A. Renal dysplasia
B. Focal segmental sclerosis
C. Horseshoe kidney
D. Renal artery stenosis

The correct answer is A

Comment: The VACTER-L acronym stands for vertebral anomalies, anal, and cardiac malformations, tracheoesophageal fistula/atresia, radial and renal anomalies, and limb malformations. The majority of experts in VACTER-L require at least three of these anomalies to establish a diagnosis. When there is esophageal atresia, the first intrauterine manifestation is polyhydramnios. Tracheoesophageal fistula can be documented at autopsy and renal dysplasia is common in these children.[1,2]

The differential diagnosis includes Baller-Gerold syndrome (certain facial features and radial aplasia or hypoplasia), CHARGE syndrome (besides choanal atresia and coloboma, there can be cardiac and genitourinary anomalies), Currarino syndrome (lumbosacral malformations, constipation, and renal abnormalities), deletion 22q11.2 syndrome (cardiac, vertebral, and renal anomalies), Fanconi anemia (radial hypoplasia/aplasia, thumb anomalies, and hematological conditions), Feingold syndrome (hypoplastic thumb, renal, and cardiac congenital disease), Fryns syndrome (congenital diaphragmatic hernia, cardiac disease, and hypoplastic thumb), MURCS association (müllerian duct, renal agenesis, and cervical vertebral defects), oculoauriculo-vertebral syndrome (vertebral anomalies hypoplasia of maxilla and mandible and ear anomalies), Pallister-Hall syndrome (abnormal digits and imperforate anus), Townes-Brocks syndrome (thumbs, auricular, and anal anomalies), and VACTER-L with hydrocephalus. A careful physical examination and family history are helpful to narrow down which conditions are most likely in a patient with features suggestive of VACTER-L association. For example, autosomal dominant inheritance of certain features may suggest Townes-Brocks syndrome, and the presence of other features not typically seen in VACTER-L association may hint toward other disorders, such as pigmentary abnormalities in Fanconi anemia or hypocalcemia in deletion 22q11.2 syndrome. A panel of experts published an excellent article about the approach to confirm suspected VACTER-L. According to them, the initial workup should include a complete family history and physical examination, a supine anteroposterior chest radiograph, supine anteroposterior and lateral views of the entire vertebral column, including sacral views, and a transthoracic echocardiogram to look for congenital heart disease. In patients with increased oral secretions, choking with feeds, or respiratory distress, an attempt to pass a nasogastric tube will help confirm or exclude esophageal atresia. Anorectal malformations can be detected by physical examination in the majority of cases, but to better determine the extent of anomalies, an abdominal ultrasound should be performed. Radial and thumb anomalies are usually detected by simple inspection, but radiologic examination of the affected extremity will better delineate the malformation. To exclude Fanconi anemia, a complete blood cell count is extremely helpful.

Clinical Presentation 9

The constellation of kidney dysplasia, skeletal malformations of the thorax, and ocular and cerebral anomalies in Joubert syndrome is seen in which of the following symptoms?

A. Short rib syndrome
B. Meckel syndrome
C. VACTER-L anomalies
D. Bardet-Biedl syndrome

The correct answers are A, B, and D

Comment: Short rib syndrome is one of the lethal osteochondrodysplasias and has been traditionally divided into four types (I, Saldino-Noonan; II, Majewski; III, Verma-Naumoff; and IV, Beemer-Langer).[1-3]

These autosomal recessive, skeletal ciliopathies are characterized by a narrow thorax resulting from short ribs, cleft lip, and/or cleft palate, cystic renal dysplasia, congenital hepatic fibrosis, pancreatic cysts, ocular and cerebral anomalies, and abnormal genitalia. Polydactyly is variably present. The histology of the kidneys and liver is undistinguishable from the findings in patients with Meckel and Joubert syndromes.

Clinical Presentation 10

Retinitis pigment Ida is the cardinal manifestation in which of the following syndrome?

A. Joubert syndrome
B. Short rib sundry
C. Bardot-Biedl syndrome
D. Prune belly syndrome

The correct answer is C

Comment: The cardinal manifestations of Bardet-Biedl syndrome are retinitis pigmentosa, obesity, renal dysplasia, polydactyly, learning disability, and hypogenitalism. The diagnosis may be confirmed later as a young adult if the patient presents in childhood only with truncal obesity and learning disabilities but has normal vision and lacks polydactyly or syndactyly and hypogonadism. However, as patients age, visual and renal problems become more severe and virtually 100% of individuals with Bardet-Biedl syndrome will develop poor vision. The possibility of renal insufficiency increases with age. It is inherited in an autosomal recessive manner. Interfamilial and intrafamilial phenotypic variability exist. Prenatal diagnosis in affected families can be made by fetal ultrasound examination with the detection of polydactyly and cysts in the kidneys. Once the affected gene has been detected in a family, it is possible to look for the known gene. Presently, 18 genes have been associated with Bardet-Biedl syndrome: *BBS1*, *BBS2*, *ARL6* (*BBS3*), *BBS4*, *BBS5*, *MKKS* (*BBS6*), *BBS7*, *TTC8* (*BBS8*), *BBS9*, *BBS10*, *TRIM32* (*BBS11*), *BBS12*, *MKS1* (*BBS13*), *CEP290* (*BBS14*), *WDPCP* (*BBS15*), *SDCCAG8* (*BBS16*), *LTZFL1* (*BBS17*), and *BBIP1* (*BBS18*). Histologically, the kidneys show extensive replacement of parenchyma by round cysts lined by flat to cuboidal epithelium. The glomeruli are preserved. Persistent fetal lobulations have been described, suggesting a defect in renal maturation.[1,2]

Clinical Presentation 11

The assumption of hypoplastic lower extremities, vertebrae, sacrum, neural tube, bilateral renal agenesis or dysplasia, and imperforate anus are constant findings in which of the following syndromes?

A. VACTER-L
B. Potter syndrome
C. Caudal dysplasia syndrome
D. Joubert syndrome

The correct answer is C

Comment: This syndrome is characterized by hypoplastic lower extremities, caudal vertebrae, sacrum, neural tube, and urogenital system. There may also be an imperforate anus. Renal anomalies include bilateral renal agenesis, renal dysplasia, and horseshoe kidney. Frequently, placentas have a single umbilical artery and less commonly have amnion nodosum secondary to oligohydramnios.[1,2] These patients may also have congenital heart disease and their mothers frequently have pregestational diabetes mellitus. The association of polysplenia and caudal dysplasia has been reported.

Infants of diabetic mothers have three to four times the incidence of congenital malformations than that in the general population. They can have skeletal, neurologic, genitourinary and digestive tract maldevelopment, and caudal dysplasia syndrome. The brain and proximal spinal cord are normal in children with caudal dysplasia. Surviving children usually have a normal intelligence but tend to have lower extremity difficulties as well as urinary problems and may require extensive intervention by pediatric orthopedics and urologists. Prenatal diagnosis can be made by fetal ultrasound and parental counseling should be offered depending on the severity of malformations.

Clinical Presentation 12

Which of the following therapeutic interventions is inappropriate for patients with autosomal dominant polycystic kidney disease (ADPK)?

A. Administration of lipid-lowering drugs
B. Administration of angiotensin-converting enzyme inhibitors
C. Dietary salt and protein restrictions
D. Administration of arginine-vasopressin-receptor inhibitor
E. Forced fluids
F. None of the above

The correct answer is F

Comment: ADPK is a relatively common condition that affects 1 of every 400 to 1000 live births and accounts for approximately 10% of patients with chronic renal failure requiring dialysis or transplant. ADPK should be considered a systemic disorder that mainly affects adult patients who can also develop hepatic and pancreatic cysts, chronic hypertension, intracranial aneurysms, and cardiac valve anomalies, especially mitral valve prolapse. The likelihood of renal failure increases progressively with age after 40 years, rising to 25% by age 50 years, 40% at 60 years, and 75% at age 70 years. The kidneys of adult patients contain multiple round cysts of variable size filled with urine and blood, becoming extremely large and extending up to 10 times their normal weight. Histology reveals completely disorganized renal parenchyma with large cystically dilated tubules and occasional glomeruli and fibrotic interstitium with chronic inflammation.[1,2]

For many years, ADPK was considered an untreatable renal disease leading to chronic renal failure and required either dialysis or transplant, but more recently there is some hope of a better treatment by early administration of an arginine-vasopressin (AVP)-V2 receptor inhibitor in individuals with subclinically detected disease. The rationale behind this therapy is that the collecting ducts and distal nephrons (that are the more severely affected by cysts in ADPK) are sensitive to vasopressin. This receptor is the main hormonal regulator of adenyl cyclase activity in collecting ducts. To avoid dehydration, mammals live under the constant action of AVP on the distal nephron and collecting duct. When the individual drinks large volumes of water, plasma AVP levels decrease enough to make the urine more dilute than plasma; therefore, during most of the day, cyst epithelial cells undergo stimulation to secrete fluid. The circulating levels of AVP are likely elevated in patients with ADPK to compensate for the reduced concentrating capacity of the affected kidneys and the AVP effect leads to cyst formation. The administration of an AVP receptor inhibitor delays the cyst formation but does not help the regeneration of tubular epithelium; therefore, it is critical to start treatment as early as possible to prevent cyst formation. Other recommendations are to drink plenty of fluids, up to 3 L/day for adults and proportionately less for children, avoid caffeine, decrease salt and protein intake, add angiotensin-converting enzyme inhibitors or angiotensin-receptor blockers to lower blood pressure and decrease the amount of fat ingested. In addition, prescribe a cholesterol-lowering agent.[1,2]

Clinical Presentation 13

Which of the following distinguishes autosomal recessive polycystic kidney (ARPK) from autosomal dominant polycystic kidney (ADPK) disease?

A. Bilateral enlarged kidneys
B. Hypertension
C. Abnormal renal function
D. Hepatic fibrosis
E. Polyuria

The correct answers are D and E

Comment: Autosomal recessive polycystic kidney (ARPK) disease is currently considered a primary ciliopathy that equally affects the kidneys and liver. ARPK has an incidence of 1:20,000 to 1:40,000 live births and a heterozygous carrier rate of 1 in 70. It occurs as a result of a mutation in a single gene named Polycystic Kidney and Hepatic Disease (*PKHD1*). Severely affected fetuses are born with oligohydramnios, Potter face, and some will develop respiratory insufficiency, but many survive the neonatal period. Of all neonatal survivors, approximately 40% have severe hepatic and renal disease. Of the remaining children, 30% present with severe renal and mild hepatobiliary disease and the other 30% with severe hepatobiliary problems and mild renal disease.[1,2]

The renal pathology is extremely characteristic because it is always bilateral, the organ is enlarged but maintains its reniform shape, and when opened it transudates a large amount of urine. Histologically, the cysts are elongated and their long axis is perpendicular to the capsule. The hepatic manifestations are congenital hepatic fibrosis (CHF), which is indistinguishable from the CHF found in other ciliopathies such as Meckel, short rib, or polysplenia. Secondary to liver fibrosis, autosomal dominant polycystic kidney (ADPK) disease develop portal hypertension, esophageal varices, hemorrhoids, upper gastrointestinal bleeding, splenomegaly, and hypersplenism.[1,2]

Genetic studies have demonstrated that ARPK is associated with two genes (*PKD1* and *PKD2*). The former produces the severe form of the disease and its gene product, polycystin-1, is a receptor-like integral membrane protein that seems to be involved in cell-cell matrix interactions and also plays a role in calcium homeostasis through its physical interaction with polycystin-2, the protein product of *PKD2*.[1,2]

Parents of a child born with ARPK who are obligate carriers may be offered preimplantation genetic diagnosis using single-cell multiple displacement amplification products for PKHD1 haplotyping, which significantly decreases the problem of allelic dropout. This specific protocol uses whole-genome amplification of single blastomeres, multiple displacement amplification, and haplotype analysis with 20 novel polymorphic short-tandem repeat markers from the *PKHD1* gene and flanking sequences.[1,2]

Once the child is born with the disease, the current treatment is symptomatic. However, in cases of severe renal and hepatobiliary disease, the combined renal-liver transplant looks promising because the outcome of liver transplant has improved recently and it has been proven that if left unattended, CHF may lead to ascending cholangitis, sepsis, portal hypertension, and gastrointestinal bleeding. All of these complications could impact the ultimate outcome of liver transplant months or years after renal transplant. The future seems more promising for these patients because there are several preclinical trials that hopefully will discover new treatment modalities to block fluid transfer into the tubular epithelial cells and decrease or completely block cyst formation.[1,2]

Clinical Presentation 14

VACTR-L and CHARGE syndromes share many major clinical features.

Which of the following is the least common feature of CHARGE syndrome?

A. Renal anomalies
B. Immune system disorders
C. Scoliosis
D. Polydactyl
E. None of the above
F. All of the above

The correct answer is F

Comment: CHARGE syndrome is a disorder that affects many areas of the body. CHARGE is an abbreviation for several of the features common in the disorder including coloboma, heart defects, atresia choanae (also known as choanal atresia), growth retardation, genital abnormalities, and ear abnormalities. The pattern of malformations varies among individuals with this disorder, and the multiple health problems can be life-threatening in infancy. Affected individuals usually have several major characteristics or a combination of major and minor characteristics.[1,2]

The major characteristics of CHARGE syndrome are common in this disorder and occur less frequently in other disorders. Most individuals with CHARGE syndrome have a gap or hole in one of the structures of the eye (coloboma), which forms during early development. A coloboma may be present in one or both eyes and may impair a person's vision, depending on its size and location. Some affected individuals also have abnormally small or underdeveloped eyes (microphthalmia). In many people with CHARGE syndrome, one or both nasal passages are narrowed (choanal stenosis) or completely blocked (choanal atresia), which can cause difficulty breathing. Affected individuals frequently have cranial nerve abnormalities. The cranial nerves emerge directly from the brain and extend to various areas of the head and neck, controlling muscle movement and transmitting sensory information. Abnormal function of certain cranial nerves can cause swallowing problems, facial paralysis, a sense of smell that is diminished (hyposmia) or completely absent (anosmia), and mild to profound hearing loss. People with CHARGE syndrome also typically have middle and inner ear abnormalities, which can contribute to hearing problems, and unusually shaped external ears.

Affected individuals frequently have hypogonadotropic hypogonadism, which affects the production of hormones that direct sexual development. As a result, males with CHARGE syndrome are often born with an unusually small penis (micropenis) and undescended testes (cryptorchidism). Abnormalities of external genitalia are seen less often in affected females. Puberty can be incomplete or delayed in affected males and females. Another minor feature of CHARGE syndrome is tracheoesophageal fistula, which is an abnormal connection (fistula) between the esophagus and the trachea. Most people with CHARGE syndrome also have distinctive facial features, including a square-shaped face and differences in appearance between the right and left sides of the face (facial asymmetry). Affected individuals have a wide range of cognitive function, from normal intelligence to major learning disabilities with absent speech and poor communication.

Less common features of CHARGE syndrome include kidney abnormalities, immune system problems, abnormal curvature of the spine (scoliosis or kyphosis), and limb abnormalities, such as extra fingers or toes (polydactyly) and missing fingers or toes.[1,2]

Clinical Presentation 15

Which of the following renal structural abnormalities are reported in DiGeorge syndrome?

A. UPJ obstruction
B. Vesicoureteral reflux (VUR)
C. A genesis of the kidney
D. Multicystic dysplasia

The correct answers are A, B, C, and D

Comment: DiGeorge syndrome, also known as 22q11.2 deletion syndrome, is a disorder caused when a small part of chromosome 22 is missing. This deletion results in the poor development of several body systems.[1]

The term *22q11.2 deletion* syndrome covers what once were thought to be separate conditions, including DiGeorge syndrome, velocardiofacial syndrome, and other disorders that have the same genetic cause, though features may vary slightly.

Medical problems commonly associated with 22q11.2 deletion syndrome include heart defects (VSD, ASD, tetralogy of Fallot, and truncus arteriosus), poor immune system function, hypoparathyroidism, hypoplastic or absence of thymus gland, hypothyroidism, distinct facial features (low-set ears, short width of eye openings, hooded eyes, enlarged nose tip, long face), autism, attention deficit hyperactivity disorders, a cleft palate, complications related to low levels of calcium in the blood, and delayed development with behavioral and emotional problems.

The number and severity of symptoms associated with 22q11.2 deletion syndrome vary. However, almost everyone with this syndrome needs treatment from specialists in a variety of fields. In children, hypoplasia or agenesis of the kidney is the most common feature (17%), followed by multicystic dysplasia, obstructive hydronephrosis (10%), and vesicoureteral reflux (4%).

Clinical Presentation 16

A 17-year-old boy with a rapidly progressive form of immunoglobulin A (IgA) nephropathy is placed on regular hemodialysis therapy for end-stage kidney disease. His brother, aged 22 years, and an older adopted brother, aged 24 years, both offer to donate a kidney. Both potential donors are healthy and have completely normal pretransplant medical evaluations.

The older adopted brother is a two-antigen mismatch, whereas the younger brother is also a two-antigen mismatch (single haplotype match) with the patient.

Which ONE of the following choices would you recommend to the patient?

A. Renal transplantation is not appropriate because of the high risk of recurrence of IgA nephropathy and subsequent graft failure.
B. Renal transplantation from the adopted sibling is preferred because of a lower risk of recurrence of IgA nephropathy and a superior graft survival.
C. Renal transplantation from the adopted sibling is preferred because of a lower risk of recurrence of IgA nephropathy and equivalent graft survival.
D. Renal transplantation should be delayed until a bilateral nephrectomy of the recipient is performed.
E. Renal transplantation from a cadaver donor is preferred; neither sibling should be used as a donor.

The correct answer is B

Comment: In recent years, major genome-wide association studies have provided significant insight into the genetic basis of IgA nephropathy. Patients typically have high levels of aberrantly O-glycosylated IgA1 molecules, which become targets of an autoantibody response, leading to immune complex formation.[1–3] These deposit in the mesangium and spark an unhindered immune response, ultimately leading to fibrosis and kidney failure.

To date, genome-wide association studies for IgA nephropathy have successfully identified many risk loci with candidate genes involved in antigen processing and presentation, gut mucosal immunity, IgA biology, and dysregulation of the alternative complement pathway.

An overall genetic risk can be computed with these genome-wide significant susceptibility variants and has been shown to inversely correlate with the age of diagnosis. Interestingly, the IgA nephropathy genetic risk score is strongly associated with global pathogen diversity, suggesting that the selective pressure from environmental factors may account for variation in risk allele frequency and the geographic variation in disease prevalence among world populations.[1]

There is a significant variability of up to 30% in the incidence of recurrence of IgA nephropathy after transplantation. Recurrence is associated with a higher risk of graft failure and is more common in younger patients with rapidly progressive, crescentic disease in their native kidneys.[2]

Because the risk of allele frequency in disease prevalence among the general population is considerably lower than related donor kidneys, transplantation from the adopted sibling is preferred for transplantation in IgA patients with end-stage renal disease.[3,4]

Clinical Presentation 17

A 15-year-old girl was admitted for evaluation of bilateral nephrolithiasis, which was detected incidentally by plain radiography and abdominal ultrasonography during the evaluation of abdominal pain. The patient had no history of polyuria, polydipsia, or urinary tract infection. Consanguinity was not present between her parents. Family history was positive for nephrolithiasis in her uncle and cousin.

On admission, the results of the physical examination were normal. Her height was 156 cm (between the 10th and 25th percentile, weight 58 kg (fourth percentile), and blood pressure 110/67 mm Hg.

Laboratory investigation revealed a normal complete blood cell count. Urinalysis revealed microhematuria (25 red blood cell/μL and trace proteinuria). Urine specific gravity was 1.015, with a pH of 5.0. BUN was 77 mg/dL, creatinine 1.4 mg/dL, sodium 143 mEq/, potassium 4.3 mEq/L, chloride 110 mEq/L, bicarbonate 19.9 mEq/, calcium 9.1 mg/dL, phosphorus 4.0 mg/dL, magnesium 1.1 mg/dL, uric acid 8.0 mg/dL, and alkaline phosphatase 88 U/L. Arterial blood gas revealed a pH of 7.34, PCO_2 30 mm Hg, bicarbonate 19.5 mEq/L, and a base excess of −6.4. Estimated GFR was 67 mL/min/0.73 m^2. Serum parathyroid hormone (PTH) levels was elevated at 101 ng/mL, 25 (OH) vitamin D 15.1 ng/mL, and 1,25(OH)2 vitamin D 19.0 μg/mL. Urinary calcium excretion (7.2 mg/kg/day); magnesium to creatinine ratio (0.31), oxalate, (0.6 mg/kg/day), and uric acid (8.7 mg/kg/day) were increased. Tubular reabsorption of phosphate was normal (>91%). Urine protein electrophoresis showed tubular and glomerular proteinuria (26 mg/m^2/h). Urinary amino acid excretion was normal. Repeat renal ultrasound revealed bilateral diffuse hyperechogenicity of pyramids, which is typical for medullary nephrocalcinosis.

What is the MOST likely diagnosis in this patient?

A. Bartter syndrome
B. Gitelman syndrome
C. Vitamin D intoxication
D. Familial hypomagnesemia hypercalciuria and nephrocalcinosis (FHHNC)
E. Dent disease

The correct answer is D

Comment: The constellation of clinical and laboratory findings, including a positive family history of nephrolithiasis, hypomagnesemia, hypermagnesemia, hypercalciuria, and medullary nephrocalcinosis, are consistent with the diagnosis of FHHNC.[1] Bartter and Gitleman syndromes were ruled out because of normal blood pH and the absence of hypokalemia and metabolic alkalosis. Patients with Dent disease usually have low plasma parathyroid and elevated 1,25(OH)2 vitamin D levels.

FHHNC is a rare autosomal recessive tubular disorder that causes medullary nephrocalcinosis.[2] In addition to presenting the characteristic triad included in the name of the disease, affected individuals may present clinically with polydipsia, polyuria, recurrent urinary tract infections, vomiting, abdominal pain, convulsion, and carpopedal spasm.

Urinary tract infections are the most common clinical manifestation (43%), followed by polyuria and polydipsia (27%). Some patients show extrarenal symptoms, such as hearing impairment or ocular abnormalities. The most important biochemical findings of FHHNC syndrome are hypomagnesemia, hypermagnesemia, and hypercalciuria. Hyperuricemia, hypocitraturia, and elevated PTH levels are also present. The primary defect is impaired reabsorption of magnesium and calcium in the loop of Henle. This defect is due to a mutation in the *CLDN16* gene that encodes the paracellular protein claudin-16, which is located in the tight junctions of the thick ascending limb of the loop of Henle. Consequently, patients with FHHNC should not only present with typical clinical and biochemical data; they should also be screened for mutation of the *CLDN16* gene.

Clinical Presentation 18

A previously healthy 15-year-old boy was referred for the evaluation of recurrent, painless gross hematuria of 2 weeks' duration. The patient denied abdominal or back pain, had no dysuria, fatigue, or fever, and a complete review of systems was unremarkable except for the bright red urine. There was no history of trauma, sore throat, sinusitis, symptoms or evidence of other infections, or bleeding diathesis. His past medical history was unremarkable, with no history of urinary tract infections and no previous episodes of hematuria. He had been a full-term normal delivery and his mother recalled there being no issues with his antenatal ultrasound. The patient came to the clinic with both parents, who denied a history of hematuria or cystic kidney disease in any members of the family. The patient's father had been recently diagnosed with hypertension and was on medication.

On physical examination, the patient's weight and height were greater than the 50th percentile for height and weight. Vital signs were unremarkable and blood pressure was normal at 118/74 mm Hg. Physical examination was normal with no evidence of bruising or rashes, absence of hepatosplenomegaly, no palpable renal masses, and a normal genital examination. He had a normal hemoglobin (16 mg/dL) and white blood count. His electrolytes were normal and his BUN was 15 mg/dL with a creatinine of 0.9 mg/dL. The coagulation profile was unremarkable: partial thromboplastin time was 29 seconds (normal range, 22–37 seconds), the prothrombin time was 13.1 seconds (normal range, 12–15 seconds), and the international normalized ratio was 1.1 (normal range, 0.86–1.14). Urine analysis had a specific gravity of 1.025, 3+ blood, 1+ protein, many red blood cells, three to five white blood cells per high-power field, and one to two hyaline casts. Urine culture was negative. Complements were normal C3 was 91 (normal range, 75–180 mg/dL) and C4 was 19 mg/dL (normal range, 15–50 mg/dL) with negative antinuclear antibody and negative antineutrophil cytoplasmic antibody. A renal ultrasound was remarkable for multiple small cysts involving the upper pole of the left kidney without an associated discrete mass. The remainder of the renal parenchyma was unremarkable with normal-sized kidneys for his height (right, 12.2 cm; left, 13.2 cm), normal cortical thickness, normal echogenicity, and normal corticomedullary differentiation with no other cysts. The patient underwent a CT scan with and without contrast with delayed phases, which confirmed a left upper pole cystic lesion filling nearly the entire upper pole of the left kidney without involvement of the urinary collecting system. The lower pole of the left kidney had multiple minute subcentimeter cysts that had not been evident on ultrasound; the right kidney was completely normal. The renal parenchyma surrounding the cysts was functioning as evidenced by the normal contrast enhancement. There were no suspicious lymph nodes and no homogeneous tumor mass visualized. There were no cysts visualized in the liver.

What is the differential diagnosis and what additional diagnostic tests would you perform?

A. ADPK disease
B. Multicystic nephroma
C. Unilateral multiocular dysplastic kidney
D. Wilms tumor

The correct answers are A, B, and C

Comment: The differential diagnosis in patients presenting with unilateral multicystic renal lesions is multilocular cystic nephroma, unilateral renal cystic disease, segmental multicystic dysplastic kidney disease, and ADPK disease. The therapy for multilocular cystic nephroma is radical nephrectomy because it cannot be differentiated from more aggressive neoplasms such as the cystic variant of Wilms tumor and cystic renal cell carcinoma, which makes it crucial to carefully consider other diagnoses first. The lack of suspect lymph nodes and homogeneous tumor mass as well as the presence of cysts in other areas of the patient's affected kidney made the diagnosis of cystic nephroma less likely. Unilateral renal cystic disease is a less well-known nonfamilial and nonprogressive entity.[1] Segmental multicystic dysplastic kidney disease was unlikely in our patient because, on the CT scan, there was normal contrast enhancement in the renal tissue adjacent to the cysts and a lack of evidence of duplication of the collecting system. Regardless of the potential diagnosis, in most cases, unilateral multicystic kidney in children usually incurs considerable morbidity for the child, including partial to full nephrectomies and open biopsies.

Our patient presented with a multicystic lesion in the upper pole of his left kidney with completely normal contralateral kidney. Both parents underwent a renal ultrasound to evaluate the presence of cysts. His father had bilaterally enlarged kidneys with numerous cysts. A genetic testing was done for ADPK disease and the patient had a deletion in the *PKD1* gene on chromosome 16.

ADPK disease is the clinical manifestation of a genetic defect that is typically a bilateral renal cystic disease of adults because children are most often asymptomatic.[1,2] Most of these children have bilateral renal cystic disease, but 17% have been identified with an initial presentation of a unilateral cystic kidney.[2]

Clinical Presentation 19

A 7-year-old girl was admitted to our hospital for further evaluation of bilateral nephrolithiasis and nephrocalcinosis. Her past medical history was remarkable for polyuria/polydipsia that had persisted for the past 5 years and recurrent urinary tract infections. A dimercaptosuccinic acid scan performed 4 years previously was normal. At the age of 4 years, her urinary calcium/creatinine level was 0.4 mg/mg (normal, <0.21 mg/mg) and she was started on potassium citrate treatment, which she was still on at the time of presentation. Her parents were nonconsanguineous and she had a healthy sister. Physical examination revealed a healthy child with a height of 114.5 cm (50th–75th percentile) and a weight of 22 kg (50th–75th percentile). The physical examination was unremarkable; her blood pressure was 100/60 mm Hg. Laboratory tests at admission revealed a normal complete blood cell count; urinalysis revealed pH 6, specific gravity of 1005 to 1010, and protein (+1) with a few leukocytes observed in the microscopic examination. Other laboratory findings were blood pH 7.46, PCO_2 34 mm Hg, HCO_3 24 mEq/L, urea 58 mg/dL, serum creatinine 0.9 mg/dL, sodium 140 mEq/L, potassium 4.3 mmol/L, uric acid 6.9 mg/dL, magnesium 1.3 mg/dL, calcium 10.3 mg/dL, phosphorus 4.4 mg/dL, alkaline phosphatase 281 U/L, PTH 108.4 pg/mL (normal, 15–65 pg/mL), and 25(OH)D 25.5 ng/mL (normal 20–32 ng/mL). Calcium excretion was 6.9 mg/kg/ day (normal <4 mg/kg/day), and protein excretion was 7 mg/m^2/h (normal < 4 mg/m^2/h). Urinary oxalate/creatinine was 0.072 mEq/mEq/L (normal, <0.08 mmol/mmol), citrate/creatinine was 0.25 mEq/L/mEq (normal, 0.3–0.7 mEq/mEq), cystine/creatinine was 3.25 μEq/mEq creatinine (normal, 4–22 μmEq/mEq/creatinine), uric acid/GFR was 0.416 mg/dL (normal, <0.56 mg/dL GFR), ratio of phosphorus tubular maximum to glomerular filtration was 4.27 (normal, 2.8–4.4), fractional sodium reabsorption was 0.5% (normal, <1%), and fractional potassium reabsorption was 13.7% (normal, <15%).

Excretion of amino acids was within the normal range in the urine. The GFR calculated using the Schwartz formula was 69.6 mL/min/1.73 m^2, and creatinine clearance calculated on 24-hour collected urine was 60 mL/min/1.73 m^2. Renal ultrasound revealed bilateral diffuse hyperechogenicity of the pyramids, which is typical for medullary nephrocalcinosis. Ophthalmologic examination revealed bilateral maculopathy characterized by sharply demarcated areas of depigmentation and atrophy in both macular areas and bilateral irregularity in the retinal pigment epithelium.

What is the most likely diagnosis for this patient?

A. Vitamin D intoxication
B. FHHNC
C. Williams-Beuren syndrome
D. Hyperparathyroidism
E. Dent disease

The correct answer is B

Comment: FHHNC was the most likely diagnosis in our patient. The most striking finding was bilateral medullary nephrocalcinosis, which was demonstrated in the renal ultrasound performed after recurrent urinary tract infections. Nephrocalcinosis refers to diffuse deposition of calcium in the kidney resulting from increased urinary calcium, oxalate, or urate.[1] Medullary nephrocalcinosis may be associated with several disorders including idiopathic hypercalcemia, hypervitaminosis D, Williams-Beuren syndrome, primary neonatal hyperparathyroidism, antenatal Bartter syndrome, Dent disease, Lowe syndrome, cystinosis, renal tubular acidosis, medullary sponge kidney, and FHHNC.[2] None of the clinical or laboratory findings was supportive of the diagnoses other than FHHNC. The patient fulfilled the diagnostic criteria for FHHNC, including hypomagnesemia, hypercalciuria, and nephrocalcinosis.[3] Besides the laboratory findings of the diagnostic triad, hyperuricemia, hypomagnesuria, impaired GFR, and sometimes hypocitraturia are also common in FHHNC, as seen in our case.

Patients with FHHNC usually present during early childhood with recurrent urinary tract infections, polyuria/polydipsia, isosthenuria, and renal stones in addition to vomiting, abdominal pain, tetanic episodes, or generalized seizures. Our patient had a history of recurrent urinary tract infections, polyuria/polydipsia, isosthenuria, and renal stones, but no episodes of seizures resulting from electrolyte imbalance.

The underlying genetic defect in FHHNC is a mutation in either the *CLDN16* or the *CLDN19* gene.[1–5] *CLDN16* and *CLDN19* encode tight junction proteins claudin-16 and claudin-19, respectively, which are both important for renal magnesium reabsorption in the thick ascending limb of Henle.[1–4] Claudin-19 is also expressed at high levels in the retina. Thus, both

CLDN16 and *CLDN19* mutations result in a similar renal phenotype, whereas *CLDN19* mutations cause additional ocular involvement.[4]

The ocular manifestations associated with *CLDN19* mutations include macular colobomata, nystagmus, chorioretinitis, and myopia.[5] In addition to the classical findings of FHHNC, ophthalmological examination revealed bilateral maculopathy in our patient. This additional finding led us to search for a mutation in the *CLDN19* gene. As expected, a homozygous truncating mutation (W169X) in *CLDN19* was identified in our patient.

Familial hypomagnesemia with hypercalciuria and nephrocalcinosis generally has a poor prognosis, ending up with end-stage renal disease, and a definitive cure can only be achieved by renal transplantation.[5] Treatment with magnesium salts, thiazides, and potassium citrate do not influence the progression of the disease but may decrease calcium excretion and formation of renal stones and nephrocalcinosis.[5] We planned to continue on potassium citrate and add magnesium salts and thiazides to the treatment in addition to regular ophthalmological examinations.

Clinical Presentation 20

A 14-month-old female child presented with a 1-day history of urinary retention. As for the past medical history, the mother noted chronic constipation since the age of 2 months, which was treated by laxatives. On presentation, the patient was alert and active without signs of peripheral edema. On admission, she had normal vital signs, a blood pressure of 100/80 mm Hg, a body weight of 9 kg, and normal height for age.

On physical examination, the patient had abdominal distension and diminished deep tendon reflexes in the lower limbs. Biochemical investigations showed a normal kidney function with a serum creatinine of 0.3 mg/dL, normal electrolyte concentrations, and normal liver function tests. Complete blood count was normal except for hemoglobin of 8 mg/dL. The girl had a Foley catheter inserted and instantaneously passed urine. Urine analysis showed a specific gravity of 1.020, a pH of 5, and absence of protein, erythrocytes, and leukocytes.

Renal sonography showed a huge pelvic mass extending to the upper part of the abdomen, 20 × 10 cm in size, and with liquid fillings within the mass. A CT scan of the abdomen revealed a heterogeneous mass with soft tissue components in its lower part, extending to the perineum and causing significant mass effect on the surrounding structures. Based on the radiological images, further biochemical investigations were performed. Serum β-HCG level was normal (<0.1 IU/L), whereas alpha fetoprotein was increased to 18,837 IU/mL (0-5.79) and lactate dehydrogenase to 2000 IU/L. The child underwent abdominal surgery to remove the mass. Tissue specimens were sent to histopathology.

What is the diagnosis and what should be done next?

A. Polycystic ovaries
B. Hematometra
C. Leiomyoma
D. Malignant teratoma (according to images and alpha fetoprotein)

The correct answer is D

Comment: Our patient presented with chronic constipation from the age of 14 months, which was treated with laxatives. Only after acute urinary retention had developed were further investigations initiated. Histopathologic studies established the diagnosis. The alpha fetoprotein level returned to normal after tumor removal. A CT scan of the abdomen and chest demonstrated secondary deposits in both lungs. A bone scintography was normal. Because the mass involved the sacrococcygeal bone and infiltrated the surrounding tissues, parts of the sacrum and coccyx needed to be removed, and chemotherapy was started.

Sacrococcygeal teratoma are seen in 1:35,000 live births, with a female-to-male ratio of 3:1.[1] Both benign and malignant forms of sacrococcygeal teratomas have been described in children <4 years of age. The clinical presentation depends on the child's age at the time of diagnosis and tumor localization. It is most often diagnosed prenatally by ultrasound or during the neonatal period and may be clinically silent.[2] In older children, the tumor often presents as a palpable mass that might compress the rectum and bladder, with subsequent complications such as constipation and urinary retention.[3]

In children with malignant abdominal teratoma, urinary retention might be secondary to nervous system involvement, especially in cases of intramedullary infiltration, or from urethral compression and consecutive urinary retention. If late diagnosis is made, hydronephrosis might even occur. Next to teratoma, other tumors such as ependymomas and congenital ependymoblastoma can occur in the sacrococcygeal regions, which might result in similar findings. In our case, urinary retention was most likely from both intramedullary involvement and urethral compression.

Clinical Presentation 21

A 3.5-kg male term newborn was delivered spontaneously to a 25-year-old mother after an uneventful pregnancy and discharged 1 day after birth. The newborn presented with cough and respiratory insufficiency on postnatal day 12, concurrently with an upper respiratory tract infection in his older brother. The patient's physical examination on admission was normal except for wheezing and desaturation. Posteroanterior chest radiograph of the infant revealed right paracardiac consolidation and resistant consolidate lesion in posterior mediastinal region on right lateral decubitus chest radiography after medical treatment with inhaler salbutamol, oxygen, and antibiotic therapy for 10 days.

His physical examination was normal (weight 4210 g [50th percentile], length 52 cm [25th percentile], and head circumference 37 cm [50th percentile] on postnatal day 22), except for diminished ventilation on right lower chest on admission. Blood gas analysis and complete blood count were within normal ranges. Biochemical evaluation for renal and liver function were all normal (Na 139 mEq/L, potassium 4.4 mEq/L, bicarbonate 20 mEq/L, BUN 8 mg/dL, and creatinine 0.2 mg/dL). Urine output was measured as 3 mL/kg/h. Echocardiography revealed normal cardiac structure.

How could this intrathoracic mass be investigated?

A. Thoracic Doppler ultrasound
B. Thoracic CT scan with contrast
C. Thoracic MRI
D. Intravenous pyelogram

The correct answers are A, B, C, and D

Comment: The patient's lesion in the lung did not respond to antibiotic treatment, which eliminated pneumonia or atelectasis. Diaphragmatic hernia, teratoma, mediastinal neuroblastoma, intra- or extralobar pulmonary sequestration, bronchopulmonary foregut malformations, such as cystic adenomatoid malformation or bronchogenic cysts, and intrathoracic kidney can cause this radiographic appearance. These pathologies should be considered in the differential diagnosis.[1–4]

A CT scan of the thorax performed because of the consolidated appearance on radiography revealed the presence of the right kidney within the thorax. Right and left renal veins formed a common vascular structure and drained into the enlarged azygos vein, and bilateral accessory renal arteries were observed. The right kidney was above the level of the hemidiaphragm, with dimensions of 65 × 30 × 34 mm, and parenchymal thickness was measured at 7 mm on the ultrasonographic image. The left kidney was observed at its normal location, with dimensions of 63 × 23 × 24 mm and a parenchymal thickness of 7.5 mm.

Patients with a suspected intrathoracic mass require further evaluation, including Doppler ultrasound, CT scan of the thorax with intravenous contrast, or MRI.[4] These studies may delineate the lesion and its associated vasculature and determine whether any communication with the tracheobronchial tree exists.[2,4] An intravenous pyelogram can be performed in such cases with suspected ectopic kidneys.

All patients should be evaluated for associated congenital disorders, in particular cardiac anomalies.[2] Rotational irregularities with the hilum facing inferiorly, distorted shape, elongated urethra, high origin of renal vessels, and medial deviation of the lower renal pole can be associated with congenital intrathoracic kidney.

Clinical Presentation 22

A 5-month-old male infant was referred to our hospital because of a decrease in urinary output and difficulty breathing. The patient had been diagnosed with acute pyelonephritis when he presented with fever and vomiting 45 days previously at another medical center, where he was hospitalized and treated with several broad-spectrum antibiotics (amikacin, ceftriaxone, piperacillin, tazobactam, meropenem, and vancomycin) because of urosepsis. An ultrasound (US) scan performed at that time showed an increase in bilateral renal length and parenchymal echogenicity and the presence of millimetric echogenicities in the renal pelvis.

Two days before his referral to our hospital, urinary output progressively decreased, and he started to gain weight. He showed no signs of fever, vomiting, or diarrhea, and there was no change in urine color. According to his medical history, he was born at 26 weeks of gestation and had a birth weight of 680 g; there was no consanguinity between his parents. He was hospitalized in the neonatal intensive care unit for 2.5 months. He had been intubated for 45 days during that time and an umbilical catheter had been placed. He had been fed with formula in addition to breast milk. Apart from vaccination for hepatitis B, he had not been vaccinated for other diseases. On physical examination at the time of admission to our hospital's emergency service, he had hypertension (100/60 mm Hg; age-specific 95th percentile 87/68 mm Hg), tachycardia (152 beats/min), and tachypnea (72 /min). His height and weight were below the 3rd percentile after adjustment for age (length, 43 cm; weight, 2.7 kg). A diffuse edema on the eyelids and lower extremities, fine rales at the base of both hemithoraxes, and a 3/6 pansystolic murmur at all foci were detected. He had severe abdominal distention, and both kidneys were readily palpable. No genitourinary abnormalities were detected.

Laboratory examinations yielded the following results: hemoglobin 9.0 g/dL (normal, 12–16 g/dL), leukocytes 21.700/mm^3 (normal, 4800–10,800/mm^3) (absolute neutrophil count, 15.500/mm^3), thrombocytes 203.000/mm^3 (normal, 150,000–450,000/mm^3), C-reactive protein 21.7 mg/dL (normal, 0–0.5 mg/dL), procalcitonin 32 ng/mL (normal, 0–0.5 mg/dL), blood urea nitrogen 55 mg/dL (normal, 4–18 mg/dL), and creatinine 3.8 mg/dL (normal, 0.2–0.87 mg/dL). The estimated GFR was calculated as 6.8 mL/m^2/min using the Schwartz formula. The infant had hyponatremia (130 mEq/L), hyperkalemia (5.2 mEq/L), hyperuricemia (13 mg/dL), and decompensated metabolic acidosis (pH 7.18, PCO_2 22, HCO_3 10.2, base excess −14). The results of the urinalysis were: pH 6, density 1018, leukocyte esterase 3+, nitrite 1+; 12 leukocytes/high-power field on microscopic examination; no bacteria were seen.

What is the etiology of renal failure in this patient?

A. Bilateral upper tract obstruction caused by fungus ball
B. Congenital hydronephrosis
C. Vesicoureteral reflux (VUR)
D. Acute tubular necrosis

The correct answer is A

Comment: The ultrasound scan showed that both kidneys were large for his age (left kidney, 72 mm; right kidney, 73 mm), and it was difficult to differentiate cortex and medulla. Bilateral hydronephrosis, graded according to the Society for Fetal Urology, was grade 3, which means that the renal pelvis dilated beyond the sinus, and calyces were uniformly dilated, with a renal pelvic anteroposterior diameter of 10 mm. Multiple echogenic particles within both renal pelvises without an acoustic shadow, compatible with bilateral renal fungus balls, were seen. An antegrade pyelography revealed no passage of contrast agent to the ureter because of obstruction of fungus balls. The reason for acute kidney injury (AKI) in our case was bilateral urinary system obstruction caused by fungus balls. Both urine and blood cultures were positive for *Candida albicans*. A urine specimen taken from the renal pelvis via nephrostomy was also positive for *C. albicans*. The patient had a history of intubation, central catheterization, total parenteral nutrition, long-term and broad-spectrum antibiotic usage in addition to prematurity and low birth weight, all of which are risk factors for the development of renal candidiasis.

The patient was administered intravenous furosemide and sodium bicarbonate at the emergency service; however, lung auscultation signs did not improve and his metabolic acidosis was resistant to medical treatment at the second hour following admission. As a result, it was decided to initiate renal replacement therapy. A peritoneal dialysis catheter was placed and dialysis was performed in the intensive care unit. At hour 16 following the initiation of peritoneal dialysis, his rales completely disappeared and the acidosis was corrected. Because of the presence of bilateral urinary system obstruction, bilateral nephrostomy catheters were placed to provide urinary drainage, after which renal failure resolved rapidly.

In addition to intravenous lipid formula amphotericin B treatment, amphotericin B was also administered through both nephrostomy catheters twice a day. Although fluconazole is the first-choice antifungal agent in treatment of renal candidiasis, it is not recommended in patients with renal failure or hydronephrosis because adequate urinary concentration cannot be achieved.[1] Despite the effectiveness of amphotericin B, it was not used in systemic treatment because of its nephrotoxic side effects. Weekly urinary microscopic examinations, urine cultures, and US examinations were performed to monitor the effectiveness of the treatment. On US examination performed on day 12 of treatment, the echogenic mass and obstruction findings had completely disappeared and the left nephrostomy catheter was withdrawn. After 3 weeks of antifungal treatment, no more yeast was observed in urine microscopy and culture. However, it is recommended to continue antifungal treatment for an additional 3 to 6 weeks after negative conversion of the culture.[2,3] Despite sterility under culture, on US, the echogenic appearance of the right kidney persisted; therefore, streptokinase was administered via the nephrostomy catheter twice daily (5 mL, 3000 U/mL). At the eighth week of treatment, the echogenic appearance in the right pelvis was still present. However, it was decided that this might persist for a long time and that the nephrostomy catheter might present a risk for new infections, so the catheter was withdrawn at the eighth week of treatment and antifungal treatment was discontinued.[4] The patient has been under follow-up with antibiotic prophylaxis for the past 13 months. During this period, no urinary tract infections have developed, and urine microscopic examinations performed at intervals were normal. Pelvicalyceal dilatation detected on US totally disappeared 5 months after treatment.

Clinical Presentation 23

A female neonate was born at 32 weeks of gestation with intrauterine growth retardation. Antenatal US at 20 weeks was normal, but at 31 weeks a repeat US showed oligohydramnios, and the fetus was small for dates, although the kidneys were reported to be normal. The pregnancy was otherwise uncomplicated, and the mother did not take any medications antenatally.

The patient was born at 32 weeks weighing 1354 g (9th–25th percentile) by spontaneous vaginal delivery. No resuscitation was needed. On examination at birth, clitoromegaly was noted but was felt to be in keeping with the gestation of the infant. On day 1, oliguria (urine output, 0.1 mL/kg/h) was noted and the plasma creatinine was elevated at 1.2 mg/dL. The oliguria persisted and the plasma creatinine increased to 3.1 mg/dL by day 4. The plasma albumin was very low at 0.7 g/dL, but liver function tests were normal. Urinalysis on day 6 showed heavy proteinuria (4083 mg/mmol creatinine) and microscopic hematuria. Renal ultrasound showed slightly enlarged kidneys (both 4.2 cm in length) with a globular configuration, echogenic cortex, and decreased corticomedullary differentiation. The kidneys were not dysplastic, nor did they demonstrate any evidence of reduced venous or arterial flow on Doppler. Manual peritoneal dialysis was commenced on day 7 of life.

What test will be the most likely to establish underlying diagnosis?

A. CT scan
B. Genetic karyotype
C. VCUG
D. Diuretic renogram scan

The correct answer is B
Comment: Oliguric renal failure from birth is unusual in the absence of a hypoxic-ischemic or toxic insult that causes AKI. Antenatal oligohydramnios and intrauterine growth retardation are reliable antenatal markers, making CKD more likely despite normal size kidneys. Proteinuria associated with AKI from acute tubular necrosis is not usually in the nephrotic range, and urine protein-creatinine measurement of >4 g/mmol should stimulate further exploration of a congenital nephrotic syndrome as an underlying cause. The oligohydramnios at 31 weeks of gestation suggest a low intrauterine GFR from a particularly aggressive sclerosing process.

Reevaluation of the genital appearance prompted karyotype analysis, revealing a 46, XY pattern, leading to a diagnosis of Denys-Drash syndrome (DDS). This diagnosis was subsequently confirmed with targeted analysis of *WT1*, which led to the identification of a heterozygous missense variant c.1097 G>A, p (Arg366His) in exon 8.

Denys-Drash syndrome is a triad of nephropathy (typically diffuse mesangial sclerosis), gonadal dysgenesis (with undermasculinized external genitalia in a 46, XY individual), and a propensity to Wilms tumor.[1,2] It is caused by heterozygous mutations of *WT1* on chromosome 11p13, which encodes a zinc finger DNA transcription protein involved in the development of kidneys, urogenital tract, and other organs.[3] Consistent with its critical role in early embryonic development, *WT1* mutations are also associated with other phenotypes, including Frasier syndrome, Meacham syndrome, and isolated presentation of nephrotic syndrome or Wilms tumor. DDS is a rare disorder and the incidence is unknown. The vast majority of patients with DDS have a *WT1* missense mutation within exons 8 or 9 of the gene.[1,4] Most missense mutations in these exons affect the zinc-finger domains and impair the DNA binding capacity of *WT1*.

Clinical Presentation 24

A 17-year-old White male presented with intermittent gross hematuria for 3 months and an episode of bilateral flank pain 2 weeks before the clinic visit. He had no history of trauma, dysuria, frequency, urinary tract infections, or passage of kidney stones. Initial workup showed normal serum creatinine of 0.7 mg/dL, normal complete blood count, normal C3, negative antinuclear antibody, and negative urine culture. Urine analysis showed 1+ blood with 51 to 100 red blood cells/hpf, no red blood cell casts, crystals, or protein. Urine calcium/creatinine ratio was 0.19 mg/mg and the urine protein/Cr ratio 0.14 mg/mg.

Doppler renal US performed at a local hospital showed normal renal artery blood flow. The right and left kidneys measured 11.1 cm and 11.2 cm, respectively, and there was no evidence of mass, hydronephrosis, or stones, and the bladder was normal.

His medical history was significant for HLA-B27 ankylosing spondylitis, for which he was followed by rheumatology on Humira 40 mg subcutaneously every 7 days. His family history was significant because his mother had had ankylosing spondylitis and kidney stones. Physical examination showed a healthy-appearing male with normal blood pressure 126/74 mm Hg and a body mass index of 22.92 kg/m^2 (75th percentile) in no apparent distress and unremarkable examination without any flank tenderness, rash, or lower extremity edema. Because there was a family history of stones, he was advised to hydrate a minimum of 3 L/day and to monitor for recurrence of symptoms.

The patient returned for a follow-up appointment 4 months later and reported intermittent episodes of gross hematuria at baseball practice, with no episodes of flank pain or proteinuria (urine dipsticks were being used at home). Evaluation was unremarkable except for microscopic hematuria; therefore, continued observation was planned. Four months later, he was seen at another hospital's emergency room with severe left-sided flank pain associated with vomiting, gross hematuria, and with the passage of blood clots. Spiral CT did not show any stones, and he was sent home after a few hours of observation as the symptoms resolved with hydration and analgesia.

What is the diagnosis and what would you order to confirm your diagnosis?

A. Nutcracker syndrome
B. Nephrolithiasis
C. Acute pyelonephritis
D. Acute cholangitis

The correct answer is A

Comment: In patients with severe symptoms such as severe flank pain, gross hematuria in the absence of hydronephrosis pyelonephritis, kidney stone, or cholangitis should raise the possibility of nutcracker syndrome. A CT angiography of the abdomen and pelvis in our patient showed a dilated left renal vein with narrowing as it crosses between the abdominal aorta and the superior mesenteric artery along with opacification of the gonadal vein, which confirmed the diagnosis.

There are no agreed-on diagnostic criteria for Doppler renal US. The gold standard for diagnosing nutcracker syndrome is left renal vein venography because it allows measurement of the venous pressure gradient between the left renal vein and inferior vena cava and can visualize any collateral veins. A pressure gradient ≥3 mm Hg is considered to be elevated. With the availability of CT angiography[1] and magnetic resonance angiography, it is easy to make the diagnosis of nutcracker syndrome without the need for a more invasive venogram.

Nutcracker syndrome, also known as left renal vein entrapment syndrome, occurs when the left renal vein is compressed between the abdominal aorta and the superior mesenteric artery. Nutcracker syndrome can present with hematuria (microscopic or gross) accompanied by groin or flank pain occurring after physical activity.[2] The proposed pathogenesis of nutcracker syndrome includes an acute aorta-superior mesenteric artery angle, an abnormal branching or origin of the superior mesenteric artery from the aorta, an abnormal course of the left renal vein (coursing behind the aorta or a higher course), and excessive fibrous tissue at the origin of the superior mesenteric artery.[3]

Clinical Presentation 25

A 16-year-old female was the only child born to nonconsanguineous parents of Turkish background. She showed normal development and had an unremarkable history. She was admitted with right first-finger pain, weakness, and lack of appetite of 10 days' duration. The family history was not significant for a systemic disease. On physical examination, she looked pale. She weighed 41 kg (fifth percentile) and was 153 cm tall (eighth percentile). Blood pressure was 110/70 mm Hg. There was no evidence of arthritis. The rest of the physical examination was unremarkable. Baseline laboratory test values were as follows: white blood cells 14,700/μL, hemoglobin 7.4 g/dL, hematocrit 21.1%, and platelets 242,000/μL. Urea, creatinine, and uric acid levels were 103 mg/dL, 1.2 mg/dL, and 11.3 mg/dL, respectively, and measured creatinine clearance was 42 mL/min/1.73 m^2. Daily urine output was normal (1.5–2.4 mL/kg/h), with a urine osmolarity of 350 mOsm/L. Tubular reabsorption of phosphate was 80% (normal range, ≥85%), and fractional excretion of uric acid was 1.6% to 2.5% (normal range, >14% ± 5.3%). Urine analysis did not show glycosuria, proteinuria, aminoaciduria, hypercalciuria, hypercitraturia, or ketonuria. There were no red and white blood cells. Urine culture showed no growth. Renal US demonstrated bilateral renal parenchymal hyperechogenicity with normal dimensions and without ureteral dilatation or renal cysts. Voiding cystourethrography was normal. Dimercaptosuccinate (DMSA) renal scintigraphy demonstrated a low renal uptake and a high background activity. She was diagnosed as having moderate chronic renal failure of unknown etiology. A renal biopsy was performed and 70 glomeruli were sampled; 50% were globally sclerosed. The remaining glomeruli were unremarkable, and no deposition of crystalloid was observed. The biopsy revealed chronic interstitial nephritis and moderate to marked tubular atrophy and interstitial fibrosis, especially in neighboring sclerosed glomerulus. The blood vessels were unremarkable. Direct immunofluorescence studies showed no significant immunoglobulin or complement deposition.

Which diseases should be considered in the differential diagnosis of this clinical picture?

A. Partial hypoxanthine-guanine phosphoribosyltransferase deficiency
B. Medullary cystic kidney disease type 2 (MCKD2)
C. Familial juvenile hyperuricemic nephropathy (FJHN)
D. None of the above

The correct answers are A, B, and C

Comment: The clinical differential diagnosis of renal failure in conjunction with hyperuricemia includes partial hypoxanthine-guanine phosphoribosyltransferase deficiency, MCKD2, and FJHN.[1]

Hypoxanthine-guanine phosphoribosyl-transferase deficiency is an X-linked disorder that results in the overproduction of uric acid. The patient's female gender and the absence of neurological symptoms, history of nephrolithiasis, or urate granulomas on renal biopsy argued against partial hypoxanthine-guanine phosphoribosyltransferase deficiency. On the other hand, renal US did not demonstrate renal cysts; therefore, the diagnosis of MCKD2 was ruled out. The most likely etiology of the hyperuricemic chronic renal disease could be FJHN. This clinical picture is an autosomal-dominant disorder characterized by hyperuricemia, low fractional renal urate excretion, progressive chronic interstitial nephritis, and chronic renal failure. Renal impairment usually appears between 15 and 40 years of age, leading to end-stage renal disease within 10 to 20 years. This syndrome was first described in 1960 in a family with gout, hyperuricemia, and renal disease. However, presentation is not always with gout, and unusually for gout, FJHN affects young men, women, and children equally.[2]

FJHN is caused by mutations in the uromodulin gene (*UMOD*) located at 16p11.2-12 that encodes for uromodulin or Tamm-Horsfall glycoprotein, the most abundant protein in normal urine. Several mutations in the *UMOD* gene have been identified in some families. Thus, to achieve exact diagnosis, the patient was tested for *UMOD* mutations by polymerase chain reaction amplification of genomic DNA and bidirectional automated DNA sequencing of all exons in the coding region of the *UMOD* gene. Genetic testing detected three novel missense amino acid mutations in codon 317 (Cys to Ser), codon 125 (Thr to Arg), and codon 488 (Gly to Arg), consistent with *UMOD*-associated kidney disease. In addition, two single-nucleotide substitutions (IVS5+50C>T and IVS9-8C>A) were also detected in the *UMOD* gene that did not result in amino acid changes. The parents were also tested for *UMOD* mutations: father (IVS9-8C>A) and mother (IVS5+50C>T) showed single-nucleotide substitutions. Based on these molecular genetic findings, a diagnosis of FJHN was established.[3] On the other hand, immunohistochemical staining for *UMOD* could be performed, and intracellular *UMOD* inclusions could be detected by light and electron microscopy. Furthermore, on electron microscopy, the inclusions may appear as abundant fibrillar or granular storage material within bundles of endoplasmic reticulum.

In FJHN, it has been suggested that intracellular *UMOD* overload impairs sodium reabsorption by the thick ascending limb of Henle, leading to defective urine-concentrating capacity. The resultant volume depletion may be compensated by increased proximal tubular reabsorption of sodium, which in turn may promote heightened proximal tubular urate reabsorption and reduced secretion, similar to the mechanism responsible for hyperuricemia in patients receiving loop diuretics. The cause of the chronic renal disease is not completely understood. *UMOD* mutations potentially cause disruption of the molecule's stable tertiary structure, resulting in altered protein folding, accumulation within the endoplasmic reticulum, and impaired trafficking. Retention in the endoplasmic reticulum may lead to formation of the intracellular *UMOD* aggregates observed in kidney biopsies and is likely a key step in the pathogenesis of FJHN.[4]

Clinical Presentation 26

A 16-year-old female was admitted to our hospital for further evaluation of bilateral nephrolithiasis, which was detected incidentally by plain radiography and abdominal US during the evaluation of abdominal pain in a local hospital. The patient had no history of polyuria, polydipsia, or urinary tract infection. Consanguinity was not present between her parents. Her family history revealed nephrolithiasis in her uncle and cousin. On admission, the results of the physical examination were normal. Her height was 153 cm (between the 10th and 25th percentiles), weight 42.3 kg (<third percentile), and her blood pressure was 100/60 mm Hg.

The laboratory findings were as follows: complete blood cell count was normal. Urinalysis revealed microhematuria (20 erythrocytes/μL) and proteinuria (30 mg/dL) and urine density and pH were 1015 and 5, respectively. Blood urea was 67 mg/dL, creatinine 1.3 mg/dL, Na 146 mmol/L, K 4.1 mmol/L, Cl 109 mmol/L, Ca 9.0 mg/dL (normal, 8.6–10.2 mg/dL), P 3.9 mg/dL (normal, 2.6–4.5 mg/dL), alkaline phosphatase 90 U/L (normal, 47–119 U/L), uric acid 7.9 mg/dL (normal, 2.4–5.7 mg/dL), and Mg 1.2 mg/dL (normal, 1.6–2.6 mg/dL). Arterial blood gas analysis showed a pH of 7.37, a PCO_2 of 30 mm Hg, a bicarbonate level of 19.9 mmol/L, a base excess of −6.6, and the anion gap was calculated as 17 mmol. Serum PTH level was 95 ng/mL (normal, 15–65 ng/mL), and 25 (OH) and 1,25(OH)2 vitamin D levels were 16.0 ng/mL (normal, 10–40 ng/mL) and 18.4 μg/L (normal, 10–50 μg/L), respectively.

The patient's 24-hour urinary excretions Ca (7 mg/kg/day) and Mg (2 mg/kg/day) were elevated. Two-hour urine oxalate (0.5 mg/kg/day), uric acid (8.6 mg/kg/day), and phosphorus (ratio of phosphorus tubule maximum to GFR 3.1 mg/dL) were normal and urinary excretion of citrate was undetectable. Urine protein electrophoresis revealed tubular and glomerular proteinuria

(26 mg/m^2/h) (albumin 61.4%, α_1-globulin 11.4%, α_2-globulin 6.9%, β-globulin 10.7%, γ-globulin 9.6%). Urinary excretion of amino acids was within the normal range. The GFR was calculated (with 24-hour urine collection) to be 65 mL/min/1.73 m^2.

A symmetric opaque appearance with uniform distribution bilaterally was detectable on the plain radiography scan and the renal US scan revealed bilateral diffuse hyperechogenicity of the pyramids, typical for medullary nephrocalcinosis.

What is the most likely diagnosis in this patient?

A. Bartter syndrome
B. Gitelman syndrome
C. Dent disease
D. FHHNC

The correct answer D

Comment: Our patient's main problem was the presence of medullary nephrocalcinosis (NC). Nephrocalcinosis is defined as calcification located in the renal parenchyma. It can be divided into two forms, medullary and cortical,[1] with the former usually a bilateral process with symmetric involvement.[1] Medullary NC is the most common form and occurs in various disorders.[1] Based on clinical and laboratory findings, we easily ruled out Cushing syndrome, malignancy, sarcoidosis, sickle cell disease, idiopathic hypercalcemia, chronic pyelonephritis, hypervitaminosis D, hyperparathyroidism, hyper-/hypothyroidism, and drug-associated NC. Renal tubular acidosis, primary hyperoxaluria, and purine/pyrimidine pathway disorders were also not considered realistic diagnoses because of normal acid-base parameters and the excretion of amino acids, oxalate, and uric acid.[1,2]

The patient was investigated further for diseases that cause hypercalciuria in addition to NC. Bartter syndrome was ruled out because of normal acid-base parameters. The absence of hypokalemia and metabolic alkalosis also excluded Gitelman syndrome. Patients with classic Dent disease generally have low PTH and elevated 1,25(OH) vitamin D levels with low-molecular-weight proteinuria. Our patient has elevated PTH and normal vitamin D levels with both tubular and glomerular proteinuria; the latter could be secondary to chronic renal failure.

After making these differential diagnostic steps as well as taking the presence of hypomagnesemia, hypomagnesuria, and hypercalciuria into consideration, we suggested a rare disease, FHHNC, as the most probable cause of the medullary NC in our patient. In most cases, FHHNC is caused by loss-of-function mutations in the *CLDN16* gene encoding claudin-16 (formerly called paracellin-1), renal tight junction protein expressed in the thick ascending limb of the loop of Henle and in the distal convoluted tubule. In families with FHHNC and severe ocular involvement, the disease has been shown to be caused by a mutation in the *CLDN19* gene encoding claudin-19, another important tight junction protein that is expressed in renal tubules and the eye. Our patient was then investigated for the presence of hearing and ocular abnormalities. The results of the ophthalmologic examination and audiograms were normal. Blood samples were taken from both the patient and her parents for genetic diagnosis of the FHHNC. A homozygous Arg216His mutation in the *CLDN16* gene was detected in our patient. Both parents were heterozygous for this mutation. Once the genetic diagnosis was made, the patient was put on a low-salt diet, with high fluid intake, oral magnesium citrate (1 mmol/kg/day), and hydrochlorothiazide (2 mg/kg/day). There was no significant change in her renal function and severity of nephrocalcinosis within the 3 months of follow-up with medications.

FHHNC is a rare autosomal recessive tubular disorder that causes medullary nephrocalcinosis.[3] In addition to presenting the characteristic triad included in the name of the disease, affected individuals may present clinically with polydipsia, polyuria, recurrent urinary tract infections, vomiting, abdominal pain, convulsion, and carpopedal spasm.[4] Urinary tract infections are the most common clinical manifestation (43%), followed by polyuria and polydipsia (27%).[4] Some patients show extrarenal symptoms, such as hearing impairment or ocular abnormalities. The most important biochemical findings of FHHNC syndrome are hypomagnesemia, hypermagnesemia, and hypercalciuria. Hyperuricemia, hypocitraturia, and elevated PTH levels are also present.[5] The primary defect is the impairment of the reabsorption of magnesium and calcium in the loop of Henle. This defect is due to a mutation in the *CLDN16* gene that encodes the paracellular protein claudin-16, which is located in the tight junctions of the thick ascending limb of the loop of Henle.[4] Consequently, patients with FHHNC should not only present with typical clinical and biochemical data; they should also be screened for mutation of the *CLDN16* gene.[6]

The clinical course of FHHNC is heterogeneous. It is frequently associated with progressive renal failure with a variable progression rate, but the reason for this clinical variability has not yet been clarified.[7,8] The most important aim of treatment should be the reduction of urinary calcium excretion. Hydrochlorothiazide is effective in diminishing calcium excretion in children with hypercalciuria. Oral magnesium supplements and citrate, both well-known inhibitors of renal nephrocalcinosis and lithiasis, may also be given to the patients.[7]

Despite calcium and magnesium substitution, normal serum values could not be achieved in our patient. Medical treatment does not appear to influence the progression of the disease and, as a result, the overall prognosis of FHHNC is poor. A definitive cure can be achieved by renal transplantation.[5]

Clinical Presentation 27

The first male child of nonconsanguineous parents was born at 36 weeks' gestation after a pregnancy complicated by oligohydramnios related to bilateral hypoplastic and cystic fetal kidneys. There was no known family history of kidney disease. Renal ultrasound on day 3 of life confirmed bilaterally small (<fifth percentile) cystic kidneys with no other urinary tract abnormalities. Serum creatinine at birth was 250 µmol/L, which improved to 200 µmol/L over the first 3 weeks of life and stabilized at this level. Electrolyte abnormalities and anemia associated with chronic kidney disease were managed with supplemental bicarbonate, calcitriol, and erythropoietin. Clinically, the child remained well over the first 2 years of life, although developmental progress was delayed and was associated with mild hypotonia on physical examination.

Despite intensive nutritional support via nasogastric feeding (100% estimated energy requirement) and correction of biochemical abnormalities, the patient continued to experience suboptimal weight gain and growth failure. By 3 years of age, his weight was 10.7 kg (–2.92 standard deviation score [SDS]) and height was 84.5 cm (–3.03 SDS), with creatinine unchanged (200 µmol/L). Investigations including fecal elastase excluded pancreatic insufficiency and endocrine pathology. Serum bicarbonate, calcium, phosphate, and PTH levels were all regularly monitored and remained within clinically recommended limits. He had significantly delayed skeletal maturity, with a bone age of 2 years, 8 months, at a chronological age of 3 years, 9 months (>2 SDS below the mean).

He was initially assessed at age 3 years for commencement of recombinant human growth hormone (rhGH), but this was declined by the parents. At the age of 4 years, 2 months, because of persistent poor growth velocity (3 cm/year), rhGH at a dose of 7.5 mg/m^2/week was commenced. Postprandial and fasting hyperglycemia was noted following commencement of rhGH, and an oral glucose tolerance test (OGTT) showed a plasma glucose level of 976 mg/dL at 120 minutes, indicating impaired glucose tolerance. A continuous glucose monitoring system was initiated for 7 days and demonstrated hyperglycemic excursions overnight and postprandial hyperglycemia with a maximum measured glucose concentration of 589 mg/dL. We suggest that an OGTT should be considered in patients with renal cysts and diabetes (RCAD) before commencing rhGH therapy along with regular monitoring of glycemic indices after commencing treatment.

What is the underlying etiology of hyperglycemia in this patient?

A. Metabolic syndrome
B. rhGH therapy
C. Cushingoid syndrome
D. RCAD

The correct answer is D

Comment: The present patient had RCAD syndrome diagnosed as part of an investigation of his developmental delay at 3 years of age and thus had known potential for the development of hyperglycemia before commencing rhGH therapy. Fasting glucose and glycated hemoglobin levels before starting rhGH were normal, and we postulate that rhGH acted as the trigger for hyperglycemia in this child. However, an OGTT was not performed before starting treatment and, given the development of hyperglycemia within a short time frame, preexisting impaired glycemic control cannot be completely excluded.

Growth hormone has well-recognized diabetogenic properties with effects on lipid and glucose metabolism and is also believed to promote gluconeogenesis.[1,2]

RCAD also referred to as maturity-onset of diabetes in the young, type 5, is an autosomal dominant disorder resulting from mutations in *HNF1*β and is the most commonly identified genetic cause of congenital anomalies of the kidney and urinary tract.[3] *HNF1*β (located on chromosome 17q12) is involved in tissue-specific regulation of gene expression in various organs but is particularly influential in the embryonic development of the kidney.[3] In addition to cysts, other renal manifestations that have been reported include cystic dysplasia, familial hypoplastic glomerulocystic kidney disease, solitary kidney, oligomeganephronia, hyperuricemic nephropathy with gout, renal magnesium wasting, horseshoe kidney, and hydronephrosis/hydroureter.[4]

Given the potential β-cell dysfunction and changes in insulin sensitivity associated with RCAD, patients with this condition may be expected to be more susceptible to diabetogenic stimuli. Waller and colleagues reported on a 14-year-old boy with posttransplant diabetes.

It has been recommended that an OGTT should be considered in patients with RCAD before starting rhGH therapy along with regular monitoring of glycemic indices after commencing treatment.

Clinical Presentation 28

A 15-year-old boy was referred to our clinic for determined high blood urea (188 mg/dL) and creatinine (4.8 mg/dL) in blood examinations. There was no consanguinity between the parents and his family did not have any genetic renal disease. He had a 12-year-old healthy brother.

In his medical history, he was described by his parents as very healthy until a year ago. However, he had nocturnal enuresis some nights until the age of 12 years but was not taken to a doctor. He was not visiting the toilet unless his parents prompted him (only two to three times in a day) but had not had daytime wetting or recurrent urinary tract infection. One year ago, he complained of progressive leg pain, weakness, and a struggle to walk. He was examined by a pediatric neurologist and an orthopedist, who did some x-ray investigations, MRI scans of the brain and spinal column, and electromyography. He was taken to a rehabilitation program by his doctors without a specific diagnosis but his symptoms had worsened over recent months. They did not consider a renal-related disease because he did not have any complaints suggesting urinary system disease and there was no family history of genetic renal disease. His parents described him as an ambitious and perfectionist adolescent boy. He was very successful in his education, but this had worsened over the past year. He had to give up basketball because of leg pain and weakness.

On admission to our clinic, he seemed slightly pale and his weight and height were between the 10th and 25th percentiles. Blood pressure was 100/60 mm Hg. He had a walking disorder and valgus knee deformity but no neurologic abnormality. In laboratory examinations, estimated creatinine clearance rate by the Schwartz formula was 13.7 mL/min/1.73 m^2 and he was therefore diagnosed with end-stage renal disease. Anemia (hemoglobin, 9.0 g/dL), metabolic acidosis (pH 7.30 and bicarbonate 18 mmol/L), severe hyperparathyroidism (PTH, 1949 pg/mL; N, 15–65), and urinary tract infection were also found. Specific treatment was started for each of the findings. Wrist radiograph showed osteoporosis and deformation of ulna and radius after a possible minor fracture. The bone findings and hyperparathyroidism were associated with severe renal osteodystrophy. Abdominal US revealed bilateral small kidneys with severe hydroureteronephrosis and overloaded and thickened bladder.

Which further investigation would you order?

A. Cystoscopy
B. VCUG
C. Intravenous pyelogram
D. CT scan of the kidney

The correct answer is B

Comment: A VCUG demonstrated bilateral grade 5 vesicoureteral reflux and bladder with trabeculation. Cystoscopy excluded posterior ureteral valve or obstruction. The spine and spinal cord were seen as normal on MRI. The urodynamic study showed high detrusor pressure (74 cm H_2O on micturition) and dyssynergia between the detrusor and the ureteral sphincter.

The patient had functional bladder outlet obstruction without any neurological abnormalities; therefore, he was diagnosed with Hinman syndrome. He did not have any complaints associated with gastrointestinal retention. His smiling was not diagnostic for urofacial syndrome and his family did not have any genetic renal diseases. The urologist started self-clean intermittent catheterization four to six times per day for bladder emptying. Recently, the patient has started antibiotic prophylaxis and is continuing supportive treatment for renal insufficiency. We are currently preparing him for our peritoneal dialysis program.

Hinman syndrome involves a nonneurogenic neurogenic bladder and the most severe form of dysfunctional voiding disorder. The bladder-sphincter discoordination causes damage to the bladder and upper urinary tract if it is not diagnosed early and treated adequately.[1] This case emphasizes the following important message: nighttime wetting is not a benign condition in every child. Parental awareness should be raised about voiding disorders, so that it may be possible to prevent important renal diseases such as Hinman syndrome. We hope that in the future, the definition of mutations will generate new classifications for these diseases. If we can gain more insight into the pathophysiological mechanism of Hinman syndrome, more effective therapies could emerge.

Clinical Presentation 29

A 17-month-old girl was referred to our unit for recurrent urinary tract infections. She had an intermittent low-grade fever, anorexia, abdominal pain, fatigue, malaise, weight loss, and night sweating of a 2-month duration. Although several courses of antibiotics (cefixime, trimethoprim-sulphathiazole, nitrofurantoin) were prescribed for urinary tract infections, pyuria persisted. There was no family history of renal anomalies or renal tumors.

At presentation, she had a temperature of 37.7°C, a pulse rate of 90 beats/min, and a blood pressure of 102/58 mm Hg (50th–75th percentile). Her weight was below the third percentile. She looked pale. Physical examination revealed tenderness over the left back area with no palpable mass. Systemic examination was otherwise normal. No congenital anomalies such as aniridia, hemihypertrophy, or cryptorchidism were noted.

Blood investigation revealed leukocytosis (14.900 × 10^3/μL). C-reactive protein (11 mg/dL) and erythrocyte sedimentation rate (31 mm/h) were raised. The rest of the hematology and biochemical parameters were within the normal limits. Immunologic investigations (serum immunoglobulins and HIV serology) were normal. Urinalysis showed a specific gravity of 1.015 and a pH of 6 with moderate leukocyte esterase (+2). Nitrites, blood, and protein were negative on the urine dipstick. Urine sediment revealed 10 to 15 white cells per high-powered field. Urine and blood cultures were negative.

Abdominal US revealed an atrophic left kidney with a 20-mm mass lesion with a hypoechogenic solid and cystic area. Doppler US examination showed no vascular color coding within the mass. Vesicoureteral reflux was not detected on voiding cystourethrography. CT performed before admission at a different medical center revealed the mass had central hypodense and peripheral hyperdense qualities. MRI of the abdomen and pelvis (with and without contrast) showed a disclosed atrophic left kidney with a mass located in the middle, near the pelvicalyceal system. On T2, an intermediate signal, and on T1-weighted images, MRI showed a peripheral low and central high signal. Contrast-enhanced studies showed a slight enhancement of the mass. Multiple pathologic lymph nodes were seen near the mass and paraaortic region.

What would be the differential diagnosis of renal mass in this child?

A. Hydronephrosis
B. Xanthogranulomatous pyelonephritis (XP)
C. Wilms tumor
D. Neuroblastoma

The correct answers are A, B, C, and D

Comment: The patient presented with a renal mass. Based on age, she was at high risk for developing a renal tumor. Clear-cell sarcoma occurs before 4 years of age. Wilms tumors are the most common renal masses occurring in those younger than age 5 years. Rhabdoid tumors and congenital mesoblastic nephroma are seen in infants. On the other hand, renal cell carcinoma is more likely to be diagnosed after 15 years of age.[1]

Xanthogranulomatous pyelonephritis is a rare, severe, and atypical form of chronic renal parenchymal infection, often mimicking neoplastic renal disorder.[2] It is important to distinguish this entity in children that it may be misdiagnosed as childhood renal neoplasm, especially Wilms tumor.[3]

Clinical features are usually associated with nonspecific signs and symptoms such as weight loss, malaise anorexia, recurrent febrile episodes, and abdominal pain, as in adults.[3] The most common symptoms are flank pain and fever. Wilms tumor has similar signs and symptoms such as malaise, pain, hypertension, and microscopic or gross hematuria.[1]

Conventional MRI is useful in the characterization of solid and cystic renal masses, congenital abnormalities, renal vascular disease, and posttraumatic conditions.[2] MRI is sensitive for identifying the accumulation of lipid-laden foamy macrophages as high-intensity signals on T1-weighed images. The hypodense lesion in T2-weighted MRI is in favor of XP as opposed to the hyperintense tumoral masses. The "bear paw" sign, which describes water density–rounded areas in renal parenchyma with calyceal dilatation and abscess cavities with pus and debris can be seen with XP.[4] In this case, the renal pelvis and calyxes are dilated and enlarged mimicking the toe pads of a bear's paw. The bear paw pattern metaphorically describes the replacement of the renal parenchyma by hypoattenuating masses that are cellular infiltration of lipid-laden macrophages.[4] Renal scintigraphy with technetium-99m dimercaptosuccinic acid (99mTc-DMSA) may be used to evaluate and confirm differential renal function.

Clinical Presentation 30

A 10-year-old boy born from a nonconsanguineous marriage with a normal birth history presented with congenital bilateral cataracts and delayed milestones. Later, he developed psychomotor retardation, dysmorphic facial features, and behavioral disturbances (irritability), which progressively worsened. There was a change in gait followed by frequent falls and multiple fractures at 4 years of age. Renal impairment was detected at the age of 6 years.

On examination, he had frontal bossing, normally placed large ears, deep-set eyes, hypermetropia, deformation of teeth, and enamel hypoplasia. His height and weight were within 3 standard deviations. Systemic examination showed a pigeon-shaped chest with the prominence of costochondral junctions and Harrison sulcus present at the anterior aspect of the chest, and he had 60% IQ with diminished deep tendon reflexes and tone decreased in all four limbs. Lower limbs were externally rotated and knock knee and genu valgus deformity were present. The presence of hypotonia, congenital cataract, and features of renal rickets led to a high suspicion of Lowe syndrome in this patient.

On investigations, he had a hemoglobin of 9.2 g/dL, a total leukocyte count of 8200/mm^3 with 69% polymorphs, and 8% lymphocytes. His blood urea was 87 mg, creatinine 1.8 mg, serum calcium 8.2 mg/dL, serum phosphorous 3.6 mg/dL, and liver function tests were normal. Arterial blood gas analysis showed normal anion gap metabolic acidosis. Urine routine analysis showed pH 6.0, specific gravity 1.01, sugar +1, and protein +2. Genetic analysis showed normal karyotyping. His urinary biochemical parameters revealed elevated alanine 7076 μmol/L, citrulline 720 μmol/L, and lysine 2500 μmol/L, and were positive for cysteine and tyrosine. Brain MRI of the patient demonstrated white matter abnormalities, particularly in the periventricular area. Radiographs of the wrists and long bones demonstrated changes that are typical of rickets, including metaphyseal splaying and fraying and osteopenia. His treatment included cataract extraction and physical and speech therapy. He was given drugs that addressed his behavioral problems, correction of the renal tubular acidosis, and consequent bone diseases. A missense mutation (c.1427C>T) in exon 14 of the *OCRL* gene was observed in our patient.

What is the most likely diagnosis?

A. Zellweger syndrome
B. Lowe syndrome
C. Smith-Lemli-Opitz syndrome
D. Dent disease
E. Cataract-dental syndrome (Nance-Horan syndrome)

The correct answer is B

Comment: Lowe syndrome (oculocerebrorenal syndrome) is characterized by congenital cataracts and glaucoma, severe intellectual disability, hypotonia with diminished to absent reflexes, and renal abnormalities. Fanconi syndrome is followed by progressive renal impairment. End-stage renal disease usually does not occur until the third to fourth decades of life.[1]

Lowe syndrome is transmitted as an X-linked recessive trait. Despite the X-linked inheritance pattern, Lowe syndrome has occurred in a few females. The defective gene codes for inositol polyphosphate 5-phosphatase, *OCRL1*, are involved with cell trafficking and signaling.

Light microscopy of the kidney is normal early in the disorder, with endothelial cell swelling and thickening and splitting of the glomerular basement membrane seen by electron microscopy. In the proximal tubule cells, there is a shortening of the brush border and enlargement of the mitochondria.[1]

Cataracts are present at birth and kidney and brain abnormalities are associated with intellectual disabilities.

Almost all boys with Lowe syndrome have developmental and intellectual disability that can range from mild to severe. Seizures occur in approximately half of those by 6 years of age, and behavioral problems are present in some boys with Lowe syndrome. A fraction of affected males develop keloids on the corneas of one or both eyes during late childhood and adolescence. These growths are progressive and can lead to blindness.

Renal Fanconi syndrome is one of the most common kidney involvements in patients with Lowe syndrome. The GFR usually begins to fail during the second decade of life and slowly progresses to end-stage renal failure by 30 to 40 years of age.

Other signs frequent in boys with Lowe syndrome include short stature, dental cysts and abnormal dentin formation of the teeth, skin cysts, and vitamin D deficiency that can lead to soft bones, skeletal changes (rickets), bone fractures, scoliosis, and noninflammatory degenerative joint disease. Some patients have shown a delayed bleeding diathesis following surgery, characterized by normal hemostasis and clot formation, only to be followed a few hours later by sudden recurrence of bleeding. This may be an important consideration with any surgery but especially both cataract surgery and glaucoma surgery in which bleeding inside the eye may have considerable consequences.

Disorders with similar symptoms to Lowe syndrome include congenital rubella, Zellweger syndrome, cataract-dental syndrome (Nance-Horan syndrome), Smith-Lemli-Opitz syndrome, and Dent disease.

Clinical Presentation 31

A 3-year-old girl was referred for evaluation of recurrent urinary tract infections. She had intermittent low-grade fever, anorexia, abdominal pain, fatigue, malaise, weight loss, and night sweating of a 4-month duration. Urinary tract infections reoccurred despite prophylactic antibiotic therapy. There was no family history of renal anomalies or renal tumors.

On examination, she had a temperature of 37.7°C, a pulse rate of 90 beats/min, and a blood pressure of 102/58 mm Hg (50th–75th percentile). Her weight was below the third percentile. She looked pale. Physical examination revealed tenderness over the left back area with no palpable mass. Systemic examination was otherwise normal. No congenital anomalies were noted such as aniridia or hemihypertrophy.

Blood investigation revealed leukocytosis (14.900/mm^3). C-reactive protein (11 mg/dL) and erythrocyte sedimentation rate (31 mm/h) were raised. The rest of the hematology and biochemical parameters were within the normal limits. Immunologic investigations (serum immunoglobulins and HIV serology) were normal. Urinalysis showed a specific gravity of 1.015 and a pH of 6 with moderate leukocyte esterase (+2). Nitrites, blood, and protein were negative on the urine dipstick. Urine sediment revealed 10 to 15 white cells per high-powered field. Urine and blood cultures were negative. Abdominal US revealed an atrophic left kidney with a 20-mm mass lesion with a hypoechogenic solid and cystic area. Doppler US examination showed no vascular color coding within the mass. Vesicoureteral reflux was not detected on voiding cystourethrography. CT performed before admission at a different medical center revealed the mass had central hypodense and peripheral hyperdense qualities. MRI of the abdomen and pelvis (with and without contrast) showed disclosed atrophic left kidney with a mass located in the middle, near the pelvicalyceal system. On T2, an intermediate signal, and on T1-weighted images, MRI showed peripheral low and central high signal. Contrast-enhanced studies showed slight enhancement of the mass. Multiple pathologic lymph nodes were seen near the mass and paraaortic region.

What is your diagnosis?

A. Wilms tumor
B. Rhabdoid tumor

C. Clear-cell sarcoma
D. X.
E. Rhabdoid tumor

The correct answer is D

Comment: Wilms tumors are the most common renal masses younger than age 5 years. Clear-cell sarcoma occurs before age 4 years. Rhabdoid tumors and congenital mesoblastic nephroma are seen in infants. XP is very rare in childhood and often mistaken for renal malignancies. XP should be kept in mind if there is a history of recurrent urinary tract infection and flank tenderness.[1]

The hypodense lesion in T2-weighted MRI is in favor of XP as opposed to the hyperintense tumoral masses.[2,3] "Bear paw sign," which describes water density–rounded areas in renal parenchyma with calyceal dilatation and abscess cavities with pus and debris can be seen with XP.[4] In this case, the renal pelvis and calyxes are dilated and enlarged, mimicking the toe pads of a bear's paw. The bear paw pattern metaphorically describes the replacement of the renal parenchyma by hypoattenuating masses that are cellular infiltration of lipid-laden macrophages.[1] Renal scintigraphy with technetium-99m dimercaptosuccinic acid (^{99m}Tc-DMSA) may be used to evaluate and confirm differential renal function. The nuclear scans usually show a nonfunctioning or poorly functioning kidney in XP.

XP is the result of chronic renal infection. Most commonly, organisms associated with XP are *Proteus mirabilis*, *Escherichia coli*, *Staphylococcus aureus*, *Klebsiella*, and *Pseudomonas*. Urine cultures is positive in most of the patients; cultures may be negative in 25% of cases. Sterile urine culture in our case may be undertaken before antibiotic therapy. The inflammatory process can be localized or diffuse and generally unilateral.[2] Most of the XP are unilateral and diffuse in form. A predilection of left kidney, as in our case, has been reported.[3] Complications are flank pain and rarely abscess formation in the psoas, nephrocutaneous, or colonic fistula and paranephric abscess.[4]

Laboratory tests that have been reported in XP are anemia, leukocytosis, thrombocytosis, and increased inflammatory markers (ESR, C-reactive protein levels).[5] Ultrasound imaging will reveal enlargement of the entire kidney and hypoechoic renal areas of calyceal dilatation and parenchymal destruction. The true preoperative diagnosis may be difficult in children but it seems to be possible by the help of dynamic contrast-enhanced MRI.[1]

The management of diffuse and focal XP is different. Nephrectomy is the standard approach for diffuse disease but partial nephrectomy is recommended whenever possible especially for bilateral XP.[4] There are reports of a few patients recovering with antibiotic therapy with the focal form of XP.[5] In this child, a complete nephrectomy was performed because the kidney was nonfunctional. The prognosis for the affected child is excellent.[5]

Clinical Presentation 32

A 3-year-old girl was admitted because of abdominal distention over the past 2 months. She was the first child of consanguineous parents. Her family history was unremarkable. Her weight was 14.0 kg (16th percentile), height was 96 cm (sixth percentile), and blood pressure was 108/62 mm Hg. Her cardiovascular and respiratory examinations were unremarkable. Her abdomen was distended; on percussion, there was periumbilical tympani with dullness in the flanks. There was no organomegaly or edema. Laboratory investigation revealed a white blood cell count of 511,000/mm^3, hemoglobin 12.5 g/dL, platelets 320,000/mm^3, urea 20 mg/dL, serum creatinine 0.2 mg/dL, and electrolytes and urine analysis were normal. In addition, liver function tests and albumin were normal. The structure and diameters of the liver and spleen were normal on abdominal US. Intra-abdominal-free fluid was present. The length of the right kidney measured 82 mm, the left kidney was 88 mm, and the parenchymal thickness was 10 mm. Renal echogenicity was increased in both the right and left kidneys, and corticomedullary differentiation was lost. Multiple, subcortical, anechoic cysts were present. The largest cysts measured 45 mm in diameter on the right kidney and 16 mm in diameter on the left kidney. There was no dilatation of the collecting system. Patient was hospitalized with a differential diagnosis of ascites and renal cysts. Paracentesis of the ascites excluded infection (because culture was negative), chylous ascites (because fluid was clear with low triglycerides at 12 mg/dL), pancreatitis (amylase, 9.8 IU/L), and urine leakage (ascites urea 23, mg/dL; creatinine, 0.14 mg/dL). The fluid was a transudate (density, 1006; ascites to serum protein ratio, 0.3; ascites to serum lactate dehydrogenase [LDH] ratio, 0.4). The serum ascites albumin gradient was >1.2 g/dL. Cytology of the fluid revealed a few lymphocytes. Viral serology and echocardiographic examination were unremarkable.

Abdominal MRI revealed a normal hepatobiliary system and multiple subcortical cysts separated, which were hypointense without enhancement in T1-weighted and hyperintense in T2-weighted images. The cysts resulted in indentations to the renal parenchyma. There was right-sided pleural effusion which was 13-mm thick and also abdominal-free fluid.

What is the likely diagnosis?

A. Renal lymphangiomatosis (RL)
B. Autosomal recessive polycystic kidney disease
C. Autosomal dominant polycystic kidney disease
D. Urinoma

The correct answer is A

Comment: Renal lymphangioma is a rare and benign renal malformation. It is believed that a developmental malformation of the intrarenal, perirenal, and peripelvic lymphatics causes accumulation of lymph as parenchymal edema or subcapsular and/or hilum cysts.[1,2] This condition has also been termed renal lymphangioma, peripelvic lymphangiectasia, renal sinus polycystic disease, and renal hygroma.[3] The age of the patient at presentation varies and there is no sex predilection.

The diagnosis of RL can be made according to characteristic radiologic findings. The radiologic features of RL on US, MRI, or CT are well-defined.[3] RL can be unilateral/focal or bilateral/diffuse. There are two radiologic manifestations.[4] In the first pattern, cystic lesions in the renal sinus may be seen. The second pattern reveals lobular perinephric fluid with multiple septations and less apparent renal sinus cysts. US examination may reveal enlarged kidneys, increased renal parenchymal echogenicity, loss of corticomedullary differentiation, and anechoic cysts. On CT, thin-walled, fluid-filled cysts with attenuation on the cyst walls are evident. The cysts on MRI appear as hypointense without enhancement on postcontrast images in T1-weighted and hyperintense in T2-weighted images. Diagnostic aspiration of the cysts or ascites can be performed but is not necessary for diagnosis. The characteristic of the aspirated fluid is usually the same as those for transudate (nonchylous and unremarkable for urea, protein, triglyceride, and LDH). The fluid may however have elevated renin and lymphocyte content.[2]

Autosomal recessive polycystic kidney disease is the most common differential diagnosis in pediatric patients, especially when ascites is present. Other differential diagnoses include autosomal dominant polycystic kidney disease, Wilms tumor, lymphoma, and urinoma.[1]

Treatment is not required for the majority of asymptomatic cases. Diuretic treatment has proven effective in cases with ascites and pleural effusion.[5] Although recurrence is possible, percutaneous aspiration and sclerotherapy of the cysts have been successfully performed in symptomatic cases.[6]

Clinical Presentation 33

A fetal ultrasound examination in the 37th week of gestation revealed a tumor mass in the upper left abdomen of a female fetus. A fetal MRI examination confirmed a solid mass in the upper pole of the left kidney. The course of the pregnancy was otherwise uneventful. The mother's medical history and the family history were unremarkable; there was no evidence of any abuse of noxious substances during pregnancy. The baby was born spontaneously in the 41st week of gestation without any other signs of abnormality, the physical examination was normal, and laboratory tests were within normal range.

After birth, a postpartum ultrasonographic and MRI examination showed a solid tumor (35 × 27 mm) in the upper pole of the left kidney. Compared with the other kidney, the upper calyx group could not be clearly delineated. Compression or infiltration of adjacent structures was not detected. The laboratory tests revealed normal values for renal function. Serum sodium was 134 mEq/L, potassium 4.1 mEq/L, chloride 99 mEq/L, bicarbonate 19 mEq/L, BUN 12 mg/dL, creatinine 0.3 mg/dL, total protein 5.4 g/dL, calcium 9.5 mg/dL, and phosphorous 4.4 mg/dL. Urinalysis showed pH 6.5, with a specific gravity of 1.014 with no blood or protein on dipstick.

On day 20 after birth, a laparoscopic tumor nephrectomy was performed. Macroscopically, the cut surface in the upper pole of the 16-g left kidney had a gray-tan to white appearance. The tumor tissue was poorly demarcated from the surrounding tissues. The microscopic examination displayed kidney parenchyma with minimal chronic inflammatory infiltrates, merging into a lesion composed of bundles of spindle cells with no to mild atypia and islands of metaplastic cartilage. Immunohistochemical staining for Wilms Tumor-Gene 1 (*WT1*) showed nonspecific cytoplasmic staining and no nuclear staining.

Which differential diagnosis has to be considered?

A. Congenital mesoblastic nephroma (CMN)
B. Wilms tumor/nephroblastoma
C. Teratoma
D. Neuroblastoma

The correct answers are A and B

Comment: The antenatal discovery of tumor in the upper pole of the left kidney with no metaplastic cartilage is typical for a CMN. Wilms tumor/nephroblastoma is the most frequent kidney tumor in childhood, and this diagnosis has to be considered.[1] Additional immunohistochemical staining is helpful to distinguish CMN from Wilms tumor with heterologous differentiation.[1,2]

Congenital mesoblastic nephroma represents 3% of all pediatric kidney tumors.[3] It is the most common kidney neoplasm diagnosed in the first 3 months of life, and it is frequently detected antenatally, as described in our case.[4] The malignant potential of the tumor is low.

CMN is classified into three histological subtypes: classic, cellular, and mixed type.[5] Classic CMN is composed of braiding bundles of spindle cells and frequent metaplastic cartilage with no capsular boundaries. The tumor often infiltrates the surrounding perirenal fat tissue and parenchyma.[6,7] Cellular CMN also presents bundles of spindle cells but has a stronger hemangiopericytoma pattern and a higher mitotic activity than the classic type. In contrast, the cellular type less frequently infiltrates the perirenal fat and/or kidney parenchyma. Mixed CMN shows, as the name indicates, a mixture of both the previously mentioned types.

Total nephrectomy is curative for most patients with stage I/II disease. Stage III tumors of the classic and mixed histologic subtypes are also indicated for nephrectomy alone. Stage III tumors of the cellular type treated only surgically have a higher rate of relapse than the other histologic subtypes, requiring chemotherapy or radiotherapy in some cases. However, because of limited data, there are no specific recommendations for adjuvant chemotherapy.[7,8] The known side effects of radiotherapy particularly in these very young patients limit this treatment modality to selected cases with aggressive tumors not responding to chemotherapy.[8]

Clinical Presentation 34

A 5-year-old boy was referred for treatment because of a long-standing history of polyuria/polydipsia of more than 3 L/day and failure to thrive. He woke up three to four times during the night to drink. The mother reported feeding problems, including vomiting, since he was 5 months old. The results of biochemical tests at 13 months of age had been normal, with plasma sodium of 143 mmol/L and creatinine of 0.3 mg/dL. His family history was remarkable for a 1-year-old brother having similar symptoms. In addition, a maternal uncle had a long-standing history of polyuria. Physical examination was unremarkable. The boy had a healthy appearance, his height and weight were at the second percentile, and blood pressure was 74/52 mm Hg. Repeat renal function biochemistry results were all in the normal range, with sodium at 142 mmol/L and creatinine at 0.4 mg/dL. Urine albumin was <3 mg/L. The patient underwent a water deprivation test, leading to a maximum urine osmolality of 269 mOsm/kg with a concomitant plasma osmolality of 305 mOsm/kg. A subsequent dose of 0.3 mcg desmopressin acetate 1-deamino-8-D-arginine vasopressin (DDAVP) given intravenously failed to increase the urine osmolality further. A renal ultrasound was normal.

What is the cause of hydronephrosis?

A. UPJO
B. VUR
C. Nephrogenic diabetes insipidus (NDI)
D. Posterior ureteral valve (PUV)

The correct answer is C

Comment: This patient suffered from primary X-linked NDI, confirmed by genetic testing that identified a previously described mutation, R106C, in the gene encoding the arginine vasopressin receptor 2 (*AVPR2*).[1] Polyuria and hydronephrosis in this boy could have been explained by primary hydronephrosis with secondary NDI or vice versa. However, the family history was not consistent with a secondary NDI, and the bladder trabeculation was not explained by high urine flow.

The US showed severe hydronephrosis on the left and moderate hydronephrosis on the right, which is due in part to the high urinary flow consequent to his NDI. Importantly, it also shows a trabeculated, thickened bladder wall. This finding is suggestive of primary urinary tract obstruction, an additional cause for his hydronephrosis. In this boy, the obstructive uropathy was due to a PUV.

The key diagnostic tests are urodynamic assessment and cystoscopy (a micturating cystourethrogram is also a reasonable option). The trabeculated appearance of the bladder raised the suspicion of a bladder outlet or urethral obstruction. An obstructive pattern on subsequent urodynamic investigations confirmed this suspicion. In a boy, this must prompt consideration of PUV. Given his age, it was decided to proceed directly to cystoscopy, rather than pursuing specific diagnostic imaging such as a micturating cystourethrogram.

Hydronephrosis is a recognized complication of primary NDI and thought to be secondary to the high urine flow.[2–4] The danger, however, is to automatically assume this causality because these conditions can also occur independently in the same patient. Although both are rare diseases, with an estimated incidence of 1 in 5000 (PUV) and 1 in 1,000,000 (X-linked NDI) boys, they are not mutually exclusive, and cooccurrence was indeed reported previously, albeit without genetic confirmation of the NDI because the underlying gene was not known at the time.[2–4] Here, the key finding suggesting a separate cause for the hydronephrosis was the trabeculated appearance of the bladder on ultrasound.

An interesting aspect is the normal plasma creatinine level in this boy, as the increased urine output from the NDI would be expected to aggravate pressure damage to the kidneys in the setting of urethral obstruction. Indeed, the ultrasound is consistent with reduced cortical mass in the left kidney with less than 5% divided function on a nucleotide scan (not shown). It is unclear why the left kidney has experienced more damage, but it may have buffered most of the back pressure, thus protecting the right kidney.

References

Clinical Presentation 1

1. Arlen AM, Nawaf C, Kirsch AJ. Prune belly syndrome: current perspectives. *Pediatric Health Med Ther.* 2019;10:75–81. https://doi.org/10.2147/PHMT.S188014.
2. Lopes RI, Baker LA, Denes FT. Modern management of and update on prune belly syndrome. *J Pediatr Urol.* 2021;17:548–554.

Clinical Presentation 2

1. Schutgens RBH, Wanders RJA, Heymans HSA, et al. Zellweger syndrome: biochemical procedures in diagnosis, prevention and treatment. *J Inherit Metab Dis.* 1987;10:33–45. https://doi.org/10.1007/BF01812845.
2. Bose M, Yergeau C, D'Souza Y, et al. Characterization of severity in Zellweger spectrum disorder by clinical findings: a scoping review, meta-analysis and medical chart review. *Cells.* 2022;11:1891.

Clinical Presentation 3

1. Jelin A. Renal agenesis. *Am J Obstet Gynecol.* 2021;225:PB25–PB30.
2. Pahlavan F, Niknejad F, Sajadi H, et al. Unilateral kidney agenesis and other kidney anomalies in infertile men with congenital bilateral absence of vas deferens: a cross-sectional study. *Int J Fertil Steril.* 2022;16:152–155.

Clinical Presentation 4

1. Husain M, Hajini F, Bhatt A. Duplicated pyelocaliceal system with partial duplication of ureter. *BMJ Case Rep.* 2013;2013:bcr2013009115. https://doi.org/10.1136/bcr-2013-009115.
2. Yener S, Pehlivanoğlu C, Akis Yıldız Z, et al. Duplex kidney anomalies and associated pathologies in children: a single-center retrospective review. *Cureus.* 2022;14:e25777.

Clinical Presentation 5

1. Karnak I, Woo LL, Shah SN, Sirajuddin A, Kay R, Ross JH. Prenatally detected ureteropelvic junction obstruction: clinical features and associated urologic abnormalities. *Pediatr Surg Int.* 2008;24:395–402.
2. Jackson L, Woodward M, Coward RJ. The molecular biology of pelvi-ureteric junction obstruction. *Pediatr Nephrol.* 2018;33:553–571.

Clinical Presentation 6

1. Pareklar S, Kapadnid S, Sanghvi B, et al. Meckel-Gruber syndrome: a rare and lethal anomaly with review of literature. *J Pediatric Neurosci.* 2013;8:154–157. https://doi.org/10.4103/1817-1745.117855.
2. Hartill V, Szymanska K, Sharif SM, et al. Meckel–Gruber syndrome: an update on diagnosis, clinical management, and research advances. *Front Pediatr.* 2017;5:244. https://doi.org/10.3389/fped.2017.00244.
3. Hetty BP, Alva N, Patil S. Meckel Gruber syndrome (dysencephalia splanchnocystica). *J Contemp Dent Pract.* 2012;13:713–715.

Clinical Presentation 7

1. Joubert M, Jean-Jacques E, Robb JP, et al. Familial agenesis of the cerebellar vermis. A syndrome of episodic apnea, abnormal eye movements, ataxia, and retardation. *Neurology.* 1969;19:813–825.
2. Assadi F. Lack of NPHP2 mutations in a newborn infant with Joulert syndrome-related disorder presenting as end-stage renal disease. *Pediatr Nephrol.* 2007;22:750–752.

Clinical Presentation 8

1. Solomon BD, Baker LA, Bear KA, et al. An approach to the identification of anomalies and etiologies in neonates with identified or suspected VACTERL (vertebral defects, anal atresia, tracheo-esophageal fistula with esophageal atresia, cardiac anomalies, renal anomalies, and limb anomalies) association. *J Pediatr.* 2014;164:451–457.

2. Reinicke T, Costantino CL, Anderson DJ, et al. A network of anomalies prompting VACTERL workup in a trisomy 21 newborn. *Cureus*. 2022;14:e21290.

Clinical Presentation 9

1. Cidecyan D, Rodriguez MM, Haun RL, et al. New findings in short rib syndrome. *Am J Med Genet*. 1993;46:255–259.
2. Thiel C, Kessler K, Giessl A, et al. NEK1 mutations cause short-rib polydactyly syndrome type Majewski. *Am J Hum Genet*. 2011;88:106–114.
3. Fanh Y, Li S, Yi D. Genetic analysis and prenatal diagnosis of short-rib thoracic dysplasia 3 with or without polydactyly caused by compound heterozygous variants of *DYNC2H1* gene in four Chinese families. *Front Genet*. 2023;14:1075187. https://doi.org/10.3389/fgene.2023.1075187.

Clinical Presentation 10

1. Green JS, Parfrey PS, Harnett JD, et al. The cardinal manifestations of Bardet–Biedl syndrome, a form of Laurence–Moon–Biedl syndrome. *N Engl J Med*. 1989;321:1002–1009.
2. Forsythe E, Keny J, Bacchelli C, et al. Managing Bardet-Biedl syndrome-now and in the future. *Front Pediatr*. 2018;6:23. https://doi.org/10.3389/fped.2019.00023.

Clinical Presentation 11

1. Bruce JH, Romaguera RL, Rodriguez MM, et al. Caudal dysplasia syndrome and sirenomelia: are they part of a spectrum? *Fetal Pediatr Pathol*. 2009;28:109–131.
2. Kylat RI, Bader M. Caudal regression syndrome. *Children (Basel)*. 2020;7(11):211. https://doi.org/10.3390/children7110211.

Clinical Presentation 12

1. Torres VE. Vasopressin antagonists in polycystic kidney disease. *Semin Nephrol*. 2008;28:306–317.
2. Rastogi A, Ameen KM, Al-Baghdadi M, et al. Autosomal dominant polycystic kidney disease: updated perspectives. *Ther Clin Risk Manag*. 2019;15:1041–1052.

Clinical Presentation 13

1. Tobin JL, Beales PL. The nonmotile ciliopathies. *Genet Med*. 2009;11:386–402.
2. Sweeney WE, Avner ED. Pathophysiology of childhood polycystic kidney diseases: new insights into disease-specific therapy. *Pediatr Res*. 2014;75:148–157.

Clinical Presentation 14

1. Hale CL, Niederriter AN, Green GE, Martin DM. Atypical phenotypes associated with pathogenic CHD7 variants and a proposal for broadening CHARGE syndrome clinical diagnostic criteria. *Am J Med Genet A*. 2016;170A:344–354. https://doi.org/10.1002/ajmg.a.37435.
2. Bergman JE, Janssen N, Hoefsloot LH, Jongmans MC, Hofstra RM, van Ravenswaaij-Arts CM. CHD7 mutations and CHARGE syndrome: the clinical implications of an expanding phenotype. *J Med Genet*. 2011;48:334–342. https://doi.org/10.1136/jmg.2010.087106.

Clinical Presentation 15

1. McDonald-McGinn DM. 22q11.2 deletion syndrome: a tiny piece leading to a big picture. *Am J Med Genet A*. 2018;176:2055–2057. https://doi.org/10.1002/ajmg.a.40653.

Clinical Presentation 16

1. Prakash S, Gharavi AG. Assessing genetic risk for IgA nephropathy. *Clin J Am Soc Nephrol*. 2021;16:182–184. https://doi.org/10.2215/CJN.19491220.
2. Chadban SJ, Ahn C, Axelrod DA, et al. KDIGO clinical practice guideline on the evaluation and management of candidates for kidney transplantation. *Transplantation*. 2020;104:S11–S103. https://doi.org/10.1097/TP.0000000000003136 PMID: 32301874.
3. Voiculescu A, Ivens K, Hetzel GR, et al. Kidney transplantation from related and unrelated living donors in a single German centre. *Nephrol Dial Transplant*. 2003;18:418–425. https://doi.org/10.1093/ndt/18.2.418.
4. Simmons RL, Thompson EJ, Kjellstrand CM, et al. Parent-to-child and child-to-parent kidney transplants. Experience with 101 transplants at one centre. *Lancet*. 1976;1:321–324. https://doi.org/10.1016/s0140-6736(76)90082-9.

Clinical Presentation 17

1. Hoppe B, Kemper MJ. Diagnostic examination of the child with urolithiasis or nephrocalcinosis. *Pediatr Nephrol.* 2008;25:403–413. https://doi.org/10.1007/s00467-008-1073-x.
2. Kang JH, Choi HJ, Cho HY, et al. Familial hypomagnesemia with hypercalciuria and nephrocalcinosis associated with CLDN16 mutations. *Pediatr Nephrol.* 2005;20:1490–1493.

Clinical Presentation 18

1. Fick GM, Duley IT, Johnson AM, et al. The spectrum of autosomal dominant polycystic kidney disease in children. *J Am Soc Nephrol.* 1994;4:1654–1660.
2. Fick-Brosnahan G, Johnson AM, Strain JD, et al. Renal asymmetry in children with autosomal dominant polycystic kidney disease. *Am J Kidney Dis.* 1999;34:639–645.

Clinical Presentation 19

1. Alon US. Nephrocalcinosis. *Curr Opin Pediatr.* 1997;9:160–165.
2. Hoppe B, Kemper MJ. Diagnostic examination of the child with urolithiasis or nephrocalcinosis. *Pediatr Nephrol.* 2010;25:403–413.
3. Weber S, Schneider L, Peters M, et al. Novel paracellin-1 mutations in 25 families with familial hypomagnesemia with hypercalciuria and nephrocalcinosis. *J Am Soc Nephrol.* 2001;12:1872–1881.
4. Hou J, Renigunta A, Konrad M, et al. Claudin-16 and claudin-19 interact and form a cation-selective tight junction complex. *J Clin Invest.* 2008;118:619–628.
5. Naeem M, Hussain S, Akhtar N. Mutation in the tight- junction gene claudin 19 (CLDN19) and familial hypomagnesemia, hypercalciuria, nephrocalcinosis (FHHNC) and severe ocular disease. *Am J Nephrol.* 2011;34:241–248.

Clinical Presentation 20

1. Rescorla FJ, Sawin RS, Coran AG, et al. Long-term outcome for infants and children with sacrococcygeal teratoma. *J Pediatr Surg.* 1998;33:171–176.
2. Killen DA, Jackson LM. Sacrococcygeal teratoma in the adult. *Arch Surg.* 1964;88:425–433.
3. Bale PM. Sacrococcygeal developmental abnormalities and tumors in children. *Perspect Pediatr Pathol.* 1984;8:9–56.

Clinical Presentation 21

1. Bagłaj M. Late-presenting congenital diaphragmatic hernia in children: a clinical spectrum. *Pediatr Surg Int.* 2004;20:658–669.
2. Eber E. Antenatal diagnosis of congenital thoracic malformations: early surgery, late surgery, or no surgery? *Semin Respir Crit Care Med.* 2007;28:355–366.
3. Laberge JM, Puligandla P, Flageole H. Asymptomatic congenital lung malformations. *Semin Pediatr Surg.* 2005;14:16–33.
4. Williams HJ, Johnson KJ. Imaging of congenital lung lesions. *Paediatr Respir Rev.* 2002;3:120–127.

Clinical Presentation 22

1. Triolo V, Gari-Toussaint M, Casagrande F, et al. Fluconazole therapy for Candida albicans urinary tract infections in infants. *Pediatr Nephrol.* 2002;17:550–553.
2. Karlowicz MG. Candidal renal and urinary tract infection in neonates. *Semin Perinatol.* 2003;27:393–400.
3. Rikken B, Hartwig NG, Hoek J. Renal Candida infection in infants and neonates: report of four cases. Review of literature and treatment proposal. *Curr Urol.* 2007;1:113–120.
4. Benjamin DK Jr, Fisher RG, McKinney RE Jr, et al. Candidal mycetoma in the neonatal kidney. *Pediatrics.* 1999;104:1126–1129.

Clinical Presentation 23

1. Denys P, Malvaux P, Van Den Berghe H, et al. Association of an anatomopathological syndrome of male pseudohermaphroditism, Wilms' tumor, parenchymatous nephropathy and XX/XY mosaicism. *Arch Fr Pediatr.* 1967;24:729–739.
2. Drash A, Sherman F, Hartmann WH, et al. A syndrome of pseudohermaphroditism, Wilms'tumor, hypertension, and degenerative renal disease. *J Pediatr.* 1970;76:585–593.
3. Call KM, Glaser T, Ito CY, et al. Isolation and characterization of a zinc finger polypeptide gene at the human chromosome 11 Wilms' tumor locus. *Cell.* 1990;60:509–520.

4. Royer-Pokora B, Beier M, Henzler M, et al. Twenty-four new cases of WT1 germline mutations and review of the literature: genotype/phenotype correlations for Wilms tumor development. *Am J Med Genet A*. 2004;127A:249–257.

Clinical Presentation 24

1. Kim KW, Cho JY, Kim SH, et al. Diagnostic value of computed tomographic findings of nut cracker syndrome: correlation with renal venography and renocaval pressure gradients. *Eur J Radiol*. 2011;80:648–654.
2. Beinart C, Sniderman KW, Saddekni S, et al. Left renal vein hypertension: a cause of occult hematuria. *Radiology*. 1982;145:647–650.
3. He Y, Wu Z, Chen S, et al. Nutcracker syndrome—how well do we know it? *Urology*. 2014;83:12–17.

Clinical Presentation 25

1. Tinschert S, Ruf N, Bernascone I, et al. Functional consequences of a novel uromodulin mutation in a family with familial juvenile hyperuricaemic nephropathy. *Nephrol Dial Transplant*. 2004;19:3150–3154.
2. Nasr SH, Lucia JP, Galgano SJ, et al. Uromodulin storage disease. *Kidney Int*. 2008;73:971–976.
3. Scolari F, Caridi G, Rampoldi L, et al. Uromodulin storage diseases: clinical aspects and mechanisms. *Am J Kidney Dis*. 2004;44:987–999.
4. Vylet'al P, Kublova M, Kalbacova M, et al. Alterations of uromodulin biology: a common denominator of the genetically heterogeneous FJHN/MCKD syndrome. *Kidney Int*. 2006;70:1155–1169.

Clinical Presentation 26

1. Dyer RB, Chen MY, Zagoria RJ. Abnormal calcifications in the urinary tract. *Radiographics*. 1998;18:405–424.
2. Navarro O, Daneman A, Kooh SW. Asymmetric medullary nephrocalcinosis in two children. *Pediatr Radiol*. 1998;28:687–690.
3. Kang JH, Choi HJ, Cho HY, et al. Familial hypomagnesemia with hypercalciuria and nephrocalcinosis associated with CLDN16 mutations. *Pediatr Nephrol*. 2005;20:1490–1493.
4. Peru H, Akin F, Elmas S, Elmaci AM, Konrad M. Familial hypomagnesemia with hypercalciuria and nephrocalcinosis: report of three Turkish siblings. *Pediatr Nephrol*. 2008;23:1009–1012.
5. Kari JA, Farouq M, Alshaya HO. Familial hypomagnesemia with hypercalciuria and nephrocalcinosis. *Pediatr Nephrol*. 2003;18:506–510.
6. Hoppe B, Kemper MJ. Diagnostic examination of the child with urolithiasis or nephrocalcinosis. *Pediatr Nephrol*. 2010;25:403–413. https://doi.org/10.1007/s00467-008-1073-x.
7. Kuwertz-Bröking E, Fründ S, Bulla M, et al. Familial hypomagnesemia–hypercalciuria in 2 siblings. *Clin Nephrol*. 2001;56:155–161.
8. Knoers NV. Inherited forms of renal hypomagnesemia: an update. *Pediatr Nephrol*. 2009;24:697–705.

Clinical Presentation 27

1. Moller N, Jorgensen JO. Effects of growth hormone on glucose, lipid, and protein metabolism in human subjects. *Endocr Rev*. 2009;30:152–177.
2. Hwang DY, Dworschak GC, Kohl S, et al. Mutations in 12 known dominant disease-causing genes clarify many congenital anomalies of the kidney and urinary tract. *Kidney Int*. 2014;85:1429–1433.
3. Shields BM, Hicks S, Shepherd MH, et al. Maturity-onset diabetes of the young (MODY): how many cases are we missing? *Diabetologia*. 2010;53:2504–2508.
4. Bellanne-Chantelot C, Chauveau D, Gautier JF, et al. Clinical spectrum associated with hepatocyte nuclear factor-1beta mutations. *Ann Intern Med*. 2004;140:510–517.

Clinical Presentation 28

1. Hinman F, Bauman FW. Vesical and ureteral damage from voiding dysfunction in boys without neurologic or obstructive disease. *J Urol*. 1973;109:727–732.

Clinical Presentation 29

1. Kissane JM, Dehner LP. Renal tumors and tumor-like lesions in pediatric patients. *Pediatr Nephrol*. 1992;6:365–382.
2. Korkes F, Favoretto RL, Bróglio M, et al. Xanthogranulomatous pyelonephritis: clinical experience with 41 cases. *Urology*. 2008;71:178–180.

3. Shah K, Parikh M, Gharia P, et al. Xanthogranulomatous pyelonephritis mimicking renal mass in 5-month-old child. *Urology*. 2012;79:1360–1362.
4. Zugor V, Schott GE, Labanaris AP. Xanthogranulomatous pyelonephritis in childhood: a critical analysis of 10 cases and of the literature. *Urology*. 2007;70:157–160.

Clinical presentation 30

1. Bökenkamp A, Ludwig M. The oculocerebrorenal syndrome of Lowe: an update. *Pediatr Nephron*. 2016;31:2201–2212. https://doi.org/10.1007/s00467-016-3343-3.

Clinical Presentation 31

1. Cakmakci H, Tasdelen N, Obuz F, et al. Pediatric focal xanthogranulomatous pyelonephritis: dynamic contrast-enhanced MRI findings. *Clin Imaging*. 2002;26:183–186.
2. Hyla-Klekot L, Paradysz A, Kucharska G, et al. Successfully treated bilateral xanthogranulomatous pyelonephritis in a child. *Pediatr Nephrol*. 2008;23:1895–1896.
3. Shah K, Parikh M, Gharia P, et al. Xanthogranulomatous pyelonephritis mimicking renal mass in 5-month-old child. *Urology*. 2012;79:1360–1362.
4. Korkes F, Favoretto RL, Bróglio M, et al. Xanthogranulomatous pyelonephritis: clinical experience with 41 cases. *Urology*. 2008;71:178–180.
5. Gupta S, Araya CE, Dharnidharka VR. Xanthogranulomatous pyelonephritis in pediatric patients: case report and review of literature. *J Pediatr Urol*. 2010;6:355–358.

Clinical Presentation 32

1. Varela JR, Bargiela A, Requejo I, Fernandez R, Darriba M, Pombo F. Bilateral renal lymphangiomatosis: US and CT findings. *Eur Radiol*. 1998;8:230–231. https://doi.org/10.1007/s003300050368.
2. Jeon TG, Kong do H, Park HJ, et al. Perirenal lymphangiomatosis. *World J Mens Health*. 2014;32:116–119. https://doi.org/10.5534/wjmh.2014.32.2.116.
3. Bagheri MH, Zare Z, Sefidbakht S, et al. Bilateral renal lymphangiomatosis: sonographic findings. *J Clin Ultrasound*. 2009;37:115–118. https://doi.org/10.1002/jcu.20488.
4. Gupta R, Sharma R, Gamanagatti S, et al. Unilateral renal lymphangiectasia: imaging appearance on sonography, CT and MRI. *Int Urol Nephrol*. 2007;39:361–364. https://doi.org/10.1007/s11255-006-9039-z.
5. Nassiri AA, Lotfollahi L, Bakhshayeshkaram M, et al. Renal lymphangiectasia: a curious cause of pleural effusion. *Tanaffos*. 2016;14:213–216.
6. Kashgari AA, Ozair N, Zahrani Al, et al. Renal lymphangiomatosis, a rare differential diagnosis for autosomal recessive polycystic kidney disease in pediatric patients. *Radiol Case Rep*. 2017;12:70–72. https://doi.org/10.1016/j.radcr.2016.11.016.

Clinical Presentation 33

1. van den Heuvel-Eibrink MM, Grundy P, Graf N, et al. Characteristics and survival of 750 children diagnosed with a renal tumor in the first seven months of life: a collaborative study by the SIOP/GPOH/SFOP, NWTSG, and UKCCSG Wilms tumor study groups. *Pediatr Blood Cancer*. 2008;50:1130–1134. https://doi.org/10.1002/pbc.21389.
2. Ooms A, Vujanic GM, D'Hooghe E, et al. Renal tumors of childhood-a histopathologic pattern-based diagnostic approach. *Cancers (Basel)*. 2020;12:729. https://doi.org/10.3390/cancers12030729.
3. Pettinato G, Manivel JC, Wick MR, et al. Classical and cellular (atypical) congenital mesoblastic nephroma: a clinicopathologic, ultrastructural, immunohistochemical, and flow cytometric study. *Hum Pathol*. 1989;20:682–690. https://doi.org/10.1016/0046-8177(89)90156-1.
4. Furtwaengler R, Reinhard H, Leuschner I, et al. Mesoblastic nephroma–a report from the Gesellschaft fur Padiatrische Onkologie und Hamatologie (GPOH). *Cancer*. 2006;106:2275–2283. https://doi.org/10.1002/cncr.21836.
5. Sandstedt B, Delemarre JF, Krul EJ, et al. Mesoblastic nephromas: a study of 29 tumours from the SIOP nephroblastoma file. *Histopathology*. 1985;9:741–750. https://doi.org/10.1111/j.1365-2559.1985.tb02860.x.
6. Argani P, Ladanyi M. Recent advances in pediatric renal neoplasia. *Adv Anat Pathol*. 2003;10:243–260. https://doi.org/10.1097/00125480-200309000-00001.
7. Knezevich SR, Garnett MJ, Pysher TJ, et al. ETV6-NTRK3 gene fusions and trisomy 11 establish a histogenetic link between mesoblastic nephroma and congenital fibrosarcoma. *Cancer Res*. 1998;58:5046–5048.

8. Gooskens SL, Houwing ME, Vujanic GM, et al. Congenital mesoblastic nephroma 50 years after its recognition: a narrative review. *Pediatr Blood Cancer*. 2017;64. https://doi.org/10.1002/pbc.26437.

Clinical Presentation 34

1. Bichet DG, Birnbaumer M, Lonergan M, et al. Nature and recurrence of AVPR2 mutations in X-linked nephrogenic diabetes insipidus. *Am J Hum Genet*. 1994;55:278–286.
2. Nakada T, Miyauchi T, Sumiya H, et al. Non-obstructive urinary tract dilatation in nephrogenic diabetes insipidus. *Int Urol Nephrol*. 1990;22:419–427.
3. Uribarri J, Kaskas M. Hereditary nephrogenic diabetes insipidus and bilateral nonobstructive hydronephrosis. *Nephron*. 1993;65:346–349.
4. van Lieburg AF, Knoers NV, Monnens LA. Clinical presentation and follow-up of 30 patients with congenital nephrogenic diabetes insipidus. *J Am Soc Nephrol*. 1999;10:1958–1964.
5. Yoo TH, Ryu DR, Song YS, et al. Congenital nephrogenic diabetes insipidus presented with bilateral hydronephrosis: genetic analysis of V2R gene mutations. *Yonsei Med*. 2006;47:126–130.

CHAPTER 3

Chronic Kidney Disease

Clinical Presentation 1

A 4-year-old boy was admitted to the pediatric intensive care unit (PICU) with a 3-day history of nonprojectile vomiting and fever. The patient was also experiencing loss of consciousness on admission and suffered a convulsion on the day after admission, with a concomitant sustained decrease in blood pressure and urine output. His urine output was <1 mL/kg/h.

On examination, he had generalized edema, and his weight was 21 kg, temperature 40.1°C, blood pressure 68/41 mm Hg, respirations 19 breath/min, and heart rate 110 beats/min. He had multiple organ dysfunction syndrome (MODS) including acute kidney injury (AKI), disseminated intravascular coagulation, acute myocardial injury, acute liver injury, and meningitis.

Laboratory data included white cell count (WBC) of 21.2 × 106/dL, hemoglobin 9.2 g/dL, platelets 152 × 103/dL, sodium 129 mEq/L, chloride 101 mEq/L, potassium 5.6 mEq/L, calcium 8.5 mg/dL, phosphorus 6.1 mg/dL, blood urea nitrogen (BUN) 54 mg/dL, and creatinine 4.5 mg/dL. Arterial blood gas analysis showed pH 7.15, HCO_3^- 9 mEq/L, and pCO_2 32 mm Hg. Liver function studies included alanine transaminase 12,982 U/L, aspartate transaminase 14,782 U/L, total bilirubin 1.13 mg/dL, direct bilirubin 0.11 mg/dL, albumin 2.6 g/dL, creatinine phosphokinase 25175 U/L, C-reactive protein 11 mg/dL, activated partial thromboplastin time 65/s, prothrombin time 29.1/s, and international normalized ratio 5.74. Blood, urine, and spinal fluid cultures grew gram-positive *Staphylococcus* bacteria. He was started on epinephrine infusion 4 µg/min and phenobarbital for the management of hypotension and control of seizures, respectively.

Which form of renal replacement therapy is most appropriate for this patient?

A. Initiate continuous cyclic peritoneal dialysis.
B. Initiate continuous renal replacement therapy (CRRP), continuous venovenous hemofiltration (CVVH).
C. Initiate intermittent hemodialysis.
D. Initiate CRRP, continuous venovenous hemodialysis (CVVHD).
E. Initiate CRRP, continuous venovenous hemodialysis filtration (CVVHDF).

The correct answer is B

Comment: The patient underwent treatment with CVVH, because of his altered mental status, hyponatremia, metabolic acidosis, electrolyte imbalance, oliguric AKI, and increased serum creatinine and creatinine phosphokinase levels resulting from septic shock and hepatic failure.

CVVH is the simplest and most widely used CRRT in pediatric patients and is a highly effective method of solute removal and is indicated for uremia, severe metabolic acidosis, or electrolyte imbalance with or without fluid overload. CVVH is particularly efficient at removing small and large molecules (e.g., B12, tumor necrosis factor) via convection using a pre- and/or postfilter replacement solution at about 35 mL/kg/h. Solutes can be removed in large quantities while easily maintaining a net zero or even a positive fluid balance in the patient. The amount of fluid in the effluent bag is equal to the amount of fluid removed from the patient plus the volume of replacement fluids administered. No dialysis solution is used.

CVVH adds use of pumped replacement fluids, either pre- or postfilter, to enhance middle molecule clearance by convection. The maximum patient fluid removal rate is 1000 mL/h.

Replacement solutions in CVVH are infused into the blood circuit using replacement pump 1 through the purple line of the Prismaflex set and/or replacement pump 2 through the green line of the Prismaflex set. Replacement pump 1 infuses solution pre- or postfilter, and pump 2 infuses fluid postfilter only.

The primary therapeutic goal of CVVH is water and solute removal across a semipermeable membrane to provide fluid balance and to control electrolyte balance. Continuous hemofiltration with the aid of a blood pump provides solute removal by convection.

A replacement solution is required to drive convection. This type of convection uses no countercurrent dialysate solution. It offers high-volume ultrafiltration using replacement fluid, which can be administered prefilter (or postfilter). By reducing the hematocrit at the blood inlet, predilution is believed to reduce clotting. Postdilution will require less replacement fluid to achieve a given clearance (dose). A combination of predilution, for example, by the predilution pump, and postdilution by the replacement pump would provide benefits in several areas and provide the flexibility required to treat a given patient. Predilution also means a loss between 15% and 35% of clearance (dose), depending on the flow rates. The pump guarantees adequate blood flow to maintain required ultrafiltration (UF) rates. Venous blood access is usually femoral, jugular, or subclavian using a double-lumen cannula.

Replacement solutions for CVVH can be normal saline, lactated Ringer's solution, total parenteral nutrition, routine intravenous fluids, or pharmacy-made solutions. Bicarbonate-based buffered replacement solutions are preferred for patients with hepatic failure because these patients may not be able to convert lactate to bicarbonate.

Replacement fluid is given at a rate of 2000 mL/L/1.73 m^2 (35 mL/kg/h) into the circuit either before blood reaches the membrane (predilution) or after passage over the filter membrane (postdilution).

Prefilter dilution increases the hemofilter membrane filter life. It also increases convective solute transport. Prefilter dilution reduces solute clearance and lowers anticoagulation requirements. Some of the delivered replacement fluid will be lost by hemofiltration; thus, higher UF is required given the loss of replacement fluid through the filter. In postdilution, the drug clearance equals the UF rate, whereas in predilution the replacement fluid should be considered when calculating clearance.

It is recommended to base the decision when to start CRRT not only on the severity of acute renal failure but also on the severity of other organ failure.

Initiation of CRRT is to be considered in oliguric patients despite adequate fluid resuscitation and/or a persisting steep rise in serum creatinine, in addition to persisting shock.

Potential benefits of CRRT in patients with multiple organ dysfunctions include management of fluid balance, decreasing fluid overload, removal of inflammatory mediators, enhanced nutritional support, and control of electrolyte and acid-base abnormalities.

For cases involving AKI, particular attention should be paid to water and sodium retention and blood nitrogen levels, all of which have a significant impact on the treatment and survival of infants and young children, as well as the speed of progress. The characteristics of systemic disease are also important factors.

CVVH requires blood, effluent, and replacement pumps. Dialysate is not required. Plasma water and solutes are removed by convection and ultrafiltration. The convection transport mechanism removes middle and large molecular solutes as well as large volumes of fluid simultaneously. This transport mechanism is used in CVVH and CVVHDF.

Bicarbonate-based or lactate-based replacement fluids are used (pre- or postfilter) based on the patient's clinical need. Higher replacement fluid rates increase convective clearances.

CVVHD requires the use of blood, effluent, and dialysis pump. Replacement solution is not required. Plasma water and solutes are removed by a combination of diffusion and UF. Dialysate is used to create a concentration gradient across a semipermeable membrane. This transport mechanism is used in CVVHD and CVVHDF. Through diffusion, dialysate corrects underlying metabolic imbalances. Dialysate is dependent on buffering agent, electrolytes, and glucose concentrations. Dialysate composition should reflect normal plasma values to achieve homeostasis. Bicarbonate-based solution is physiologic and replaces lost bicarbonate immediately. A bicarbonate concentration of 30 to 35 mEq/L corrects metabolic acidosis in 24 to 48 hours. It is a superior buffer in normalizing acidosis without the risk of alkalosis. Bicarbonate-based solution is also a preferred buffer for patients with liver failure. It improves hemodynamic instability with fewer cardiovascular events.

Lactate-based solution is metabolized into bicarbonate in the liver on a 1:1 in subjects with normal liver function and can sufficiently correct acidemia. However, lactate-based solution has a pH value of 5.4 and is a powerful peripheral vasodilator leading to further acidemia for patients with hypoxia, liver impairment, and preexisting lactic acidemia.

The replacement and dialysate fluids should have the same composition to reduce staff confusion and the risk for error.

CVVHDF requires the use of blood, effluent, dialysate, and replacement pumps. Both dialysate and replacement solutions are used. Plasma water and solutes are removed by diffusion, convection, and UF. In CVVHDF, removal of small molecules is achieved by diffusion through the addition of dialysate solution and removal of middle and large molecules by convection through the addition of replacement solution. This transport mechanism is used only in CVVHDF.

In general, CRRT clearance of solute is dependent on the molecule size of the solute, the sieving coefficient, and the pore size of the semipermeable membrane. The higher the UF rate, the greater the solute clearance. Small molecules easily pass through a membrane driven by diffusion and convection. Middle- and large-size molecules are cleared primarily by convection. The semipermeable membrane removes solutes with a molecular weight of up to 50,000 Da. Plasma proteins or substances that are highly protein bound will not be cleared.[1]

The sieving coefficient of a molecule is the ability of a substance to pass through a membrane from the blood compartment of the hemofilter to the fluid compartment. A sieving coefficient of 1 will allow the free passage of a substance but a sieving coefficient of 0 indicates that the substance is unable to pass. The sieving coefficient of sodium is 0.94, potassium 1.0, creatinine 1.0, and albumin 0.

It is recommended to continue CRRT as long as the criteria defining severe oliguric AKI are present. If the clinical condition improves, it may be considered to wait before connecting a new circuit to see whether renal function recovers. CRRT should be restarted in case of clinical or metabolic deterioration.[1]

CRRT may be postponed when the underlying disease is improving, other organ failure is recovering, and the slope in the serum creatinine rise declines to see if renal function is also recovering.

Establishing vascular access is a key factor for successful CRRT in children. The internal jugular vein is the primary site of choice because of a lower associated risk of complications and simplicity of catheter insertion. The femoral vein is optimal and constitutes the easiest site for insertion. The subclavian vein is the least preferred site given its higher risk of pneumonia/hemothorax and its association with central venous stenosis. The length of the catheter chosen will depend on the site used. Two single-lumen venous hemodialysis catheters can be used in infants. Recommended catheters by age are <6 months, 4 to 5 Fr single lumen; 6 to 12 months, 5 to 7 Fr double lumen; 1 to 3 years, 8 to 9 Fr double lumen; and >3 years, 8 to 12 Fr double lumen.

The semipermeable membrane is structurally designed to allow high fluid removal and molecular cutoff weight of 30,000 to 50,000 Da. The membrane provides an interface between the blood and dialysate compartment. The membrane biocompatibility minimizes severe patient reactions and decreases the complement activation.

Filters and tubing with a low prefilled volume should be used to reduce the blood volume in extracorporeal circulation and help ameliorate the decrease in effective circulating blood volume. Filters with a high-molecular-weight polymer membrane, high permeability, good biocompatibility, and small impact on the coagulation system should be selected. The use of AN69 membranes has been linked to bradykinin release syndrome among patients who are acidotic or taking angiotensin-converting enzyme inhibitors. Alternative membranes should be used in such cases. Generally, the blood volume in extracorporeal circulation should be maintained at <10 % of body weight (e.g., <30 mL in neonates, <50 mL in infants, <100 mL in children). For neonates weighing <2.5 kg, tubing can be prefilled with plasma, whole blood, or 5% albumin.[1]

For continuous modes of renal replacement therapy to be effective, in terms of both effective solute clearance and fluid removal, the extracorporeal circuits must operate continuously. Thus, preventing clotting in the CRRT circuit is a key goal to effective patient management. Because these patients may also be at increased risk of bleeding, regional anticoagulation with citrate is increasing in popularity, particularly after the introduction of commercially available CRRT machines and fluids specifically designed for citrate anticoagulation. Although regional anticoagulation with citrate provides many advantages over other systemic anticoagulants, excess citrate may lead to metabolic complications, ranging from acidosis to alkalosis, and may also potentially expose patients to electrolyte disturbances from hyper- and hyponatremia and hyper- and hypocalcemia.[1]

Transmembrane pressure should be monitored and maintained at <200 mm Hg (a transmembrane pressure >250 mm Hg may indicate clotting in the filter). Particular attention should be paid to warming the replacement fluid. The recommended flow rates are as follows: blood flow, 30 mL/min in neonates, 30 to 40 mL/min in infants/young children, 50 to 75 mL/min in children weighing <20 kg, and 75 to 100 mL/min in children weighing >20 kg; UF rate, 8 to 10 mL/min/m^2 in neonates/infants and 8 to 15 mL/min/m^2 in children (daily fluid input/output, cardiac function, and edema should be considered); and dialysates, 15 to 20 mL/min/m^2 in neonates/infants/children.[1]

A simple and easy method for estimating drug clearance as a function of total creatinine clearance when the information on the pharmacokinetics of a particular drug is not available is to add replacement fluid rate (CVVH) or dialysate flow rate (CVVHD), usually 2 L/1.73 m^2/h or 33 mL/1.73 m^2/min, to the patient's native creatinine clearance (mL/1.73 m^2/min). This value is the patient's new creatinine clearance, and drugs should be dosed accordingly.

Patients treated with continuous renal therapies in the intensive care unit are probably at risk for antibiotic underdosing and therapeutic failures.[1]

Estimation of renal function in acute injury is very challenging, but recently short-interval creatinine clearance measurements have been demonstrated.

Widely available drug databases support individualized decision-making. There is little literature to support adjusting the loading dose of antibiotics in AKI. The sum of renal creatinine clearance and CVVH ultrafiltration provides a starting point for subsequent antibiotic dosing. When available, therapeutic drug monitoring should be used, especially for drugs with low therapeutic index. Loss of macro- and micronutrients is well documented during CRRT and, in general, requires replenishing or compensating eventual deficits.[1]

The final aim should be to optimize the nutritional status of the patient and to reduce the so-called daily trauma induced by CRRT. Daily recommended energy requirements during CRRT fluctuate between 25 and 35 kcal/kg (60–70% carbohydrates and 30–40% lipids) and between 1.5 and 1.8 g/kg protein. Significant alterations of carbohydrate and lipid metabolism as well as severe electrolyte disturbances may be found in patients undergoing CRRT. Close monitoring of these metabolic parameters and their interactions is imperative. Energy requirements during CRRT are increased and should best be assessed by indirect calorimetry. However, this technique is not universally available and will need correction for the known bicarbonate/CO_2 diversion induced by CRRT. The current European Society for Clinical Nutrition and Metabolism guidelines allow us to adequately supplement important micronutrients such as amino acids (glutamine), water-soluble vitamins, and trace elements. More widespread recognition of "daily trauma" and the use of an appropriate checklist may help the bedside clinician better assess and handle nutrition deficits in CRRT patients.[1]

Clinical Presentation 2

Prophylaxis against dialysis catheter-related bacteremia includes which *one* of the following?

A. Intravenous antibiotic administration near the end of each dialysis
B. Gentamicin-citrate catheter lock
C. Ultrapure water
D. Ultrapure dialysi
E. Replacement of the catheter

The correct answer is B

Comment: Several controlled studies have shown that locking the catheter with an antibiotic or antiseptic solution can reduce the incidence of bacteremia as much as 10-fold. Although the use of ultrapure water and ultrapure dialysate is recommended in general to combat a subtle inflammatory influence of dialysis, such measures will not protect against catheter-induced sepsis. Antibiotics given to the patient near the end of the dialysis treatment have little effect on catheter biofilm because the exposure is limited to both concentration and time. Replacing the catheter will resolve the problem, but it cannot be considered a prophylactic measure.[1]

Clinical Presentation 3

A 9-year-old girl with end-stage renal disease (ESRD) resulting from immunoglobulin A (IgA) nephropathy is on peritoneal dialysis (PD) and is hypertensive. Her current weight is 48 kg, and she has no signs of volume overload and no peripheral edema, and there are no abdominal bruits. In the past 2 years of PD therapy, she has been on cycler therapy doing four 2.5% dextrose exchanges over 9 hours and a 15-hour daytime dwell with 2.5% dextrose. She was normotensive on no antihypertensives. She is adequately dialyzed in terms of small solute clearance, but over the past 2 months, she has become hypertensive (blood pressure [BP] 155/90 mm Hg) despite using 2 antihypertensive medications.

In addition to decreasing dietary sodium intake, which *one* of the options listed would be the best change in her current prescription that would *most* likely improve her BP control?

A. Change the overnight prescription to three 2.5% dextrose dwells over 9 hours and add a daytime dwell of icodextrin.
B. Continue current overnight prescription but change daytime dwell to 4.25% dextrose during the daytime.
C. Change her nightly prescription to three 2.5% dextrose dwells over 10 hours and continue 2.5% dextrose during the daytime.
D. Continue the current overnight prescription and add a 1.5% dextrose last bag fill and a 1.5% dextrose midday exchange.

E. Change overnight prescription to five 4.25% exchanges and a 4.25% daytime dextrose exchange.

The correct answer is A

It has been well documented that with glucose (dextrose)-containing fluids, the crystalloid-induced transcapillary UF is dependent on maintaining an osmotic gradient between the peritoneum and the blood, which favors the movement of fluid from the blood to the peritoneum. The peritoneal membrane functions as an impermeable membrane and allows movement of most solutes down their concentration gradients. Unfortunately, glucose (dextrose) is readily absorbed, and eventually the concentration gradient for transcapillary UF no longer exists. At that time, UF ceases and lymphatic absorption predominates.

An ideal osmotic agent for PD solutions would either not be absorbed or would only very slowly be absorbed so that the osmotic gradient is maintained throughout the dwell. Icodextrin is such a solution. Icodextrin is a polymer that induces ultrafiltration via a colloid osmotic force.[1] By substituting icodextrin for dextrose, one may be able to increase UF volume during long dwells (8–15 hours) when compared with dextrose-containing fluids. Because attention has returned to optimizing BP and volume control, it has been recognized that at times, the UF volume may be relatively sodium free. Crystalloid-induced UF is via small pores (salt and water removal) and transcellular aquapores (water removal only). Therefore, during short dwells, one may remove relatively less sodium than water. In contrast, colloid-induced UF is almost exclusively via small pores, so there is no discrepancy between the relative amounts of salt and water removed during a typical dwell with a colloid osmotic agent. These differences must be appreciated when attempting to optimize BP control in PD patients.

Clinical Presentation 4

An 18-year-old female with ESRD managed with hemodialysis develops acute substernal chest pain and requires help in choosing the least toxic form of angiography.

Which *one* of the following choices regarding this issue is *true*?

A. More than 75% of injected gadolinium can be removed by a single dialysis.
B. There is no risk from injection of radiographic contrast agents in anuric patients.
C. Iodinated radiographic contrast agents are slowly removed by dialysis.
D. Gadolinium and iodinated contrast agents are large molecules and cannot be removed by dialysis.

The correct answer is A

Comment: Hemodialyzed patients are especially prone to acute volume overload after intravenous injection of radiographic contrast agents, including aortography or contrast-enhanced magnetic resonance imaging (MRI). Recent studies have shown that both gadolinium and iodinated radiographic contrast agents are rapidly and efficiently removed by hemodialysis and hemofiltration. Average removal rates of gadolinium were 78%, 95%, 98%, and after the first to third hemodialysis sessions. Physicians must also be alert to the significantly low serum calcium levels that may last up to 4.5 days after gadolinium administration. This effect of gadolinium is apparently dose related.[1,2]

Clinical Presentation 5

A 15-year-old hemodialysis patient has developed intradialytic palpitation on several occasions. His electrocardiograph demonstrates increased QT dispersion (variation in the QT interval).

Which *one* of the following maneuvers would be most appropriate in attempting to reduce QT dispersion?

A. Increasing dialysate sodium concentration
B. Increasing dialysis time to reduce net hourly required ultrafiltration
C. Administering oxygen during the dialysis procedure
D. Increasing dialysate calcium concentration from 2.5 mg/dL to 3.5 mg/dL
E. Increasing blood flow and dialysate flow rate to increase Kt/V urea

The correct answer is D

Comment: QT dispersion, defined as the difference in duration between the longest and shortest QT interval on an electrocardiogram, is a method of approximating repolarization abnormalities. QT dispersion has been shown to independently predict cardiovascular mortality in incident dialysis patients. Intra-dialytic QT dispersion has been demonstrated to be inversely related to a dialysate calcium composition.[1,2]

Clinical Presentation 6

A 17-year-old male receiving chronic hemodialysis therapy has multiple comorbidities, including dilated cardiomyopathy, anemia despite high doses of erythropoietin, hypertension, hyperlipidemia, and generalized muscle weakness. You are considering adding L-carnitine to his medical regimen.

What is the single *most* consistent clinical effect of L-carnitine supplementation in the maintenance hemodialysis patient?

A. Improvement in myocardial function
B. Reduction in triglycerides
C. Reduction in serum cholesterol
D. Improvement in erythropoietin resistance
E. Improvement in exercise capacity and muscle weakness

The correct answer is D

Comment: L-carnitine is a readily dialyzed, low-molecular-weight metabolic intermediate. L-carnitine deficiency has been proposed as a contributor to myocardial dysfunction, hyperlipidemia, muscle weakness, and erythropoietin resistance in dialysis patients. The best evidence for the benefit of L-carnitine in maintenance dialysis patients is for the treatment of erythropoietin resistance.[1]

Clinical Presentation 7

A 19-year-old patient on chronic hemodialysis has an estimated dry weight of 85 kg. His dialysis prescription consists of the following: treatment time, 4.5 hours; dialysis access, arteriovenous fistula; blood flow, 35 mL/min; dialysis flow, 600 mL/min; dialyzer, high-flux polysulfone. His measured single pool variable volume Kt/V urea is consistently less than 1.2.

Which *one* of the following approaches will likely lead to the greatest improvement in weekly urea clearance?

A. Increasing blood flow to 400 mL/min
B. Increasing dialysate flow to 800 mL/min
C. Increasing dialysis time to 5 hours for each treatment
D. Adding fourth weekly dialysis treatment

The correct answer is D

Comment: As an index of solute clearance, Kt/V urea <1.2 serves as a generally accepted marker of inadequate dialysis doses. Patients with a large body mass are less likely to achieve an individual treatment target Kt/V urea of 1.2. Although each of the proposed solutions will increase weekly Kt/V urea, increasing the frequency of hemodialysis will have the greatest effect on weekly urea clearance by increasing the efficiency of the hemodialysis procedure.[1,2]

Clinical Presentation 8

A 17-year-old male is receiving hemodialysis therapy using a cuffed tunneled catheter. At the dialysis unit, he is found to have a low-grade fever and erythema at the catheter exit site. Two blood cultures are obtained, and mupirocin ointment is prescribed for a suspected exit-site infection. Vancomycin 1000 mg is also administered intravenously. Two days later, blood cultures are growing *Staphylococcus aureus* sensitive to both vancomycin and cephalosporins. The patient is afebrile, and there is no erythema and no drainage from the catheter exit site. He has no drug allergies.

Which *one* of the following is the most appropriate course of action?

A. Complete a 3-week course of vancomycin (500 mg) after each dialysis treatment.
B. Complete a 3-week course of cefazolin (1000 mg) intravenously with each dialysis treatment.
C. Arrange for catheter removal and exchange and complete a 3-week course of intravenous cefazolin (1000 mg) with each dialysis treatment.
D. Continue treatment with mupirocin ointment and use cefazolin (1000 mg) after each dialysis treatment for 3 weeks if the patient develops recurrent fever.

The correct answer is D

Comment: Strategies involving catheter removal coupled with a 3-week course of cefazolin intravenously have been demonstrated to be successful in achieving high cure rates. Antibiotic therapy alone results in an insufficient cure rate.[1]

Clinical Presentation 9

A 15-year-old male on dialysis has recurrent intradialytic hypotension, often necessitating that he remains in the dialysis unit until his BP has stabilized. His mother confides in you that her son is contemplating discontinuation of dialysis therapy because of this problem, and she asks if you can adjust the dialysis prescription to improve the problem.

Which *one* of the following is least effective in reducing intradialytic hypotension?

A. Sequential ultrafiltration followed by dialysis using high-sodium dialysate
B. Sequential ultrafiltration followed by hemodialysis
C. High-sodium dialysis
D. Use of sodium modeling
E. Low-temperature dialysate (35°C)
F. Administration of midodrine

The correct answer is A

Comment: Intradialytic hypotension occurs in 15% to 25% of all hemodialysis treatments. Although many strategies to prevent this complication are at least partly successful, a recent prospective crossover study did not support the use of isolated UF followed by isovolemic dialysis. Each of the other four choices has demonstrated utility in preventing dialysis hypotension, albeit a head-to-head comparison of these four strategies has not been performed in a single study.[1]

Clinical Presentation 10

Which *one* of the following statements is *most correct* concerning the use of nonsteroidal antiinflammatory drugs (NSAIDs) among chronic kidney disease (CKD) patients with type 1 diabetes mellitus?

A. Use of NSAIDs will lead to superimposed analgesic nephropathy in this population.
B. Anemia from NSAIDs will lead to superimposed analgesic nephropathy in this population.
C. Development of minimal change disease associated with NSAIDs will lead to confusion regarding proteinuria.
D. NSAIDs have been associated with AKI in the general population and with the progression of disease in those with CKD.

The correct answer is D

Comment: The management of pain in patients with CKD is challenging for many reasons. These patients have increased susceptibility to adverse drug effects from altered drug metabolism and excretion, and there are limited safety data for use in this population despite a high pain burden. NSAIDs have long been regarded as dangerous for use in patients with CKD because of the risk for nephrotoxicity; thus, alternative classes of analgesics, including opioids, have become more commonly used for pain control in this population. Given the well-established risks that opioids and other analgesics pose, further characterization of the risk posed by NSAIDs in patients with CKD is warranted. NSAID use has been associated with acute kidney injury, progressive loss of glomerular filtration rate in CKD, electrolyte derangements, and hypervolemia with worsening of heart failure and hypertension. The risk for these nephrotoxicity syndromes is modified by many comorbid conditions, risk factors, and characteristics of use, and in patients with CKD, the risk differs between levels of glomerular filtration rate. In this review, we offer recommendations for the cautious use of NSAIDs in the CKD population after careful consideration of these risk factors on an individualized basis.[1]

Clinical Presentation 11

Which *one* of the following statements is *most correct* concerning the use of NSAIDs among CKD patients with type 1 diabetes mellitus?

A. Use of NSAIDs will lead to superimposed analgesic nephropathy in this population.
B. Anemia from NSAIDs will lead to superimposed analgesic nephropathy in this population.
C. Development of minimal change disease associated with NSAIDs will lead to confusion regarding proteinuria.
D. NSAIDs have been associated with AKI in the general population and with progression of disease in those with CKD.

The correct answer is D

Comment: The risk of analgesic nephropathy from the use of NSAIDs remains controversial.[1]

Clinical Presentation 12

An 18-year-old male with chronic renal failure secondary to type 1 diabetes mellitus presents for evaluation for renal transplantation. He has a creatinine clearance of 20 mL/min and has not yet initiated dialysis. His 26-year-old brother is in the same blood group and is willing to donate a kidney.

Which *one* of the following options would you now recommend?

A. Arrange for cadaver kidney transplantation alone.
B. Arrange for simultaneous kidney-pancreas (SKP) transplantation.
C. Arrange for living donor kidney transplantation alone.
D. Arrange for donor kidney transplantation before initiating dialysis followed by pancreas after kidney transplantation.
E. Arrange for donor translation after initiating dialysis.

The correct answer is D

Comment: Recent studies have shown increased patient survival (95%) and kidney graft survival (92%) at 1 year for SKP transplantation, representing a higher kidney graft survival than that for recipients with diabetes of cadaveric kidney transplants alone. SKP transplant offers the best survival advantage and represents the treatment of choice for type 1 diabetes patients with renal failure. Patients who have received 1 to 6 months of dialysis before transplantation have had at least a 15% increase in mortality risk in comparison to those who underwent preemptive transplantation. A 75% higher risk of death was seen in those patients who were on dialysis for greater than 24 months.[1,2]

Clinical Presentation 13

A 12-year-old boy had successful renal transplant 2 years ago and now has a serum creatinine of 1.0 mg/dL. He is on prednisone, mycophenolate mofetil (MMF), and cyclosporine. He asks you about surveillance for skin cancer.

Which *one* of the following choices is the *best* for this patient?

A. Do not worry about skin cancer because he is a male subject.
B. He should undergo surveillance by dermatologists at least yearly for premalignant lesions.
C. Immunosuppression therapy should be progressively reduced or delay the incidence of skin cancer.
D. All warts should be removed to prevent malignant transfusion.
E. Patient should switch from MMF to azathioprine for better protection against transplant rejection.

The correct answer is B

Comment: Skin cancers are the most frequent malignant conditions seen in transplant recipients and can cause increased morbidity and mortality. Standard practice is to undergo surveillance aggressively to remove all basal and squamous cell carcinomas—thus, answer B is correct. There is no evidence that male subjects have less skin cancer than females. Reducing immunosuppression will result in an increased risk of rejection and probably not do much to prevent skin cancer after 2 years of immunosuppressive therapy. Viral warts do suggest some degree of overimmunosuppression. There is no evidence, however, that these warts need to be removed to prevent malignant transformation. They probably should be removed on their own merits. There is no evidence that MMF is better than azathioprine for the prevention of malignancy; in fact, there is some anecdotal evidence that the opposite is true.[1]

Clinical Presentation 14

An 8-year-old boy received a cadaveric renal transplant 2 years ago. While taking tacrolimus, sirolimus, and prednisone, he is started on clarithromycin by his primary care physician for a respiratory tract infection. One week later, he is seen in the renal transplant clinic and found to have a hemoglobin 9.6 g/dL, WBC 3200/mL, platelets 68,000/mL, and BUN of 42 mg/dL. Serum creatinine has increased from his baseline value of 1.2 mg/dL to 2.2 mg/dL, sodium 142 mEq/L, potassium 5.9 mEq/L, chloride 110 mEq/L, bicarbonate 18 mEq/L, and lactate dehydrogenase (LDH) 136 U/L. Liver function tests are normal.

Which *one* of the following diagnoses is most likely in this patient?

A. *Mycoplasma pneumonia*
B. Tacrolimus nephrotoxicity
C. Viral pneumonia
D. Sirolimus nephrotoxicity
E. Sirolimus and tacrolimus nephrotoxicity

The correct answer is E

Comment: The patient has anemia, leukopenia, thrombocytopenia, hyperkalemia, non-anion gap acidosis, and renal failure. Clarithromycin increases the levels of tacrolimus, cyclosporine, and sirolimus by decreasing their metabolism by the cytochrome P450 system; therefore, it should not be administered to transplant patients unless absolutely necessary. This is also true for erythromycin.[1]

Azithromycin does not have the same effect on the metabolism of cyclosporine, tacrolimus, or sirolimus and may be used safely in transplant patients. Very high levels of tacrolimus can cause acute renal failure because of the vasoconstriction effect on the renal arteries and may be associated with type IV renal tubular acidosis. High levels of sirolimus may cause thrombocytopenia and leukopenia. Tacrolimus and cyclosporine may cause hemolytic uremic syndrome (HUS); sirolimus does not.

Clinical Presentation 15

A 6-year-old girl received a cadaveric renal transplant 3 weeks ago and she now presents with worsening dyspnea on excretion. Her current immunosuppression therapy includes sirolimus, mycophenolate mofetil, and prednisone. Her baseline posttransplant creatinine was 0.8 mg/dL. Findings on physical examination are BP 130/86 mm Hg, pulse 100 beats/min, temperature 37°C, and oxygen saturation 90%. She is tachypneic but in no distress. Her jugular venous pressure is not increased, nor is she cyanotic. Her heart sounds are normal, but a mitral incompetence murmur (2/6) is present. Occasional fine crackles are present at both lung bases posteriorly. The abdominal examination is normal. No peripheral edema is present. Laboratory results show the following: hemoglobin 10.8 g/dL, WBC 5600/mL, platelet 178,000/mL, sodium 135 mEq/L, potassium 4.5 mEq/L, chloride 100 mEq/L, bicarbonate 26 mEq/L, and LDH 120 U/L. Liver function tests are normal. Chest x-ray and computed tomography scan show diffuse bilateral pulmonary infiltrates.

Given these findings, which *one* of the following is the *most* likely diagnosis for this patient?

A. Cytomegalovirus (CMV) pneumonitis
B. *Pneumocystis pneumonia*
C. Aspergillosis
D. Sirolimus-related pneumonitis
E. *Legionella pneumonia*

The correct answer is D

Comment: The patient is only 3 weeks postrenal transplantation. Opportunistic infections are less likely. They are, however, in the differential diagnosis. She is afebrile with a normal WBC, suggesting that this is not an infectious case.

This makes infections such as CMV and *Pneumocystis pneumonia* or others unlikely. So the correct answer is D.

Her LDH, which may be raised in *Pneumocystis pneumonia*, is normal. She has no findings on examination to suggest congestive heart failure. The patient has recently started on sirolimus. There have been several reported cases of interstitial pneumonitis in patients treated with sirolimus. The pneumonitis is not dose-related and responds to discontinuation of sirolimus, with complete resolution within 3 months in all reported cases.[1]

Clinical Presentation 16

The use of which *one* of the following immunosuppressive agents is *not* associated with hyperlipidemia?

A. Tacrolimus
B. Cyclosporine
C. Rapamycin
D. MMF
E. Prednisone

The correct answer is D

Comment: Both cyclosporine and tacrolimus can cause hyperlipidemia; however, the risk is greater with cyclosporine. Hyperlipidemia has been reported as 1 of the major side effects of sirolimus therapy (35–50%) compared with azathioprine (18%). Hyperlipidemia is also a known side effect of corticosteroids. MMF has not been associated with lipid abnormalities.[1]

Clinical Presentation 17

Posttransplantation anemia is *not* related to which *one* of the following?

A. Mycophenolate mofetil therapy
B. Angiotensin-converting enzyme (ACE) inhibitor therapy
C. Paravirus infection
D. Tacrolimus therapy
E. Sirolimus therapy

The correct answer is D

Comment: Mycophenolate mofetil has been associated with leukopenia and anemia. Both ACE inhibitors and angiotensin-receptor blockers (ARB) have been shown to cause anemia in renal transplant patients. Anemia has been infrequently reported as a side effect of sirolimus, but it has been reported. There have been many reports documenting the association between paravirus B19 as a cause of anemia in renal transplant recipients.[1–4]

Clinical Presentation 18

An 8-year-old girl with lupus nephritis and a panel reactive antibody (PRA) of 65% receives her third renal transplant. Her postoperative course is complicated by delayed graft function and her serum creatinine eventually stabilizes at 1.8 mg/dL by 6 weeks after transplantation. Her immunosuppressive medications are tacrolimus, MMF, and prednisone. At 10 months after transplantation, she presents with epigastric discomfort and dysphasia. Upper gastrointestinal endoscopy reveals a gastric lesion, which is found to be Epstein-Barr virus–related posttransplant lymphoproliferative disease (PTLD) on histology.

A. Immunosuppression should be reduced.
B. Immunosuppression should be withdrawn.
C. Rituximab should be started, and immunosuppression maintained at its current levels.
D. Immunosuppression should be reduced and valganciclovir initiated.
E. Surgical resection of the lesion should be performed.

The correct answer is A

Comment: PTLD carries a high mortality of about 70%, according to various reports, and several factors—including the number of involved organs, primary central nervous system involvement, and monoclonality—suggest a poorer prognosis. Therapeutic interventions include the reduction of immunosuppression, antiviral therapy, anti–B-cell antibodies, anti-interleukin 6 antibodies, alpha-interferon, cytotoxic T cells, chemotherapy, radiation, and surgical resection. The reduction of immunosuppression forms the cornerstone of all treatment and may be sufficient by itself, with complete remission in 63% of cases in some reports. This girl is a high immunological risk patient with localized PTLD. Withdrawal of immunosuppression will almost certainly result in acute rejection in an individual who is not at a very high risk of dying from PTLD.

Currently, many transplant programs would also administer rituximab in addition to reducing immunosuppression. Rituximab has been shown to induce remission in transplant recipients, including lung, liver, small bowel, and stem cell transplants. However, there are insufficient data to maintain immunosuppression at current levels in combination with rituximab therapy. Neither acyclovir nor ganciclovir have an effect on Epstein-Barr virus persistence associated with latent infection, and their use has not been effective in the treatment of PTLD.[1]

Clinical Presentation 19

A 6-year-old girl with biopsy-proven IgA nephropathy presents for nephrology care. Her serum creatinine has increased from 0.8 mg/dL to 2.5 mg/dL over the past 3 years. Her BP is now 155/90 mm Hg. There is no edema, rash, or arthritis on physical examination. Hemoglobin is 10.5 g/dL, potassium 5.5 mEq/L, and intact parathyroid hormone (PTH) level 150 pg/mL.

Which *one* of the following statements is *most correct*?

A. Her hemoglobin should be increased to 11 to 12 g/dL with human recombinant erythropoietin therapy to reduce the risk of congestive heart failure.
B. Her serum potassium should be reduced to <5.0 mEq/L to reduce the risk of sudden death.
C. Her intact PTH level should be reduced to 70 to 11 pg/mL to reduce the risk of fractures.
D. None of the above.

The correct answer is D

Comment: Unfortunately, none of the interventions has been shown to yield the listed clinical benefits in randomized controlled trials.[1]

Clinical Presentation 20

A 7-year-old girl presents with nephritic syndrome secondary to focal segmental glomerulosclerosis (FSGS). A kidney biopsy is diagnostic for focal and segmental glomerulosclerosis. Her current estimated glomerular filtration rate (GFR) is 60 mL/min/1.73 m^2.

Which of the following is the best predictor of her risk of progressing to ESRD?

A. The percentage of glomeruli with focal changes on biopsy
B. ACE genotyping polymorphisms
C. The extent of tubulointerstitial disease on biopsy
D. The level of plasma renin activity
E. A family history of hypertension

The correct answer is C

Comment: The two most predictive risk factors for the progression of glomerular diseases are the quantity of protein excreted in the urine and the extent of tubulointerstitial disease in a renal biopsy. There is no evidence that choice A is a predictive factor. There is no convincing evidence that the ACE genotype predicts the progression of glomerular diseases, particularly FSGS. Therefore, choice B is also incorrect. Choice D, the level of plasma renin activity, has not been demonstrated to be a predictor of renal disease progression. In fact, in most CKDs, plasma renin activity is suppressed, most likely related to volume expansion. Thus, the beneficial effects of ACE inhibitors in slowing the progression of renal disease are somewhat of a paradox. There is no evidence that a family history of hypertension predicts the progression of FSGS. Therefore, choice E is incorrect. The link between tubulointerstitial disease and progression may relate to reabsorption of proteins by proximal tubular cells, with activation of these cells and subsequent release of inflammatory mediators.[1,2]

Clinical Presentation 21

A 19-year-old female has CKD from type 1 diabetes. Her current GFR is 45 mL/min/1.73 m^2.

Which of the following is *true* regarding alterations in bone and mineral metabolism in CKD?

A. The most sensitive marker of abnormal mineral metabolism is decreased calcitriol production.
B. Elevations in PTH secretion do not occur until GFR is <20 mL/min/1.73 m^2.
C. Elevated serum phosphate inhibits the 1 hydroxylase enzyme in the kidney, leading to calcitriol synthesis.
D. An alteration in the set point for calcium occurs in the parathyroid glands, leading to increased PTH secretion for any increase in serum calcium.

The correct answer is C

Comment: This patient has stage 3 CKD. Abnormalities in calcium, phosphorous, and PTH commonly develop as GFR declines. The earliest and most sensitive marker of abnormal mineral metabolism is an elevation in serum PTH. This develops when the GFR decreases to <70 mL/min/1.73 m^2. Therefore, choice A is incorrect. Calcitriol synthesis decreases in CKD, but usually not until the GFR is <40 mL/min/1.73 m^2, and the changes are somewhat variable. Choice B is incorrect because PTH secretion occurs at an earlier stage in CKD, when the GFR is 40 to 70 mL/min/1.73 m^2. Choice C is correct because one of the mechanisms for decreased calcitriol synthesis is the inhibition of the one hydroxylase enzyme in the kidney by elevated serum phosphorous. In regard to choice D, the set point for calcium is altered in CKD, leading to increased PTH secretion for a given decrease (not increase) in serum calcium level. Choice E is incorrect because parathyroid-related bone disease (osteitis fibrosa cystica) is more common than osteomalacia.[1]

Clinical Presentation 22

An 8-year-old girl is seen in your office for evaluation of CKD. Over the past 2 years, her GFR has decreased from 47 to a current value of 19 mL/min/1.73 m^2, despite good BP control with an ACE inhibitor. Laboratory studies include serum creatinine of 4.1 mg/dL, potassium of 5.0 mEq/L, and bicarbonate of 17 mEq/L. An arterial blood gas test confirms she has a compensated metabolic acidosis.

Which of the following explanations is correct regarding metabolic acidosis in CKD patients?

A. No evidence of acidosis is seen until the bicarbonate is <15 mEq/L.
B. Acidosis stimulates albumin synthesis by the liver.
C. Acidosis suppresses PTH release.
D. Acidosis increases calcium loss from bone.
E. Acidosis stimulates skeletal muscle hypertrophy.

The correct answer is D

Comment: Buffering of hydrogen by bone is associated with the release of calcium. In addition, acidosis stimulates osteoclastic activity. Metabolic acidosis occurs when the GFR falls to 60 mL/min/1.73 m^2 and can have adverse consequences even when the serum bicarbonate is between 15 and 22 mEq/L. Option A is therefore incorrect. Option B is incorrect because acidosis suppresses albumin synthesis by the liver. Option C is incorrect because acidosis is associated with increased PTH release. Option E is also incorrect because acidosis-stimulated degradation of protein from skeletal muscle is mediated in part by increased cortisol release and decreased release of insulin-like growth factor 1.[1]

Clinical Presentation 23

A 9-year-old boy has kidney dysplasia. His BP is 135/90 mm Hg, his weight is 78 kg, and his examination is unremarkable. Laboratory tests include serum creatinine of 2 mg/dL, serum calcium of 7.6 mg/dL, serum phosphate of 5.1 mg/dL, serum albumin of 4.0 g/dL, serum intact PTH of 280 pg/mL, and calculated GFR of 46 mL/min/1.73 m^2.

Which of the following is *true* regarding therapy?

A. Dietary phosphate should be restricted to 2 g/day.
B. He should be treated with 0.25 g/day calcitriol.
C. Calcium-containing phosphate binders should be avoided.
D. Long-term therapy with aluminum hydroxide should be started at a dose of 15 mL orally with meals.
E. Sevelamer therapy would be associated with an increased risk of development of osteomalacia and bone fractures.

The correct answer is B

Comment: The patient has stage 3 CKD, and secondary hyperparathyroidism is present. Calcitriol therapy (choice B) can effectively reduce PTH secretion and is the best treatment for this patient. Dietary phosphorous restriction to 800 mg to 1000 mg should be instituted when the serum phosphorous is >4.6 mg/dL (option A is incorrect). Option C is incorrect because calcium-containing phosphate binders can be used as primary therapy but should be limited to 1500 mg/day. If vascular calcification is present, current treatment guidelines suggest the non–calcium-containing phosphate binders may be preferred. Option D is incorrect because long-term treatment with aluminum-containing phosphate binders can cause osteomalacia secondary to the deposition of aluminum in bone. Option E is incorrect because sevelamer has not been associated with osteomalacia or an increased risk of bone fractures.[1]

Clinical Presentation 24

A 17-year-old female with type 2 diabetes and CKD presents to your office for treatment recommendations. She has hypertension that is being treated with furosemide, metoprolol, and lisinopril. Her major complaint is fatigue. On examination, her BP is 140/85 mm Hg and she has 1+ peripheral edema. Her serum creatinine is 2.2 mg/dL with a calculated GFR of 32 mL/min/1.73 m^2. A spot urine protein-to-creatinine result is 4 mg/mg. Her blood sugar is 150 mg/dL.

Which of the following choices is most *correct* regarding this patient?

A. Carefully follow hemoglobin and start recombinant erythropoietin therapy if it is <10 g/dL.
B. Check an echocardiogram and start recombinant erythropoietin therapy if left ventricular hypertrophy is present.
C. Start oral iron and recheck hemoglobin level in 1 month.
D. Start recombinant erythropoietin at 10,000 units subcutaneously once weekly along with oral iron.
E. Transfuse 2 units of packed red blood cells.

The correct answer is E

Comment: The patient has stage 3 CKD secondary to diabetic nephropathy. In addition to a decrease in her GFR, she has significant proteinuria. In an analysis of the MDRD study that did not enroll those with diabetes, patients with more than 1 g of protein per 24 hours had a slower rate of progression with the lowered BP goal of a mean arterial pressure of 92 mm Hg. Based on this study, on JNC-VI recommendations, and on expert opinion, the best option is E for lowering her target BP to 125 to 130/75 to 80 mm Hg. Option A is incorrect because there are no data demonstrating that more intensive glycemic control in type 2 diabetes with established nephropathy can allow the progression of their kidney disease. HbA1c levels, however, have been independently associated with a faster rate of decline of GFR in patients with established diabetic nephropathy. Option B is incorrect because the patient has a high risk of progression to ESRD. Option C is incorrect because no J-shaped curve—that is, a worse cardiovascular or renal outcome with progressively lower BP—has been demonstrated in those with diabetes. Option D is incorrect because the addition of an ARB to an ACE inhibitor can reduce proteinuria in some studies but has never been demonstrated to slow the progression of kidney disease. In contrast, in nondiabetic kidney disease, the COOPERATE study demonstrated combination therapy can slow progression.[1]

Additional laboratory tests performed on the patient demonstrate a hemoglobin of 10.1 g/dL with a serum iron of 92 mg/dL, a transferring saturation of 23%, and a ferritin of 130 ng/mL.

Clinical Presentation 25

Which of the following is *true* regarding therapy in this patient?

A. Treatment of anemia is associated with a higher rate of hospitalization.
B. Treatment of anemia can prevent the development of left ventricular failure.
C. Erythropoietin can accelerate the progression of kidney disease.

The correct answer is B

Comment: Option B is correct because studies have demonstrated that treatment of anemia can prevent the development of left ventricular hypertrophy. Option A is incorrect because treatment of anemia is associated with lower rates of hospitalization. Option C is incorrect because many studies have shown treatment with erythropoietin has no effect on the progression of kidney disease. Option D is incorrect because adverse consequences of anemia occur when hemoglobin levels are greater than 8 g/dL. Option E is incorrect but remains controversial. In a study by Hayashi et al., left ventricular mass index progressively decreased as hemoglobin was normalized, suggesting target hemoglobin should be higher than 11 g/dL.[1,2]

Clinical Presentation 26

A 19-year-old male has developed progressive kidney failure from type 1 diabetes diagnosed at age 7 years. His BP is currently 125/75 mm Hg on treatment with an ACE inhibitor, beta-blocker, and loop diuretic. Laboratory studies include a serum creatinine of 2.4 mg/dL, serum cholesterol of 298 mg/dL, serum albumin of 2.8 g/dL, calculated GFR of 40 mL/min/1.73 m^2, and a 24-hour urinary protein excretion of 5.3 g.

Which of the following is *true* regarding the therapy of this patient?

A. Dietary protein restriction would be of no benefit in slowing the progression of his kidney disease.
B. Dietary protein restriction is most effective in slowing progression in patients with the lowest GFR.
C. An initial reduction in proteinuria with dietary protein restriction in conjunction with aggressive BP control with agents that inhibit the renin-angiotensin system would be associated with a slower rate of progression.
D. Dietary protein restriction of 0.6 g/kg/day would likely be associated with a decrease in serum albumin.

The correct answer is C

Comment: The results of clinical trials of dietary protein restriction on slowing the progression of kidney disease have been mixed. In the primary analysis of the MDRD study, no beneficial effect of dietary protein restriction was seen, although there are a number of limitations of this trial. Nonetheless, other trials have demonstrated a beneficial effect in slowing the development of ESRD. Those with diabetes tend to have a more beneficial response in comparison to those without diabetes. Therefore, option A is incorrect. Option B is also incorrect because a post hoc analysis of the MDRD study showed the greatest beneficial effect of protein restriction in the patients with the highest initial levels of GFR. Option C is incorrect because the MDRD study demonstrated that an initial reduction in proteinuria was associated with a slower rate of progression. Option D is incorrect because this level of protein restriction should not have a negative impact on nutritional parameters.[1,2]

Clinical Presentation 27

A 19-year-old female is seen in your office for evaluation of elevated serum creatinine. She currently has hypertension. A kidney biopsy performed 2 years ago showed membranous glomerulonephritis. There was severe tubulointerstitial disease, and 10 to 15 glomeruli were globally sclerosed. At that time, her serum creatinine was 2.1 mg/dL, her calculated GFR using the Schwartz formula was 27 mL/min/1.73 m^2, serum cholesterol was 320 mg/dL, and she had a 24-hour urinary excretion of protein of 8.2 g.

Which of the following is true regarding her risk of developing progressive kidney failure?

A. Few glomerular were globally sclerosed; therefore, her renal prognosis is good.
B. The severity of tubulointerstitial disease is a good predictor of kidney disease progression.

C. Proteinuria is not a risk factor for the progression of kidney disease.
D. On the basis of the amount of proteinuria, she is unlikely to respond to an ACE inhibitor.

The correct answer is A

Comment: This patient has stage 4 CKD secondary to membranous glomerulonephritis. Tubulointerstitial disease accompanies most glomerular disease, and its severity is a major risk for subsequent renal disease progression. Therefore, option B is incorrect because the severity of tubulointerstitial disease is a stronger predictor of progression than the low number of globally sclerosed glomeruli in this patient. Option C is incorrect because proteinuria is another major risk factor for renal disease progression in almost all studied diseases. Option D is incorrect because the patients with the highest levels of proteinuria have the greatest response to ACE inhibitor therapy.[1]

Clinical Presentation 28

A 15-year-old male is seen in your office for an elevated serum creatinine level. He has focal segmental glomerulosclerosis diagnosed by renal biopsy at age 9 years when he presented with nephritic syndrome. On examination, his BP is 140/90 mm Hg, his pulse is 94 beats/min, and his weight is 68 kg. He has 2+ peripheral edema. Laboratory studies include a serum creatinine of 3.7 mg/dL compared with a value of 2.4 mg/dL 1 year ago. Urinalysis shows 4+ protein, negative for blood, and 0 to 2 red blood cells/high-power field. His 24-hour urine protein excretion is 6.2 g.

Which of the following statements is true regarding the pathophysiology of renal disease progression in this patient?

A. Increases in single-nephron GFR would not occur because of the presence of glomerulosclerosis.
B. Proteinuria can lead to glomerular scarring but has not been a pathogenic factor in the development of tubulointerstitial disease.
C. Increased ammonia genesis in surviving nephrons can lead to complement activation and enhanced tubulointerstitial disease.
D. Plasma renin activity is likely to be elevated and be a major factor in the pathogenesis of his hypertension.
E. Increased glomerular size blunts the adverse effects of the increased pressures and flows in the glomerulus.

The correct answer is C

Comment: Adaptations occur in surviving nephrons in an attempt to compensate for the loss of renal mass. One of these adaptations is increased ammoniagenesis. Ammonia can activate complement, which can be a risk factor in the development of tubulointerstitial disease. Option A is incorrect because the degree of glomerular involvement is heterogeneous and increases in single-nephron GFR is an adaptation that would occur in the less-damaged glomeruli. Option B is incorrect because reabsorption of protein in proximal tubule cells with their subsequent activation is felt to be a mechanism leading to tubulointerstitial disease. Option E is incorrect because it presents a paradox in thinking about chronic polycystic kidney disease (PKD). Plasma renin activity is suppressed in most chronic kidney diseases, yet inhibition of angiotensin II is a major renal protective strategy. The hypertension seen in kidney disease is related to mechanisms other than activation of the renin-angiotensin system.[1]

Clinical Presentation 29

A 7-year-old girl is found to have microscopic hematuria on a routine physical examination. Her mother and a maternal aunt are on hemodialysis for ESRD secondary to polycystic kidney disease. On examination, her BP is 115/65 mm Hg, pulse is 80 beats/min, and weight is 43 kg. Her serum creatinine is 0.4 mg/dL, and urinalysis shows specific gravity of 1.017, no protein, trace blood, and 5 to 10 red blood cells/high-power field. A spot urine protein/creatinine is 0.15 mg/mg. Estimated GFR by Schwartz study is 92 mL/min/1.73 m^2. Kidney ultrasound is normal.

Which of the following is true regarding her condition?

A. She does not have CKD because her BP, serum creatinine, and protein excretion are all normal.
B. She has CKD based on the finding of microscopic hematuria.
C. eGFR should be measured by 125 I-iothalamate clearance to accurately stage her CKD.
D. Estimated GFR by the Schwartz equation is inaccurate in children with CKD.

The correct answer is B

Comment: The presence of microscopic hematuria fits the definition of CKD (stage 1). Her calculated GFR based on the Schwartz equation is 90 mL/min/2.73 m^2, consistent with stage 2 CKD. Option A is incorrect for these reasons. Option C is incorrect because there is no evidence that the Schwartz study equation is not accurate in CKD patients. Option C is incorrect because measuring GFR by 125 I-iothalamate clearance is not clinically necessary.[1]

Clinical Presentation 30

A 14-year-old African American male presents with edema. His BP is 150/100 mm Hg. He is found to have a serum creatinine of 2.8 mg/dL and a urinary protein excretion of 16 g/24 hours. A renal biopsy shows focal and segmental glomerulosclerosis. He is started on an ACE inhibitor and a loop diuretic. One week later, his BP is 125 mm Hg, his urinary protein excretion has decreased to 3 g/day, but his serum creatinine has increased to 3.2 mg/dL.

Which of the following should be recommended?

A. Stop the ACE inhibitor, switch to a beta-blocker, and evaluate for renal artery stenosis.
B. Stop the loop diuretic.
C. Continue the current antihypertensive medication and recheck serum creatinine in 1 week.
D. Stop the ACE inhibitor and switch to an ARB.

The correct answer is C

Comment: This patient has responded to treatment with an ACE inhibitor with a decrease in BP and urinary protein excretion. His serum creatinine, however, has increased from 2.8 to 3.2 mg/dL. This is an approximate 13% increase in serum creatinine. ACE inhibitors are commonly associated with an increase in creatinine following initiation therapy because of a preferential effect on dilating the efferent arteriole. If the increase in serum creatinine is less than 30%, the ACE inhibitor can be continued with a recheck of serum creatinine. Option A is incorrect, for the reasons discussed previously. In patients with bilateral renal artery disease, serum creatinine can certainly go up on an ACE inhibitor, but it is usually more than a 30% increase, and it tends to be persistent. Option B is incorrect because it is unlikely that the loop diuretic is causing the increase in serum creatinine in the absence of evidence of volume depletion. Option D is incorrect because ARB and an ACE inhibitor are both likely to have a similar effect on an increase in serum creatinine.

Option E is incorrect because there is no evidence that steroids and cyclophosphamides are indicated in the treatment of this disease.[1]

Clinical Presentation 31

A 13-year-old male has biopsy-proven IgA nephropathy. His hypertension has been controlled with a loop diuretic, ACE inhibitors, and an ARB. Currently, his serum creatinine is 4.3 mg/dL and his 24-hour urinary protein excretion is 4.1 g. A fasting lipid profile shows the following values: cholesterol 244 mg/dL, triglyceride 270 mg/dL, high-density lipoprotein 45 mg/dL, and low-density lipoprotein (LDL) 16 mg/dL.

Which *one* of the following statements is true regarding his dyslipidemia?

A. Treatment with a statin can lower serum cholesterol but has no effect on LDL cholesterol.
B. Target LDL cholesterol should be <140 mg/dL.
C. The addition of a cholesterol absorption inhibitor (ezetimibe) to a statin has no additional benefit on lowering LDL cholesterol compared with the statin alone.
D. Treatment with a statin has been associated with a reduction in proteinuria.
E. Statin therapy in this patient has been demonstrated to decrease the time to a first major vascular event.

The correct answer is C

Comment: Treatment with a statin can lower both serum cholesterol, as well as LDL cholesterol, and is indicated in this patient with significant CKD.

There is evidence that the addition of ezetimibe cholesterol absorption inhibitor to a statin does have additional benefits in lowering LDL compared with the already being treated with an ACE inhibitor or ARB can decrease proteinuria and statin alone (SHARP study). Treatment with a statin in patients with CKD who are already being treated with ACE inhibitor or ARB can decrease proteinuria and stabilize creatinine clearance.[1]

Clinical Presentation 32

A 4-year-old girl is admitted to the hospital with failure to thrive. On examination, she is cachectic and has 2+ lower extremity pitting edema. Her serum creatinine is 1.0 mg/dL. A random spot urine protein-to-creatinine ratio is 2.6 g/g. A complete 24-hour urine collected during the second hospital day reveals 1.6 g of protein and 453 creatinine.

Which *one* of the following statements is *true*?

A. The patient has nephrotic range proteinuria.
B. There is contradictory information presented regarding whether or not the patient has nephrotic range proteinuria.
C. There is insufficient information to determine whether or not the patient has nephrotic range proteinuria.
D. The random spot urine protein-to-creatinine ratio is misleading because of the low creatinine production.
E. It is not valid to use protein-to-creatinine ratios to assess proteinuria when the serum albumin is low.

The correct answer is D

Comment: The patient's spot urine protein-to-creatinine ratio is misleading because the patient is cachectic and produces only approximately 453 mg of creatinine per day. Other mechanisms besides nephritic syndrome (such as malnutrition) are needed to account for this patient's low albumin and creatinine.[1]

Clinical Presentation 33

A 6-year-old boy was diagnosed with hypertension 2 years ago. His current serum creatinine is 2.3 mg/dL and his estimated GFR is 37 mL/min/1.73 m^2. His 24-hour urinary protein excretion is 0.6 g.

Which *one* of the following choices is *true* regarding his therapy?

A. Target mean arterial pressure of 92 mm Hg is more effective in preventing the progression of his kidney disease than a mean arterial pressure of 102 mm Hg.
B. A kidney biopsy is necessary for guiding therapy.
C. An ACE inhibitor is more effective than a beta-blocker in slowing the progression of kidney disease.
D. The type of antihypertensive does not affect kidney disease outcomes.
E. A dihydropyridine calcium channel blocker (CCB) is more effective than a beta-blocker in slowing the decline in GFR.

The correct answer is C

Comment: Previous studies examined the effects of BP lowering on the progression of hypertensive kidney disease. Patients were treated with either a beta-blocker, ACE inhibitor, or a dihydropyridine CCB. None of the drugs was associated with a difference in GFR slope. ACE inhibitors, however, decreased the risk of developing the clinical composite outcome by 22% compared with the beta-blocker and by 38% compared with the CCB. Thus, answers A, D, and E are incorrect. Answer B is incorrect because biopsies have demonstrated typical hypertensive nephrocalcinosis in patients with a clinical diagnosis of hypertension.[1]

Clinical Presentation 34

Which *one* of the following is *true* regarding cardiovascular disease (CVD) in patients with CKD?

A. Microalbuminuria is not a risk factor for CVD.
B. Most patients with CKD will die of CVD before they reach ESRD.
C. CKD is a risk factor for CVD but not for stroke or peripheral vascular disease.
D. A higher prevalence of CKD is a risk factor for CVD but not for stroke or peripheral vascular disease.

The correct answer is B

Comment: The presence of CKD is an independent predictor of CVD. The risk holds even mild elevation in the serum creatinine, or small decreases in GFR, and not for a serum creatinine greater than 3 mg/dL. Therefore, answer D is incorrect. Microalbuminuria is an independent risk factor for CVD and may be a more general marker of disordered function of the vascular endothelium. In a study of the Medicare population, Collins et al. demonstrated that patients with a diagnosis of CKD were 5 to 10 times more likely to die than to reach ESRD. Therefore, answer B is incorrect. Not only is CKD a risk factor for CVD, but recent analyses have also shown that the presence of CKD is a risk for both cerebral and peripheral vascular disease.[1,2]

Clinical Presentation 35

A 10-year-old girl has progressive kidney failure from biopsy-proven FSGS. Her current serum creatinine is 3.7 mg/dL and estimated GFR is 16 mL/min/1.73 m^2. The urine protein-to-creatinine ratio is 4560 mg/g. Other medical problems include hypertension, currently treated with furosemide 40 mg orally twice daily and lisinopril 40 mg once daily. Her BP is 160/85 mm Hg.

Which *one* of the following statements is correct?

A. The diastolic BP is the best predictor of renal outcome.
B. Target systolic BP should be 110 mm Hg to 129 mm Hg.
C. Systolic BP <110 mm Hg has been associated with a lower risk of kidney disease progression.
D. The addition of a dihydropyridine CCB should be avoided because of the risk of accelerating the progression of her renal disease.
E. Studies have proven that the level of BP does not affect the rate of loss of kidney function in hypertensive African Americans.

The correct answer is B
Comment: This patient has stage 4 CKD secondary to FSGS. Significant proteinuria is present and his BP is elevated. Controlling BP can slow the progression of kidney failure, although the exact target BP remains somewhat controversial. In a meta-analysis of 11 randomized control trials that compared the efficacy of antihypertensive treatment with or without an ACE inhibitor for patients with nondiabetic kidney disease, it was demonstrated that a systolic BP between 110 and 129 mm Hg was associated with the lowest risk of kidney disease progression. In this analysis, the systolic BP was not predictive of progression. Systolic BP less than 110 mm Hg was associated with a higher risk for kidney disease progression, making answers A and C incorrect. Dihydropyridine CCBs should not be the drugs of first choice in the setting of CKD because these drugs have been associated with greater amounts of proteinuria compared with ACE inhibitors or ARBs. When used in combination with an ACE or ARB, however, dihydropyridine CCBs can effectively lower BP and do not limit the antiproteinuric effects of the ACE inhibitor or ARB.[1]

Clinical Presentation 36

A 15-year-old healthy teenager was referred for further evaluation of persistent asymptomatic proteinuria of 2 years' duration. Urine dipstick examinations varied from 1+ to 3+ for protein throughout this period. Family history was noncontributory. Repeated physical examinations had been normal. Serum electrolytes, BUN, creatinine, protein, cholesterol, C3, C4, and antinuclear antibody (ANA) levels had been normal. A 24-hour urine protein excretion of 870 mg was clearly abnormal and prompted the referral. A renal ultrasound revealed a solitary left kidney. Urinalysis revealed clear yellow urine with a pH of 5.0 specific gravity 1.025, 2+ protein, and a negative sediment.

What treatment would you advise?

A. Prednisone alone
B. Prednisone and cyclosporine
C. Prednisone and cyclophosphamide
D. Prednisone plus mycophenolate mofetil
E. ACE inhibitor

The correct answer is E
Comment: Evaluation of proteinuria should begin with a careful history and thorough physical examination, urine microscopic examination, and determination of the amount of protein

excretion rate. The protein excretion rate has been traditionally measured using 24-hour urine collections. However, the collection of 24-hour urine is often cumbersome, and spot urinary protein-to-creatinine ratio (PCR), expressed in g/g or mg/mg, has become a simple and attractive yet reliable alternative. A spot urine PCR has been found to have a significant linear correlation with a 24-hour urine PCR. Furthermore, because the PCR compares urinary protein concentration with urinary creatinine concentration, urinary dilution or concentration does not influence this value.

Orthostatic proteinuria is diagnosed when the PCR is greater than 0.3 in a urine specimen tested during daytime activity but less than 0.3 when the urine is collected after the nighttime recumbent position.

Isolated persistent proteinuria lasting more than 6 months or proteinuria complicated with hematuria, hypertension, or abnormal renal function usually associated with glomerular lesions or congenital kidney and urinary tract anomalies such as unilateral kidney agenesis, obstructive hydronephrosis, and reflux nephropathy, which often require further evaluations including renal ultrasonography and voiding cystourethrogram.

If proteinuria is associated with glomerulonephritis, then referral to a pediatric nephrologist is warranted for possible renal biopsy indication.

Isolated persistent proteinuria (<1.0 g/day) not associated with hypertension, hematuria, or renal dysfunction can be treated with ACE inhibitors or ARBs with close follow-up.[1]

Clinical Presentation 37

ACE inhibitors are valuable in the treatment of CKD but must be stopped in 2 months if:

A. Serum creatinine exceeds 30% above baseline.
B. Hypercalcemia occurs (serum calcium >11 mg/dL).
C. Edema occurs.
D. Significant anemia occurs.

The correct answer is A

Comment: Renin-angiotensin system inhibitors are considered first-line agents for hypertensive patients with progressive CKD.

Stopping renin-angiotensin system inhibition in patients with CKD increases GFR and is associated with higher absolute risks of mortality and major adverse cardiovascular events, but also with a lower absolute risk of initiating renal replacement therapy.[1]

Clinical Presentation 38

A 14-year-old female develops gross hematuria and nonoliguric renal failure 5 days after the onset of severe, purulent tonsilitis. She had received azithromycin because of a penicillin allergy. Her urinalysis revealed 4+ proteinuria, >100 dysmorphic erythrocytes, 10 to 15 leukocytes per high-power field, and several red blood cell casts. The serum creatinine was 4.6 mg/dL. A renal biopsy revealed 20 glomeruli, two of which showed segmental crescents and one that showed global glomerulosclerosis. The remainder showed mild mesangial hypercellularity. The interstitium revealed moderate focal inflammation and edema. Many tubular lumina were filled with erythrocytes, and the lining epithelial cells showed focal detachment and necrosis or apoptosis. The immunofluorescence study was positive for diffuse mesangial IgA and IgG deposits along with C3 and focal deposits of fibrin/fibrinogen. Three days after the renal biopsy, her serum creatinine is 8.0 mg/dL.

What would you do next (select all that apply)?

A. Start 1.0 g/day intravenous methylprednisolone for 3 days, mycophenolate mofetil 2.0 g/day, and hemodialysis only as needed.
B. Start 1 mg/kg oral prednisone per day and 1.0 g/m^2 intravenous cyclophosphamide.
C. Start 1.0 mg/kg oral prednisone per day with oral cyclosporine.
D. Start 2.0 mg/kg prednisone with mycophenolate mofetil.

The correct answer is A

Comment: Rapidly progressive glomerulonephritis (RPGN), characterized by a rapid development of nephritis with loss of kidney function in days or weeks, is typically associated histologically, with crescents in most glomeruli, and is a challenging problem, particularly in low-resource settings. RPGN is a diagnostic and therapeutic emergency requiring prompt evaluation and treatment to prevent poor outcomes. Histopathologically, RPGN consists of four major categories, anti-glomerular basement membrane (GBM) disease, immune complex mediated, pauci-immune disorders, and idiopathic/overlap disorders. Clinical manifestations include gross hematuria, proteinuria, oliguria, hypertension, and edema. Diagnostic evaluation, including renal function tests, electrolytes, urinalysis/microscopy, and serology including (anti-GBM antibody, antineutrophil cytoplasmic antibody) starts simultaneously with management. An urgent renal biopsy is required to allow specific pathologic diagnosis as well as to assess disease activity and chronicity to guide specific treatment. The current guidelines for the management of pediatric RPGN are adopted from adult experience and consist of induction and maintenance therapy. Aggressive combination immunosuppression has markedly improved outcomes; however, nephrotic syndrome, severe acute kidney injury requiring dialysis, presence of fibrous crescents, and chronicity are predictors of poor renal survival. RPGN-associated with postinfectious glomerulonephritis usually has a good prognosis in children without immunosuppression, whereas immune-complex-mediated glomerulonephritis and lupus nephritis are associated with poor prognosis with development of end-stage kidney disease in more than 50% and 30%, respectively.[1]

Clinical Presentation 39

A 17-year-old male with a rapidly progressive form of IgA nephropathy is placed on regular hemodialysis therapy for end-stage kidney disease. His brother, aged 22 years, and an older adopted brother, aged 24 years, both offer to donate a kidney. Both potential donors are healthy and have completely normal pretransplant medical evaluations.

The older adopted brother is a two-antigen mismatch, whereas the younger brother is also a two-antigen mismatch (single haplotype match) with the patient.

Which *one* of the following choices would you recommend to the patient (select all that apply)?

A. Renal transplantation is not appropriate because of the high risk of recurrence of IgA nephropathy and subsequent graft failure.
B. Renal transplantation from the adopted sibling is preferred because of a lower risk of recurrence of IgA nephropathy and a superior graft survival.
C. Renal transplantation from the adopted sibling is preferred because of a lower risk of recurrence of IgA nephropathy and equivalent graft survival.
D. Renal transplantation should be delayed until bilateral nephrectomy of the recipient is performed.
E. Renal transplantation from a cadaver donor is preferred; neither sibling should be used as a donor.

The correct answer is B

Comment: In recent years, major genome-wide association studies have provided significant insight into the genetic basis of IgA nephropathy. Patients typically have high levels of aberrantly O-glycosylated IgA1 molecules, which become targets of an autoantibody response, leading to immune complex formation. These deposit in the mesangium and spark off an unhindered immune response, ultimately leading to fibrosis and kidney failure.

To date, genome-wide association studies for IgA nephropathy have successfully identified many risk loci with candidate genes involved in antigen processing and presentation, gut mucosal immunity, IgA biology, and dysregulation of the alternative complement pathway.

An overall genetic risk can be computed with these genome-wide significant susceptibility variants and has been shown to inversely correlate with age of diagnosis. Interestingly, the IgA nephropathy genetic risk score is strongly associated with global pathogen diversity, suggesting that the selective pressure from environmental factors may account for variation in risk allele frequency and the geographic variation in disease prevalence among world populations.[1]

There is significant variability of up to 30% in the incidence of recurrence of IgA nephropathy after transplantation. Recurrence is associated with a higher risk of graft failure and is more common in younger patients with rapidly progressive, crescentic disease in their native kidneys.[2]

Because the risk of allele frequency in disease prevalence among the general population is considerably lower than related donors, kidney transplantation from the adopted sibling is preferred for transplantation in IgA patients with ESRD.[3,4]

Clinical Presentation 40

You are asked to see a 16-year-old female in the emergency department with hypercalcemia and kidney failure. She notes the onset of mild polyuria and nocturia 6 to 8 months earlier. Headache, constipation, and malaise became apparent approximately 6 weeks earlier. She began using a tanning salon 4 weeks before. Yesterday, she visited her mother, who noted that she was "not herself" and seemed confused. Her mother brought her to the emergency room for evaluation. Medical history is significant for passing a single kidney calculus 2 years before. She has a 1-year history of mild hypertension, for which was treated with hydrochlorothiazide, 50 mg/d. She does not smoke or drink alcohol. She denies the use of any other medications or over-the-counter supplements. She denies any hormonal therapy and avoids all dairy products. On examination, she appears in no acute distress. Her blood pressure is 140/92 mm Hg; pulse, 86/minute; respiratory rate, 12/minute; body temperature, 37°C; body weight, 62.5 kg; and height, 159 cm. Heart rate is regular with no murmurs, the lungs are clear, the abdomen is soft with no masses, and there is no pitting edema. Neurological examination shows mild depression and some cognitive dysfunction. Laboratory studies show the following: hematocrit, 46%; leukocyte count, 5.6×10^9/L; BUN, 61 mg/dL; serum creatinine, 3.0 mg/dL; serum sodium, 140 mEq/L; serum potassium, 3.9 mEq/L; serum chloride, 101 mEq/L; serum bicarbonate, 22 mEq/L; serum calcium, 13.8 mg/dL; serum phosphate, 3.9 mg/dL; serum magnesium, 1.9 mg/dL; and serum albumin, 4.2 g/dL. Urinalysis shows trace protein, no glucose, no blood, 2 to 4 hyaline casts per high-power field, but no erythrocytes or leukocytes.

Which of the following treatment modalities would you like to order now (select all that may apply)?

A. Calcitonin
B. Intravenous saline solution
C. Surgical consult
D. Mitramycin
E. Pamidronate/zoledronate

The correct answers are A, B, and E

Comment: The initial treatment of symptomatic hypercalcemia should have three elements to provide some efficacy, both initially and several days later. Virtually all patients with significant hypercalcemia have some element of extracellular fluid volume contraction. For this reason, it is important to start therapy with intravenous saline (option B).[1,2]

Calcitonin is effective in approximately 70% of patients. It is safe and relatively nontoxic, and it acts to lower serum calcium within several hours. For this reason, it should be the initial agent of choice to provide some benefit before the more potent bisphosphonates become maximally effective (option A). It typically loses its effectiveness within hours in most patients. For this reason, it is important to begin therapy with a bisphosphonate at this time, as well (option E).

Bisphosphonates block the hypocalciuric effect of PTH. They act by interfering with the metabolic activity of osteoclasts; they are cytotoxic to osteoclasts. Pamidronate, zoledronic acid, and etidronate are the currently available agents that are recommended for the treatment of malignancy-associated hypercalcemia. Zoledronate appears to be the most efficacious, with a maximum effect occurring in 48 to 72 hours.[1,2]

Clinical Presentation 41

Pediatric kidney transplant recipients are different from adult recipients regarding primary kidney diseases, surgical techniques, drug metabolism, adherence to medications, growth and neurocognitive development, and immunization needs before transplantation.

According to the Recommendation, Assessment, Development and Evaluation (GRADE) approach, which of the following statements is *not* recommended for the management of pediatric kidney transplant recipients (select all that apply)?

A. Lymphocyte-depleting therapy (thymoglobulin, antithymocyte globulin) with a dose of 1.5 mg/kg for induction in kidney transplant recipients with high immunologic risk (PRA > 80%), multiple blood transfusions, and those with a history of graft rejections within the first year after transplantation.

B. Screening for diabetes by oral glucose tolerance test in candidates who are not known to have diabetes.

C. All kidney transplant recipients should be vaccinated against tetanus, hepatitis B, meningococcal, pneumococcal, *Haemophilus influenza*, poliomyelitis, influenza, mumps (hepatitis B virus surface antigen), hepatitis B surface antibody, and hepatitis B core antibody.

D. Screening patients for HIV infection with HIV serology tests.

E. All kidney transplant recipients should receive prophylaxis with daily sulfamethoxazole-trimethoprim 5 mg/kg (trimethoprim component) to a maximum dose of 800/160 mg/d for 6 months after transplantation and also for 6 weeks during and after treatment of acute rejection.

F. Patients with recurrent antineutrophil cytoplasmic antibody-associated vasculitis or anti-GBM disease.

G. Treatment with an ACE inhibitor or an ARB in patients with recurrent glomerulonephritis and proteinuria.

H. Interleukin 2 receptor antagonist (basiliximab) for induction in patients with low immunological risk PRA (<20% and no donor specific antigen [DSA]) or intermediate risk (PRA between 20% and 80%, with no DSA) with a dose of 1.5 mg/kg or 12 mg/m^2 (maximum, 20 mg) diluted with 50 mL 0.9% saline, injected intravenously over 20 to 30 minutes, 2 hours before transplantation, and repeated on third and fourth posttransplantation days.

I. Lymphocyte-depleting therapy (thymoglobulin, antithymocyte globulin) with a dose of 1.5 mg/kg for induction in kidney transplant recipients with high immunologic risk (PRA > 80%), multiple blood transfusions, and those with a history of graft rejections within the first year after transplantation.

The correct answers are F and G

Comment: A recent systematic review on the evaluation and management of pediatrics examined 317 citations, of which 132 papers were selected for analysis and 62 were included in final analysis.[1] The studies are categorized on the basis of GRADE. The overall quality of evidence is categorized as high (A), moderate (B), low (C), or poor (D). The strength of a recommendation was determined as level 1 (recommended) or level 2 (suggested). The ungraded statements were determined on the basis of common sense to provide general advice on the basis of study design and all intervention outcomes of interest are as follows: A, B, C, or D translating to high, moderate, low, and very low, respectively.

Of 115 statements, 56 (48.6%) were graded 1 (we recommend), 34 (29.5%) were graded 2 (we suggest), and 25 (21.7%) were ungraded statements. Altogether, only 22 (19.1%) of the recommendations achieved the “A” or “B” level.

Using the GRADE system, in our clinical presentation, options A, B, C, D, and E are categorized as A and highly recommended.[1] Options F and G are categorized as poor (D) and are not recommended. Options H and I are categorized as moderate (B) and are suggested.

Clinical Presentation 42

A 12-year-old boy treated with hemodialysis presents with a serum calcium level of 10.7 mg/dL, phosphate of 5.9 mg/dL, iPTH level of 1065 pg/mL, and a parathyroid gland weight of 5.0 g as determined by ultrasonography. Previous attempts with oral calcitriol therapy to suppress PTH had produced a 15% fall in PTH levels.

Which of the following treatments should be ordered next?

A. Aggressive use of sevelamer to lower serum phosphate level.
B. Intravenous calcitriol (1.0 μg) at the time of dialysis treatment.
C. Intravenous 25 (OH) vitamin D.
D. Parathyroidectomy.

The correct answer is D

Comment: The indications for parathyroidectomy include: (1) hypercalcemia and hyperphosphatemia in the presence of very high PTH level (>800 pg/mL) with failure to lower PTH levels after 6 to 8 weeks of vitamin D analog and/or calcimimetics therapy; (2) fractures and tendon avulsions; (3) calcific arteriolopathy; and (4) hypertrophied gland and weight >4.0 g as determined by ultrasonography.[1]

Clinical Presentation 43

A 7-year-old boy with dialysis-dependent ESRD and chronic hip pain had an MRI scan that revealed aseptic necrosis attributed to previous glucocorticoid therapy for asthma. Two hours after the MRI, he had his scheduled hemodialysis treatment. His predialysis serum calcium was 5.4 mg/dL, phosphorus 5.6 mg/dL, and albumin 3.6 g/dL. He has been closely followed for moderate secondary hyperparathyroidism and has received vitamin D supplementation.

Which is the *most* likely explanation for these findings?

A. Gadodiamide (Omniscan)-induced spurious hypocalcemia.
B. Parathyroid infarction.
C. Gadopentetate (Magnevist)-induced spurious hypocalcemia.
D. Inadvertent barium administration.

The correct answer is A

Comment: Gadodiamide binds with colorimetric agents used in assaying serum calcium and produces spurious hypocalcemia. Parathyroid infarct is a rare event. Gadopentetate does not produce the same effect. Barium administration is associated with hypokalemia, and barium sulfate used in radiologic studies does not enter the circulation. A defective laboratory instrument is always possible, but gadodiamide predictably produces this artificial finding.[1]

Clinical Presentation 44

A 19-year-old female patient has been treated with hemodialysis for the past 14 years after rejection of a cadaver transplant. Her original disease was Henoch-Schoenlein purpura. She now presents with ascending pain and weakness in her hands and feet. There are prominent contractures of her extremities that have caused her to become bedridden over the past 4 months. Her major problems associated with hemodialysis had been hyperphosphatemia (7–8.5 mg/dL) and hypercalcemia (10–11 mg/dL) after vitamin D therapy. Her PTH levels are mildly elevated at 56 pg/mL, although they have been substantially higher in the past. A workup for collagen vascular disease, including vasculitis, has been negative, as have Lyme titer and thyroid function tests. Blood glucose has never been elevated. Electromyography and nerve conduction studies are normal. Muscle biopsy shows atrophy and intramuscular calcification.

What is the most likely cause of this condition?

A. Uremic myopathy
B. Mitochondrial myopathy
C. Scleroderma
D. Calcific uremic arteriopathy
E. Recurrent Henoch Schonlein purpura (HSP)

The correct answer is D

Comment: In its most florid form, calcific vasculopathy may be manifested as calciphylaxis. A small fraction of patients with ESRD, particularly those treated with dialysis, develop deep skin ulcerations in association with calcification of subcutaneous arterioles. Uremic peripheral neuropathy is a distal, symmetrical, mixed sensorimotor. It occurs more commonly in men, and it is independent of the underlying disease. There is no specific myopathy associated with uremia.

Arthralgia and myalgias characterize diffuse scleroderma. Early diffuse cutaneous systemic sclerosis includes arthritic symptoms. A specific myopathy is not seen. Recurrent HSP does not manifest a specific myopathic picture, as seen in this case.[1]

Clinical Presentation 45

A 14-year-old male patient begins hemodialysis treatments under your care. His original disease was FSGS. Physical examination is unremarkable. His serum calcium is 9.7 mg/dL, phosphate 6.1 mg/dL, and PTH 340 pg/mL. To optimize his management, you initiate therapy with sevelamer hydrochloride to maintain his serum phosphate level within an acceptable range.

Which of the following statements BEST describes the likely response of this patient to sevelamer hydrochloride in comparison with calcium acetate?

A. Sevelamer hydrochloride will be more effective in reducing serum phosphate levels.
B. Calcium acetate will be more effective in reducing serum phosphate levels.
C. Sevelamer hydrochloride will be effective at reducing PTH levels.
D. Sevelamer hydrochloride use will result in less hyperchloremia as a later complication.

The correct answer is D

Comment: Sevelamer hydrochloride (Renagel) significantly lowers serum phosphorous in hemodialysis patients but with minimal effects on serum calcium in comparison to treatment with standard calcium-based phosphate binders. Patients with the highest PTH levels (>300 pg/mL) experienced the greatest reduction in PTH. The effect on PTH levels, however, may be inconsistent.[1]

Clinical Presentation 46

An 18-year-old female maintained on hemodialysis for the past 6 years because of congenital kidney dysplasia presents with a large necrotic lesion on the skin of her upper thigh. She is obese, has mild glucose intolerance and poorly controlled hypertension, and has been receiving large doses of iron dextran and erythropoietin for resistant anemia as well as enalapril for hypertension. Her serum phosphate level has ranged from 6 to 9 mg/dL, serum albumin from 2.2 to 2.9 g/dL, and serum calcium from 8.8 to 9.0 mg/dL. Serum magnesium is 2.6 mg/dL, alkaline phosphatase 165 IU/L, and serum PTH 450 pg/mL. A biopsy of her skin lesion reveals medial calcification and intimal hyperplasia of the small arteries and fat necrosis.

Which of her clinical characteristics is a key risk factor for this condition?

A. Iron dextrin therapy
B. Hypertension
C. Hypomagnesemia
D. Hyperphosphatemia
E. Erythropoietin therapy

The correct answer is D

Comment: Hyperphosphatemia is the strongest predictor of calciphylaxis in patients receiving hemodialysis treatment. There is a 3.5-fold increase in the risk of calciphylaxis associated with each 1-mg/dL increase in the serum phosphate concentrations. Body mass index, diabetes, hypertension, hypomagnesemia, aluminum, and higher dosages of erythropoietin and iron dextran are not independent predictors of calciphylaxis.[1]

Clinical Presentation 47

A 9-year-old patient with a 5-year history of chronic hemodialysis for the treatment of FSGS begins to complain of bone pain and muscle weakness. The workup of the patient revealed the following: serum calcium 9.2 mg/dL, PO_4 5.2 mg/dL, intact PTH level 250 pg/mL, and plasma aluminum 433 g/dL. Bone mineral density was reduced with a total *Z* score (standard deviation from the mean of a healthy, age- and gender-matched reference population) of −1.25.

Which of the following should be done now?

A. Bone biopsy
B. 1,25 (OH)2 vitamin D measurement
C. Bone-specific alkaline phosphatase measurement
D. Procollagen-carboxy-terminal propeptide level
E. 2-microglobulin level

The correct answer is A

Comment: This patient's clinical picture is consistent with low turnover bone disease; therefore, aluminum toxicity must be considered. In the presence of significant aluminum exposure, bone biopsy seems indicated in the following cases: before parathyroidectomy and before starting long desferrioxamine treatment, given the risks of deafness and fatal mucormycosis as complications of treatment. Bone alkaline phosphatase is not sensitive enough to distinguish between low and normal turnover. Procollagen-carboxy-terminal propeptide is not a specific indicator of bone disease because it is not well-controlled with bone histology.[1]

Clinical Presentation 48

A 12-year-old male patient on maintenance hemodialysis is referred to you from an outside hospital for help with treating his renal osteodystrophy. The patient has been poorly compliant with his phosphate binders and has multiple PTH measurements in the 1400 pg/mL range. He has also had a fractured fibula after minor trauma. The referring nephrologist has tried to suppress the patient's PTH levels with intravenous calcitriol but has produced hypercalcemia to 12.5 mg/dL on several occasions.

In reviewing a number of treatment options, which would you recommend to the patient?

A. 22-oxacalcitriol because it will likely prove more beneficial than calcitriol
B. Paricalcitol because it will likely prove more beneficial than calciferol
C. Parathyroidectomy should be performed.
D. 1-Alfa-hydroxyvitamin D2 because it will likely prove more beneficial than calcitriol
E. 1-Alfa hydroxyvitamin D3 because it will likely prove more beneficial than calcitriol

The correct answer is C

Comment: The indications for parathyroidectomy, 2 of which apply to this patient, have classically included (1) hypercalcemia and hyperphosphatemia in the presence of very high PTH levels (>800 pg/mL), as in this patient, with concurrent resistance to pharmacologic control; (2) fractures and tendon avulsions; (3) when the estimated weight of a parathyroid gland exceeds 1 g; and (4) calcific arteriolopathy, which some experts have considered to be an absolute indication.[1]

Clinical Presentation 49

A 10-year-old boy was referred to you for evaluation and treatment of persistent postrenal transplant hypophosphatemia. He has been treated with cyclosporine and prednisone but has complained of some persistent muscle aches. Physical examination was unremarkable except for mild proximal muscle weakness in the lower extremities. He is on no medications except for his immunosuppressive agents. Laboratory values revealed the following: creatinine 1.2 mg/dL, calcium 9.6 mg/dL, phosphate 2.1 mg/dL, intact PTH 38 pg/mL, and fractional excretion of phosphate 28%.

Which of the following is the most likely cause of his renal phosphate wasting?

A. PTH
B. Cyclosporine
C. Phosphatonin
D. 1,25 (OH)2 D3
E. Glucocorticoids

The correct answer is C

Comment: Green et al. studied the mechanism of posttransplant hypophosphatemia and found that sera from hypophosphatemic posttransplant patients inhibited PO_4 transport in vitro in a PTH-independent mechanism. This finding is consistent with the concept that there are PTH-independent humoral agents (phosphating) that dramatically reduce PO_4 reabsorption, and they may underline disorders of phosphate transport, as seen in oncogenic osteomalacia.[1]

Cyclosporine does not produce phosphate wasting, nor does 1,25 (OH)2 D3. Glucocorticoids are phosphaturic but do not produce the severe degree of phosphate wasting seen in this case.

Clinical Presentation 50

Which *one* of the following statements is *true* regarding the effective prevention of hyperphosphatemia in patients receiving adequate dialysis therapy?

A. Calcitriol administration does not alter dietary phosphate absorption.
B. Avoiding processed foods will reduce phosphate absorption.
C. Avoiding meat-derived phosphate will be more beneficial than avoiding plant-derived phosphate.
D. $CaCO_3$ is less effective than sevelamer hydrochloride for the control of serum phosphorus.

The correct answer is C

Comment: Any evaluation of dietary phosphorus adequacy should consider not only the content of phosphorus in food but also the bioavailability of phosphorus because most phosphorus in plants is in the form of phytate. Because humans do not have the phytase enzyme that is required to degrade phytate and to release phosphorus, phytate is poorly digested in the human gastrointestinal tract and therefore limits phosphorus absorption from plant sources. Phosphorus in meat is well-absorbed because it is found mostly as intracellular organic compounds that are easily hydrolyzed in the gastrointestinal tract, releasing inorganic phosphorus for absorption.[1]

Clinical Presentation 51

A 15-year-old male is evaluated for muscle weakness and bone pain over the past 5 months. Physical examination reveals marked proximal myopathy but no other abnormalities. Laboratory studies reveal the following: calcium 10.2 mg/dL, phosphorous 1.2 mg/dL, immunoreactive PTH 23 pg/mL (normal, 10–65 pg/mL), 1,25 (OH)2 vitamin D 8 pg/mL (normal, 10–55 pg/mL), and tubular reabsorption of phosphate 75% (normal, 90%). A computed tomography scan shows a 3-cm × 4-cm tumor of the right thigh.

The tumor is removed and the patient fully recovers.

Which of the following is involved in the pathogenesis of hyperphosphaturia in this patient?

A. PTH-related protein
B. Overproduction of fibroblast growth factor 23 (FGF-23)
C. Overproduction of stanniocalcin
D. Calcitonin
E. 25 OH vitamin D

The correct answer is B

Comment: Recent evidence suggests that the tumor product responsible for the phosphaturic action is FGF-23, a member of a large family of proteins involved in regulating fibroblast function. In oncogenic osteomalacia, there is an overproduction of FGF-23. In hereditary X-linked hypophosphatemic rickets, there is a mutation in an endopeptidase that normally inactivates FGF-23 and prevents high levels of the cytokine from migrating from bone to act systemically and in the kidney. In autosomal dominant hypophosphatemic rickets, there are mutations in the gene encoding FGF-23 so that it is functional.[1]

References

Clinical Presentation 1

1. Assadi F, Ghane Sharbaf F, eds. *Pediatric Continuous Renal Replacement Therapy: Principles and Practice.* New York, NY: Springer; 2016. https://doi.org/10.1007/978-3-319-26202-4.

Clinical Presentation 2

1. Allon M. Prophylaxis against dialysis catheter-related bacteremia with a novel antimicrobial lock solution. *Clin Infect Dis.* 2003;36:1539–1544.

Clinical Presentation 3

1. Konings C, Kooman JP, Schonck M, et al. Effect of icodextrin on volume status, BP and echocardiographic parameters: a randomized study. *Kidney Int.* 2004;63:1556–1563.

Clinical Presentation 4

1. Marenzi G, Marana I, Lauri G, et al. The prevention of radiocontrast-agent-induced nephropathy by hemofiltration. *N Engl J Med.* 2003;349:1333–1340.
2. Okada S, Katagiri K, Kumazaki T, et al. Safety of gadolinium contrast agent in hemodialysis patients. *Acta Radiol.* 2001;42:339–348.

Clinical Presentation 5

1. Beaubien ER, Pylypchuk GB, Akhtar J, et al. Value of corrected QT interval dispersion in identifying patients initiating dialysis at increased risk of total and cardiovascular mortality. *Am J Kidney Dis.* 2002;39:834–842.
2. Nappi SE, Virtanen VK, Saha HHT, et al. QT dispersion increases during hemodialysis with low-calcium dialysate. *Kidney Int.* 2000;57:2117–2122.

Clinical Presentation 6

1. Hurot JM, Cucherat M, Haugh M, et al. Effects of L-carnitine supplementation in maintenance hemodialysis patients: a systematic review. *J Am Soc Nephrol.* 2002;13:708–714.

Clinical Presentation 7

1. Depner TA. Daily hemodialysis efficiency: an analysis of solute kinetics. *Adv Ren Replace Ther.* 2002;8:227–235.
2. Frankenfield DL, McClellan WM, Helgerson SD, et al. Relationship between urea reduction ratio, demographic characteristics, and body weight for patients in 1996 National ESRD Core Indicators Project. *Am J Kidney Dis.* 1999;33:584–591.

Clinical Presentation 8

1. Beathard GA. Management of bacteremia associated with tunneled-cuffed hemodialysis catheters. *J Am Soc Nephrol.* 1999;10:1049–1051.

Clinical Presentation 9

1. Dheenan S, Henrich WL. Preventing dialysis hypotension: a comparison of usual protective measures. *Kidney Int.* 2001;59:1175–1181.

Clinical Presentation 10

1. Baker M, Perazella MA. NSAIDs in CKD: are they safe? *Am J Kidney Dis.* 2020;76(4):546–557. https://doi.org/10.1053/j.ajkd.2020.03.023.

Clinical Presentation 11

1. Baker M, Perazella MA. NSAIDs in CKD: are they safe? *Am J Kidney Dis.* 2020;76(4):546–557. https://doi.org/10.1053/j.ajkd.2020.03.023.

Clinical Presentation 12

1. Becker BN, Odorico JS, Becker YT, et al. Simultaneous pancreas-kidney and pancreas transplantation. *J Am Soc Nephrol.* 2001;12:2527 –2527.
2. Rayhill SC, D'Alessandro AM, Odorico JS, et al. Simultaneous pancreas-kidney transplantation and living donor renal transplant in patients with diabetes: is there a difference in survival? *Ann Surg.* 2000;231:417–423.

Clinical Presentation 13

1. Euvrad S, Kanitakis J, Claudy A. Skin cancer after organ transplantation. *N Engl J Med.* 2003;348:1681–1689.

Clinical Presentation 14

1. Kahan BD, Napoli KL, Podbielski J, et al. Therapeutic drug monitoring for optimal renal transplant outcomes. *Transplant Proc.* 2001;33:1278–1285.

Clinical Presentation 15

1. Singer SJ, Tiernan R, Sullivan EJ. Interstitial pneumonitis associated with sirolimus therapy in renal transplant recipients. *N Engl J Med.* 2000;343:1815–1816.

Clinical Presentation 16

1. Kendrick E. Cardiovascular disease and the renal transplant recipient. *Am J Kidney Dis.* 2001;38:S36–S43.

Clinical Presentation 17

1. Ersoy A, Dilek K, Usta M, et al. Angiotensin-II receptor antagonist losartan reduces microalbuminuria in hypertensive renal transplant recipients. *Clin Transplant.* 2002;16:202–205.
2. Hernandez D, Lacalzada J, Salido E, et al. Regression of left ventricular hypertrophy by lisinopril after renal transplantation: role of ACE gene polymorphism. *Kidney Int.* 2000;58:889–897.
3. MacDonald AS. A worldwide, phase III, randomized, controlled, safety and efficacy study of a sirolimus/cyclosporine regimen for prevention of acute rejection in recipients of primary mismatched renal allografts. *Transplantation.* 2001;71:271–280.
4. Yango A, Morrissey P, Gohl R, Wahbeh A. Donor-transmitted paravirus infection in a kidney transplant recipient presenting as pancytopenia and allograft dysfunction. *Transpl Infect Dis.* 2002;4:163–166.

Clinical Presentation 18

1. Assadi F, Hooman N, Seyedzadeh A, et al. Revisiting the management of pediatric kidney transplants, a multicenter analysis. *Iran J Kidney Dis.* 2022;16(6):319–329.

Clinical Presentation 19

1. Dillon JJ. Treating IgA nephropathy. *J Am Soc Nephrol.* 2001;12:846–847.

Clinical Presentation 20

1. Hels CN. Suicide of the nephron. *Lancet.* 2001;357:136–137.
2. Nath K. The tubulointerstitium in progressive renal disease. *Kidney Int.* 1998;54:992–1456.

Clinical Presentation 21

1. National Kidney Foundation. K/DOQI clinical practice guidelines for chronic kidney disease: evaluation, classification, and stratification. *Am J Kidney Dis.* 2002;39(2 Suppl 1):S1–S266.

Clinical Presentation 22

1. Caravaca F, Arrobas M, Pizarro JL, et al. Metabolic acidosis in advanced renal failure: differences between diabetic and nondiabetic patients. *Am J Kidney Dis.* 1999;33:892–898.

Clinical Presentation 23

1. Slatopolsky E, Burke SK, Dillon MA, et al. Renagel, a nonabsorbed calcium-and aluminum-free phosphate binder, lowers serum phosphorus and parathyroid hormone. *Kidney Int.* 1999;55:299–307.

Clinical Presentation 24

1. Levin A, Thompson C, Ethier J, et al. Left ventricular mass index increase in early renal disease: impact of decline in hemoglobin. *Am J Kid Dis.* 1999;34:125–134.
2. Ritz E, Orth SR. Nephropathy in patients with type 2 diabetes mellitus. *N Engl J Med.* 1999;341:1127–1151.

Clinical Presentation 25

1. Hayashi T, Suzuki A, Shoji T, et al. Cardiovascular effect of normalizing the hematocrit level during erythropoietin therapy in predialysis patients with chronic renal failure. *Am J Kidney Dis.* 2000;36:250–356.
2. Levin A, Thompson CR, Ethier J, et al. Left ventricular mass index increase in early renal disease: impact of decline in hemoglobin. *Am J Kidney Dis.* 1999;34:125–134.

Clinical Presentation 26

1. Levey AS, Greene T, Beck GJ, et al. Dietary protein restriction and the progression of chronic renal disease: what have all of the results of the MDRD study shown? *J Am Soc Nephrol.* 1999;10:2436–2439.
2. Pedrini MT, Levey AS, Lau J, et al. The effect of dietary protein restriction on the progression of diabetic and non-diabetic renal disease: a meta-analysis. *Ann Intern Med.* 1996;124:267–637.

Clinical Presentation 27

1. Keane WF. Proteinuria: its clinical importance and role in progressive renal disease. *Am J Kidney Dis.* 2000;35:S97–S105.

Clinical Presentation 28

1. Hales CN. Suicide of the nephron. *Lancet.* 2001;357:136–137.

Clinical Presentation 29

1. Ecder T, Edelstein CL, Fick-Brosnahan GM, et al. Diuretics versus angiotensin-converting enzyme inhibitors in autosomal dominant polycystic kidney disease. *Am J Nephrol.* 2002;21:98–103.

Clinical Presentation 30

1. Bakris GL, Weir MR. Angiotensin-converting enzyme inhibitor-associated elevations in serum creatinine. Is this a cause for concern? *Arch Intern Med.* 2000;160:685–693.

Clinical Presentation 31

1. Baigent C, Landry M. Study of Heart and Renal Protection (SHARP). *Kidney Int.* 2003;63:S207–S210.

Clinical Presentation 32

1. Hogg RJ, Portman RJ, Millimer D. Evaluation of proteinuria and nephritic syndrome in children: recommendations from a pediatric nephrology panel established at National Kidney Foundation conference on proteinuria, albuminuria, risk, detection, and elimination (PARDE). *Pediatrics.* 2000;105:1242–1249.

Clinical Presentation 33

1. Wright JT, Glassock R, Herbet I, et al. Effect of BP lowering and antihypertensive drug class on progression of hypertensive kidney disease: results from the AASK trial. *JAMA.* 2002;288:2421–2431.
2. Fogo AG. Hypertensive risk factors in kidney disease in African Americans. *Kidney Int.* 2003;63:2331–2341.

Clinical Presentation 34

1. Collins AJ, Li S, Gilbertson DT, et al. Chronic kidney disease and cardiovascular disease in Medicare population. *Kidney Int.* 2003;87:S24–S31.

2. Ritz E, McClellan W. Overview: increased cardiovascular risk in patients with minor renal dysfunction: an emerging issue with far-reaching consequences. *J Am Soc Nephrol.* 2004;15:513–516.

Clinical Presentation 35

1. Barkis GL, Weir MR, Seic M, et al. Differential effects of calcium antagonist subclasses on markers of nephropathy progression. *Kidney Int.* 2004;65:1991–2002.

Clinical Presentation 36

1. Mazaheri M, Assadi F. Simplified algorithm for evaluation of proteinuria in clinical practice: how should a clinician approach? *Int J Prev Med.* 2019;10:35. https://doi.org/10.4103/ijpvm.IJPVM_557_18.

Clinical Presentation 37

1. Assadi F. Rising serum potassium and creatinine concentrations after prescribing renin-angiotensin-aldosterone system blockade: how much should we worry? *World J Pediatr.* 2021;17(5):552–554. https://doi.org/10.1007/s12519-021-00455-8.

Clinical Presentation 38

1. Naik RH, Shawar SH. Rapidly progressive glomerulonephritis. In: *StatPearls.* Treasure Island, FL: StatPearls Publishing; 2023.

Clinical Presentation 39

1. Prakash S, Gharavi AG. Assessing genetic risk for IgA nephropathy. *CJASN.* 2021;16(2):182–184. https://doi.org/10.2215/CJN.19491220.
2. Chadban SJ, Ahn C, Axelrod DA, et al. KDIGO clinical practice guideline on the evaluation and management of candidates for kidney transplantation. *Transplantation.* 2020;104(4S1 Suppl 1):S11–S103. https://doi.org/10.1097/TP.0000000000003136.
3. Voiculescu A, Ivens K, Hetzel GR, et al. Kidney transplantation from related and unrelated living donors in a single German centre. *Nephrol Dialysis Transplant.* 2003;18(2):418–425. https://doi.org/10.1093/ndt/18.2.418.
4. Simmons RL, Thompson EJ, Kjellstrand CM, et al. Parent-to-child and child-to-parent kidney transplants. Experience with 101 transplants at one centre. *Lancet.* 1976;1(7955):321–324. https://doi.org/10.1016/s0140-6736(76)90082-9.

Clinical presentation 40

1. Carroll MF, Schade DS. A practical approach to hypercalcemia. *Am Fam Physician.* 2003;67(9):1959–1966.
2. Assadi F. Disorders of divalent metabolism. In: Assadi F, ed. *Clinical Decisions in Pediatric Nephrology: A Problem Solving Approach to Clinical Cases.* New York, NY: Springer; 2008:98–124.

Clinical Presentation 41

1. Assadi F, Hooman N, Seyedzadeh A, et al. Revisiting the management of pediatric kidney transplants, a multicenter analysis. *Iran J Kidney Dis.* 2022;16(6):319–329.

Clinical Presentation 42

1. Ritz E. Which is the preferred treatment of advanced hyperparathyroidism in a renal patient? II. Early parathyroidectomy should be considered as the first choice. *Nephrol Dial Transplant.* 1994;9:1819–1821.

Clinical Presentation 43

1. Choyke PL, Knopp MV. Pseudohypocalcemia with MR imaging contrast agents: a cautionary tale. *Radiology.* 2003;227:627–628.

Clinical Presentation 44

1. Kunis CL, Markowitz GS, Liu-Jarin X, et al. Painful myopathy and end-stage renal disease. *Am J Kidney Dis.* 2001;37:1098–1104.

Clinical Presentation 45

1. Bleyer AJ, Burke SK, Dillon M, et al. A comparison of the calcium-free phosphate binder sevelamer hydrochloride with calcium acetate in the treatment of treatment of hyperphosphatemia in dialysis patients. *Am J Kidney Dis.* 1999;33:694 –670.

Clinical Presentation 46

1. Mazhar AR, Johnson RJ, Gillen D, et al. Risk factors and mortality associated with calciphylaxis in end-stage renal disease. *Kidney Int.* 2001;60:324–332.

Clinical Presentation 47

1. Ferreria MA. Diagnosis of renal osteodystrophy: when and how to use biochemical markers and non-invasive methods; when bone biopsy is needed. *Nephrol Dial Transplant.* 2000;5:S8–S14.

Clinical Presentation 48

1. Schomig M, Ritz E. Management of disturbed calcium metabolism in uremic patients: 2. Indications for parathyroidectomy. *Nephrol Dial Transpl.* 2000;5:25–29.

Clinical Presentation 49

1. Green J, Debby H, Lederer E, et al. Evidence for a PTH-independent humeral mechanism in post-transplant hypophosphatemia and phosphaturia. *Kidney Int.* 2000;60:1182–1196.

Clinical Presentation 50

1. Uribarri J, Calvo MS. Hidden sources of phosphorus in the typical American diet: does it matter in nephrology? *Semin Dial.* 2004;16:186–188.

Clinical Presentation 51

1. Jonsson KB, Zahradnik R, Larsson T, et al. Fibroblast growth factor 23 in oncogenic osteomalacia and x-linked hypophosphatemia. *N Engl J Med.* 2003;348:1656–1663.

CHAPTER 4

Fluid, Electrolytes, and Acid-Base Disorders

Clinical Presentation 1

A 16-year-old girl with a history of chronic asthma was admitted to the hospital for treatment of status asthmaticus and hyperventilation. A physical examination revealed a well-developed female in respiratory stress. She was afebrile. Blood pressure was 116/72 mm Hg, pulse rate 79 beats/min, and respiratory rate 32 breaths/min. Expiratory wheezing was head bilaterally. Serum electrolytes (mEq) were sodium 138, potassium 3.2, bicarbonate 16, and chloride 115. Urine sodium was 51 mEq/L, potassium 39 mEq/L, and chloride 63 mEq/L. Urine pH was 6.1 and specific gravity 1.029 with no blood or protein. Serum creatinine was 0.6 mg/dL and blood urea nitrogen (BUN) 22 mg/dL.

She was treated with repeated doses of inhaled albuterol sulfate and intravenous theophylline and methylprednisolone. Oxygen was administered by nasal prongs at a flow rate of 4.0 L/min.

Which *one* of the following choices best describes her acid-base disturbance (select all that apply)?

A. Chronic respiratory alkalosis
B. Simple metabolic acidosis (dRTA-1)
C. Mixed metabolic acidosis (dRTA-1) and respiratory alkalosis
D. Insufficient data to interpret the acid-base disorder

The correct answer is A

Comment: The history of chronic asthma, hyperventilation, low serum bicarbonate concentration, and a positive urine anion gap together suggest the presence of chronic respiratory alkalosis.[1,2]

Further, the patient's serum bicarbonate of 16 mEq/L corresponds to a PCO_2 of 20 to 22 mm Hg, as in chronic respiratory alkalosis, and for each 10 mm Hg drop in the pCO_2 below 40 mm Hg, the serum bicarbonate level decreases by about 5 mEq/L.[1]

Clinical Presentation 2

A 12-year-old boy was found to have hyponatremia during a regular health check-up.

His past medical history is significant for intracranial hemorrhage at 10 years of age, following a motor vehicle accident. He underwent surgical repair and has done well since then. He is taking no medications.

His blood pressure is 112/64 mm Hg, heart rate 87 beats/min, respiratory rate 19 breaths/min, and temperature 37°C. Clinically, he appears to nonedematous.

Baseline serum sodium is 128 mEq/L, potassium 3.5 mEq/L, chloride 105 mEq/L, bicarbonate, 24 mEq/L, glucose 97 mg/dL, BUN 21 mg/dL, creatinine 0.7 mg/dL, and uric acid 3.5 mg/dL. Urine and blood osmolarity are 120 and 271 mOsm/kg, respectively. Urinary sodium is 62 mEq/L, potassium 30 mEq/L, and chloride 51 mEq/L. A 24-hour urine output is 1250 mL The fractional excretion of urate is 8%.

Which *one* of the following options would be the most appropriate treatment (select all that apply)?

A. Fluid restriction
B. Increase salt and water intake
C. Free access to fluid
D. Fludrocortisone (Florinef)

The correct answer is C

Comment: Hyponatremia, hyperosmolality, and normovolemia in a setting of normal fractional excretion of urate (FEurate) at baseline strongly suggest the presence of reset osmostat (RO). Hyponatremia in the RO requires no therapy (option C).

Patients with the syndrome of inappropriate antidiuretic hormone (ADH) secretion (SIADH) renal/cerebral salt wasting (R/CSW) and RO have similar clinical and laboratory characteristics including hyponatremia (Na <135 mEq/L), hypo-osmolality (<275 mOsm/kg), normal renal function, elevated urine osmolality (<100 mOsm/kg), and decreased serum uric acid level. All may have no clinical evidence of edema at the time of presentation.[1–5]

It is therefore important to distinguish these three syndromes from one another because they are treated with opposite treatment strategies.

For R/CSW, the patient is treated with fluids and sodium supplementation to restore the extracellular fluid (ECF) volume contraction. For SIADH, the patient is fluid restricted to remove the excess free water. For patients with RO, no therapy is needed because their ECF volume is intact and renal response to water and sodium is normal.[2,5]

The use of FEurate can accurately differentiate these three syndromes from one another.[2,4,5]

The key difference is that in SIADH, the initial FEurate is abnormally elevated (>10%) and returns to baseline value only when hyponatremia is corrected.[1–3]

In R/CSW, the FEurate persistently remains elevated (>10%) even after the correction of hyponatremia.[2,3]

In RO, unlike SIADH and R/CSW, the baseline FEurate is normal (between 4% and 10%).[2,3,5] Hyponatremia resulting from hypoaldosteronism is associated with non-gap hyperkalemic metabolic acidosis, FEurate is low (<4%), and the ECF volume is depleted. Therapy with a mineralocorticoid such as Florinef along with sodium supplements are indicated to correct hyponatremia.

Clinical Presentation 3

A 14-year-old girl was admitted because of severe dehydration following decreased appetite, low-grade fever, and frequent episodes of vomiting. She denied thirst.

Her past medical history was significant for frequent episodes of hypernatremic dehydration following upper respiratory or gastrointestinal infections. Family history was unremarkable.

The blood pressure (BP) was 90/65 mm Hg, pulse 149/min, respirations 28/min, and temperature 37°C. Her weight was 38 kg (<fifth percentile) and height 145 cm (<fifth percentile). There was severe developmental delay. Neurological examination revealed right hemiparesis, wide-based gait, and mild spasticity of the left arm. Fundoscopic examination was intact.

Laboratory data on admission (mEq/L) were Na 176, K 5.5, Cl 145, and HCO_3 15. BUN was 98 g/dL, creatinine 2.1 mg/dL, glucose 143 g/dL, Ca 9.4 mg/dL, Mg 3.4 mg/dL, phosphorus 2.6 mg/dL, total protein 7.4 g/dL, albumin 3.2 g/dL, and uric acid 6.6 mg/dL.

Serum and urine osmolality were 398 and 832 mOsm/kg H_2O, respectively. Urine pH was 5.0 with trace protein and no blood. The urine sediment showed two to three red blood cells and two to four white blood cells per high-power field. Tests for liver and endocrine functions were normal.

The patient was rehydrated with intravenous fluids and within 48 hours, her serum Na fell to 156 mEq/L, serum creatinine to 0.6 mg/dL, and BUN to 15 mg/dL. A magnetic resonance imaging (MRI) scan of the brain showed dilated lateral and their ventricles and left cerebral atrophy.

Which of the following would be the *most* likely the cause of hypernatremia in this patient (select all that apply)?

A. Nephrogenic diabetes insipidus (DI)
B. Central DI
C. Reset hypernatremia (osmostat)
D. Hyperosmolar hyperglycemic state
E. Primary hyperaldosteronism

The correct answer is C

Comment: The major findings in this patient were recurrent episodes of hypernatremic dehydration and absence of thirst with a plasma osmolality as high as 398 mOsm/kg H_2O. The patient was able to concentrate her urine (832 mOsm/kg H_2O). Volume expansion with water hypernatremia and hyperosmolarity and increased urine flow because of suppression of endogenous ADH.

These findings are consistent with an isolated defect in the osmoregulation of thirst as the cause of essential hypernatremia or RO (option C).[1,2]

The following criteria are necessary to establish this diagnosis[1,2]:

A. recurrent episodes of severe hypernatremic dehydration
B. absence of thirst
C. normal ADH response to both osmotic and volume challenges
D. correction of hypernatremia with fluid loading

Differentiation of reset hypernatremia from nephrogenic or central DI is important because management differs according to diagnosis. In patients with RO, vasopressin therapy is inappropriate and may lead to water intoxication.

Clinical Presentation 4

A 5-year-old girl complains of profound weakness and polyuria. She is taking no medications. She is the first child of a nonconsanguineous healthy parents.

On examination, her height was 105 cm and weight 16 kg, both below 15th percentiles for her age and gender. Her BP is 97/64 mm Hg. Serum electrolytes (mEq/L) are sodium 138, potassium 2.5, chloride 95, and bicarbonate 37. Urea nitrogen and serum creatinine levels are 18 and 0.5 mg/dL, respectfully. A 24-hour urine sample contained sodium 90, potassium 60, and chloride 103 (mEq/L). The urinary calcium to creatinine ratio was elevated at 0.6 mol/mol. Plasma renin activity and aldosterone level were elevated. Urinalysis was negative for glucose and protein but positive for 1+ blood. Abdominal ultrasound showed normal-sized kidneys with bilateral nephrocalcinosis.

You suspect Bartter syndrome and order a genetic test, which reveals mutations in the *SLC12A1* gene, confirming type 1 Bartter syndrome.

Treatment with potassium supplementations, K-sparing diuretic, angiotensin-converting enzyme inhibitor, and indomethacin, all in high doses, did not lower her elevated BP or improve electrolyte abnormalities.

In addition to standard theory, which *one* of the following would be the most appropriate treatment (select all that apply)

A. Acetazolamide 5 mg/kg/day
B. Amiloride 0.5 mg/kg/day
C. NH4CL 15 mg/kg/day
D. MgSO4 500 mg every 6 hours
E. Propranolol 0.5 mg/kg/day
F. Hydrochlorothiazide 1 mg/kg/day

The correct answer is A

Comment: A recent randomized, open-label, crossover controlled trial examined the efficacy and safety of adding acetazolamide into standard therapy consisting of a potassium-sparing diuretic (spironolactone), RAAS inhibitors (enalapril), and cyclooxygenase inhibitors (indomethacin) supplemented with large doses of potassium in 22 children with genetically proven Bartter syndrome resistant to the standard therapy. The study results concluded that acetazolamide in combination with standard therapy significantly improved renal responses to indomethacin plus enalapril and spironolactone without any drug-related adverse events.[1]

Clinical Presentation 5

A 14-year-old girl complained of easy fatigability and generalized muscle weakness. Her history was otherwise unrevealing, and she denied vomiting or the use of any medications. Physical examination revealed a thin, anxious girl with a normal blood pressure. Her examination was otherwise unremarkable. Her serum sodium was 141 mEq/L; potassium, 2.1 mEq/L; chloride, 85 mEq/L; bicarbonate, 45 mEq/L; calcium, 9.5 mg/ dL (reference range, 8.5–10.3 mg/dL); phosphate, 3.2 mg/dL (reference range, 2.8–4.5 mg/dL); magnesium, 1.2 mg/dL (reference range, 1.8–2.3 mg/dL); and albumin, 4.6 g/dL (reference range, 3.5–5.0 g/dL). The fractional excretion of magnesium was 6.5%, the urine chloride was 56 mEq/L, and the urine calcium-creatinine ratio was 3.2 (reference range, <0.22).

The fractional excretion of magnesium was 6.5%, the urine chloride was 56 mEq/L, and the urine calcium-creatinine ratio was 3.2 (reference range, <0.22).

What is the most likely diagnosis (select all that apply)?

A. Primary hyperaldosteronism
B. Loop diuretic abuse
C. Apparent mineralocorticoid excess (AME)
D. Bartter syndrome

The correct answer is D

Comment: The findings of hypokalemia, metabolic alkalosis, and normal BP suggest the diagnosis of secondary hyperaldosteronism caused by surreptitious vomiting, diuretic abuse, or Bartter syndrome. Measurement of urinary chloride, calcium, and magnesium is useful in the differentiation between these disorders. The urinary chloride concentration is typically less than 15 mEq/L in hypovolemia resulting from surreptitious vomiting. In contrast, a urinary chloride greater than 15 mEq/L suggests diuretic abuse, Bartter syndrome, or Gitelman syndrome. Measurement of urine calcium will help distinguish between Bartter syndrome and Gitelman syndrome. Screening urine for diuretics is indicated if surreptitious ingestion is suspected. Measurement of the urinary magnesium will help distinguish between gastrointestinal and renal losses as the major contributor.

Bartter syndrome can cause hypokalemia, metabolic alkalosis, renal magnesium wasting, and hypomagnesemia without hypertension in a manner similar to that of loop diuretics. Bartter syndrome is caused by mutations in a furosemide-sensitive ion transport mechanism in the loop of Henle and is associated with hypercalciuria. A diuretic screen is the only way to distinguish Bartter syndrome from diuretic abuse (option D).[1,2]

Clinical Presentation 6

A 16-year-old boy noted the onset of blurring of vision several weeks ago. Indirect ophthalmoscopy revealed white, fluffy retinal lesions located close to retinal vessels and associated with hemorrhage. Cytomegalovirus (CMV) retinitis was diagnosed, and he was begun on intravenous therapy with foscarnet 120 mg/kg twice per day. This was to be continued for 2 weeks followed by maintenance therapy with 90 mg/kg once daily. He complained of several episodes of numbness and tingling, particularly around his mouth, with the first several treatments. This morning he experienced a generalized seizure immediately following completion of his treatment. Laboratory studies showed hematocrit 28%, white blood cells (WBC) 4600 cells/μL; BUN 28 mg/dL; creatinine 1.4 mg/dL; sodium 136 mEq/L; chloride 106 mEq/L; potassium 4.0 mEq/L; CO_2 23 mEq/L (calcium 9.0 mg/dL [phosphate 3.5 mg/dL] and albumin 4.5 g/dL). Urinalysis revealed pH 7.0, specific gravity 2.013; trace protein, and small blood.

His clinicians are concerned and confused. His symptoms sound like hypocalcemia, but his serum calcium concentration and serum albumin level are normal.

What would you recommend be done next (select all that apply)?

A. Measure a parathyroid hormone (PTH) level.
B. Measure the serum ionized calcium at the end of the next infusion.
C. Reduce the foscarnet dose.
D. Measure a calcidiol level.
E. Measure serum magnesium level.
F. Measure serum potassium level.
G. Order an electrocardiogram.

The correct answers are B, C, E, and F

Comment: Foscarnet is an antiviral drug used to treat CMV and CMV-associated ophthalmic retinitis in individuals who are unable to tolerate ganciclovir or those who have drug-resistant CMV and fail ganciclovir. It also has approval as a treatment option in immunocompromised patients with the herpes simplex virus who exhibit resistance to acyclovir, the gold-standard therapy for herpes simplex virus.[1]

Although there are multiple adverse effects of foscarnet, the most notable are nausea associated with the infusion of the drug, electrolyte derangements, and reduced renal function. Of these three significant adverse effects, reports of renal insufficiency are relatively more common events in patients receiving this drug.[2]

Foscarnet affects the renal tubular cells via direct cytotoxic mechanisms, and the degree of drug-induced toxicity directly correlates to the dosage administered. Along with the renal tubular damage, foscarnet can also cause crystal nephropathy with the deposition of crystals in the glomerular capillaries.

Electrolyte derangement is another adverse effect of foscarnet and often presents as hypocalcemia and hypomagnesemia. Hypocalcemia may be due to the formation of the foscarnet and calcium ion complex, or it may result from foscarnet-induced hypomagnesemia, which leads to both hypocalcemia (from a hypomagnesemia-induced hypoparathyroidism state) and hypokalemia (from excess renal potassium wasting).

The less commonly reported adverse events resulting from foscarnet administration include seizures.

Clinical Presentation 7

A 17-year-old girl presented initially with a 3-year history of aching in her bones affecting her arms and legs. More recently, she had noted the onset of muscle weakness so that her gait had become cautious and she used her arms to rise from a sitting position. She has no significant medical history and she does not smoke or drink alcohol. She denies the use of any medications. Her most recent office visit was 5 years ago, at which time there were no abnormal physical or laboratory findings. On examination, she appeared in no acute distress. BP was 143/85 mm Hg, pulse 76, respiratory rate 12, temperature 98.6°F, weight 62.5 kg, and height 159 cm. The heart had regular beats without murmurs, the lungs were clear, and the abdomen was soft without masses. There was no edema. There was moderate proximal muscle weakness. Laboratory data showed hematocrit 46%, BUN 8 mg/dL, serum creatinine 1.0 mg/dL, sodium 140 mEq/L, potassium 3.9 mEq/L, chloride 101 mEq/L, CO_2 28 mEq/L, calcium 9.0 mg/dL, phosphate 1.9 mg/dL, magnesium 1.8 mg/dL, and albumin 4.2 g/dL.

Which of the following studies should be done first in attempting to distinguish the diagnosis (select all that apply)?

A. PTH level
B. 24-hour urine phosphate collection
C. 24-hour urine creatinine collection
D. 24-hour urine calcium collection
E. Serum calcidiol level

The correct answers are B and C
Comment: The 24-hour urine phosphate and creatinine excretion results were 800 mg and 1250 mg, respectively. The fractional phosphate excretion was 43%.

Which of the following conditions should now be considered in the differential diagnosis (select all that apply)?

A. Primary hyperparathyroidism
B. Poor phosphate intake and diarrhea
C. Fanconi syndrome
D. X-linked hypophosphatemic rickets
E. Oncogenic osteomalacia
F. Excess ingestion of phosphate-binding antacids
G. Vitamin D deficiency

The correct answers are D and E
Further laboratory studies revealed: serum 25 (OH) D 26 ng/mL (normal, 15–50 ng/mL); 1,25 (OH)2 D 10 pg/mL (normal, 15–60 pg/mL); PTH 3 pmol/L (normal, 1–5 pmol/L); uric acid 5 mg/dL; urine glucose negative; urine amino acid negative; and urine uric acid 50 mg/dL (normal, 10–80 mg/dL).

What is the most likely diagnosis now?

A. Fanconi syndrome
B. Hereditary hypophosphatemic rickets

C. Oncogenic osteomalacia
D. Vitamin D deficiency

The correct answer is C

Comment: Oncogenic osteomalacia, referred to as tumor-induced osteomalacia (TIO), is a rare endocrine disorder in which a small bony or soft tissue mesenchymal tumor causes hypophosphatemia via secretion of fibroblast growth factor 23 (FGF23).[1,2] The latter causes hypophosphatemia via two mechanisms: (1) reduction of renal tubular phosphate reabsorption leading to phosphaturia and (2) impairment of hydroxylation of 25-hydroxyvitamin D to 1,25-dihydroxyvitamin D, thus reducing intestinal phosphorus absorption. As a result of chronic hypophosphatemia, patients develop osteomalacia and associated insufficiency fractures.

The diagnosis of TIO should be considered in patients who have musculoskeletal pain with hypophosphatemia, with or without insufficient fractures. Diagnostic testing should include quantification of the tubular reabsorption of phosphorus, which is reduced in the presence of FGF23; additional diagnostic laboratory and imaging studies are useful for the evaluation of TIO. The differential diagnosis of hypophosphatemia includes X-linked hypophosphatemia (consider with younger age of onset, suggestive family history, and dental anomalies), proximal renal tubulopathies (consider with multiple electrolyte abnormalities; may be genetic or acquired), and dietary-related hypophosphatemia (consider in patients with low intake or refeeding syndrome).[2]

Presence of hypocalcemia, hypokalemia, and proximal renal tubular acidosis (RTA) may suggest Fanconi syndrome.

If there is a discordance between 25 (OH) vitamin D and 1,25 (OH)2 vitamin D, this would suggest the presence of interfering FGF23, favoring the diagnosis of oncogenic osteomalacia.

Elevated PTH would result in hypophosphoremia and hypercalcemia.

Clinical Presentation 8

A 19-year-old man presents to the emergency department with acute abdominal pain. Two days ago, he noted the onset of steady right upper quadrant pain. The pain radiates in a band-like fashion to the back and is relieved somewhat by bending forward. He has also experienced nausea and vomiting for the past 10 hours. He has had multiple hospitalizations in the past with similar presentation. He has been having loose, greasy, foul-smelling stools that are difficult to flush for the past month. Current medications include Dilantin and phenobarbital with a history of generalized seizures over the past several years. The patient appears restless and is in significant pain. His BP is 127/67 mm Hg; pulse 110, respiratory rate 25 with shallow respirations, temperature 101°F; weight 60 kg; and height 163 cm. The chest is clear. There is abdominal distention, tenderness, or guarding. The liver and spleen are not palpable. There is no edema. The neurologic examination is within normal limits. Laboratory studies show hematocrit 33%, WBC 4600/mm^3, BUN 8 mg/dL, serum creatinine 1.0 mg/dL, sodium 135 mEq/L, potassium 3.3 mEq/L, chloride 106 mEq/L, CO_2 21 mEq/L, calcium 6.9 mg/dL, phosphate 3.1 mg/dL, albumin 3.7 g/dL, and amylase 330 U/L (normal, <130 U/L). Abdominal flat plate showed nephrocalcinosis. Urinalysis was within normal limits.

Which of the following may be contributing to the hypocalcemia (select all that apply)?

A. Hypophosphatemia
B. Hypomagnesemia
C. Hypermagnesemia
D. Low calcidiol
E. Extravascular deposition of calcium

The correct answers are C, D, and E

Comment: Hypocalcemia has many causes. It can result from inadequate PTH secretion, PTH resistance, vitamin D deficiency or resistance, abnormal magnesium metabolism, and extravascular deposition of calcium, which can occur in several clinical situations.[1,2]

The diagnostic approach to hypocalcemia involves confirming, by repeat measurement, the presence of hypocalcemia and distinguishing among the potential etiologies. The diagnosis may be obvious from the patient's history; examples include chronic kidney disease and postsurgical hypoparathyroidism.

Clinical Presentation 9

A 12-year-old boy presents in the office complaining of slowly progressive pain in his right chest. The pain began about 2 months ago and is described as being similar to a toothache. It is unrelated to exercise or position. It initially responded to nonsteroidal anti-inflammatory drugs, but they are no longer effective. Review of systems reveals that he has noted some urinary urgency and frequency over the past 4 months and has had nocturia for 3 months. He has also noted in the past several weeks that he has episodes of tingling around his mouth and occasional cramps in his hands and legs.

On physical examination, vital signs are normal, the chest is clear, and there is tenderness over the fourth rib in the midline. There are no murmurs and the abdomen is soft and nontender. There is no edema. Laboratory studies showed hematocrit 34%, WBC 5600/mm^3, BUN 20 mg/dL, creatinine 1.6 mg/dL, sodium 140 mEq/L, potassium 4.0 mEq/L, chloride 106 mEq/L, CO_2 25 mEq/L; calcium 6.9 mg/dL, phosphate 3.3 mg/dL, and albumin 3.7 mg/dL. Urinalysis results are within normal limits.

Which of the following do you expect to find (select all that apply)?

A. Elevated PTH
B. Low PTH
C. Elevated alkaline phosphatase
D. Low alkaline phosphatase
E. High calcitriol
F. Low calcidiol

The correct answers are C and E

Comment: Vitamin D is a fat-soluble vitamin used by the body for normal bone development and maintenance by increasing the absorption of calcium, magnesium, and phosphate. A circulating level of 25-hydroxyvitamin D greater than 30 ng/mL is required to maintain a healthy level of vitamin D. Vitamin D deficiency can lead to an array of problems, most notably rickets in children and osteoporosis in adults.[1]

Vitamin D deficiency is now more prevalent than ever and should be screened in high-risk populations. Many conflicting studies are now showing an association between vitamin D deficiency and cancer, cardiovascular disease, diabetes, autoimmune diseases, and depression. This section reviews the evaluation and management of vitamin D deficiency and explains the role of the interprofessional team in improving care for patients with this condition.

Certain malabsorption syndromes such as celiac disease, short bowel syndrome, gastric bypass, inflammatory bowel disease, chronic pancreatic insufficiency, and cystic fibrosis may lead to vitamin D deficiency. Lower vitamin D intake orally is more prevalent in the elderly population.

Decreased exposure to the sun as seen in individuals who have dark skin or have prolonged hospitalizations can also lead to vitamin D deficiency.[1]

Individuals with chronic liver disease such as cirrhosis can have defective 25-hydroxylation leading to deficiency of active vitamin D. Defect in 1-alpha 25-hydroxylation can be seen in hyperparathyroidism, renal failure, and 1-alpha hydroxylase deficiency.

Medications such as phenobarbital, carbamazepine, dexamethasone, nifedipine, spironolactone, clotrimazole, and rifampin induce hepatic p450 enzymes, which activate degradation of vitamin D.

Last, end-organ resistance to vitamin D can be seen in hereditary vitamin D–resistant rickets.

Vitamin D deficiency is evaluated by the measurement of serum 25-hydroxyvitamin D. Optimal serum levels of 25-hydroxyvitamin D is still a matter of controversy.[1]

The International Society for Clinical Densitometry and International Osteoporosis Foundation recommends minimum serum levels of 25-hydroxyvitamin D of 30 ng/mL to minimize the risk of fall and fractures in older individuals.

In patients in which vitamin D deficiency has been diagnosed, it is important to evaluate for secondary hyperparathyroidism and levels of PTH and serum calcium should be measured.

Clinical Presentation 10

A 2-year-old girl was referred for evaluation of polyuria and polydipsia. She was the third child of related parents. Both parents and her two older siblings are healthy, and none of the relatives was known to have polydipsia, polyuria, or hypertension. There was no history of vomiting or diarrhea. On examination, her height and weight are below the 10th percentile. Blood pressure is elevated at 125/69 mm Hg. No other abnormal findings were noted. Urinalysis showed a specific gravity of 1.010 and pH 8.0 without hematuria or proteinuria. Serum sodium was 138 mEq/L, potassium 2.7 mEq/L, chloride 89 mEq/L, bicarbonate 30 mEq/L, BUN 10 mg/dL, and creatinine 0.4 mg/dL. Serum aldosterone, cortisol, progesterone, deoxycorticosterone, and plasma renin levels were normal. Treatment with various combinations of labetalol, hydralazine, nifedipine, and spironolactone, all at high doses, failed to control the elevated blood pressure. Renal ultrasound and captopril-enhanced renal scan were normal.

What further investigation should be performed to establish the diagnosis (select all that apply)?

A. Contrast cystogram
B. Arteriogram measurement of urinary catecholamines
C. Amiloride therapy
D. Abdominal computed tomography (CT) scan with contrast

The correct answer is C

Comment: Liddle syndrome is a genetic disorder characterized by hypertension with hypokalemic metabolic alkalosis, hyporeninemia, and suppressed aldosterone secretion that often appears early in life. It results from inappropriately elevated sodium reabsorption in the distal nephron. Liddle syndrome is caused by mutations to subunits of the epithelial sodium channel (ENaC). Among other mechanisms, such mutations typically prevent ubiquitination of these subunits, slowing the rate at which they are internalized from the membrane and resulting in an elevation of channel activity. A minority of Liddle syndrome mutations, though, result in a complementary effect that also elevates activity by increasing the probability that ENaC channels within the membrane are open. Potassium-sparing diuretics such as amiloride and triamterene reduce ENaC activity, and in combination with a reduced sodium diet can restore normotension and electrolyte imbalance in Liddle syndrome patients and animal models. Liddle syndrome can be diagnosed clinically by phenotype and confirmed through genetic testing.[1,2]

Liddle syndrome differentiates from other genetic diseases with a similar phenotype, and what is currently known about the population-level prevalence of Liddle syndrome is discussed here. This review gives special focus to the molecular mechanisms of Liddle syndrome.

Treatment of Liddle syndrome is typically through the use of a potassium-sparing diuretic, such as amiloride or triamterene.[1,2] Both diuretics work by blocking the activity of ENaC, and their efficacy in Liddle syndrome cases has been shown to be enhanced with dietary salt restriction (<2 g NaCl per day). These diuretics can correct the elevated BP as well as the hypokalemic metabolic alkalosis seen in Liddle syndrome.

Clinical Presentation 11

You are asked to see a 17-year-old female with acute postoperative hyponatremia. The patient had been in a good health until yesterday when she fell and sustained a compound wrist fracture. It was recommended that surgery be performed immediately. A urinary tract catheter was placed and she received prophylactic antibiotics and was taken to the operating room. Current medications include oxcarbazepine for trigeminal neuralgia and Inderal for hypertension. On examination, she appears restless and confused and is complaining of significant pain in her right wrist. Her temperature is 98°F, pulse 110, and respiratory rate 25. The chest is clear. There is no abdominal distention, tenderness, or guarding. There is no organomegaly. There is no edema. The neurological examination in within normal limits except for mild to moderate confusion. Laboratory study shows serum sodium 118 mEq/L, potassium 4.3 mEq/L, chloride 78 mEq/L, CO_2 26 mEq/L, BUN 12 mg/dL, and creatinine 0.9 mg/dL. Urinalysis shows trace protein, negative glucose, no blood, red blood cells, or WBCs. Urine sodium is 41 mEq/L, urine osmolality 489 mOsmol/kg, and plasma osmolality 240 mOsmol/kg.

Her fluid intake over the past 6 hours during surgery and recovery was 4 L of 0.45% saline. There was little estimated blood loss and she has made 100 mL of urine.

What is the likely cause of this condition?

A. SIADH secretion
B. Adrenal I insufficiency
C. Dilutional hyponatremia
D. Hypothyroidism

The correct answer is A

Comment: True (hypoosmolal) hyponatremia is associated with a reduction in serum osmolality and is further classified as euvolemic, hypervolemic, and hypovolemic.

Euvolemic hyponatremia accounts for 60% of all cases of hyponatremia. The most common cause of euvolemic hyponatremia is SIADH.[1–3]

The criteria necessary for a diagnosis of SIADH include:

1. Decreased measured serum osmolality (<275 mOsm/kg H_2O)
2. Clinical euvolemia
3. Urinary osmolality >100 mOsm/kg H_2O
4. Urinary Na >40 mmol/L with normal dietary sodium intake
5. Normal thyroid and adrenal function
6. Normal renal functions
7. Exclude use of diuretic agents within the week before evaluation
8. No hypokalemia
9. No acid-base disorders

Supporting diagnostic criteria for SIADH include serum uric acid less than 3.5 mg/dL, BUN <10 mg/dL, fractional urine sodium excretion >1%, fractional urea excretion >55%, failure to improve or worsening of hyponatremia after 0.9% saline infusion, and correction of hyponatremia with fluid restriction.[1–3]

Clinical Presentation 12

You are asked to see a 2-year-old boy who has congestive heart failure (CHF). His medications include digoxin and furosemide. On examination, he is lethargic and in mild respiratory distress, with BP of 100/54 mm Hg and irregular pulse of 104°F. Rales are present one-quarter of the way up his lung fields, and there is 2+ ankle edema. Laboratory studies reveal the following: sodium 125 mEq/L, potassium 3.3 mEq/L, chloride 95 mEq/L, CO_2 24 mEq/L, BUN 11 mg/dL, creatinine 0.8 mg/dL, serum osmolarity 230 mOsmol/kg, and urine osmolality 600 mOsmol/kg.

Which of the following statements concerning his hyponatremia are true?

A. He most likely has SIADH secretion.
B. Hyponatremia can easily be managed with water restriction.
C. A plasma concentration below 125 mEq/L typically represents near end-stage cardiac disease.
D. The hyponatremia is due to a decrease in cardiac output (effective volume depletion), which indicates a baroreceptor response and neurohumoral stimulation.

The correct answers are C and D

Comment: Hyponatremia has been identified as a risk factor for increased morbidity and mortality in patients with congestive heart failure (CHF) and other edematous disorders and can lead to severe neurologic derangements. Low cardiac output and BP associated with CHF triggers a compensatory response by the body that activates several neurohormonal systems designed to preserve arterial blood volume and pressure. Hyponatremia in patients with CHF is primarily caused by increased activity of arginine vasopressin (AVP). AVP increases free-water reabsorption in the renal collecting ducts, increasing blood volume and diluting plasma sodium concentrations. Hyponatremia may also be triggered by diuretic therapy used in the management of symptoms of CHF.

At an early stage of CHF, retention of sodium and water causes expansion of extracellular fluid volume and peripheral edema, but not hyponatremia. However, at late-stage CHF, patients exhibit an impairment in the renal excretion of water (aquaresis or water diuresis), predisposing them to the development of hyponatremia. An increase in the antidiuretic hormone in this late stage imposes an aquaretic defect, which, in combination with the use of potent diuretics and severe salt restriction, frequently leads to dilutional hyponatremia.[1,2]

Clinical Presentation 13

An 18-year-old female (60 kg) presents to the emergency department with severe pain in her mouth. She had dental work done 5 days ago and now had developed a tooth abscess. She has been taking a variety of pain pills and has been unable to eat solid food for several days. Her past medical history was significant for a postpartum hemorrhage complicated with hypotension 2 years ago. Laboratory data revealed sodium 124 mEq/L, chloride 74 mEq/L, potassium 3.9 mEq/L, CO_2 28 mEq/L, BUN 12 mg/dL, and creatinine 0.9 mg/dL. Urinalysis showed trace protein, glucose negative, and no blood, RBC, or WBC. Urine sodium was 11 mEq/L and urine osmolality was 400 mOsm/kg.

What orders would you like to write?

A. Restrict free water to <1000 mL/day.
B. Oral surgery consult
C. Intravenous saline, 3 L / 24 hours
D. Hypertonic saline

The correct answer is A

Comment: SIADH involves the continued secretion or action of AVP despite normal or increased plasma volume. The resulting impairment of water secretion and consequent water retention produce the hyponatremia (i.e., serum Na^+ <135 mmol/L) with concomitant hypo-osmolality (serum osmolality <280 mOsm/kg) and high urine osmolality that are the hallmarks of SIADH.[1]

The key to understanding the pathophysiology, signs, symptoms, and treatment of SIADH is the awareness that hyponatremia results from an excess of water rather than a deficiency of sodium.

Differentiating SIADH from reset hyponatremia renal salt wasting (RSW) has been extremely difficult to accomplish, in part because of significant overlapping clinical findings between both syndromes. All three syndromes are associated with intracranial diseases; have normal renal, thyroid, and adrenal function; are hyponatremic and hypouricemic; and have concentrated urines, with high urinary sodium >40 mEq/L. The baseline fractional excretion of urate is also high in SIADH and RSW, but normal in reset hyponatremia.[1–3]

The only clinical difference is the state of the patient's ECV, being euvolemic or hypervolemic in SIADH, hypovolemic in RSW, and euvolemic in reset hyponatremia.

This diagnostic dilemma between SIADH and RSW can be resolved by repeating the fractional excretion of urate after correction of hyponatremia. In SIADH the fractional urate excretion returns to normal value (<10%), whereas in RSW, it remains persistently high (>11%).[1,2]

Clinical Presentation 14

You are asked to see a 15-year-old male with a serum sodium level of 123 mEq/L. He was in a good state of health until 4 months ago when he developed a persistent cough. He subsequently experienced a 10-kg weight loss. Shortness of breath developed 5 days ago. A chest x-ray showed a right pleural effusion, and he was admitted for further evaluation. On examination, he appeared cachectic in no apparent acute distress. BP was 110/72 mm Hg without orthostatic hypotension, pulse 68, respiratory rate 18, temperature 98.6°F, weight 62 kg, and height 159 cm. His heart had regular rhythm with no murmurs. Chest was dull to percussion with diminished breathing sounds at the right base. There was no edema. The remainder of the physical examination was normal. Laboratory study showed serum sodium 126 mEq/L, potassium 3.5 mEq/L, chloride 91 mEq/L, CO_2 24 mEq/L, BUN 6 mg/dL, and creatinine 0.7 mg/dL. Urine osmolality was 305 and serum osmolality 250 mOsm/kg.

What are the causes of hyponatremia in this patient (select all that apply)?

A. Dilutional hyponatremia because of hyperglycemia
B. Pseudohyponatremia because of hyperlipidemia
C. SIADH secretion
D. Adrenal insufficiency
E. RO

The correct answers are C and E

Comment: Hyponatremia is the most common electrolyte abnormality seen in hospitalized patients, with 15% to 20% of patients having a sodium level <135 mmol/L. The differential diagnosis for hyponatremia is broad, and a systematic and logical approach is needed to identify the cause.

RO is an uncommon and underrecognized cause of hyponatremia that does not require any treatment. This diagnosis needs to be considered when the hyponatremia workup suggests SIADH, but the hyponatremia is not amenable to fluid restriction, salt administration, or diuretic treatment.[1–3]

Diagnosing RO is a diagnosis of exclusion. Individuals must be euvolemic, and a thorough exclusion of other causes of euvolemic hyponatremia (e.g., hypothyroidism, cortisol deficiency, medications) must take place. A key feature of RO is that individuals should be able to concentrate and dilute the urine appropriately. Thus, a water challenge should result in dilute urine (e.g., <100 mOsm/kg) and a water deprivation test should result in concentrated urine. Sometimes, a patient given a diagnosis of SIADH will be proven to reset the osmostat when it becomes apparent that fluid restriction does not successfully raise the serum sodium level.

RO classically occurs in neurologic conditions such as epilepsy and paraplegia, in addition to pregnancy, malignancy, and malnutrition. It has also been observed in healthy individuals.

Hyponatremia in the SIADH results from ADH-induced retention of ingested or infused water. Although water excretion is impaired, sodium handling is intact because there is no abnormality in volume-regulating mechanisms such as the renin-angiotensin-aldosterone system or atrial natriuretic peptide.[1]

Clinical Presentation 15

A 14-year-old boy presents to the emergency department with severe vomiting and the recent onset of chest pain. The patient has a history of peptic ulcer disease. Vomiting began 48 hours ago and continued until the present time without improvement. Fifteen minutes before arriving in the emergency room, the patient developed the sudden onset of left-sided pleuric chest pain, shortness of breath, and hemoptysis. Physical examination revealed a tachypneic male in acute distress with a respiratory rate of 30 and complaining of chest pain. The remainder of the examination was normal. Laboratory data revealed sodium 140 mEq/L, potassium 3.0 mEq/L, chloride 92 mEq/L, CO_2 36 mEq/L, BUN 30 mg/dL, creatinine 1.3 mg/dL, calcium 10.0 mg/dL, phosphate 3.5 mg/dL, blood ketones negative, glucose 90 mg/dL, and plasma osmolarity 280 mOsoml/kg. The chest x-ray showed marked pleural effusion on the left pleural chest with the left lower lobe infiltrate.

The blood gas revealed a pH of 7.69 with a pCO_2 of 30 mm Hg, an HCO_3 of 35 mEq/L, and a pO_2 of 47 mm Hg.

What is (are) the acid-base diagnosis(es) (select all that apply)?

A. Metabolic alkalosis
B. Respiratory alkalosis
C. Mixed metabolic alkalosis and respiratory alkalosis
D. None of the above

The correct answer is C

Comment: The constellation of high blood pH, high serum bicarbonate concentration, and pCO_2 above 40 mm Hg suggests the presence of a mixed metabolic and respiratory alkalosis. Metabolic alkalosis is caused by persistent vomiting over the past 48 hours. Respiratory alkalosis is likely from hyperventilation as a result of shortness of breath secondary to chest pain.[1]

Clinical Presentation 16

A 19-year-old female is brought to the emergency room by her roommate because of increasing weakness. They both had been having low-grade fever and severe diarrhea for 4 days. Laboratory studies reveal sodium 140 mEq/L, potassium 2.4 mEq/L, chloride 115 mEq/L, CO_2 15 mEq/L, BUN 21 mg/d, creatinine 1.5 mg/dL, glucose 88 mg/dL, calcium 10.0 mg/dL, phosphate 3.5 mg/dL, magnesium 1.8 mg/dL, and plasma osmolality 284 mOsm/kg.

What do you estimate her arterial pH to be?

A. 7.20 to 7.24
B. 7.25 to 7.29
C. 7.30 to 7.34
D. 7.40 to 7.44
E. 7.45 to 7.49

The correct answer is C

Comment: The acid-base diagnosis is uncomplicated hyperchloremic acidosis resulting from severe diarrhea. This would allow you to estimate her pCO_2 from the Winter formula, which applies only when simple (uncomplicated) metabolic acidosis is present.

The expected fall can be estimated using the following equation:

$$\text{delta } pCO_2 = 1.2 \times \text{delta } HCO_3^- \text{ or } 12 \text{ mm Hg.}$$

Then, the predicted pCO_2 compensation can be estimated as the difference between normal pCO_2 and the expected fall in pCO_2 [normal pCO_2 (40)] – delta [pCO_2 (12)] or 28 mm Hg.

The H^+ can then be calculated with the modified Henderson-Hasselbach equation:

$$H^+ = 24 \times pCO_2/HCO_3^-$$

The H^+ value obtained is 45 mEq/L, which is equivalent to a pH of 7.35 (every 0.1 fall in pH is equivalent to 10 mEq/L rise in plasma H^+ concentration).[1]

Clinical Presentation 17

A 16-year-old young man was admitted for elective surgery for a small-bowel carcinoid tumor. Nephrology was consulted for evaluation of persistent hypokalemia and metabolic alkalosis. The patient denied abdominal pain, headache, fever, vomiting, or diarrhea. He did not use over-the-counter or herbal medications. Home medications included omeprazole 20 mg and a daily and a monthly octreotide injection. In the hospital, he was receiving omeprazole 20 mg daily.

On physical examination, the patient's temperature was 37.3°C, heart rate was 90 beats/min, blood pressure was 155/95 mm Hg, respiration rate was 14 breaths/min, and oxygen saturation was 97% on room air. Cardiac examination findings were unremarkable. Lungs were clear bilaterally. His abdomen was soft with no visceromegaly or tenderness. There was no edema. There were no focal neurologic findings. Laboratory studies showed serum sodium 144 mmol/L, potassium 2.8 mmol/L, chloride 9 mmol/L, bicarbonate 33 mmol/L, BUN 16 mg/dL, creatinine 0.8 mg/dL, calcium 7.9 mg/dL, albumin 3.8 mg/dL, and glucose 96 mg/dL. Arterial blood gas pH was 7.52, PCO_2 38 mm Hg, HCO_3^- 32 mmol/L, plasma renin 1.06 ng/mL (reference, 0.25–5.82), plasma aldosterone 1 ng/dL (reference, 3–16), plasma cortisol 41.8 mcg/dL (reference, 6–26), and plasma corticotropin (adrenocorticotropic hormone [ACTH]) 92 pg/mL (reference, 6–50). In a 24-hour urine collection, cortisol was 1062 nmol/L (reference, 4–50 nmol/L), creatinine 1.08 g, potassium 105 mmol, and chloride 62 mmol.

What is the *most* likely cause of hypokalemia in this patient?

A. Liddle syndrome
B. Hyperaldosteronism
C. AME
D. Ectopic ACTH-dependent Cushing syndrome from carcinoid tumor

The correct answer is D

Comment: Hypokalemia is generally from either urinary or gastrointestinal tract losses, a shift from the extracellular to intracellular fluid compartment, or, in rare cases, decreased oral intake.[1,2] In this patient, renal losses were thought to be most likely, given the elevated urinary potassium concentration.[1]

Metabolic alkalosis is often classified as chloride responsive (urine chloride <20 mmol/L or less) or chloride resistant (urine chloride >20 mmol/L or more). When urine chloride excretion is greater than 20 mmol/L, the metabolic alkalosis is usually saline responsive. In metabolic alkalosis, urine chloride concentration may be a more accurate indicator of intravascular volume depletion than urine sodium concentration because bicarbonaturia in early stages of development of a chloride-depletion metabolic alkalosis results in sodium and potassium excretion in urine (as accompanying cations with bicarbonate). Thus, urine sodium and potassium concentrations may be elevated in the first 24 to 72 hours of volume depletion and then decline subsequently. Urine chloride concentration will remain low because of ongoing sodium and chloride reabsorption in the proximal tubule from activation of the renin-angiotensin-aldosterone axis and other factors in response to volume depletion.[2]

This patient developed chloride-resistant metabolic alkalosis (urine chloride >20 mmol/L). Given the presence of hypertension along with urine potassium excretion >20 mmol/L and low levels of both serum renin and aldosterone, the differential diagnosis includes Liddle syndrome, syndrome of AME, Cushing syndrome, congenital adrenal hyperplasia, and excessive licorice use.[1–3] Liddle syndrome, syndrome of AME, and congenital adrenal hyperplasia were unlikely given the patient's age. Given the patient's elevated morning cortisol level, markedly increased 24-hour urine cortisol excretion, and high serum corticotropin (ACTH) level, ACTH-dependent Cushing syndrome was diagnosed. ACTH-dependent Cushing syndrome could be due to either an ACTH-secreting pituitary tumor or an ectopic ACTH-secreting tumor. Findings from MRI of the pituitary gland and CT of the chest were unremarkable. Computed tomography of the abdomen revealed peritoneal nodules consistent with his history of recurrent carcinoid tumor. Ectopic ACTH-dependent Cushing syndrome, most likely from the active carcinoid tumor, was diagnosed. There are a few case reports that describe Cushing syndrome attributed to the presence of a carcinoid tumor.

Cortisol has the capacity to bind mineralocorticoid receptors in principal cells of the cortical collecting duct.[4] Normally, this is limited by conversion of cortisol to cortisone, which is unable to bind to the mineralocorticoid receptor, by the enzyme 11b-hydroxysteroid dehydrogenase type 2. Excess production of cortisol, as seen in our patient, saturates the enzyme, allowing cortisol to persist and activate mineralocorticoid receptors. This causes translocation of epithelial sodium channel proteins into the luminal membrane, increasing basolateral adenosine triphosphatase sodium/potassium pump activity and increasing renal outer medullary potassium channel activity, leading to sodium reabsorption and hypertension, hypokalemia, and metabolic alkalosis. Ideally, treatment in such patients is complete resection of the nonpituitary ACTH-secreting tumor. Unfortunately, the peritoneal carcinoid metastases were not resectable, and our patient's metabolic alkalosis and hypertension were treated with the mineralocorticoid receptor antagonist spironolactone. After being treated with spironolactone 50 mg daily for 4 weeks, the patient's blood pressure had improved to 118/77 mm Hg, serum potassium concentration had increased to 3.9 mmol/L, and serum bicarbonate concentration was 25 mmol/L.[3,4]

Clinical Presentation 18

A 19-year-old schoolteacher with no significant medical history or medication use presented with 3 months of lower back pain, proximal muscle weakness that limited his ability to stand, urinary frequency, and nocturia. Although denying dry mouth, dry eyes, or polydipsia, he describes frequent photophobia during this period.

On physical examination, blood pressure was 110/70 mm Hg and pulse rate 72 beats/min. He had tenderness over his ribs bilaterally and painful restriction to flexion and extension of the ankle and knee joints. Proximal muscle strength in the upper and lower limbs was 4/5, deep tendon reflexes were present as a normal ankle jerk, superficial reflexes were normal, and there was no sensory deficit. Serum laboratory studies include the following values: serum sodium 132 mmol/L, potassium 2.8 mmol/L, chloride 98 mmol/L, bicarbonate 18 mmol/L, creatinine 1.7 mg/dL, estimated glomerular filtration rate (GFR) 50 mL/min/1.73 m^2, glucose (fasting) 96 mg/dL, albumin 4.6 g/dL, calcium 6.8 mg/dL, phosphorous 3.1 mg/dL, ceruloplasmin 23 mg/mL (reference, 13–36 mg/mL), arterial blood gas pH 7.27, and PCO_2 47.8 mm Hg. Urinalysis showed pH 6.0, specific gravity 1.030, albumin 2+, and glucose 2+. The 24-hour urine contained 1.9 g protein, 250 potassium, 450 calcium, and 1.3 g phosphate. In addition, serological tests for antinuclear antibodies and antibodies Ro and La were negative. An ultrasound of the abdomen showed kidney sizes of 9.84.5 cm (right) and 9.64.3 cm (left); there was normal echo texture and corticomedullary differentiation.

What is the most likely diagnosis and what treatment is indicated?

A. Proximal tubular acidosis (RTA-2)
B. Nephropathic cystinosis–intermediate type
C. Distal renal tubular acidosis (RTA-1)
D. Tubulointerstitial nephritis

The correct answer is B

Comment: The features of polyuria, metabolic acidosis, hypokalemia, hypophosphatemia, glycosuria, and proteinuria suggest Fanconi syndrome.[1] This diagnosis is confirmed by the demonstration of generalized aminoaciduria and tubular proteinuria and should be followed by identification of the underlying cause. In adults, the major causes of Fanconi syndrome are monoclonal gammopathies, amyloidosis, membranous nephropathy, focal segmental glomerulosclerosis, and tubulointerstitial nephritis.[2] The other feature in this patient was photophobia. Sjögren syndrome presents classically with distal renal tubular acidosis and photophobia, although without the other abnormalities seen in Fanconi syndrome. Tubulointerstitial nephritis with uveitis also may present with proximal tubular dysfunction and photophobia, but most commonly is a diagnosis of exclusion in adolescent girls.[2]

Photophobia with Fanconi syndrome is suggestive of cystinosis.[3–5] In classic nephropathic cystinosis, Fanconi syndrome appears at 6 to 12 months of age and end-stage renal disease develops at 9 years. It accounts for 95% of reported patients. Forms with late onset, as occurred in this patient, account for 5% of all cases of cystinosis. The late-onset forms are of two phenotypes. Intermediate cystinosis, also called late-onset or juvenile cystinosis, has the same features as the nephropathic form, but patients may retain kidney function into their 30s. Ocular or nonnephropathic cystinosis, previously called benign or adult cystinosis, is characterized by only ocular findings, with all systemic manifestations lacking.[3]

Measuring the cystine usually makes the diagnosis content of peripheral leukocytes or cultured fibroblasts. The diagnosis can also be made through recognition of cystine crystals in corneal stoma, imparting a polychromatic luster on slit-lamp examination, as in this patient. Rectangular or hexagonal cystine crystals may be found in a bone marrow or kidney biopsy specimen.[4] Because cystine crystals are water-soluble, these are not retained in tissue sections after routine histological preparation with aqueous solutions. The bone marrow biopsy specimen in this patient did not show cystine crystals. The kidney biopsy specimen included eight glomeruli. Glomeruli were of normal size with patent glomerular capillaries. There was neither thickening nor irregularity of the capillary wall. Mesangial cellularity was normal. The interstitium was edematous with lymphocytic infiltrate. Cystine crystals also were not identified in the kidney biopsy specimen. *CTNS*, the gene implicated in cystinosis, encodes the protein cystinosis and maps to chromosome 17p13.[4,5]

Oral cysteamine therapy is recognized as the treatment of choice for patients with nephropathic cystinosis who have not undergone a transplant. Cysteamine depletes lysosomal cystine by a multistep mechanism. First, it enters into the lysosomal compartment through a specific transporter and reacts with cystine to form the mixed disulfide cysteamine-cysteine; this compound in turn exits the lysosomes through an intact lysine transporter, and when in the cytoplasm, is reduced by glutathione to cysteamine and cysteine. Cysteamine has the marked odor and taste of thiols and binds to oral mucosa and dental fillings. This patient, after 9 months of treatment with cysteamine, 50 mg/kg/day, had a serum creatinine level of 1.8 mg/dL. His joint pains, rib tenderness, and proximal muscle strength have improved.[1–5]

Clinical Presentation 19

A 10-year-old girl was evaluated for uncontrolled hypertension, progressive weakness, and fatigue. High BP was diagnosed at the age of 8 years during a routine clinic visit. Her BP was poorly controlled, first on atenolol therapy, and then on candesartan and amlodipine therapy. Her course also has been notable for persistent hypokalemia, with potassium values ranging from 2.8 to 3.2 mmol/L. On physical examination, the patient's BP was 150/105 mm Hg and pulse rate was 88 beats/min. Grade II retinopathy was present. Serum laboratory data included the following values: sodium 138 mmol/L, potassium 2.9 mmol/L, bicarbonate 33 mmol/L, creatinine 0.7 mg/dL, estimated GFR 97 mL/min/1.73 m^2, and magnesium 1.64 mmol/L. Urinalysis showed pH 6.0; specific gravity 1019; negative glucose, ketone, and nitrite; and 2+ protein; urinary sediment was unremarkable. Twenty-four hour urinary protein excretion ranged between 518 and 1409 mg. Echocardiography showed mild concentric left ventricular hypertrophy. Twenty-four-hour urinary excretion of free cortisol and metanephrines was normal. After felodipine and doxazosin were substituted for amlodipine and candesartan, plasma renin activity (PRA) was increased at 39.94 ng/mL/h (reference range, 1.50–5.70 ng/mL/h) and aldosterone level in the upright position was very high at 92.9 ng/dL (reference, 3.8–31.3 ng/dL).

What is the *most* likely diagnosis and how do you treat it?

A. Renin-secreting tumor
B. High renin essential hypertension
C. Renovascular hypertension
D. Hyperaldosteronism

The correct answer is A

Comment: Between 12% and 20% of patients with essential hypertension have PRA greater than the upper limit of the renin-sodium profile of normotensive control patients; however, less than 30% of these patients with high-renin essential hypertension have PRA exceeding 11 ng/mL/h, independent of daily sodium excretion.[1] Therefore, one would anticipate encountering no more than 3.5% to 6% of all patients with PRA greater than this value. The persistence of unusually high PRA despite treatment with a blocker rendered the hypothesis of high-renin essential hypertension less likely in this case. High PRA may also suggest renovascular or malignant hypertension.[2–5] In a recently published series of malignant hypertension, 76% of patients had

PRA greater than 4.9 ng/mL/h with 25% greater than 20 ng/mL/h.[2] However, patients with malignant hypertension usually present with a dramatic clinical picture and significant target-organ damage, including kidney damage and advanced retinopathy, neither of which was observed in our patient. Finally, the hypothesis of a renin-secreting tumor of the juxtaglomerular apparatus (TJGA) should be considered despite the rarity of this disease.[2]

The captopril test has been used as a screening test for renovascular hypertension; however, remarkable variability exists in the diagnostic PRA cutoff values. Renal Doppler ultrasonography, CT, and magnetic resonance renal angiography have greater diagnostic accuracy for renovascular hypertension compared with the captopril test. Renal Doppler ultrasonography and CT renal angiography were performed in our patient and excluded renovascular disease. Abdominal CT with contrast injection also was performed for suspected TJGA.[2–5]

Abdominal CT identified a 2.2-cm mass at the level of the corticomedullary junction between the middle and lower third of the left kidney, with very weak contrast enhancement in the late parenchymal phase. This location and these features are consistent with TJGA. Renal CT with contrast injection has almost 100% sensitivity for the detection of TJGA. Selective renal arteriography failed to identify these tumors, which usually appear as small hypovascular area as within the renal parenchyma in approximately 60% of patients, when this procedure was performed systematically. Renal vein sampling has at best 50% to 60% sensitivity in detecting renin lateralization, possibly because of the superficial location of these tumors draining through pericapsular veins rather than the main renal veins, variable blood dilution by extrarenal veins, or secretory intermittence.

The diagnosis was TJGA, and conservative surgery with tumor enucleation was performed. Serum potassium and BP values normalized within 7 days after surgery. At the 6-month follow-up, the patient remained normotensive (24-hour mean BP, 115/76 mm Hg). Serum potassium level was 4.6 mEq/L, upright PRA was 0.67 ng/mL/h, aldosterone level was 9.0 ng/dL, and 24-hour proteinuria decreased to 60 mg of protein.

Clinical Presentation 20

A 15-year-old presented to the emergency department with 4 days of progressive muscular weakness. Weakness developed first in his legs and hands, progressed to his arms and thighs, and finally involved his torso. He denied nausea, vomiting, diarrhea, tingling or numbness in his legs and arms, recent strenuous exertion, and alcohol use. His medical history included diabetes mellitus type 2, hypertension, and hyperlipidemia. He had bilateral leg swelling for 6 to 8 months, for which he was treated with furosemide. He denied chest pain, shortness of breath, orthopnea, or decrease in urinary output. Physical examination was significant for increased BP of 182/92 mm Hg, symmetrical flaccid paralysis with areflexia in all extremities, and bilateral pedal edema. Laboratory investigations showed the following values: sodium, 140 mmol/L; potassium, 1.8 mmol/L; chloride, 92 mmol/L; bicarbonate, 35 mmol/L; serum urea nitrogen, 25 mg/dL; serum creatinine, 1.7 mg/dL; estimated GFR, 43.2 mL/min/1.73 m2, albumin, 2.8 g/dL, calcium, 7.8 mg/dL, and creatine kinase, 2980 U/L. Urine electrolyte values were as follows: potassium, 51.9 mmol/L, and osmolality, 500 mOsm/kg. Serum osmolality was 298 mOsm/kg. Calculated transtubular potassium gradient was 17.2. Further testing showed PRA of 0.31 ng/mL/h (reference range for nonhypertensive upright adults, 0.65-5.0 ng/mL/h); serum aldosterone (upright, 8:00 a.m.), 3 ng/dL (reference ranges, <28 ng/dL); thyroid-stimulating hormone, 0.70 mIU/mL (reference range, 0.34–4.82 mIU/mL); and cortisol, 12.61 g/dL (347.9 nmol/L [reference range, 3.09–16.6 nmol/L]).

What is (are) the differential diagnosis(es) of hypokalemia in this patient (select all that apply)?

A. Cushing syndrome
B. Liddle syndrome

C. Hyperaldosteronism
D. Licorice and carbenoxolone ingestion

The correct answers are A, B, C, and D
Comment: This patient had hypertension, hypokalemia, and bilateral symmetrical muscle weakness associated with low aldosterone and renin levels. Decreased potassium intake is rarely the sole cause of hypokalemia, because urinary excretion of potassium can be decreased efficiently to 15 mEq/day. Hypokalemia caused by transcellular shift is transient, as seen with thyrotoxic periodic paralysis or hypokalemic periodic paralysis. Hypokalemia is more commonly caused by either increased gastrointestinal loss or urinary loss. In our patient, gastrointestinal loss could be excluded because the patient denied diarrhea. To explore the cause of hypokalemia from urinary losses associated with hypertension, PRA will narrow the differential diagnosis: (1) increased PRA: secondary hyperaldosteronism (renovascular hypertension, diuretics, renin-secreting tumor, malignant hypertension, and coarctation of the aorta); and (2) low PRA: primary hyperaldosteronism, Cushing syndrome, exogenous mineralocorticoids, Liddle syndrome, and licorice and carbenoxolone ingestion.[1–3]

Plasma aldosterone levels and PRA are the most helpful laboratory tests to make the diagnosis. Both plasma aldosterone concentration and PRA were less than the reference range, which excluded the possibility of primary and secondary hyperaldosteronism. The serum cortisol level was normal; however, the increased transtubular potassium gradient suggested urinary loss of potassium. Careful history taking showed that the patient was ingesting bags of licorice, which led to this mineralocorticoid excess state.[2,3]

Licorice is made from the root of Glycyrrhiza glabra. Metabolized to glycyrrhetic acid, it inhibits the enzyme 11-hydroxysteroid dehydrogenase 2 (encoded by the *HSD11B2* gene), which converts active cortisol to locally inactive cortisone at the renal tubule. The accumulated cortisol has mineralocorticoid-like activity that acts on the receptor in the distal convoluted tubules, causing sodium retention and potassium wasting, and leads to a state of hypertension and hypokalemia.

The licorice-induced mineralocorticoid effect is usually reversible on cessation of licorice ingestion. It also responds to spironolactone therapy. Dexamethasone may be considered because it suppresses endogenous cortisol production and thus decreases cortisol-mediated mineralocorticoid activity. The time required for correction of the potassium deficit after stopping licorice ingestion varies from days to weeks because of the large volume of distribution and long biological half-life of glycyrrhetinic acid. This patient was admitted to the intensive care unit, and after 3 days of receiving continuous supplements, serum potassium level normalized and clinical symptoms improved. He was discharged on an oral potassium supplement therapy and advised not to eat licorice. At 2 weeks' follow-up, his BP was 140/60 mm Hg, and chemistry test results included the following values: potassium, 4.5 mmol/L; serum creatinine, 1.0 mg/dL; and estimated GFR, 79.7 mL/min/1.73 m^2 off potassium supplements.

Clinical Presentation 21

A 19-year-old woman with type 1 insulin-dependent diabetes is admitted to the hospital with a soft-tissue infection of the palate. The initial laboratory data include the following: serum sodium 140 mmol/L, potassium 3.8 mmol/L, chloride 110 mmol/L, bicarbonate 23 mmol/L, and glucose 147 mg/dL.

The patient eats sparingly because of pain on swallowing. To minimize the risk of hypoglycemia, her insulin is withheld. Repeat blood tests are obtained 36 hours later: serum sodium 135 mmol/L, potassium 5.0 mmol/L, chloride 105 mmol/L, bicarbonate 15 mmol/L, glucose 270 mg/dL, anion gap 15 mmol/L, ketone 4+ arterial pH 7.32, and PCO_2 30 mm Hg.

Why is the anion gap only slightly elevated despite the presence of hypokalemia and ketoacidosis?

A. Beta-hydroxybutyrate and acetoacetate excretion in urine
B. Laboratory error
C. Increased serum sulfates and phosphates concentration
D. Ethylene glycol ingestion

The correct answer is A
Comment: The acidemia is due to retention of H^+ ions from ketoacidosis; the associated anions (b-hydroxybutyrate and acetoacetate) were presumably excreted in the urine, resulting in only a minor elevation in the anion gap. The patient should be given insulin with glucose. This will correct the ketoacidosis without the risk of hypoglycemia.[1,2]

Clinical Presentation 22

A 12-year-old girl complains of easy fatigability and weakness for 1 year. She has no other symptoms. The physical examination is unremarkable, including a normal BP. The following laboratory tests have been repeatedly present during this time: serum sodium 141 mmol/L, potassium 2.1 mmol/L, chloride 85 mmol/L, bicarbonate 45 mmol/L, urine sodium 80 mmol/L, and potassium 170 mmol/L.

What is the likely diagnosis?

A. Bartter syndrome
B. Liddle syndrome
C. Hyperaldosteronism
D. AME

The correct answer is A
Comment: The differential diagnosis of unexplained hypokalemia, urinary potassium wasting, and metabolic alkalosis includes surreptitious diuretic use or vomiting (during the phase of bicarbonate excretion in which both sodium and potassium excretion are increased) or some form of primary hyperaldosteronism.[1,2] The normal BP in this patient excludes all of the causes of the last condition other than Bartter syndrome.

The urine chloride concentration should be measured next. A value <25 mmol/L is highly suggestive of vomiting (which was present in this case), whereas a higher value is consistent with diuretic use or Bartter syndrome. The last two conditions can usually be distinguished by a urinary assay for diuretics.

Clinical Presentation 23

A 19-year-old man is found to be hypertensive and hypokalemic. A resident taking a careful history discovers that the patient is extremely fond of licorice.

Which of the following genetic defects produces a similar syndrome?

A. Mutation in the gene for the inwardly rectifying potassium channel (ROMK)
B. Mutation in the gene for the basolateral chloride channel CLCNKB
C. Mutation in the gene for the sodium-chloride cotransporter
D. Mutation in the gene for 11-b-hydroxysteroid dehydrogenase
E. A chimeric gene with portions of the 11-b-hydroxylase gene and the aldosterone synthesis gene

The correct answer is D

Comment: Aldosterone, the most important mineralocorticoid, increases sodium reabsorption and potassium secretion in the distal nephron. Excessive secretion of mineralocorticoids or abnormal sensitivity to mineralocorticoid hormones may result in hypokalemia, suppressed plasma renin activity, and hypertension.[1–3] The syndrome of AME is an inherited form of hypertension in which 11-b-hydroxysteroid dehydrogenase is defective.[1] This enzyme converts cortisol to its inactive metabolite, cortisone. Because mineralocorticoid receptors themselves have similar affinities for cortisol and aldosterone, the deficiency allows these receptors to be occupied by cortisol, which normally circulates at much higher plasma levels than aldosterone. Licorice contains glycyrrhetinic acid and mimics the hereditary syndrome because it inhibits 11-b-hydroxysteroid dehydrogenase.

Clinical Presentation 24

A 17-year-old young man presents to the emergency room with profound weakness of the lower and upper extremities on waking in the morning.

He has no history of prior episodes and denies weight loss, change in bowel habits, palpitations, heat intolerance, or excessive perspirations. He is not taking medications, including laxatives or diuretics, and denies drug or alcohol use. Blood pressure is 150/100 mm Hg; heart rate, 110 per minute, respiratory rate, 20 breaths per minute; and body temperature, 36.9°C. There is a symmetric flaccid paralysis with areflexia in the lower and upper extremities. The remainder of the physical examination is unremarkable. Laboratory studies show serum levels of sodium, 142 mmol/L, potassium, 1.8 mmol/L, chloride, 104 mmol/L, bicarbonate, 24 mmol/L, calcium, 10 mg/dL, phosphate, 1.2 mg/dL, magnesium, 1.6 mg/dL, glucose, 132 mg/dL, urea nitrogen, 15 mg/dL, and creatinine, 0.8 mg/ dL. Urine potassium is 1.8 mEq/L, creatinine is 146 mg/dL, and osmolality is 500 mOsm/kg of H_2O.

What is the best treatment for this patient?

A. Potassium chloride in dextrose 5% in water, 120 mEq over 6 hours
B. Potassium chloride in hypertonic saline solution, 120 mEq over 6 hours
C. Potassium phosphate in normal saline, 120 mEq over 6 hours
D. Amiloride, 10 mg, orally
E. Propranolol, 200 mg, orally

The correct answer is E

Comment: Hypokalemic periodic paralysis may be familial with autosomal dominant inheritance, or it may be acquired in patients with thyrotoxicosis.[1] Thyroid hormone increases sodium-potassium-ATPase activity on muscle cells, and excess thyroid hormone may thus increase sensitivity to the hypokalemic action of epinephrine or insulin, mediated by sodium-potassium-ATPase.[1,2]

Treatment of paralytic episodes with potassium may be effective; however, this therapy may lead to posttreatment hyperkalemia as potassium moves back out of the cells. Propranolol has been used to prevent acute episodes of thyrotoxic periodic paralysis and it may also be effective in acute attacks, without inducing rebound hyperkalemia.[1,2]

Clinical Presentation 25

A 13-year-old young woman complains of profound weakness and polyuria. She is taking no medications and has no gastrointestinal complaints. Pertinent clinical findings include a blood pressure of 90/50 mm Hg with orthostatic dizziness. Laboratory studies show plasma/serum levels of sodium, 140 mmol/L; potassium, 2.5 mmol/L; chloride, 110 mmol/L; bicarbonate, 33 mmol/L; urea nitrogen, 25 mg/dL; and creatinine, 0.7 mg/dL. A 24-hour urine sample contained sodium, 90 mmol/L; potassium, 60 mmol/L; chloride, 110 mmol/L; and calcium, 280 mg/L. Plasma renin activity and aldosterone levels are elevated.

These findings are most suggestive of which *one* of the following?

A. Gitelman syndrome
B. Licorice ingestion
C. Bartter syndrome
D. Adrenal adenoma
E. Liddle syndrome

Correct answer is C

Comment: This patient is an example of classic Bartter syndrome, characterized by early onset of metabolic alkalosis, renal potassium wasting, polyuria, and polydipsia without hypertension.[1,2] Symptoms may include vomiting, constipation, salt craving, and a tendency to volume depletion. Growth retardation follows if treatment is not initiated. Unlike in patients with Gitelman syndrome, calcium excretion is elevated. Adrenal adenoma, licorice ingestion, and Liddle syndrome are all causes of hypokalemic metabolic alkalosis, but these disorders are associated with hypertension.[1,2]

Clinical Presentation 26

A 16-year-old young woman has been referred for evaluation of hypokalemia. She has no significant past medical history and does not smoke or drink alcohol, and she denies the use of any medications. Family history is negative, but she is not sure if her parents or siblings have been diagnosed with hypertension. She avoids bread, pasta, and desserts. She denies the use of licorice, but she does eat grapefruit. Her most recent clinic visit had been 3 years earlier, at which time there were no abnormal physical or laboratory findings. Recently, the patient has begun to note occasional fatigue and muscle weakness during exercise. She also experiences occasional abdominal pain for which she saw her physician.

The physical examination is generally unremarkable, without edema, but with mild lower extremity muscle weakness. Her body mass index is 25.1 kg/m^2; blood pressure, 152/92 mm Hg with little postural change; pulse rate, 84 beats/min; respiration rate, 12 breath/min; and body temperature, 37°C. Laboratory studies show blood levels of sodium, 142 mmol/L; potassium, 2.9 mmol/L; carbon dioxide, 29 mmol/L; chloride, 106 mmol/L; urea nitrogen, 12 mg/dL; and creatinine, 0.8 mg/dL. Urinalysis shows a specific gravity of 1.030 and is otherwise negative with unremarkable sediment.

What further studies would you like to obtain at this time?

A. Spot urine for potassium-creatinine ratio
B. 24-hour urine for potassium and creatinine
C. Serum aldosterone
D. Serum cortisol
E. Spot urine for anion gap

The correct answer is A

Comment: The first step is the evaluation of urinary potassium excretion. A urinary potassium-creatinine ratio value exceeding 1.5 is evidence of inappropriate urinary potassium excretion in the face of hypokalemia and helps rule out diarrhea or laxative abuse as the cause.[1,2]

Clinical Presentation 27

The random urinary potassium-creatinine ratio value is 2.1 in the previous case.

Which of the following have we ruled out as a likely cause of the hypokalemia with this measurement?

A. Excess gastrointestinal losses
B. Excess urinary losses
C. Lower gastrointestinal tract potassium loss
D. Surreptitious diuretic abuse

The correct answer is C
Comment: The urinary potassium excretion is inappropriate for someone with hypokalemia. This indicates that the likely cause is not lower gastrointestinal loss of potassium. The upper gastrointestinal loss could still be a proximate cause because the predominant mechanism for hypokalemia in that situation is renal from secondary hyperaldosteronism and bicarbonate in the tubular fluid acting as a nonabsorbable anion. The actual potassium loss from gastric losses is not very much, as potassium concentration is only 5 mEq/L to 10 mEq/L in gastric fluid.[1,2]

Which of the following conditions remain in the differential diagnosis of this patient (select all may apply)?

A. Bartter syndrome
B. Gitelman syndrome
C. Diuretic abuse
D. Primary hyperaldosteronism
E. Secondary hyperaldosteronism
F. AME
G. Liddle syndrome

Correct answers are D, E, F, and G
Comment: The presence of hypertension and mild metabolic alkalosis indicates that all causes of primary and secondary hyperaldosteronism, as well as Liddle syndrome and the various forms of AME, have to be considered. Blood pressure would not be typically elevated with Bartter or Gitelman syndrome, but the abuse of diuretics in hypertensive patients should still be considered.[3,4]

Clinical Presentation 28

Which of the following studies would you like to order at this time (select all that may apply)?

A. Serum cortisol concentration
B. Diuretic screen concentration
C. Plasma aldosterone concentration
D. Plasma renin activity
E. Plasma magnesium concentration

The correct answers are C and D
Comment: Because we are considering the causes of hypokalemia associated with metabolic alkalosis and hypertension, measurements of plasma aldosterone concentration and plasma renin activity are necessary to differentiate the various conditions.[1,2]

Hypomagnesemia is not a cause of hypertension, nor is diuretic abuse. Diuretic abuse in a hypertensive patient might be a possibility, but it would be worthwhile to first document an elevated level of both renin and aldosterone. A plasma cortisol measurement may be of value later, but it should not be the initial test in trying to make this differentiation.

Clinical Presentation 29

Serum aldosterone level is 2.2 ng/dL (reference, 4–31 ng/dL) and plasma renin activity is less than 0.1 ng/mL/h (reference, 0.5–4 ng/mL/h).

Which of the following conditions remain under diagnostic consideration (select all that apply)?

A. Primary hyperaldosteronism
B. Liddle syndrome
C. Renovascular hypertension
D. Diuretic abuse
E. Syndrome of AME
F. Cushing syndrome
G. Deoxycorticosterone-acetate secreting tumor
H. Renin-secreting tumor

The correct answers are B and E
Comment: The data are clearly consistent with suppressed levels of aldosterone and renin. The differential diagnosis therefore now consists of conditions associated with no aldosterone-mediated mineralocorticoid excess.

Diuretic abuse and primary or secondary hyperaldosteronism are no longer considerations because all would have elevated levels of aldosterone.

Diuretic abuse and secondary hyperaldosteronism, renovascular hypertension, and renin-secreting tumors would also be associated with elevated plasma renin activity.[1,2]

Clinical Presentation 30

At this point, it might be valuable to review the patient's history.

Which of the following aspects of the patient's history might have significance to her laboratory data (select all that apply)?

A. Social history
B. Dietary history
C. Family history
D. Current medications
E. History of present illness

The correct answers are B and C
Comment: Two aspects of the dietary history are very important. She denies ingesting licorice but apparently ingests large amounts of grapefruit. Acquired AME is seen with ingestion of licorice and grapefruit. Dietary flavonoids present in licorice and in grapefruit inhibit the enzyme 11-b-hydroxysteroid dehydrogenase, allowing cortisol to occupy the mineralocorticoid receptor.[1,2]

Clinical Presentation 31

A decision is made to treat the patient. She is started on spironolactone, 400 mg/day. She returns 10 days later. Her blood pressure is 160/90 mm Hg and her serum sodium is 140 mmol/L; potassium, 3.1 mmol/L; chloride, 107 mmol/L; and bicarbonate, 30 mmol/L. She is then switched to amiloride and returns 2 weeks later. At this point, blood pressure is 127/78 mm Hg.

What is the likely diagnosis?

A. Grapefruit-induced hypokalemia
B. Congenital syndrome of AME
C. Liddle syndrome
D. Gitelman syndrome
E. Bartter syndrome

The correct answer is C
Comment: The differential response to amiloride is indicative of Liddle syndrome.[1,2] The mechanism of AME caused by either a genetic defect or an acquired abnormality in 11-b hydroxysteroid dehydrogenase (resulting from licorice or grapefruit in the latter case) is enhanced mineralocorticoid activity by virtue of occupation of the mineralocorticoid receptor by glucocorticoids. Thus, the symptoms should respond to receptor occupant ion by spironolactone. In contrast, Liddle syndrome is due to enhanced activity of the sodium channel, which is unaffected by spironolactone but is blocked by amiloride.[1,2]

Clinical Presentation 32

A 15-year-old boy presented with 3 weeks of dyspnea and cough with blood-tinged mucus. Computed tomography of the chest revealed a large mediastinal mass, and bronchoscopy with biopsy confirmed small cell lung carcinoma. There were no adrenal or brain metastases. On admission, laboratory values included potassium of 2.5 mmol/L and serum bicarbonate of 40 mmol/L. He was treated with normal saline solution infusion and potassium supplementation and was then discharged. The patient was readmitted with agitation, confusion, and hypoxia. On examination, he was hypertensive with a systolic BP of 160 to 170 mm Hg. Potassium level was 2.0 mmol/L, serum bicarbonate level was 55 mmol/L, and sodium level was 149 mmol/L; he had normal kidney function. Early-morning cortisol level was elevated at 47 mg/dL, and 24-hour urinary cortisol level was 7859 (reference, 4–50) mg/dL. Both low- and high-dose dexamethasone suppression tests failed to suppress his cortisol level. Other laboratory tests showed an aldosterone level 1.0 ng/dL and low plasma renin activity. Arterial blood gas revealed pH of 7.65, PCO_2 of 64.3 mm Hg, and PO_2 of 56 mm Hg. Urinalysis showed specific gravity of 1.008 and urine osmolality of 266 mOsm/kg. He had polyuria during admission, with urine output of 6.3 L/day. Hypokalemia persisted despite appropriate potassium supplementation.

What is the cause of this patient's polyuria and what is the appropriate treatment for this patient?

A. Primary aldosteronism
B. Renin-secreting tumor
C. Nephrogenic DI resulting from ectopic ACTH syndrome
D. AME

The correct answer is C

Comment: Hypokalemia can arise from a transcellular shift or increased renal and gastrointestinal losses. This patient's metabolic abnormalities persisted despite avoidance of diuretics, lack of gastrointestinal losses, and appropriate potassium supplementation. The triad of hypertension, severe hypokalemia, and metabolic alkalosis can be seen in various conditions that can be differentiated based on the patient's renin-angiotensin-aldosterone system profile. Suppressed PRA, increased plasma aldosterone concentration (PAC), and PAC:PRA ratio 20[3] is characteristic of primary hyperaldosteronism.[1] Elevation of both PRA and PAC levels suggests secondary hyperaldosteronism (i.e., renovascular hypertension, diuretic use, or a renin-secreting tumor). Alternatively, suppression of both PRA and PAC levels should prompt investigation for alternative causes of severe hypokalemia and metabolic alkalosis, such as congenital adrenal hyperplasia, Liddle syndrome, or states of AME.

This patient had suppressed PRA and PAC levels, which in the clinical context of lung cancer led to the diagnosis of ectopic ACTH syndrome.[2,3]

Under normal conditions, excess cortisol is converted to its inactive metabolite cortisone by the kidney by the enzyme 11-b-hydroxysteroid dehydrogenase. Excessive amounts of active cortisol can overwhelm the capacity of this enzyme, resulting in cross-reactivity with renal mineralocorticoid receptors. This can lead to an acquired form of AME with severe hypokalemia and metabolic alkalosis. Suppression of plasma renin and aldosterone release occurs by negative feedback inhibition. Additionally, ectopic ACTH causes increased secretion of the mineralocorticoid-like hormones, such as 11 deoxycorticosterone and corticosterone, which can potentially lead to a greater degree of hypokalemia and metabolic alkalosis compared to adrenal-limited Cushing syndrome.

The differential diagnosis of polyuria includes central or nephrogenic diabetes insipidus and psychogenic polydipsia.[4,5] An osmotic load, water load, or a mix of both can drive polyuria. Osmotic diuresis is characterized by high urine osmolality (>300 mOsm/kg) and can be seen in hyperglycemia, high-protein enteral nutrition, and urea or mannitol administration. Pure water diuresis presents with low urine osmolality (<100 mOsm/kg) and results from increased free water excretion in the absence of antidiuretic hormone, reduced antidiuretic hormone responsiveness, or free water intoxication (psychogenic polydipsia). This patient's urine osmolality of 266 mOsm/kg is most consistent with mixed polyuria. Given his normal kidney function and solute and water intake, the cause was thought to be DI. His severe and prolonged hypokalemia (a known cause of renal tubular dysfunction) likely resulted in defective urine concentrating ability and partial nephrogenic diabetes insipidus. Lack of brain metastases made central diabetes insipidus less likely. Of note, he had only mild hypernatremia, likely from an intact thirst mechanism and the ability to maintain free water intake.

Complete removal of an ACTH-secreting tumor is the optimal treatment of ectopic ACTH syndrome. Because this patient had a nonresectable tumor, the hypercortisolism was treated medically with an adrenal enzyme inhibitor (ketoconazole, 200 mg, three times daily). This led to near normalization of serum cortisol levels. Additionally, given concern for hypokalemia-induced nephrogenic DI, he was treated with a potassium-sparing diuretic (amiloride, 5 mg/day) with subsequent improvement in all electrolyte level derangements. His urine output also improved to 1.0 L/day.[1–5]

Clinical Presentation 33

A 15-year-old White girl presented to the emergency department with a 2-day history of generalized body weakness, abdominal pain, and an inability to move her extremities. She reported poor appetite, fatigue, dizziness, generalized joint pains, back pain, nausea, and two episodes of vomiting. She denied having a history of diarrhea, dysuria, blood in the urine, changes in urine output, and frequent or urgent urination. She also denied having a history of recent upper respiratory symptoms, headaches, chest pain, difficulty breathing, or leg or joint swelling. There was no history of seizures, rash, syncope, speech difficulty, lightheadedness, or numbness. She denied recent intense exercise, starvation, high-carbohydrate and/or low-potassium diet, and ingestion of illicit drugs or alcohol.

Her past medical history was significant for a history of medullary sponge kidneys (MSK) and RTA diagnosed 2 years ago when being worked up for generalized muscle weakness. She reported having had three previous episodes of similar presentations over the past 2 years and was told that she had low serum potassium levels. All three episodes necessitated a hospital admission lasting for about a day and the episodes resolved with intravenous potassium supplements and hydration. The patient's mother was unsure of what the serum potassium levels had been between those episodes. The patient had been placed on daily potassium and bicarbonate supplements for the past year but had not been taking it for the past 2 months. She was born at full term with a birth weight of 7.33 kg. Her growth and development were appropriate with no history of failure to thrive or repeated hospitalizations for dehydration episodes. There was no history of deafness, polyuria, or bone loss. There was no history suggestive of autoimmune disorders. She was sexually active with one male partner and had no history of sexually transmitted disease. Her family history was insignificant for consanguinity, similar problems, low serum potassium, or any other renal diseases.

On physical examination, her vitals were as follows: BP 114/56 mm Hg manually in the right upper extremity with an adequate sized cuff (95th percentile BP: 126/82 mm Hg), pulse 100 beats/min, respiratory rate 16 breath/min, temperature 36.6°C, weight 58.9 kg (70th percentile), height 157 cm (20th percentile), body mass index 24 kg/m^2 (82nd percentile), and SpO_2 99% on room air. She was alert and oriented. She was otherwise well developed and well nourished. Extraocular movements were normal. There was no periorbital edema. There was no moon facies. There was no cervical adenopathy. She did have mild neck tenderness with restricted neck movements. Speech was not slurred. Heart sounds were normal with regular rhythm and with no murmurs. Lungs were clear to auscultation with symmetric chest expansion and no use of accessory muscles. Abdomen examination showed mild generalized tenderness. Bowel sounds were normal. There was marked tenderness in both lower extremities. Deep tendon reflexes were present but diminished and the muscle strength was two in all four extremities. Tone was diminished in all four extremities, more so in the lower extremities. Pain sensation was intact. There were no cranial nerve deficits.

Laboratory investigations showed normal complete blood count and liver function test. Initial arterial blood gas showed pH 7.18, PCO_2 28 mm Hg, PO_2 129 mm Hg, bicarbonate 10 mmol/L, and base excess −18 mmol/L. Initial serum electrolytes showed serum Na+ 140 mmol/L, K+ less than 1 mmol/L, Cl^- 116 mmol/L, bicarbonate 13 mmol/L, BUN 17 mg/dL, creatinine 1.19 mg/dL, calcium 8.1 mg/dL, P 1.5 mg/dL, which later increased to 4 mg/dL, magnesium 2.6 mg/dL, lactate <0.3 mmol/L, anion gap 11, albumin 3.6 g/dL, and serum osmolality of 290 mOsm/kg. Urine osmolality was 400 mOsm/kg, spot urine sodium 68 mmol/L, spot urine potassium 20 mmol/L, spot urine creatinine 24 mg/dL, spot urine calcium 12 mg/dL, spot urine protein 16 mg/dL, and positive urine myoglobin. Transtubular potassium gradient (TTKG) was elevated at 14.5 (value >2 during hypokalemia indicates renal loss). Spot urine calcium to creatinine ratio was 0.5. Initial urinalysis showed pH of 7.5 (which remained persistently at 7-7.5 on repeat tests), specific gravity 1.008, no glucose, no ketones, no protein, 164 WBCs per high-power field (HPF), positive blood with 10 red blood cells per HPF, many bacteria, and large leukocyte esterase and negative nitrites. Urine culture was negative. Urine toxicology was negative. Urine anion gap was +4. Urine electrophoresis showed nonselective proteinuria. Blood culture showed no growth. Plasma renin activity was 1.5 ng/mL/h and serum aldosterone was 1.8 ng/dL. Serum 25 hydroxy vitamin D level was 28 ng/mL, intact PTH was 52 pg/mL, and she had a normal thyroid profile. Lupus serologies were negative. Total creatine kinase level was elevated at 1392 U/L. Electrocardiography showed evidence of normal sinus rhythm, with a rate of 98 beats/min with a normal axis but generalized ST segment depression and T-wave inversion with QT 432 ms. Renal sonogram showed a right kidney of 12.4 × 4.2 × 4.3 cm and a left kidney measuring 11.7 × 4.1 × 4.3 cm. A CT scan of the abdomen and pelvis without contrast agent was performed.

She was admitted to the pediatric intensive care unit and aggressive electrolyte replacement and acidosis correction were initiated. Acidosis and electrolytes improved with replacement of potassium acetate, potassium phosphate, and bicarbonate infusions. After treatment, her venous blood gas showed pH 7.37, PCO_2 41 mm Hg, PO_2 34 mm Hg, bicarbonate 24 mEq/L, and a base deficit of 1.4 mEq/L. Serum bicarbonate, creatinine, and potassium on discharge were 24 mmol/L, 1.03 mg/dL, and 3.4 mmol/L, respectively. Muscle weakness and pain also resolved. The patient was discharged in stable condition on potassium and bicarbonate supplements.

What is the *most* likely diagnosis?

A. Hypokalemic familial periodic paralysis (HFPP)
B. Primary hypoaldosteronism
C. Pseudohyperaldosteronism
D. MSK

The correct answer is D

Comment: Hypokalemic paralysis, as the name implies, encompasses paralysis, muscle weakness, and is seen with severe hypokalemia.[1,2] Various causes of such are mentioned previously. However, the most important challenge is to differentiate between the recurrent paralyzes caused by RTA, mainly the distal type, and that caused by HFPP, an entirely different condition.[3,4] The latter can be caused either by hypokalemia (most commonly) or by hyperkalemia. Hypokalemia in HFPP is not due to loss of potassium as observed in distal RTA (dRTA), but to abnormalities in its redistribution between intra- and extracellular compartments. Often, the predisposing factors are strenuous exercise, high-carbohydrate diet, and other triggers. They usually have normal physical growth unlike patients with dRTA. Acidosis is not a typical feature and nephrocalcinosis is not observed. Mutations in two genes encoding subunits of skeletal muscle voltage-gated calcium or sodium channels (*CACNL1A3* and *SCN4A*) have been identified in hypokalemic HFPP. Most of the cases are hereditary, mostly autosomal dominant (AD), but acquired cases can occur with thyrotoxicosis. Management in hypokalemic HFPP involves administration of potassium supplements and/or potassium-sparing diuretic; bicarbonate is not required because it may worsen the paralysis by redistributing potassium intracellularly. This is in opposition to hypokalemia in dRTA, where both potassium and bicarbonate supplements are required.

dRTA is characterized by an impaired capacity of the distal tubules to secrete hydrogen ions and hence ammonium secretion. Urine anion gap provides a rough estimate of urinary ammonium excretion. Besides normal serum anion gap and hyperchloremic metabolic acidosis, patients with dRTA have an abnormally high urine pH 5.5[3] for the degree of systemic acidemia in addition to positive urine anion gap.[4] The most common cause of dRTA in children is primary, mostly familial; it can be either AD or autosomal recessive. AD dRTA is mainly due to mutations causing defects in the kidney anion exchanger (kAE1) in the distal tubule a-intercalated cells. The autosomal recessive form of dRTA is mainly the result of mutations causing defects in beta subunit of H+ ATPase in the apical membrane of a-intercalated cells. Most of the children have some degree of growth failure. In adults, dRTA can be associated with hypergammaglobulinemia, autoimmune conditions (e.g., systemic lupus erythematous, rheumatoid arthritis), and drugs (e.g., lithium, amphotericin B, ifosfamide). Other secondary causes of dRTA are hypercalciuric conditions (e.g., hyperparathyroidism, vitamin D intoxication, sarcoidosis). Hypercalciuria is common in dRTA because of effects of chronic acidosis on both bone resorption and the renal tubular reabsorption of calcium. Hypercalciuria eventually leads to nephrocalcinosis and nephrolithiasis. Association of nephrocalcinosis with MSK has been described.

Our patient had a known diagnosis of MSK and typical features of bilateral diffuse medullary nephrocalcinosis. Patients with MSK can have medullary nephrocalcinosis along with renal tubular acidification defects; both proximal and dRTA have been described.[3] The latter is thought to be due to tubular disruption by cysts. MSK is a congenital disorder manifested by the formation of medullary cysts secondary to dilatation of the collecting ducts in the pericalyceal region of the renal pyramids. The gold standard test to diagnose MSK is an intravenous urography. Another diagnostic modality may be a CT scan with contrast showing persistence of the contrast enhancement in the renal collecting tubules and may be as useful as an intravenous pyelogram. MSK is usually diagnosed incidentally when being worked up for another condition. However, growth failure can be associated with it and hence may be diagnosed in patients as early as age 5 or 12 years. In fact, most cases of dRTA described in the literature in association with MSK presented with growth failure. Severe hypokalemia in dRTA has been described in association with MSK and nephrocalcinosis. Our patient had recurrent hypokalemic paralysis secondary to dRTA but presented with normal growth. Evaluation of her growth charts before the diagnosis of dRTA and before being on potassium and bicarbonate supplements revealed normal height and weight. This may suggest an incomplete dRTA; however, we do not have an ammonium chloride test to confirm this.

dRTA is commonly associated with varying degrees of hypokalemia. However, the exact mechanism of hypokalemia is not very clear. The accepted hypothesis is that when H+ secretion is impaired, there is simultaneous amplification of potassium secretory mechanisms involving the potassium channel, ROMK, or the epithelial sodium channels. However, some forms of dRTA can present with normal or even high serum potassium. Also, the autosomal recessive form of dRTA usually presents with more severe hypokalemia and acidosis compared with the AD form. The primary form of dRTA can present sporadically as in our patient (most likely) because there was no similar family history or history of consanguinity. However, we could not perform mutation analysis of the kAE1 or H+ ATPase because the patient was lost to follow-up.

TTKG is an index of potassium secretary activity in the distal tubules. There is a positive correlation between aldosterone activity and the TTKG; a high TTKG value during hypokalemia generally reflects increased aldosterone production or increased distal tubule response to aldosterone. TTKG lower than 6 (in adults) and lower than 4 (in children) indicates an inappropriate renal response to hyperkalemia, whereas value greater than 2 during hypokalemia generally points to renal loss. Hence, the expected value of the TTKG must be interpreted per the serum concentration of potassium. Our patient had inappropriately high TTKG in the setting of hypokalemia. The possible causes include hyperaldosteronism or pseudohyperaldosteronism. Her serum aldosterone level was not elevated. Additionally, the CT scan of the abdomen showed no adrenal lesions. Hypokalemia in association with hyperaldosteronism secondary to adrenal tumor has been described. Causes of pseudohyperaldosteronism including Cushing syndrome, AME, or licorice ingestion were unlikely given normal physical examination and normotension and no alkalosis.[1–4]

Clinical Presentation 34

A 16-year-old male is admitted to the hospital with worsening dyspnea and 8-kg weight gain and is diagnosed with acute decompensated heart failure. He has a history of hypertension, type 2 diabetes, chronic kidney disease (CKD) GFR stage III, albuminuria (3+), and ischemic cardiomyopathy with ejection fraction 30%. He is adherent to prescribed medications, including losartan, furosemide (40 mg twice daily), atorvastatin, and insulin. His BP is 162/92 mm Hg and heart rate 104 beats/min. Physical examination reveals an S3 gallop, bilateral crackles, and pitting edema (3+). Admission laboratory data include serum sodium level of 132 mEq/L, serum potassium level of 5.2 mEq/ L, serum urea nitrogen level of 63 mg/dL, and serum creatinine level of 4.1 mg/dL (baseline, 1.4 mg/dL).

Which of the following is the next best step in management?

A. Prescribe furosemide intravenous (IV) infusion.
B. Prescribe metolazone.
C. Prescribe dapagliflozin.
D. Prescribe isolated ultrafiltration.
E. Discontinue losartan.

The correct answer is A

Which of the following is the most appropriate diuretic regimen for discharge?

A. Furosemide 120 mg twice daily and metolazone 10 mg daily.
B. Furosemide 80 mg twice daily
C. Furosemide 160 daily
D. Bumetanide 4 mg daily
E. Bumetanide 4 mg twice daily

The correct answer is B

Comment: The patient was initially prescribed a furosemide loading dose of 80 mg IV to rapidly achieve a therapeutic serum level, followed by a maintenance dose of 5 mg/h (120 mg/day) IV to maintain a steady state; this management strategy has effectively achieved decongestion. This dose is equivalent to 240 mg/day orally, which should be given as 120 mg twice daily to avoid postdiuretic sodium reabsorption. However, because this patient's signs and symptoms of acute decompensated heart failure and AKI resolved and 2.4 L/day urine output is no longer necessary, a lower oral dose of furosemide, such as 80 mg twice daily, may be appropriate. Furosemide 120 mg twice daily with metolazone 10 mg/day would further increase diuresis and could cause hypovolemia and/or hypokalemia. Similarly, bumetanide 4 mg orally twice daily, which is equivalent to furosemide 160 mg IV twice daily or 320 mg orally twice daily, would also risk hypovolemia. Unless sodium intake can be severely restricted, neither furosemide nor bumetanide should be dosed once daily.[1]

Clinical Presentation 35

A 15-year-old male was admitted to the hospital with myalgias and generalized weakness. Two weeks before, he had abdominal pain, decreased oral intake, nausea, and vomiting. He denied diarrhea. One week before admission, he developed muscle weakness that worsened until he was unable to get out of bed without assistance. His medical history was unremarkable. His only reported medication was over-the-counter ibuprofen for chronic back pain, 2400 to 3200 mg daily for several months. He denied alcohol or solvent abuse. On physical examination, he was alert and oriented. His vital signs were normal. He was unable to raise his upper or lower extremities against gravity and had decreased deep tendon reflexes with intact superficial sensations. The rest of his examination findings were unremarkable. Initial laboratory workup showed normal blood cell counts, severe hypokalemia (potassium, 1.8 mEq/L), and metabolic acidosis. The electrocardiogram showed flattened T waves in lateral leads. He received 120 mEq of potassium overnight, and 12 hours after admission, his serum potassium level increased to 2.1 mEq/L.

What is the most likely diagnosis in this patient?

A. Type 1 renal tubular acidosis (dRTA)
B. Bartter syndrome

C. Hyperaldosteronism
D. Type II renal tubular acidosis (proximal RTA)
E. Gitelman syndrome

The correct answer is A

Comment: Hypokalemia is likely secondary to reversible type 1 renal tubular acidosis, likely from ibuprofen use.[1]

A systematic approach to hypokalemia can help narrow the differential diagnosis in this case.

Hypokalemia can result from shifts of potassium from the extracellular to the intracellular space (internal balance) or from potassium depletion resulting from losses into the gastrointestinal tract or urine (external balance). Severe hypokalemia with paralysis from an intracellular potassium shift can be due to hypokalemic periodic paralysis (hereditary or thyrotoxic) or exogenous insulin or catecholamines. In our patient, the relatively high urinary potassium excretion, the need for large doses of potassium during replacement, and the clinical course made us conclude that he was potassium depleted. The causes of potassium depletion include vomiting, diarrhea, RTA, toluene toxicity, diuretic use, Bartter and Gitelman syndromes, and acquired or hereditary hypertensive renal potassium wasting disorders.[1]

The expected renal response to hypokalemia would be to limit urinary potassium excretion. A patient has abnormal urinary losses during hypokalemia if potassium excretion surpasses 30 mEq in a 24-hour urine collection or a random urine potassium-creatinine ratio is >13 mEq/g. Our patient had 30 mEq of potassium per gram of creatinine in the urine on admission and 112 mEq of potassium in the 24-hour urine collection (while getting potassium repletion). Urinalysis was normal with a pH of 7.0.[1]

The cause of renal potassium wasting can be determined from the associated acid–base disturbance and blood pressure. Our patient had a normal anion gap metabolic acidosis. Therefore, we need not consider the various causes of hypertensive or normotensive renal potassium wasting with metabolic alkalosis.[1]

Normal anion gap metabolic acidosis and potassium wasting could be caused by RTA, toluene toxicity, or diarrhea. RTA with hypokalemia can be seen in type 1 (distal) or type 2 (proximal) RTA. Proximal RTA typically has mild hypokalemia, an acid urine pH (unless treated), and other proximal tubular abnormalities (Fanconi syndrome) that were absent in our patient. Severe hypokalemia and alkaline urine pH are features of distal RTA. Inhaling solvent fumes, such as glue sniffing or paint huffing, results in systemic absorption of toluene, which is oxidized to benzoic acid and then conjugated with glycine to form hippuric acid. These hippurate anions are then secreted into the tubular lumen with sodium and potassium (along with ammonium, which raises the urine pH), causing a very similar picture to distal RTA. In addition to urine potassium and pH, other relevant urine parameters include the urinary osmoles (sodium, potassium, urea, and glucose), which enable us to calculate the urinary osmolar gap, the difference between measured urine osmolarity and calculated urine osmolarity (2 × [Na + K]) + [urea] + [glucose]), which serves as a surrogate of ammonium excretion.[1]

A normal anion gap metabolic acidosis caused by diarrhea or solvent abuse is associated with high rates of urine ammonium excretion; the rate of urine ammonium excretion is not high in RTA. Urine ammonium is not routinely measured by clinical laboratory tests, but it can be estimated from the gap between measured and calculated urine osmolality; urine ammonium excretion is approximately equal to half the urine osmolar gap. In our patient, the 24-hour urine osmolar gap was not high, and hippuric acid was not found in urine. The elevated urine pH without an increase in urinary osmolar gap is consistent with a diagnosis of dRTA.[1]

The acute onset of dRTA without nephrocalcinosis makes an acquired rather than a congenital form more likely. Autoimmune disease, most often Sjögren syndrome, is the most common cause of acquired dRTA. Serologic testing was negative for autoimmune causes, so we considered additional causes. Although ibuprofen has typically been associated with hyperkalemia, there have been several case reports of severe hypokalemia and transient distal RTA resulting from abuse of a combination drug containing ibuprofen and codeine. The pathogenesis is unclear but inhibition of carbonic anhydrase, which is present in the proximal and distal tubules, has been suggested.[1]

Consistent with the suspicion of ibuprofen being the etiologic agent, after the patient stopped treatment with the medication, his serum potassium level increased dramatically and renal losses decreased. He was discharged with a normal potassium level, and normal carbon dioxide level, and had no subsequent recurrences.[1]

Clinical Presentation 36

A 10-year-old girl, born of a nonconsanguineous marriage, presented with history of poor urinary stream, continuous dribbling, and primary enuresis. She had history of recurrent febrile urinary tract infections (UTIs) and constipation since birth. She had been prescribed antibiotics and laxatives intermittently by her primary care physician. At the age of 8 years, she was seen in a urology clinic and was found to have a solitary right kidney with hydroureteronephrosis and urinary bladder wall diverticuli on ultrasonography. She was managed as a case of dysfunctional voiding with oral alpha adrenoceptor antagonist, tamsulosin, and clean intermittent catheterization, which she discontinued after a few months. There was no history of maternal diabetes or any antenatal infection, and the parents were not informed of any abnormalities on antenatal ultrasound. Her birth and family history were noncontributory. She had age-appropriate mental, social, and motor milestones.

On examination, her height was 120 cm and weight was 19 kg (both less than the third percentile), and she was stage 1 on the Tanner sexual maturity scale. She had mild pallor and stage 1 hypertension (BP 122/80 mm Hg). She had no edema, breathlessness, or bony deformities. Her spine was normal, and she had normal-appearing external genitalia. There was hypoplasia of the left thenar eminence compared with the right hand with no restriction in the movements of left thumb at the first metacarpophalangeal and interphalangeal joints. There were no palpable lumps in the abdomen or in the inguinal region. She did not have anosmia, and hearing assessment was normal. Neurological examination was unremarkable except for weak anal tone. Perineal sensation was preserved.

Her laboratory parameters showed anemia, elevated serum creatinine, low serum bicarbonate, low vitamin D, and elevated parathormone level. Urine microscopy showed abundant WBCs, and culture grew a significant colony count of *Escherichia coli*. There was no proteinuria or hematuria. Serum electrolytes were: sodium 139 mEq/L, potassium 3.5 mEq/L, chloride 90 mEq/L, bicarbonate 14 mEq/L, BUN 22 mg/dL, creatinine 2.2 mg/dL, calcium 9.2 mg/dL, phosphorous 5.3 mg/dL, alkaline phosphatase 431 IU/L, vitamin D3 11.0 ng/mL, and intact PTH 180 pg/mL. Venous blood gas showed pH was 7.32, PCO_2 17 mm Hg, and bicarbonate 13 mEq/L.

The abdominal ultrasonography confirmed the presence of solitary right kidney (8.8 × 4.1 cm, at 50th percentile in kidney length chart) with hydroureteronephrosis, poor corticomedullary differentiation, and irregular thickening of the bladder wall. The uterus and ovaries were absent. She underwent urinary catheterization, and a UTI was treated with intravenous ceftriaxone. For constipation, she received daily enemas and later maintenance therapy with oral lactulose. After confirming a normal urine analysis, a micturating cystourethrogram (MCU) was performed, which showed an elongated bladder outline with sacculations giving a "Christmas tree" appearance. Later, MRI of the pelvis and lumbosacral spine was done, which showed a neurogenic bladder with irregular walls and sacculations, solitary right hydroureter, and solitary right gross hydronephrosis. Sagittal T2 imaging revealed a neurogenic bladder and dilated rectum with absent Müllerian structure between the two organs. There is absent coccyx and lower sacral segments. Coronal T2 imaging showed partial agenesis of the sacrum with absent lower sacral segments and coccyx. The solitary right kidney had hydronephrosis.

What is your diagnosis?

A. Neurogenic bladder
B. Ureterocele
C. Ureteropelvic junction obstruction
D. Bladder neck obstruction

The correct answer is A

Comment: This girl with a solitary kidney had urinary incontinence and constipation since birth along with recurrent UTIs, resulting in the development of CKD stage IV (estimated GFR 22 mL/min/1.73 m^2 by modified Schwartz formula). She was underweight with short stature and had hypertension, anemia, metabolic acidosis, vitamin D deficiency, and hyperparathyroidism, which are manifestations of CKD. The solitary right kidney did not show compensatory hypertrophy and had loss of corticomedullary differentiation with hydroureteronephrosis in the absence of vesicoureteric reflux. These findings and increased bladder wall thickness on ultrasound suggested presence of concomitant bladder dysfunction probably because of anatomical or functional obstruction. A patulous anus and characteristic "Christmas tree" appearance of the urinary bladder with irregular contours were suggestive of a neurogenic bladder. Both ovaries and uterus were absent. Because the patient was phenotypically female, this prompted us to consider 46, XY disorders of sexual development such as androgen insensitivity syndrome (OMIM 300068). She was in her early adolescence; hence, we could not comment on the development of secondary sexual characteristics. Patients with androgen insensitivity syndrome usually do not have extragenital anomalies.[1] The presence of genitourinary abnormalities, abnormal thumb of the left hand with loss of thenar prominence, and probable neurogenic bladder raised the suspicion of multisystem structural involvement. Patients with Kallmann syndrome may rarely have solitary kidneys with genital and skeletal abnormalities but they have associated anosmia and a family history of delayed or absent puberty.[2] Hence, we revisited our differential diagnosis to a syndrome that involved Müllerian duct agenesis, congenital anomalies of the kidney and urinary tract, and the skeletal system. We further evaluated the patient for Mayer-Rokitansky-Küster-Hauser syndrome.

Clinical Presentation 37

A 6-year-old girl who had been followed up with cerebral palsy and epilepsy was admitted because of hyponatremia on routine check-up. She had been on treatment with valproic acid and clonazepam for 1 year before her referral and the dosage of valproic acid had been increased to 40 mg/kg/daily because of short-lasting intractable seizures.

At admission, her vital signs were normal; she had no signs of dehydration or hypovolemia. Neurological examination revealed increased deep tendon reflexes and Babinski reflex. Other systemic examination findings were normal.

Laboratory investigations were as follows: glucose 97 mg/dL, creatinine 0.3 mg/dL, urea 19 mg/dL, sodium 129 mEq/L, potassium 4.4 mEq/L, calcium 9.5 mg/dL, phosphorus 4.8 mg/dL, chloride 101 mEq/L, magnesium 1.9 mg/dL, aspartate aminotransferase 39 IU/L, alanine aminotransferase 18 IU/L, and uric acid 3.2 mg/dL. Thyroid function tests were normal. Blood gas analysis revealed a pH of 7.43, bicarbonate of 23 mEq/L, and PCO_2 of 28 mm Hg. Serum level of valproic acid was 141 µg/mL (therapeutic range, 50-100 µg/mL). Urine sodium was 44 mEq/L, potassium was 17 mEq/L, and density was 1.022; urine microscopic examination was normal. Plasma osmolality was 267 mOsm/kg and urine osmolality was 256 mOsm/kg. Ultrasonographic examination of kidneys and the urinary tract was normal. Cranial CT was normal except for chronic alterations resulting from perinatal asphyxia.

What is your diagnosis for this patient?

A. Cerebral salt wasting
B. Reset hyponatremia
C. SIADH
D. Pseudohyponatremia

The correct answer is C

Comment: The clinical picture described in this patient is consistent with SIADH. SIADH observed in this patient is attributed to the increased serum levels of valproic acid (VPA) that exceeded the therapeutic range. Restricting daily fluid intake and decreasing the dose of VPA to obtain a therapeutic level was our first management strategy. After 1 week of dose adjustment, the patient's serum level of VPA decreased to 90 μg/dL (50–100 μg/dL) and sodium level increased to 137 mEq/L.

SIADH is a well-known cause of euvolemic hyponatremia and is characterized by the presence of hypo-osmolality and inappropriately increased urine osmolality (>120 mOsm/kg) in the absence of abnormal kidney function, glucocorticoid deficiency, hypothyroidism, and decreased arterial blood volume. The hallmark of the activity of ADH is considered to be inappropriate in this disorder because no exact osmotic or hemodynamic stimulus is detected for its action.[1,2] Water excretion is impaired despite the hypo-osmolality of plasma.[2,3] There is a variety of etiological causes in SIADH, such as central nervous system disorders (infection, trauma, malignancies, intracranial hemorrhage), pulmonary diseases (infections, malignancy, cystic fibrosis), and neoplasia (leukemia, lymphoma).[2] A number of drugs have also been associated with this syndrome such as cyclophosphamide, vincristine, amitriptyline, and desipramine. Among antiepileptic drugs, carbamazepine and oxcarbazepine are more commonly reported to cause SIADH.[3,4] VPA is extremely rarely reported as a cause of SIADH and all of the reported cases are in adults.[3,5,6]

Our patient was diagnosed with SIADH because of euvolemic hyponatremia and elevated urine osmolality despite low plasma osmolality, normal kidney function, and the absence of thyroid deficiency. There was no obvious clinical or laboratory evidence of malignancies or pulmonary disorders, so these possible etiological causes of SIADH were excluded. Intracranial tumors and/or hemorrhage were excluded by cranial CT. She did not have fever, vomiting, altered consciousness, or meningeal irritation signs, so meningitis was also ruled out. Although we did not obtain serum cortisol levels, we believed that adrenal insufficiency was unlikely in this patient because she was asymptomatic, her volume status and blood pressure were normal, she did not have hyperpigmentation, and she had no significant abnormality on laboratory examination other than hyponatremia. After all possible causes were excluded as described, the underlying etiology of SIADH was attributed to VPA. The concomitant use of clonazepam in our patient may raise the question of whether this drug may also be the cause of hyponatremia.

Clinical Presentation 38

A previously healthy 12-year-old boy was admitted for the evaluation of recurrent, painless gross hematuria of 2 weeks' duration. The patient denied abdominal or back pain, had no dysuria, fatigue, or fever, and a complete review of systems was unremarkable except for the bright red urine. There was no antecedent history of trauma, sore throat, sinusitis, no symptoms or evidence of other infections, and no history of bleeding diathesis. The patient denied ever having been sexually active. His past medical history was unremarkable with no history of urinary tract infections and no previous episodes of hematuria. He had been a full-term normal delivery and his mother recalled there being no issues with his antenatal ultrasound. The patient came to the clinic with both parents who denied a history of hematuria or cystic kidney disease in any members of the family. The patient's father had been recently diagnosed with hypertension and was on medication.

On physical examination, the patient was greater than the 90th percentile for height and weight with an athletic build. Vital signs were unremarkable and BP was normal for height and age at 88/64 mm Hg. Physical examination was normal with no evidence of bruising or rashes, absence of hepatosplenomegaly, no palpable renal masses, and a normal genital examination. Blood work showed a slightly low platelet count (133,000/mm^3), which likely represents a normal variant. He had a normal hemoglobin (16 mg/dL) and WBC (5700/mm^3). His electrolytes were normal and his BUN was 14 mg/dL with a creatinine of 1 mg/dL. The coagulation profile was unremarkable: partial thromboplastin time was 28 seconds (normal range, 22–37 seconds), the prothrombin time was 12.1 seconds (normal range, 12–15 seconds) and the international normalized ratio was 1.2 (normal range, 0.86–1.14). Urine analysis had a specific gravity of 1.025, 3+ blood, 1+ protein, many eumorphic red blood cells, three to five WBCs per HPF, and one to two hyaline casts. Urine culture was negative. Complements were normal (C3 was 89 mg/dL with normal in our laboratory being 75–180 mg/dL and C4 was 19 mg/dL, with normal being 15–50 mg/dL) with negative antinuclear antibody and negative antineutrophil cytoplasmic antibody. A renal ultrasound was remarkable for multiple small cysts involving the upper pole of the left kidney without an associated discrete mass. The remainder of the renal parenchyma was unremarkable with normal-sized kidneys for his height (right, 12.3 cm; left, 13.1 cm), normal cortical thickness, normal echogenicity, and normal corticomedullary differentiation with no other cysts. The patient underwent a CT scan with and without contrast with delayed phases that confirmed a left upper pole cystic lesion filling nearly the entire upper pole of the left kidney without involvement of the urinary collecting system. The lower pole of the left kidney had multiple minute subcentimeter cysts that had not been evident on ultrasound; the right kidney was completely normal. The renal parenchyma surrounding the cysts was functioning as evidenced by the normal contrast enhancement. There were no suspicious lymph nodes and no homogeneous tumor mass visualized. There were no cysts visualized in the liver.

What is the differential diagnosis?

A. Multilocular cystic nephroma autosomal dominant polycystic kidney disease
B. Neuroblastoma
C. Segmental multicystic dysplastic kidney disease
D. Unilateral renal cystic disease
E. Multicystic nephroma

The correct answer is E

Comment: The differential diagnosis in patients presenting with unilateral multicystic renal lesions is multilocular cystic nephroma, unilateral renal cystic disease, segmental multicystic dysplastic kidney disease, and cystic renal cell carcinoma. The therapy for multilocular cystic nephroma is radical nephrectomy because it cannot be differentiated from more aggressive neoplasms such as the cystic variant of Wilms tumor and cystic renal cell carcinoma, which makes it crucial for us to carefully consider other diagnoses first.

The lack of suspect lymph nodes and homogeneous tumor mass as well as the presence of cysts in other areas of the affected kidney in our patient made the diagnosis of cystic nephroma less likely. Unilateral renal cystic disease is a less well-known entity reported that is nonfamilial and nonprogressive.[1] Segmental multicystic dysplastic kidney disease was unlikely in our patient because on the CT scan there was normal contrast enhancement in the renal tissue adjacent to the cysts.

Clinical Presentation 39

A 2-year-old boy was admitted for evaluation of failure to thrive complicated by frequent bouts of dehydration and electrolyte disorders.

He was born at 36 weeks of gestation with a birth weight of 2850 g as the first living male child of consanguineous, apparently healthy parents. The pregnancy had been complicated by polyhydramnios. The mother reported two previous pregnancies, one resulting in early abortion and the other in an anencephalic neonate. After birth, the patient showed prolonged jaundice, vomiting, and dehydration with hypokalemia, and the clinical diagnosis of neonatal Bartter syndrome was made. Initial treatment included intravenous fluids to correct hypovolemia and oral potassium solutions. The further clinical course was characterized by persistent diarrhea (8–9/day stools daily) complicated by frequent episodes of dehydration and water-electrolyte imbalances leading to repeated hospitalizations. Because of the unremitting course and progressive failure to thrive, it was decided to refer the patient to our institution for further diagnosis and therapy.

A review of previous hospital records showed that the patient had needed daily potassium supplements. Because the child strongly disliked the salty flavor of potassium chloride, an oral potassium gluconate solution had been given at a dose of 8 mmol/kg/day. Medication and feeding had remained difficult and the child had never developed normal eating patterns, resulting in a dependence on continuous oral feeding by relatives with occasional intravenous alimentation; however, application by a nasogastric tube had been refused by the parents. Celiac disease had been excluded by intestinal biopsy. Medication therapy with omeprazole and domperidone was without effect. Altogether, the child had spent almost half of his life in hospitals.

On admission, at the age of 2 years, the child appeared severely malnourished, and weight (8900 g), height (81.5 cm), and head circumference (45 cm) were far below appropriate percentiles for his age. Blood pressure was 98/62 mm Hg. Apart from abdominal distension and paleness, clinical examination revealed no further abnormalities and no congenital malformations. Blood gas analysis showed severe metabolic alkalosis (pH 7.58, bicarbonate 46 mmol/L, and base excess +21 mmol/L). Serum electrolytes were as follows: potassium 2.0 mmol/L, sodium 131 mmol/L, and chloride 68 mmol/L. Further clinical observation after rehydration and during a period of minimal intravenous fluid replacement showed that the patient had a spontaneous total caloric intake of approximately 20% of his recommended dietary allowance and a spontaneous fluid intake of about 200 mL.

What is your diagnosis?

A. Bartter syndrome
B. Congenital chloride diarrhea (CLD)
C. Cystic fibrosis of the pancreas
D. Hyperaldosteronism

The correct answer is B

Comment: Chronic diarrhea and the absence of polyuria/polydipsia are untypical for patients with Bartter syndrome and cystic fibrosis of the pancreas. The findings of normal BP also rule out hyperaldosteronism.

CLD is a rare autosomal recessive disease occurring mainly in people in Arabian countries, Finland, and Poland.[1–3] It is characterized by unremitting watery diarrhea with high fecal losses of chloride, failure to thrive, and renal impairment in older children and adults if the disease is left untreated. Prenatal symptoms include polyhydramnios and dilated intestinal loops; birth is often premature, and postnatal mortality rates are high because of severe dehydration and electrolyte imbalances. The disease is caused by a defective anion exchange protein, an epithelial chloride/bicarbonate (Cl^-/HCO_3^-) exchanger located in the brush border of the ileum and colon, resulting in defective intestinal chloride absorption and secretion of HCO_3^-, with a secondary defect in sodium/hydrogen (Na^+/H^+) transport, altogether leading to intestinal losses of both sodium and water, hypochloremia, hyponatremia, and metabolic alkalosis.

Some of the clinical features of CLD may resemble Bartter syndrome, which had been suspected in this case, namely, polyhydramnios, failure to thrive, and hypochloremic metabolic alkalosis. However, all forms of Bartter syndrome are characterized by high urinary losses of Na, potassium (K), and Cl because of defective tubular reabsorption. Thus, a simple spot urine measurement may rule out Bartter, as in this case. Urinary concentrations of Na and Cl were 14 mmol/L and 15 mmol/L, respectively. However, misdiagnosis of batter syndrome in CLD patients has been described in a number of cases.[1] Differential diagnosis further includes cystic fibrosis, which (especially in hot climates) may result in high Cl losses, hypochloremic metabolic alkalosis, gastrointestinal symptoms, and failure to thrive and should be ruled out by a sweat chloride test (normal in this case).[2]

Measuring chloride in stool is a simple clinical test to confirm the clinical diagnosis of CLD. Cl concentrations of >90 mmol/L are reportedly diagnostic for the disease.[3] In this case, the value was 89 mmol/L (after rehydration and chloride substitution). However, genetic testing is now available in specialized laboratories to establish the definitive diagnosis.

Patients with CLD harbor mutations in both copies of the *SLC26A3* (solute carrier family 26, member 3, or DRA) gene on chromosome 7q31. Altogether, 36 different mutations distributed within exons 3 through 19 of the gene have been identified in patients with CLD.[4,5] However, certain founder mutations are particularly frequent in patients in Arabian countries, Finland, and Poland, and account for the majority of CLD cases. No genotype-phenotype correlation has emerged. Direct sequencing of the *SLC26A3* gene detects point and splice-site mutations and small insertions and deletions, with an overall mutation detection rate of >95%. In this case, both parents were found to harbor the heterozygous mutation c.559G>T (p. G187X), resulting in a homozygous mutation of the patient at this locus. This mutation results either in severe protein truncation or in nonsense-mediated RNA decay, with no protein produced at all. This mutation has been described in patients from Saudi Arabia and Kuwait[4]; it represents the Arab founder mutation and has apparently spread to Libya as well.

Our patient was treated with placement of a percutaneous endoscopic gastrostomy, resulting in dramatic improvement of fluid and caloric intake and instantaneous weight gain. Intravenously administered alimentation was discontinued, and at discharge from the hospital, the child needed substitution with 6 mEq/kD per day of KCl to maintain normal potassium, chloride, and bicarbonate serum levels.

Clinical Presentation 40

A 4-month-old male infant presented with recurrent episodes of hyperkalemia and acidosis since birth. He was born by normal vaginal delivery at term weighing 2.7 kg (ninth percentile) with a head circumference of 33 cm (ninth percentile) to a mother with a known history of alcohol abuse. There were no perinatal problems. The mother's antenatal ultrasound scan at 20 weeks' gestation did not identify any fetal abnormalities.

At 1 month of age, the boy was admitted to the local hospital with a week's history of "funny spells," where he had extensor posturing of his trunk and limbs and cried out. These lasted for 2 to 3 minutes at a time. There was no apparent relationship to feeding or passing bowel movements. On examination, the child was noted to be thriving, with a weight of 3.29 kg (second percentile), a head circumference of 36 cm (ninth percentile), and a length of 52 cm (ninth percentile). Blood pressure was 78/52 mm Hg. Clinical examination was unremarkable. He was not dehydrated on clinical assessment. The external genitalia appeared normal.

Initial blood investigations (performed by venipuncture) showed serum potassium 7 mmol/L, sodium 135 mmol/L, chloride 112 mmol/L, bicarbonate 19 mmol/L, urea 2.1 mmol/L, and creatinine 0.2 mg/dL. The complete blood count showed normal hemoglobin, WBC, and platelet values. Liver function tests were within normal limits. Serum glucose, calcium, phosphate, and magnesium were within the normal range. Serum ammonia, lactate, and creatinine kinase were normal. Capillary blood gas showed a mild metabolic acidosis with a base deficit of −5.2.

A working diagnosis of sepsis was originally considered, and he was treated with antibiotics intravenously. A complete septic screen was negative. Cerebrospinal fluid lactate, plasma and cerebrospinal fluid amino acids, random cortisol, thyroid function tests, and 17- hydroxyprogesterone were all within normal ranges. Serum aldosterone was entirely normal for age at 454 pmol/L (normal 300–1500 pmol/L). Plasma renin activity was low at <0.2 nmol/L per hour (normal, 1.1–2.7 nmol/L per hour). Urinary potassium was 10 mmol/L, urine osmolality 151 mmol/L, and plasma osmolality 290 mmol/L. Urinary screen for drugs and toxins was negative. An ultrasound scan of the renal tract demonstrated two normal kidneys with no evidence of hydronephrosis or hydroureter.

The child had a trial of sodium bicarbonate, fludrocortisone, and calcium resonium at 2 months of age. However, these were not sufficient to correct the hyperkalemia, which at this stage was associated with poor weight gain (3.7 kg, 0.4th percentile). He was then commenced on low-potassium-containing milk. This corrected the hyperkalemia. He was discharged home with serum potassium 3.8 mmol/L, sodium 139 mmol/L, chloride 100 mmol/L, urea 112 mg/dL, and creatinine 0.2 mg/dL.

What is the most likely diagnosis?

A. Primary aldosteronism
B. Hereditary pseudohypoaldosteronism (PHA)
C. Obstructive uropathy
D. Congenital adrenal hyperplasia

The correct answer is C

Comment: The child has presented in infancy with hyperkalemia associated with a hyperchloremic metabolic acidosis and a normal anion gap of 11 (normal, 10–14). His estimated GFR is normal. Hyperkalemia in the presence of estimated GFR >15 mL/min/1.73 m^2 is generally from an aldosterone deficiency or aldosterone resistance in the distal nephron.

The action of aldosterone on the distal nephron can be quantified using the TTKG.[1]

TTKG = [Urine K^+ × Plasma osmolarity/Urine osmolarity × Plasma K^+

A low TTKG suggests aldosterone deficiency or insensitivity. A high TTKG suggests a dietary excess of potassium. Our patient had a reduced TTKG of 2.7 in the presence of hyperkalemia (normal range in infants, 4.9–15.5), suggesting aldosterone deficiency or end-organ resistance. The differential diagnosis would thus include congenital adrenal hyperplasia or hypoplasia, hypoaldosteronism, or insensitivity to aldosterone. The presence of a normal serum aldosterone in our patient makes end-organ resistance to this mineralocorticoid the most likely cause.

There are many conditions in which aldosterone levels are normal and the primary defect resides at the level of the renal tubule, including hereditary pseudohypoaldosteronism type I (in infants) and type II (in children and adult), systemic lupus erythematosus, amyloidosis, obstructive uropathy, sickle cell nephropathy, or drugs (spironolactone, triamterene, amiloride, trimethoprim, and pentamidine).

In view of the early presentation and that the infant was not on any medication, the most likely cause of his phenotype is hereditary PHA. PHA describes conditions of apparent hypoaldosteronism despite normal-to-high circulating levels of aldosterone. There are two separate clinical syndromes of PHA.

Type I PHA reflects the apparent lack of aldosterone effect on sodium reabsorption and potassium secretion and thus features hypotension and hyperkalemia. These children have renal salt wasting and often have hyponatremia.[2] Plasma renin levels are elevated, as are plasma levels of aldosterone. The latter finding, as well as the lack of response to mineralocorticoid replacement therapy, differentiates them from infants with selective aldosterone deficiency who otherwise have a similar constellation of clinical findings. There are autosomal dominant and autosomal recessive forms of this disease, caused by mutations of the mineralocorticoid receptor and ENaC, respectively.[3] Therapy with salt supplementation is effective in treating both the salt depletion and the hyperkalemia. As in other instances of mineralocorticoid deficiency, volume contraction with decreased distal delivery of salt and water appears necessary for overt hyperkalemia to develop. Spontaneous recovery usually occurs by the age of 2 years, although episodic hyperkalemia may still occur during episodes of acute illness.[2]

PHA type II (Gordon syndrome or familial hypertension with hyperkalemia) exhibits an autosomal dominant mode of transmission and is usually seen in late childhood or adulthood. These patients also have hyperkalemia and hyperchloremic metabolic acidosis but do not exhibit renal salt wasting, have low plasma renin levels, and are usually hypertensive. Aldosterone levels are normal or high and most of these patients have a normal estimated GFR. This syndrome is also characterized by short stature, intellectual impairment, dental abnormalities, and muscle weakness.[3,4] Recent positional cloning has linked mutations of *WNK1* (on chromosome 12p) and *WNK4* (on chromosome 17q21) to type II PHA.[5] With-no-lysine [K] (WNK) kinases are a new family of large serine-threonine protein kinases with an atypical placement of the catalytic lysine.[5] Wild-type WNK1 and WNK4 inhibit the thiazide-sensitive sodium chloride cotransporter in the distal tubule. Mutations of these proteins are associated with gain of function and increased cotransporter activity, excessive chloride and sodium reabsorption, and volume expansion. Hyperkalemia, another hallmark of this syndrome, might be a function of diminished sodium delivery to the cortical collecting tubule. Sodium reabsorption provides the driving force for potassium excretion, which is mediated by the ROMK. Alternatively, the same mutations in WNK4 that result in a gain of function of the Na-Cl cotransporter might inhibit ROMK activity, resulting in hyperkalemia. Treatment consists of either a low-salt diet or thiazide diuretics, aimed at decreasing chloride intake and blocking Na-Cl cotransporter activity, respectively.[5]

The presence of hyperkalemia in association with hyperchloremic metabolic acidosis, a low serum renin, normal serum aldosterone, and an adequate GFR in this child makes PHA type II the most likely diagnosis. In this syndrome, hypertension tends to develop in the third decade, so its absence in our patient does not exclude the diagnosis. Because the condition is inherited in an autosomal dominant pattern, we proceeded to screen the child's father, who was 28 years old and asymptomatic. He was hypertensive with a BP reading of 160/90 mm Hg. His serum potassium was elevated at 6.4 mmol/L. His renal function and acid-base status were normal. The father and the infant were commenced on chlorothiazide, which led to normalization of the serum potassium (and BP in the father) and eliminated the need for dietary restriction of potassium. Initial genetic screening for *WNK1* and *WNK4* gene mutations in our patient was negative. However, further mutation studies are ongoing.

Clinical Presentation 41

A 15-year-old Chinese girl presented to the emergency department with muscle paralysis of bilateral lower extremities over the course of 1 day. She had a 2-year history of polyuria, nocturia, and rampant dental caries and calculi. She denied vomiting, diarrhea, or use of alcohol, laxatives, or diuretics, and her family history was unremarkable. Her pulse rate was 90/min, BP 112/72 mm Hg, and body temperature 36.4°C. Physical examination revealed severe dental caries and calculi with dry oral mucosa. Her thyroid gland was not enlarged. Neurologic examination disclosed symmetric flaccid paralysis with areflexia of both lower extremities. The remainder of the physical examination was unremarkable. The most striking biochemical abnormalities were profound hypokalemia (1.8 mEq/L) and hyperchloremic metabolic acidosis (pH 7.28, HCO_3^- 16.6, Na+ 141, and Cl^- 114 mEq/L). Her renal, liver, and thyroid functions were all normal (creatinine 0.9 mg/dL). Urinalysis revealed proteinuria (1+), low urine specific gravity (1.010), high K+ excretion (transtubular K+ gradient 5, 24-hour urine K+ 38 mEq/day), positive urine anion gap (Na+ 43, K+ 16, and Cl^- 39 mEq/L) and persistent alkaline urine (pH 7–7.5). Electrocardiogram revealed prolonged PR interval with flattened T wave. Abdominal ultrasonography showed bilaterally medullary nephrocalcinosis.

What is the cause of her hypokalemic paralysis?

A. dRTA
B. Hypokalemic periodic paralysis (HypoPP)
C. Proximal renal tubular acidosis
D. Bartter syndrome

The correct answer is B

Comment: This 15-year-old girl presented with hypokalemic paralysis, which can result from HypoPP resulting from an acute K^+ shift into cells or non-HypoPP from a large total body K^+ deficit. Measurements of urinary K^+ excretion and blood acid–base status can help in the differential diagnosis. Her high urinary K^+ excretion, reflected by an elevated TTKG, suggested renal K^+ wasting and non-HypoPP. Her concurrent hyperchloremic metabolic acidosis suggested a condition with both K^+ depletion and direct or indirect bicarbonate loss (renal tubular acidosis). The assessment of urine $NH4^+$ excretion by urine anion gap and/or urine osmolality gap separates RTA from non-RTA. A positive urine anion gap indicated defective $NH4^+$ excretion associated with RTA. Her persistently alkaline urine (pH >7.0) pointed to a diagnosis of distal RTA. In fact, hypokalemia is a common finding in distal RTA and results from the combination of renal Na^+ wasting, secondary hyperaldosteronism, and bicarbonaturia.

Nevertheless, the underlying cause of distal RTA must be identified. On review of her history, she had been experiencing dry mouth for the past 3 months despite a normal Schirmer test for dry eye. An exhaustive workup demonstrated elevated anti-Ro antibody, rheumatoid factor, antinuclear antibody (>1:1280), polyclonal immunoglobulin G, typical delayed salivary secretion on salivary scintigraphy, and sialo duct ectasia and typical periductal lymphocytic infiltration (focus score 3) in the salivary gland biopsy. Renal histology showed chronic tubulointerstitial nephritis with predominant lymphocytic infiltration. After ruling out other autoimmune diseases, such as systemic lupus erythematosus or juvenile arthritis, primary Sjögren syndrome (SS) was diagnosed.

SS is a chronic autoimmune disease characterized by progressive lymphocytic infiltration of exocrine glands with typical features of keratoconjunctivitis, sicca, and xerostomia.[1] Various degrees of extraglandular involvement, such as arthritis, RTA, and lymphoma, may develop before or after glandular damage.[2] SS is most prevalent in women in their fourth and fifth decades and uncommon in children or adolescents. The clinical presentations of juvenile SS are diverse.[3] Dry eye and dry mouth sensation are the most common presenting complaints in adults, but usually develop later in juveniles, reflecting the atypical presentations of juvenile SS at the outset. The nonspecific clinical picture and lack of universal diagnostic criteria mean that most patients are underdiagnosed until they experience complications.[4] Profound hypokalemia with paralysis is a rare primary manifestation of SS in children. To the best of our knowledge, only nine cases, including ours, have been reported in the literature.[5–11] All of the affected children were girls between the ages of 8 and 17 years. Of note, extraglandular involvement with distal RTA causing non-HypoPP preceded the typical sicca symptoms in these patients.

The criteria for diagnosing adult SS may be not applicable to juvenile SS because of sensitivity as low as 39%.[4] Recurrent enlargement of bilateral parotid glands, antinuclear antibody, rheumatoid factor, serum amylase, leukopenia, polyclonal hypergammaglobulinemia, erythrocyte sedimentation rate, and RTA have been introduced as new parameters to enhance the diagnosis of juvenile SS. However, the inclusion of these factors has only increased the sensitivity to 76%.[11] The insensitive criteria, combined with atypical presentations, frequently result in delayed recognition of juvenile SS. In fact, many patients with juvenile SS are not diagnosed until they experience severe glandular or extraglandular sequelae, as clearly illustrated in this and other cases.[5–11]

Impaired distal tubular H^+ secretion is by far the most common renal manifestation of SS.[5] It takes time to progress from impaired distal tubular H^+ secretion to full-blown RTA. Therefore, defective renal acidification (pH > 5.5) in response to the acid-load test and low urine citrate excretion are the earliest indices to suggest renal involvement in SS.[11] The impaired ability to concentrate (hyposthenuria) is also another marker of early primary SS.

Hypokalemia and nephrocalcinosis (or nephrolithiasis) are common but late manifestations in distal RTA because they are nearly asymptomatic (>90%) in the early stages.[2] The combination of renal Na^+ wasting, secondary hyperaldosteronism, and bicarbonaturia in distal RTA contribute to hypokalemia.[5,7] Metabolic acidosis, per se, can induce bone resorption and reduce renal tubular calcium and phosphate reabsorption, leading to increased urine calcium and phosphate excretion. This, in combination with hypocitraturia, as a result of metabolic acidosis and hypokalemia, precipitates the formation of nephrocalcinosis or nephrolithiasis.

With respect to therapy, K^+ citrate must be used to correct hypokalemia and metabolic acidosis and prevent further nephrocalcinosis. Care for oral involvement includes mechanical stimulation of the salivary glands, diet modification, regular oral hygiene, and topical fluoride. Prompt recognition and management of SS achieves a good prognosis by preventing glandular and extraglandular complications. Corticosteroids are the drugs of choice for SS with visceral involvement. In life-threatening cases, mycophenolate mofetil and novel biological therapies like rituximab and infliximab can be attempted.

Clinical Presentation 42

A 13-month-old boy presented to our pediatric emergency department with failure to gain weight for the past 3 months. He had had excessive irritability, anorexia, polyuria, and polydipsia for the past 20 days. His mother also complained that the child cries excessively during micturition. He had not passed stools for 3 days and had several episodes of nonambitious vomiting 6 hours before admission. He was born at term by cesarean section (indication, oligohydramnios). The infantile course was uneventful. He had received intramuscular injections weekly along with oral medications daily for the past 10 weeks prescribed by a general physician with no documentation of the treatment received. Intake was 500 mL of cow's milk per day along with only two servings of cereals and vegetables.

On physical examination, the patient was afebrile with a pulse rate 96/min, respiratory rate 24/min, and blood pressure 92/62 mm Hg (50th–90th percentile for age, sex, and height). His weight was at the 25th percentile and height at the 50th percentile for his age. The child had decreased skin turgor, sunken eyeballs, and dry oral mucosa (signs of some dehydration). The systemic examination was unremarkable. Laboratory results revealed hemoglobin 11.5 g/dL, total leukocyte count 11,800/mm^3, with differential leulocyte count 50% polymorphs, 46% lymphocytes, 3% eosinophils, and 1% monocytes, platelets 200,000/mm^3, erythrocyte sedimentation rate 12 mm/h, random blood sugar 98 mg/dL, blood urea 20 mg/dL, serum creatinine 0.5 mg/dL, serum Na+/K+ 142/3.6 mEq/L, serum albumin 4.3 mg/dL, and blood culture sterile. Urine microscopy showed 15 to 20 WBCs per HPF, 5 to 10 red blood cells/HPF, urine cullture sterile, and urine-specific gravity 1.005.

Urine volume was 7 mL/kg/h during the first 24 hours of admission. Early morning serum osmolality was 292 mOsm/kg and urine osmolality was128 mOsm/kg. Arterial blood gases showed pH 7.35, HCO_3^- 21 mEq/L, and PCO_2 38 mm Hg. Other laboratory investigations revealed serum calcium of 19 mg/dL (normal, 8.5–10.3 mg/dL), serum phosphate of 4.21 mg/dL (normal, 3.8–6.5 mg/dL), serum alkaline phosphatase of 419 U/L (normal, 145–420 U/L), ionized calcium of 2.47 mmol/L, spot calcium creatinine ratio of 2.85 g/g (normal, <0.53 g/g), and 24-hour urinary calcium of 4.76 mg/kg/day (normal, <4 mg/kg/day). An electrocardiogram showed sinus rhythm with a regular rate and normal intervals. There was no evidence of band keratopathy on eye examination.

Ultrasound of abdomen at admission revealed a 7-mm calculus in the left kidney. Serum amylase and lipase taken on day 3 of admission in view of persistent vomiting and abdominal pain were 111 and 1631 U/L, respectively, which increased to 367 U/L and 2520 U/L respectively over the next 48 hours.

During hospitalization, the child was treated with intravenously administered fluids (vigorous hydration with normal saline initially and then 5% dextrose solution at one-half normal strength at 1.5 times maintenance), furosemide 1 mg/kg/dose, and intravenously administered hydrocortisone at 10 mg/kg/day. For further workup intact PTH was undetectable (15–65 pg/mL), 25 (OH) D, vitamin A, and E levels were sent. Despite these therapies, the total calcium level was persistently high and did not decrease until the fifth hospital day, at which time it decreased to 16 mg/dL. Although the patient was symptomatically better, with decreased irritability and normal urine output, calcium levels continued to be alarmingly high. Therefore, the patient was given a single dose of intravenous pamidronate (0.5 mg/kg) as an infusion over 4 hours after premedication with acetaminophen and antihistaminic prophylaxis (as a precaution to prevent fever and hypersensitivity reaction, respectively). Serum calcium levels gradually normalized over the next 4 days. On hospital day 4, vitamin A levels became available, which were normal.

What was the cause of hypercalcemia?

A. Hyperparathyroidism
B. Sarcoidosis
C. Vitamin D intoxication
D. Malignancy

The correct answer is C

Comment: Our patient presented with failure to thrive, excessive irritability, recent-onset polyuria, polydipsia, and severe hypercalcemia of uncertain etiology. The child was evaluated for causes of hypercalcemia. Undetectable PTH and normal serum phosphorus levels ruled out a diagnosis of primary hyperparathyroidism. Despite there being a history of failure to gain weight for the past 3 months, counts were normal, and there was no lymphadenopathy or hepatosplenomegaly. Hence, malignancy as a cause of such as like neuroblastoma and hepatoblastoma, among others. No abdominal mass was detected during the clinical examination, and ultrasonography of the abdomen also did not reveal any such abnormality. Moreover, 1,25(OH) vitamin D and PTH-related protein levels were subsequently reported to be normal. There was no contact history of tuberculosis, and a chest x-ray did not reveal any evidence of sarcoidosis or tuberculosis.

There was no family history of kidney stones or disease. The patient had hypercalciuria and low PTH levels, thereby eliminating the possibility of familial hypocalciuric hypercalcemia because this is an autosomal dominant condition with a mutation in the calcium-sensing receptor gene (*CASR*) and the patients were found to have normal or increased PTH with a low urine calcium:creatinine ratio.[1] Within 4 days of admission, laboratory test results for vitamin D, A, and E levels became available. Vitamin A and E levels were normal, but 25(OH) vitamin D levels were markedly elevated (>450 ng/mL), suggesting that the child had probably received intramuscular vitamin D injections followed by oral calcium and vitamin D supplements, which was confirmed later. Based on the medical history and clinical and biochemical evidence, the child was diagnosed with hypervitaminosis D. The parents were instructed to restrict dairy products and use sunscreen. Intravenous hydrocortisone was replaced by oral prednisolone at a dose of 1.5 mg/kg/day. The dose was tapered gradually and stopped after 3 weeks of treatment. At discharge, his 25(OH) vitamin D level was 454 ng/mL and his total calcium concentration was 10.8 mg/dL.

The cause of nephrogenic DI in hypervitaminosis D is hypercalcemia. Two underlying mechanisms leading to nephrogenic DI have been proposed. First, calcium-sensing receptors (CaSR) expressed on the basolateral (blood) side of the thick ascending limb cells indirectly inhibits the NKCC2 cotransporter BSC1 and impairs the generation of a medullary concentration gradient. Second, this receptor is also expressed on the luminal side of the collecting duct cells and decreases aquaporin-2 expression on the apical membrane.[2]

Computed tomography of the abdomen on day 5 confirmed a left renal calculus of dense limey bile layered in the dependent portion of the gallbladder and a few calculi in the lumen, as well as calcification in the head of the pancreas. Gallstones in patients with primary hyperparathyroidism are well known, but vitamin D intoxication leading to gallstone disease has not been reported. Unlike primary hyperparathyroidism, in which both hypercalcemia and high PTH levels are known to play roles in pathogenesis,[3,4] vitamin D intoxication causes hypercalcemia, thus favoring a lithogenic milieu.

Vitamin D interplays with PTH to maintain normal serum levels of calcium. Both PTH and calcitriol increase serum calcium levels by activating osteoclastic bone resorption and increasing renal absorption of filtered calcium. Calcitriol also causes increased absorption of calcium from the intestine.[8] Normal serum levels of calcium are 8.8 to 10.3 mg/dL during childhood.[5] An overdose of vitamin D leads to hypercalcemia, hyperphosphatemia, and high calcium/phosphorus product-associated complications.[6] Following the administration of an excess of vitamin D, the vitamin can be found in the circulation for several months because it is stored in fatty tissues. Treatment of vitamin D intoxication includes removal of the exogenous source, forced diuresis by adequate hydration and loop diuretics, and the use of glucocorticoids, which decrease the production of 1,25 (OH)2 vitamin D3 and thereby decrease intestinal reabsorption of calcium. In patients with alarmingly high levels of hypercalcemia refractory to conventional therapy, intravenous pamidronate in doses of 0.5 to 1 mg/kg, or even lower doses of 0.35 mg/kg are used.[6] There have been reports of the use of oral alendronate in children with vitamin D toxicity.[7,8]

Clinical Presentation 43

A previously well 12-year-old boy presented with a 1-month history of polydipsia, polyuria, and lethargy. Over that period, he had been drinking at least 3 L of water daily, reported feeling thirsty, and needed to pass urine approximately every 30 minutes. His parents also reported that he had weight loss over the previous month with reduced appetite secondary to nausea. Of note, he had a longstanding history of drinking approximately 1 L of cow's milk daily. He had no recent acute illnesses or fevers and reported no pain, discomfort, or respiratory distress. He had been treated with azathioprine for 3 years in the past for intractable eczema. His blood glucose level checked by his general practitioner was normal.

Physical examination revealed significant bilateral inguinal lymphadenopathy and a 2-cm palpable liver edge. There were patches of dry skin attributed to previously diagnosed eczema. His cardiovascular, respiratory, neurological, ear-nose-throat, and musculoskeletal examinations were otherwise unremarkable. There was an evident bacille Calmette-Guerin scar. Vital signs were within normal limits.

Laboratory investigations revealed acute renal impairment, hypercalcemia, and a mild transaminitis: urea 15.2 mmol/L, creatinine 149 mmol/L, serum calcium 3.38 mmol/L, ionized calcium

1.78 mmol/L, serum phosphate 1.42 mmol/L, sodium 139 mmol/L, potassium 3.7 mmol/L, AST 76 U/L, ALT 114 U/L, and lactate dehydrogenase 416 U/L. Serum intact PTH levels were suppressed at <6 ng/L. Serum 25(OH)-cholecalciferol level was reduced at 38 nmol/L. Urinalysis revealed significant hypercalciuria (calcium/creatinine ratio of 2.91). Full blood count measurements were within normal limits, whereas blood film revealed only occasional atypical lymphocytes and monocytes. An abdominal ultrasound revealed bilateral hyperechogenic kidneys, which were otherwise unremarkable, and mild hepatosplenomegaly with bulky inguinal lymph nodes bilaterally with speckled hyperechogenicity. A chest radiograph revealed clear lung fields, normal-sized cardiac silhouette with no evidence of a widened mediastinum.

What is the most likely cause of his presentation?

A. Sarcoidosis
B. Tuberculosis
C. Milk-alkali syndrome
D. Vitamin A intoxication

The correct answer is A

Comment: Our patient symptoms of polyuria and polydipsia result from decreased concentrating ability, which occurs secondary to any cause of hypercalcemia. The patient had a raised serum angiotensin-converting enzyme level at 225 U/L and a biopsy of one of the enlarged inguinal lymph nodes revealed multiple noncaseating epithelioid cell granulomata, which is consistent with the diagnosis of sarcoidosis.

Initial saline hyperhydration with 0.9 % NaCl and diuresis with frusemide failed to significantly reduce the total serum and ionized calcium levels over 48 hours. Commencement of steroid treatment (prednisolone 2 mg/kg/day) led to a progressive fall in calcium levels; normalizing after 11 days of treatment.

Hypercalcemia results when the entry of calcium into the circulation exceeds its excretion into the urine or deposition into bone. This can occur when there is accelerated bone resorption, excessive gastrointestinal absorption, decreased renal excretion of calcium, or in some disorders, a combination. It is often a clue to an underlying disease process. The differential diagnoses for hypercalcemia in children are wide and include[1] primary and familial hyperparathyroidism, familial isolated hyperparathyroidism, hypercalcemia of malignancy, vitamin D intoxication, vitamin A intoxication, chronic granulomatous disorders, medications (thiazide diuretics, lithium, theophylline), hyperthyroidism, acromegaly, pheochromocytoma, adrenal insufficiency, immobilization, parenteral nutrition, and milk alkali syndrome.

In our 12-year-old patient with lymphadenopathy and hepato-splenomegaly, the hypercalcemia is likely secondary to malignancy or chronic granulomatous disease. The diagnosis of sarcoidosis was confirmed with the finding of a normal bone marrow biopsy, coupled with a raised serum angiotensin-converting enzyme level and lymph node biopsy showing multiple noncaseating epithelioid cell granulomata.[2] Supporting this is that hypercalcemia in our patient was associated with a suppressed serum PTH and PTH-related protein, increased fractional excretion of calcium, and a high 1,25-dihydroxycholecalciferol level. His presentation with polyuria is attributable to a concentrating defect secondary to hypercalcemia, which in turn led to the increased sensation of thirst. The coordinated function between the Na^+/K^+ 2 Cl cotransporter (NKCC2), the inward-rectifier potassium channel (ROMK), and chloride channels (CLC-KB) found in the cells of the thick ascending limb (TAL) of the loop of Henle is critical for salt absorption. A gradient for sodium entry across apical membranes (in which most occur through the NKCC2) is generated by the Na^+/K^+/ATPase.[3,4] Sodium and chloride ions entering the apical cell surface via the NKCC2 leave the cell through the Na^+/K^+/ATPase and CLC-KB, respectively, at the basolateral membrane. Potassium recycling via ROMK ensures that K^+ concentration in the TAL remains constant to allow proper functioning of the NKCC2. In addition, the lumen-positive voltage of the TAL resulting from potassium recycling drives absorption of a second cation (Na^+, Ca^{2+}, Mg^{2+}) through the paracellular pathway.[4] Calcium regulates salt transport by interacting with CaSR expressed on the basolateral membrane of cells of the TAL. Activation of CaSR by calcium increases 20-hydroxyeicosatetraenoic acid, which potently inhibits the NKCC2, ROMK, and Na^+/K^+/ATPase, thereby disrupting NaCl absorption.[4,5] Additionally, CaSR stimulation leads to the generation of prostaglandin E2, which contributes further to inhibition of NKCC2.[6] This is compounded by a reduced responsiveness to antidiuretic hormone secondary to downregulation of AQP2 expression caused by activation of CaSR on the luminal surface of cells in the inner medullary collecting ducts in the setting of increased distal calcium delivery.[7,8]

Sarcoidosis, the etiology of which remains unknown, is a systemic, granulomatous disease. It most commonly affects patients between 10 and 40 years of age in 70% to 90% of cases and is three to four times more common in Blacks.[9] The most common presentation in adults is with hilar lymphadenopathy, pulmonary infiltrates, and ocular and cutaneous lesions. Symptomatic sarcoidosis is rare in children. In infants and children younger than age 4 years, the most common presentation is with the triad of skin, joint, and eye involvement without the typical pulmonary disease,[10] whereas in older children, involvement of the lungs, lymph nodes, and eyes predominates. In a series of Danish children with sarcoidosis, the most common presenting features were erythema nodosum and iridocyclitis.[11] Other features of sarcoidosis include fatigue, malaise, fever, and weight loss.[1]. Although the lungs are the most frequently affected organ, the disease can affect any organ system in the body. Up to 30% of patients present with extrapulmonary disease; the most prominent sites involve the skin, eyes, reticuloendothelial system, musculoskeletal system, exocrine glands, heart, kidney, and central nervous system.[13–15] Abnormalities related to calcium metabolism are the most common renal and electrolyte abnormality observed in patients with sarcoidosis. It is due to extrarenal production of activated vitamin D (1, 25-dihydroxycholecalciferol) by activated macrophages, which leads to increased intestinal calcium absorption, which in turn leads to hypercalcemia leading to hypercalciuria and nephrocalcinosis. This is due to a markedly enhanced production of 1-alpha hydroxylase (the enzyme that converts 25-hydroxycholecalciferol to the activated form) and a lack of feedback inhibition, which would normally limit enzyme expression.[6,17] Hypovolemia resulting from hypercalcemia-induced urinary salt wasting exacerbates hypercalcemia by impairing the renal clearance of calcium.[18] Saline hyperhydration expands the extracellular fluid volume and increases the GFR leading to increased excretion of calcium in the urine. Saline administration alone can control hypercalcemia in some patients but requires careful monitoring because it can lead to fluid overload in patients who fail to excrete the administered salt and water from impaired renal function. Administration of a loop diuretic can be initiated once fluid repletion is achieved to further increase urinary calcium excretion but this approach often involves intensive administration of frusemide (1–2 mg/kg every 1–2 hours) with aggressive fluid hydration (up to 10 L daily).[19] Other renal complications of sarcoidosis include membranous nephropathy, proliferative or crescentic glomerulonephritis, focal segmental glomerulosclerosis, granulomatous interstitial nephritis, polyuria, hypertension, and a variety of tubular defects.[20,21] Treatment with glucocorticoids, which decreases inflammatory activity, leading to a reduction of calcitriol synthesis, improves calcium metabolism and lowers plasma creatinine concentration.[22] Concurrent treatment with bisphosphonates with or without calcitonin can be used to treat severe hypercalcemia.[23,24] Rarely, patients with sarcoidosis develop end-stage renal disease (most often from hypercalcemic nephropathy rather than granulomatous nephritis or glomerulopathy) requiring renal replacement therapy. The outcome of renal transplantation is not well documented. A retrospective review of 18 patients from eight French centers, with a median follow-up of 4 years, showed patient and death-censored graft survival of 94%. Sarcoidosis recurred in five patients at a median of 13 months after transplantation.[25]

Clinical Presentation 44

A 14-year-old girl presented with hypertension (160/110 mm Hg, stage 2 hypertension), excessive weight gain (4 kg), and progressive swelling of both lower limbs for 1 month. There was also a history of polyuria (urine output, 4.5 L/day) accompanied by anorexia and tiredness for the past 10 days. There was no history of vomiting, headache, recurrent respiratory infections, palpitations, orthopnea, paroxysmal nocturnal dyspnea, tetany, or diarrhea. She denied intake of drugs, traditional medicines, or steroids. The Tanner sexual maturity rating was appropriate for age, and she had attained menarche at 12 years of age. However, the menstrual periods had been irregular for the past 2 months.

On examination, her face had a rounded appearance, with extensive acneiform eruptions. She also had abdominal distension, and bilateral pitting pedal edema, but no periorbital edema. There were no neurocutaneous markers. All peripheral pulses were normally felt. The vital signs at presentation were respiratory rate 18/min, heart rate 78/min, and blood pressure 150/110 mm Hg (stage 2 hypertension). She was not found to have any significant difference between readings of BP measured in all the four limbs. She was hemodynamically stable at admission, and there were no signs of dehydration. Her weight and height were 50 kg (0.06 Z) and 151 cm (–1.56 Z), respectively. Her mother revealed that her weight was 43 kg 1 month ago. There was no palpable abdominal mass, hepatosplenomegaly, or ascites. There was no abdominal bruit. Cardiovascular and neurological examinations were normal. Investigations revealed hemoglobin 10.8 g/dL, total leukocyte count 6800/mm^3, and platelet count 260,000/mm^3. The blood urea (20 mg/dL), serum creatinine (0.38 mg/dL), sodium (143 mEq/L), calcium (9.4 mg/dL), and magnesium (2.1 mEq/L) were within normal reference ranges. However, serum potassium was very low (1.72 mEq/L; reference value, 3.5-4.5 mEq/L), and the electrocardiogram showed U waves. She was found to have metabolic alkalosis (pH 7.6, bicarbonate 45.7 mEq/L). The liver function tests were normal (serum bilirubin 0.4 mg/dL, AST 30 U/L, ALT 32 U/L, serum albumin 3.4 g/dL, alkaline phosphatase 70 U/L, international normalized ratio 0.97). The free T4 (1.03 ng/dL) and thyroid-stimulating hormone (1.92 μIU/mL) were normal. Blood glucose levels were normal (random blood glucose, 120 mg/dL). Urinalysis was unremarkable, with no microscopic hematuria or proteinuria. Urine osmolality was 310 mOsm/L. Urinary chloride was high (60 mEq/L). Renal ultrasonogram and Doppler ultrasonography for renal vessels were normal. Echocardiogram showed concentric left ventricular hypertrophy with normal ejection fraction, and ophthalmological evaluation was unremarkable.

Potassium chloride (40 mEq/L) was administered in the maintenance intravenous fluids. Treatment with amlodipine was initiated and augmented with addition of prazosin. In view of refractory hypokalemia and uncontrolled hypertension, serum cortisol, plasma ACTH, plasma renin activity, and plasma aldosterone levels were sent. Potassium chloride in the maintenance fluids was increased to 60 mEq/L through a central intravenous line, and treatment with spironolactone was initiated. This led to the correction of hypokalemia (serum potassium reached 3.6 mEq/L) and, transiently, better control of hypertension (110/70 mm Hg, which was between the 50th and 90th percentiles). The urine output normalized after the correction of hypokalemia. The repeat serum osmolality was 520 mOsm/L. However, the hypertension worsened again and required further evaluation.

What is the likely diagnosis in this patient with severe hypertension and hypokalemic metabolic alkalosis (select all that apply)?

A. Cushing syndrome
B. Congenital adrenal hyperplasia
C. Apparent mineralocorticoid excess
D. Hyperaldosteronism

The correct answer is A

Comment: Our patient had metabolic alkalosis, hypokalemia, high urinary chloride, and hypertension. Because her urinary chloride was high, and she had severe hypertension with hypokalemic metabolic alkalosis in the presence of rounded facies, we clinically suspected Cushing syndrome (CS) as a possible etiology, and she underwent estimation of serum cortisol along with plasma ACTH. The history was reviewed, and she denied any history of intake of steroids or medications containing steroids. The plasma renin activity (0.2 ng/mL/h) and plasma aldosterone level (3 ng/dL) were low (reference values: plasma renin activity, 0.9–6.6 ng/mL/h; plasma aldosterone level, 6.5–29.5 ng/dL). This led to a clinical suspicion of endogenous CS as a potential explanation for the constellation of clinical and laboratory findings encountered in this patient.

In view of a clinical suspicion of CS, she underwent estimation of serum cortisol (at 8 a.m.) along with plasma ACTH. The levels of these were found to be >75 μg/dL (reference value, 4.3–22.4 μg/dL) and 363 pg/mL (reference value, 10–60 pg/mL), respectively. This led to a diagnosis of ACTH-dependent CS. MRI of the cranium showed no evidence of pituitary or hypothalamic lesions. A contrast-enhanced CT scan of the thorax and abdomen was performed for further evaluation of the etiology of endogenous CS. This showed evidence of a tumor in the tail of the pancreas, para-aortic and celiac lymphadenopathy, evidence of metastasis to the liver, and bilateral adrenal hyperplasia. Subsequently, the patient underwent distal pancreatectomy, bilateral adrenalectomy with nodal sampling, and liver nodule excision biopsy. Histopathological examination of the excised pancreatic specimen showed monomorphic tumor cells arranged in nests and sheets that showed moderate cytoplasm, fine stippled chromatin, and moderate degree of nuclear atypia. These cells were diffusely positive for immunohistochemistry with synaptophysin and chromogranin. The Ki-67 index was 40%. Hence, the final histopathology was suggestive of a well-differentiated pancreatic neuroendocrine tumor (NET) (World Health Organization grade 3) with metastasis to celiac lymph node and liver nodule.

To summarize, she had a pancreatic NET producing ACTH, leading to endogenous CS. Postoperatively, she requires amlodipine (being tapered) and hydrocortisone. Stress dose of hydrocortisone was initiated. After a multidisciplinary tumor board discussion, oral capecitabine and temozolamide chemotherapy were initiated.

The mechanisms of hypertension in endogenous CS are multifactorial. The primary mechanism is the mineralocorticoid action exerted by supraphysiological levels of serum cortisol. Serum cortisol is known to bind to both glucocorticoid and mineralocorticoid receptors.[1] The plasma levels of cortisol in humans are 100- to 1000-fold higher than that of aldosterone, which implies that mineralocorticoid receptor (MR) can be chiefly activated by cortisol. However, this is kept in check by 11β-hydroxy steroid dehydrogenase (11β-HSD), which modulates the effect of cortisol at the tissue level. There are two isoforms of the 11β-HSD enzyme. The first isoform 11β-HSD1 catalyzes both dehydrogenation and reduction reactions and is responsible for the interconversion of cortisol and cortisone. In vivo, it predominantly functions as a reductase, converting inactive cortisone to active cortisol. It is abundantly expressed in the liver and adipose tissue. The second isoform 11β-HSD2 is active at very low cortisol concentrations and has mainly dehydrogenase activity that inactivates cortisol to cortisone. It is highly expressed in mineralocorticoid target tissues such as the renal cortex, colon, salivary, and sweat glands. This enzyme prevents cortisol from binding to MR in mineralocorticoid target tissues under physiological concentrations of cortisol. However, in cortisol excess states, the levels of cortisol would exceed the capacity of 11β-HSD to inactivate it to cortisone, thus making it available to bind to MR, mimicking excess aldosterone. This MR activation in turn results in increased renal tubular sodium reabsorption and intravascular volume expansion. Mineralocorticoid-induced hypertension is due to overactivity of epithelial Na+ (ENac).[2] MR activity also leads to ROMK channel and H+K+ATPase stimulation in the distal nephron, leading to hypokalemia and metabolic alkalosis, respectively.

There are other mechanisms involved in glucocorticoid-induced hypertension. Endothelin-1, the most potent vasoconstrictor peptide, with marked hypertensive, mitogenic, and atherogenic effects, is significantly elevated in patients with untreated active CS; an action mediated by glucocorticoids.[3] Nitric oxide is a vasodilator that is produced by the enzyme NO synthase (NOS). Glucocorticoids inhibit NOS synthesis and may lead to increased BP by reduction in peripheral vasodilation.[4] Yet another mechanism of hypertension in high cortisol states is the upregulation of sympathetic nervous system through the accentuation of the action of catecholamines. Though the catecholamine levels are normal, adrenergic receptor sensitivity towards catecholamines is increased, thereby causing an increase in vascular tone.[5] Finally, insulin resistance results from chronic glucocorticoid exposure, which culminates in sodium and water retention, causing volume expansion. It also causes increased sympathetic activity, renin-angiotensin-aldosterone system activation, and vascular hypertrophy, which results in vascular resistance and hypertension.[6] Although endogenous CS is characterized by low plasma renin activity and low aldosterone levels, this is a state of apparent mineralocorticoid excess, which leads to a partial response to spironolactone. As spironolactone is an MR blocker, it leads to control of hypertension and as well as resolution of hypokalemia.[7]

Polyuria in our index case is probably from hypokalemia, which resolved after its correction. In hypokalemia, the urinary concentrating ability of the kidney is impaired because of defective activation of renal adenylate cyclase, which further prevents antidiuretic hormone-stimulated urinary concentration.[8]

Nevertheless, the patient finally required distal pancreatectomy and bilateral adrenalectomy, which led to resolution of hypertension and the hypokalemic metabolic alkalosis.

We describe here a rare case of ACTH-dependent CS (endogenous CS) resulting from pancreatic NET (producing ACTH) leading to severe hypertension associated with hypokalemic metabolic alkalosis in a 14-year-old girl. Although pediatric nephrologists often encounter etiologies such as renovascular hypertension, and rarely other entities such as Liddle syndrome, syndrome of apparent mineralocorticoid excess in a clinical setting of severe hypertension with hypokalemic metabolic alkalosis, it is important not to miss other rare and occasional causes that may be complicated by similar metabolic disturbances. The presence of rounded facies (cushingoid facies) in our patient led to a clinical suspicion of CS as an explanation for her clinical and laboratory findings.

CS is an endocrine disorder caused by a prolonged exposure to elevated cortisol. The most common form of CS results from exogenous administration of steroids. Endogenous CS is rare. Cushing disease (CD) is the most common etiology of endogenous CS. CD is caused by ACTH-secreting pituitary tumors (microadenomas or macroadenomas).[9–12] There are a few population-based studies that have evaluated etiologies of endogenous CS.[13–15] The overall incidence of endogenous CS is 0.7 to 2.4 million people/year.[16] In children older than 7 years of age, CD is the leading cause of CS (75–90% of all cases). CD is less common in children younger than 7 years of age. Adrenal causes of CS are more common in this age group (<7 years) and include adrenal adenoma, adrenal carcinoma, and bilateral adrenal hyperplasia.[17] The incidence of ectopic ACTH-producing conditions leading to endogenous CS is less than 1%, which include small cell carcinoma of the lung, carcinoid tumors of the pancreas, bronchus, thymus, gut, medullary carcinoma of thyroid, pheochromocyomas, and NETs, especially of the pancreas.[18]

NETs are rare in children (0.75 cases per 100,000 children and adolescents per year). Although the majority of these tumors is a benign or low-grade malignancy, about 10% of NETs in children are highly malignant.[19] Less than 2% of NETs are of pancreatic origin. The usual age of presentation of these tumors is older than 10 years in majority of the children.[20] Almost 90% of pancreatic NETs are hormonally inactive and are diagnosed incidentally in the majority. Hence, the diagnosis is often delayed by an estimated period of 8 to 10 years from the time of first symptom to time of confirmed diagnosis, leading to poor prognosis.[21] Pancreatic NETs may rarely secrete ACTH, growth hormone–releasing hormone, PTH-related peptide, serotonin, and cholecystokinin, leading to the respective clinical syndromes.[22] Our index case is an ACTH-secreting pancreatic NET. These ectopic ACTH-secreting tumors result in higher amounts of serum cortisol and are supraphysiological in nature, leading to excessive apparent mineralocorticoid activity. This led to severe hypertension and hypokalemic metabolic alkalosis in our case. The positivity of histological markers (chromogranin and synaptophysin) as seen in our patient is known in NETs. The Ki-67 index is an important prognostic marker in pancreatic NETs and helps in choosing an optimal therapeutic approach as well as preoperative assessment of pancreatic NETs. Ki-67 index >2% is associated with poor prognosis with increased mortality compared with Ki-67 index <2%.[23] It is noteworthy that our patient had a Ki-67 index of 40%, implying very poor prognosis. New pathological classifications help in prognostication and the 5-year survival rates of grades I, II, and III tumors are mentioned as 96%, 73%, and 28%, respectively.[24–26] Approximately 60% of malignant pancreatic NETs have metastases to the liver and 10% to 20% of the cases can have distant metastases at the time of diagnosis.[27] Treatment of pancreatic NETs includes chemotherapy and surgical resection. Although surgery is the frontline treatment for pancreatic NETs in localized tumors, there is a significant expansion in systemic treatment options in metastatic tumors. Chemotherapy with capecitabine and temozolamide (which was used in our patient) has shown prolongation of progression-free survival.[22]

To summarize, endogenous CS is predominantly of pituitary or adrenal origin; and ectopic ACTH-dependent tumors contribute to <1% of endogenous CS cases in children and adolescents. The present case represents an exceedingly rare cause of endogenous CS. Through this case, the authors wish to create awareness regarding endogenous CS as a rare cause of severe hypertension with hypokalemic metabolic alkalosis.

References

Clinical Presentation 1

1. Assadi F. Urine anion gap can differentiate respiratory alkalosis from metabolic acidosis in the absence of blood gas results. *Pediatr Pulmonol.* 2023;19:1–3. https://doi.org/10.1002/PPUL.26392.
2. Battle D, Chin-Theodrou J, Tucker BB. Metabolic acidosis or respiratory alkalosis? Evaluation of low serum bicarbonates using the urine anion gap. *Am J Kidney Dis.* 2017;70:440–444.

Clinical Presentation 2

1. Assadi F, John EG. Hypouricemia in neonates with syndrome of inappropriate secretion of antidiuretic hormone. *Pediatr Res.* 1985;19(5):424–427. https://doi.org/10.1203/00006450-198505000-00003.
2. Assadi F, Mazaheri M. Differentiating SIADH, reset osmostat, and cerebral/renal salt eating using fractional urate excretion. *J Pediatric Endocrinol Metab.* 2020;34(1):137–140. https://doi.org/10.1515/open-2020-0379.
3. Rudolph A, Gantioque R. Differentiating between SIADH and CSW using fractional excretion of uric acid and phosphate: a narrative review. *Neurodens Med.* 2018;9:53–62.
4. Assadi F. Hyponatremia: a problem-solving approach to clinical cases. *J Nephrol.* 2012;25(4):473–480. https://doi.org/10.5301/jn.5000060.
5. Assadi FK, Agrawal R, Jocher C, John EG, Rosenthal IM. Hyponatremia secondary to reset osmostat. *J Pediatr.* 1986;108(2):262–264. https://doi.org/10.1016/s0022-3476(86)81000-9.

Clinical Presentation 3

1. Assadi FK, Johnston B, Dawson M, Sung B. Recurrent hypertonic dehydration due to selective defect in the osmoregulation of thirst. *Pediatr Nephrol.* 1989;3(4):438–442.
2. Asadi FK, Norman ME, Parks JS, Schwartz MW. Hypernatremia associated with pineal tumor. *J Pediatr.* 1977;90:605–606. https://doi.org/10.1016/s0022-3476(77)80379-x.

Clinical Presentation 4

1. Mazaheri M, Assadi F, Sadeghi-Bond S. Acetazolamide as adjunct therapy for treatment of Bartter syndrome. *Int J Urol Nephrol.* 2020;52:121–128. https://doi.org/10.1007/s11255-019-02351-7.

Clinical Presentation 5

1. Kelepouris E, Agus ZS. Hypomagnesemia: renal magnesium handling. *Semin Nephrol.* 1998;18(1):58–73.
2. Assadi F. Clinical disorders associated with altered potassium metabolism. In: Elzouki AY, Harding HA, Nazar H, Stapleton FB, Oh W, Whitley RJ, eds. *Textbook of Clinical Pediatrics.* 2nd ed. New York, NY: Springer; 2011 vol 4, Section 2842663–2270.

Clinical Presentation 6

1. Chen SJ, Wang SC, Chen YC. Challenges, recent advances and perspectives in the treatment of human cytomegalovirus infections. *Trop Med Infect Dis.* 2022;7(12):439. https://doi.org/10.3390/tropicalmed7120439.
2. Inose R, Takahashi K, Takahashi M, et al. Long-term use of foscarnet is associated with an increased incidence of acute kidney injury in hematopoietic stem cell transplant patients: a retrospective observational study. *Transpl Infect Dis.* 2022;24(2):e13804. https://doi.org/10.1111/tid.13804.

Clinical Presentation 7

1. Dahir D, Zanchetta MB, Stanciu I, et al. Diagnosis and management of tumor-induced osteomalacia: perspectives from clinical experience. *J Endocrinol Soc.* 2021;5(9):bvab099. https://doi.org/10.1210/jendso/bvab099.
2. Dadoniene J, Miglinas M, Miltiniene D, et al. Tumour-induced osteomalacia: a literature review and a case report. *World J Surg Oncol.* 2015;14:4. https://doi.org/10.1186/s12957-015-0763-7.

Clinical Presentation 8

1. Shaw NJ. A practical approach to hypocalcaemia in children. *Endocr Dev.* 2015;28:84–100. https://doi.org/10.1159/000380997.
2. Bove-Fenderson E, Mannstadt M. Hypocalcemic disorders. *Best Pract Res Clin Endocrinol Metab.* 2018;32(5):639–656. https://doi.org/10.1016/j.beem.2018.05.006.

Clinical Presentation 9

1. Bordelon PA, Cheri MV, Langan R. Recognition and management of vitamin D deficiency. *Am Fam Physician.* 2009;80(8):841–846.

Clinical Presentation 10

1. Assadi FK, Kimura RE, Subramanian U, Patel S. Liddle syndrome in a newborn infant. *Pediatr Nephrol.* 2002;17(8):609–611. https://doi.org/10.1007/s00467-002-0897-z.
2. Assadi F, Mazaheri M, Kelishadi M. The role of healthy lifestyle in the primordial prevention of metabolic syndrome throughout life: what we know and what we need to know? In: Kelishadi R, ed. *Healthy Lifestyle: From Pediatrics to Geriatrics.* New York, NY: Springer Nature; 2022:11–23.

Clinical Presentation 11

1. Assadi F. Hyponatremia: a problem-solving approach to clinical cases. *J Nephrol.* 2012;25(4):473–480. https://doi.org/10.5301/jn.5000060.
2. Assadi FK. Clinical quiz. Hyponatremia. *Pediatr Nephrol.* 1993;7(4):503–505. https://doi.org/10.1007/BF00857585. Erratum in: *Pediatr Nephrol.* 1994;8(2):256.
3. Assadi FK, John EG. Hypouricemia in neonates with syndrome of inappropriate secretion of antidiuretic hormone. *Pediatr Res.* 1985;19(5):424–497. https://doi.org/10.1203/00006450-198505000-00003.

Clinical Presentation 12

1. Adrogué HJ. Hyponatremia in heart failure. *Methodist Debakey Cardiovasc J.* 2017;13(1):40. https://doi.org/10.14797/mdcj-13-1-40.
2. Rodriguez M, Hernandez M, Cheungpasitporn W, et al. Hyponatremia in heart failure: pathogenesis and management. *Curr Cardiol Rev.* 2019;15:252–261.

Clinical Presentation 13

1. Assadi F, Mazaheri M. Differentiating syndrome of inappropriate ADH, reset osmostat, cerebral/renal salt wasting using fractional urate excretion. *J Pediatr Endocrinol Metab.* 2020;34(1):137–140. https://doi.org/10.1515/jpem-2020-0379.
2. Assadi F. Hyponatremia: a problem-solving approach to clinical cases. *J Nephrol.* 2012;25(4):473–480. https://doi.org/10.5301/jn.5000060.

3. Assadi FK, Agrawal R, Jocher C, John EG, Rosenthal IM. Hyponatremia secondary to reset osmostat. *J Pediatr*. 1986;108(2):262–264. https://doi.org/10.1016/s0022-3476(86)81000-9.

Clinical Presentation 14

1. Assadi FK, John EG. Hypouricemia in neonates with syndrome of inappropriate secretion of antidiuretic hormone. *Pediatr Res*. 1985;19(5):424–427. https://doi.org/10.1203/00006450-198505000-00003.
2. Assadi F, Mazaheri M. Differentiating syndrome of inappropriate ADH, reset osmostat, cerebral/renal salt wasting using fractional urate excretion. *J Pediatr Endocrinol Metab*. 2020;34(1):137–140. https://doi.org/10.1515/jpem-2020-0379.
3. Assadi FK, Agrawal R, Jocher C, John EG, Rosenthal IM. Hyponatremia secondary to reset osmostat. *J Pediatr*. 1986;108(2):262–264. https://doi.org/10.1016/s0022-3476(86)81000-9.

Clinical Presentation 15

1. Assadi F. A practical approach to metabolic acidosis. In: Elzouki AY, Harfi HA, Nazer H, eds. *Textbook of Clinical Pediatrics*. 2nd ed. New York, NY: Springer; 2011:2671–2676 Vol 4, Section 18.

Clinical Presentation 16

1. Assadi F. Acid-base disturbances. In: Assadi F, ed. *Clinical Decision in Pediatric Nephrology: A Problem-solving Approach to Clinical Cases*. New York, NY: Springer; 2008:69–96.

Clinical Presentation 17

1. Gennari FJ. Hypokalemia. *N Engl J Med*. 1998;339(7):451–458.
2. Rose BD, Post TW. *Clinical Physiology of Acid-Base and Electrolyte Disorders*. 5th ed. New York, NY: McGraw-Hill; 2001:551–571.
3. Lococo F, Margaritora S, Cardillo G, et al. Bronchopulmonary carcinoids causing Cushing syndrome: results from a multicentric study suggesting a more aggressive behavior. *Thorac Cardiovasc Surg*. 2016;64(2):172–181.
4. Morris DJ, Souness GW, Brem AS, et al. Interactions of mineralocorticoids and glucocorticoids in epithelial target tissues. *Kidney Int*. 2000;57(4):1370–1373.

Clinical Presentation 18

1. Van't Hoff WG. Fanconi syndrome. In: Davison AM, Cameron JS, Grunfeld JP, eds. *Oxford Textbook of Clinical Nephrology*. Oxford: Oxford University Press; 2005:961–973.
2. Vohra S, Eddy A, Levin AV, et al. Tubulointerstitial nephritis and uveitis in children and adolescents. Four new cases and a review of the literature. *Pediatr Nephrol*. 1999;13(5):426–432.
3. Servais A, Morinière V, Grünfeld J-P, et al. Late-onset nephropathic cystinosis: clinical presentation, outcome, and genotyping. *Clin J Am SocNephrol*. 2008;3(1):27–35.
4. Gahl WA, Theone JG, Schnei-der JA. Cystinosis. *N Engl J Med*. 2002;347(2):111–121.
5. Bonnardeaux A, Bichet DG. Inherited disorders of the renal tubule. In: Brenner BM, ed. *Brenner and Rector's The Kidney*. Philadelphia: Saunders Elsevier; 2008:1390–1427.

Clinical Presentation 19

1. Brunner HR, Laragh JH, Baer L, et al. Essential hypertension: renin and aldosterone, heart attack and stroke. *N Engl J Med*. 1972;286:441–449.
2. van den Born B-JH, Koopmans RP, van Montfrans GA. The renin-angiotensin system in malignant hypertension revisited: plasma renin activity, microangiopathic hemolysis, and renal failure in malignant hypertension. *Am J Hypertens*. 2007;20:900–906.
3. Wong L, Hsu THS, Perlroth MG, et al. Reninoma: case report and literature review. *J Hypertens*. 2008;26:368–373.
4. McVicar M, Carman C, Chandra M, et al. Hypertension secondary to renin-secreting juxtaglomerular cell tumor: case report and review of 38 cases. *Pediatr Nephrol*. 1993;7:404–412.
5. Vasbinder GB, Nelemans PJ, Kessels AG, et al. Diagnostic tests for renal artery stenosis in patients suspected of having renovascular hypertension: a meta-analysis. *Ann Intern Med*. 2001;135:401–411.

Clinical Presentation 20

1. Yasue H, Itoh T, Mizuno Y, et al. Severe hypokalemia, rhabdomyolysis, muscle paralysis, and respiratory impairment in a hypertensive patient taking herbal medicines containing licorice. *Intern Med*. 2007;46(9):575–578.

2. Armanini D, Fiore C, Mattarello MJ, et al. History of the endocrine effects of licorice. *Exp Clin Endocrinol Diabetes*. 2002;110(6):257–261.
3. van den Bosch AE, van der Klooster JM, Zuidgeest DMH, et al. Severe hypokalaemic paralysis and rhabdomyolysis due to ingestion of liquorice. *Neth J Med*. 2005;63(4):146–148.

Clinical Presentation 21

1. Rose BD, Post TW. *Clinical Physiology of Acid–Base and Electrolyte Disorders*. 5th ed. New York, NY: McGraw-Hill Inc; 2001:551–571.
2. Assadi F. *Clinical Decisions in Pediatric Nephrology: A Problem Solving Approach to Clinical Cases*. New York, NY: Springer; 2008:69–98.

Clinical Presentation 22

1. Thomas D, Dubose J. Disorders of acid–base balance. In: Skorecki K, Chertow GM, Marsden PA et al, eds. *Brenner & Rector's The Kidney*. 10th ed. Philadelphia: Elsevier; 2016:511–558.
2. Assadi F. *Clinical Decisions in Pediatric Nephrology: A Problem Solving Approach to Clinical Cases*. New York, NY: Springer; 2008:69–98.

Clinical Presentation 23

1. White PC. 11beta-hydroxysteroid dehydrogenase and its role in the syndrome of apparent mineralocorticoid excess. *Am J Med Sci*. 2001;322:308–315.
2. Rose BD, Post TW. *Clinical Physiology of Acid–Base and Electrolyte Disorders*. 5th ed. New York, NY: McGraw-Hill; 2001:836–856.
3. Assadi F. Diagnosis of hypokalemia: a problem-solving approach to clinical cases. *Iran J Kidney Dis*. 2008;2(3):115–122.

Clinical Presentation 24

1. Lin SH, Lin YF, Halperin ML. Hypokalaemia and paralysis. *QJM*. 2001;194:133–139.
2. Assadi F. Diagnosis of hypokalemia: a problem-solving approach to clinical cases. *Iran J Kidney Dis*. 2008;2(3):115–122.

Clinical Presentation 25

1. Assadi F. Diagnosis of hypokalemia: a problem-solving approach to clinical cases. *Iran J Kidney Dis*. 2008;2(3):115–122.
2. Shaer AJ. Inherited primary renal tubular hypokalemic alkalosis: a review of Gitelman and Bartter syndromes. *Am J Med Sci*. 2002;322:316–332.

Clinical Presentation 26

1. Gennari FJ. Hypokalemia. *N Engl J Med*. 1998;339:451–458.
2. Groeneveld JHM, Sijpkens YWJ, Lin S-H, et al. An approach to the patient with severe hypokalaemia: the potassium quiz. *QJM*. 2005;98:305–316.

Clinical Presentation 27

1. Gennari FJ. Hypokalemia. *N Engl J Med*. 1998;339:451–458.
2. Groeneveld JHM, Sijpkens YWJ, Lin S-H, et al. An approach to the patient with severe hypokalaemia: the potassium quiz. *QJM*. 2005;98:305–316.
3. Palmer BF, Alpern RJ. Metabolic alkalosis. *J Am Soc Nephrol*. 1977;8:1462–1469.
4. Assadi F. Diagnosis of hypokalemia: a problem-solving approach to clinical cases. *Iran J Kidney Dis*. 2008;2(3):115–122.

Clinical Presentation 28

1. Palmer BF, Alpern RJ. Metabolic alkalosis. *J Am Soc Nephrol*. 1977;8:1462–1469.
2. Assadi F. Diagnosis of hypokalemia: a problem-solving approach to clinical cases. *Iran J Kidney Dis*. 2008;2(3):115–122.

Clinical Presentation 29

1. Assadi F. Diagnosis of hypokalemia: a problem-solving approach to clinical cases. *Iran J Kidney Dis*. 2008;2(3):115–122.
2. Morineau G, Sulmont V, Salomon R, et al. Apparent mineralocorticoid excess: report of six new cases and extensive personal experience. *J Am Soc Nephrol*. 2006;17:3176–3184.

Clinical Presentation 30

1. Ishiguchi T, Mikita N, Iwata T, et al. Myoclonus and metabolic alkalosis from licorice in antacid. *Intern Med.* 2004;43:59–62.
2. Assadi F. Diagnosis of hypokalemia: a problem-solving approach to clinical cases. *Iran J Kidney Dis.* 2008;2(3):115–122.

Clinical Presentation 31

1. Assadi F. Diagnosis of hypokalemia: a problem-solving approach to clinical cases. *Iran J Kidney Dis.* 2008;2(3):115–122.
2. Botero-Velez M, Curtis JJ, Warnock DG. Brief report: Liddle's syndrome revisited—a disorder of sodium reabsorption in the distal tubule. *N Engl J Med.* 1994;33:178–181.

Clinical Presentation 32

1. Blumenfeld JD, Sealey JE, Schlussel Y, et al. Diagnosis and treatment of primary hyperaldosteronism. *Ann Intern Med.* 1994;121(11):877–885.
2. Martinez-Valles MA, Palafox-Cazarez A, Paredes-Avina JA. Severe hypokalemia, metabolic alkalosis and hypertension in a 54-year-old male with ectopic ACTH syndrome: a case report. *Cases J.* 2009;2:6174.
3. Jammalamadaka D, Shahnia S, Buller G. Refractory hypokalemia from ectopic adrenocorticotropic hormone secreting thymic tumor. *Webmed-Central.* 2010;1(10):WMC00912.
4. Bhasin B, Velez JCQ. Evaluation of polyuria: the roles of solute loading and water diuresis. *Am J Kidney Dis.* 2016;67(3):507–511.
5. Khositseth S, Uawithya P, Somparn P, et al. Autophagic degradation of aquaporin-2 is an early event in hypokalemia-induced nephrogenic diabetes insipidus. *Sci Rep.* 2015;5:18311.

Clinical Presentation 33

1. Gamakaranage CS, Rodrigo C, Jayasinghe S, et al. Hypokalemic paralysis associated with cystic disease of the kidney: case report. *BMC Nephrol.* 2011;12:16.
2. Fontaine B, Lapie P, Plassart E, et al. Periodic paralysis and voltage-gated ion channels. *Kidney Int.* 1996;49(1):9–18.
3. Kasap B, Soylu A, Oren O, et al. Medullary sponge kidney associated with distal renal tubular acidosis in a 5-year-old girl. *Eur J Pediatr.* 2006;165:648–651.
4. Battle D, Moorthi KM, Schlueter W, et al. Distal renal tubular acidosis and the potassium enigma. *Semin Nephrol.* 2006;26(6):471–478.

Clinical Presentation 34

1. Novak JE, Ellison D. Diuretics in states of volume overload: core curriculum 2022. *Am J Kidney Dis.* 2022;80(2):264–276. https://doi.org/10.1053/j.ajkd.2021.09.029.

Clinical Presentation 35

1. Chhabria M, Portales-Castilian, Chowdhury M, et al. A case of severe hypokalemia. Am J Kidney Dis. 2029;76:PA9–A12.

Clinical Presentation 36

1. Hughes IA, Davies JD, Bunch TI, et al. Androgen insensitivity syndrome. *Lancet.* 2012;380:1419–1428. https://doi.org/10.1016/S0140-6736(12)60071-3.
2. Kim S-H, Hu Y, Cadman S, Bouloux P. Diversity in fibroblast growth factor receptor 1 regulation: learning from the investigation of Kallmann syndrome. *J Neuroendocrinol.* 2007;20:141–163. https://doi.org/10.1111/j.1365-2826.2007.01627.x.

Clinical Presentation 37

1. Bartter FC, Schwartz WB. The syndrome of inappropriate secretion of antidiuretic hormone. *Am J Med.* 1967;42(5):790–806. https://doi.org/10.1016/0002-9343(67)90096-4.
2. Jones DP. Syndrome of inappropriate secretion of antidiuretic hormone and hyponatremia. *Pediatr Rev.* 2018;39(1):27–35. https://doi.org/10.1542/pir.2016-0165.
3. Branten AJ, Wetzels JF, Weber AM, et al. Hyponatremia due to sodium valproate. *Ann Neurol.* 1998;43(2):265–267. https://doi.org/10.1002/ana.410430219.

4. Choi SA, Kim H, Kim S, et al. Analysis of antiseizure drug-related adverse reactions from the electronic health record using the common data model. *Epilepsia.* 2020;61(4):610–616. https://doi.org/10.1111/epi.16472.
5. Miyaoka T, Seno H, Itoga M, et al. Contribution of sodium valproate to the syndrome of inappropriate secretion of antidiuretic hormone. *Int Clin Psychopharmacol.* 2001;16(1):59–61. https://doi.org/10.1097/00004850-200101000-00008.
6. Beers E, van Puijenbroek EP, Bartelink IH, van der Linden CM, Jansen PA. Syndrome of inappropriate antidiuretic hormone secretion (SIADH) or hyponatraemia associated with valproic acid: four case reports from the Netherlands and a case/non-case analysis of vigibase. *Drug Saf.* 2020;33(1):47–55. https://doi.org/10.2165/11318950-000000000-00000.

Clinical Presentation 38

1. Curry NS, Chung CJ, Gordon B. Unilateral renal cystic disease in an adult. *Abdom Imaging.* 1994;19:366–368.

Clinical Presentation 39

1. Choi M, Scholl UI, Ji W, et al. Genetic diagnosis by whole exome capture and massively parallel DNA sequencing. *Proc Natl Acad Sci U S A.* 2009;106:19096–19101.
2. Sojo A, Rodriguez-Soriano J, Vitoria JC, et al. Chloride deficiency as a presentation or complication of cystic fibrosis. *Eur J Pediatr.* 1994;153:825–828.
3. Holmberg C. Congenital chloride diarrhea. *Clin Gastroenterol.* 1996;15:583–602.
4. Hoglund P, Auranen M, Socha J, et al. Genetic background of congenital chloride diarrhea in high-incidence populations: Finland, Poland, and Saudi Arabia and Kuwait. *Am J Hum Genet.* 1998;63:760–768.
5. Makela S, Kere J, Holmberg C, Hoglund P. SLC26A3 mutations in congenital chloride diarrhea. *Hum Mutat.* 2002;20:425–438.

Clinical Presentation 40

1. Rees L, Webb NJA, Brogan PA. Hyperkalemia. In: Rees L, Webb NJA, Brogan PA, eds. *Oxford Specialist Handbooks in Paediatrics.* Oxford: Oxford University Press; 2007:88–91.
2. Tannen RL. Primary defects in tubular secretion of potassium. In: Kokko JP, Tannen RL, eds. *Fluids and Electrolytes.* 3rd ed. Philadelphia: W. B. Saunders; 1996:169–171.
3. Wilson FH, Disse-Nicodeme S, Choate KA, et al. Human hypertension caused by mutations in WNK kinases. *Science.* 2001;293:1107–1112.
4. Proctor G, Linas S. Type 2 pseudohypoaldosteronism: new insights into renal potassium, sodium, and chloride handling. *Am J Kidney Dis.* 2006;48:674–693.
5. Garovic VD, Hilliard AA, Turner ST. Monogenic forms of low-renin hypertension: Gordon's syndrome. *Nat Clin Pract Nephrol.* 2006;2:624–630.

Clinical Presentation 41

1. Fox RI. Sjögren's syndrome. *Lancet.* 2005;366:321–331.
2. Garcia-Carrasco M, Ramos-Casals M, Rosas J, et al. Primary Sjogren syndrome: clinical and immunologic disease patterns in a cohort of 400 patients. *Medicine (Baltimore).* 2002;81:270–280.
3. Ostuni PA, Ianniello A, Sfriso P, Mazzola G, Andretta M, Gambari PF. Juvenile onset of primary Sjögren's syndrome: report of 10 cases. *Clin Exp Rheumatol.* 1996;14:689–693.
4. Stiller M, Golder W, Döring E, Biedermann T. Primary and secondary Sjögren's syndrome in children: a comparative study. *Clin Oral Investig.* 2000;4:176–182.
5. Ohlsson V, Strike H, James-Ellison M, et al. Renal tubular acidosis, arthritis and autoantibodies: primary Sjogren syndrome in childhood. *Rheumatology.* 2006;45:238–240.
6. Skalova S, Minxova L, Slezak R. Hypokalaemic paralysis revealing Sjogren's syndrome in a 16-year old girl. *Ghana Med J.* 2008;42:124–128.
7. Chang YC, Huang CC, Chiou YY, et al. Renal tubular acidosis complicated with hypokalemic periodic paralysis. *Pediatr Neurol.* 1995;13:52–54.
8. Zeng Y, Huang W, Wang L-Zea. A case report of pediatric Sjogren's syndrome presenting with renal tubular acidosis. [Chinese]. *Clin Focus.* 2002;17:355.
9. Liu DM, Li M-Z. A case of primary Sjogren's syndrome. [Chinese]. *J Appl Clin Pediatr.* 2003;8:45.
10. Zhang LL, Li L, Lin MY. One case report of pediatric Sjogren's syndrome presenting with renal tubular acidosis. [Chinese]. *J Appl Clin Pediatr.* 1994;9:310–311.

11. Pessler F, Emery H, Dai L, et al. The spectrum of renal tubular acidosis in paediatric Sjögren syndrome. *Rheumatology*. 2006;45:85–91.

Clinical Presentation 42

1. Fuleihan G-H. Familial benign hypocalciuric hypercalcemia. *J Bone Miner Res*. 2002;17:51–56.
2. Khanna A. Acquired nephrogenic diabetes insipidus. *Semin Nephrol*. 2006;26:244–248.
3. Broulik PD, Haas T, Adamek S. Analysis of 645 patients with primary hyperparathyroidism with special references to cholelithiasis. *Int Med*. 2005;44:917–921.
4. Bhadada SK, Bhansali A, Shah VN, et al. High prevalence of cholelithiasis in primary hyperparathyroidism: a retrospective analysis of 120 cases. *Indian J Gastroenterol*. 2011;30:100–101.
5. Blank S, Scanlon KS, Sinks TH, et al. An outbreak of hypervitaminosis D associated with the over fortification of milk from a home-delivery dairy. *Am J Public Health*. 1995;85:656–659.
6. Vanstone MB, Oberfield SE, Shader L, et al. Hypercalcemia in children receiving pharmacologic doses of vitamin D. *Pediatrics*. 2012;129:e1060–e10631.
7. Chatterjee M, Speiser PW. Pamidronate treatment of hypercalcemia caused by vitamin D toxicity. *J Pediatr Endocrinol Metab*. 2007;20:1241–1248.
8. Sezer RG, Guran T, Paketçi C, et al. Comparison of oral alendronate versus prednisolone in treatment of infants with vitamin D intoxication. *Acta Paediatr*. 2008;101:e122–e125.

Clinical Presentation 43

1. Khairallah W, Fawaz A, Brown EM, et al. Hypercalcemia and diabetes insipidus in a patient previously treated with lithium. *Nat Clin Pract Nephrol*. 2013;3(7):397–404.
2. American Thoracic Society. The joint statement of the American Thoracic Society (ATS), The European Respiratory Society (ERS), and the World Association of Sarcoidosis and other Granulomatous Disorders (WASOG). Statement on sarcoidosis. *Am J Respir Crit Care Med*. 1999;160(2):736–755.
3. Greger R, Schlatter E. Properties of the basolateral membrane of the cortical thick ascending limb of Henle's loop of rabbit kidney: a model for secondary active chloride transport. *Pflugers Archiv*. 1983;396:325–334.
4. Gamba G, Friedman PA. Thick ascending limb: the Na(+):K (+):2Cl (-) co-transporter, NKCC2, and the calcium-sensing receptor, CaSR. *Pflugers Arch*. 2009;458(1):61–76.
5. Amlal H, Legoff C, Vernimmen, et al. Na(+)-K+(NH4+)-2Cl- cotransport in medullary thick ascending limb: control by PKA, PKC, and 20-HETE. *Am J Physiol*. 1996;271:C455–C463.
6. Wang D, An S, Wang W. CaR-mediated COX-2 expression in primary cultured mTAL cells. *Am J Physiol*. 2011;281:F658–F664.
7. Sands JM, Naruse M, Baum M, et al. Apical extracellular calcium/polyvalent cation-sensing receptor regulates vasopressin-elicited water permeability in rat kidney inner medullary collecting duct. *J Clin Invest*. 1997;99:1399–1405.
8. Earm JH, Christensen BM, Frøkiaer J, et al. Decreased aquaporin-2 expression and apical plasma membrane delivery in kidney collecting ducts of polyuric hypercalcaemic rats. *J Am Soc Nephrol*. 1998;9(12):2181–2193.
9. Iannuzzi MC, Rybicki BA, Teirstein AS. Sarcoidosis. *N Engl J Med*. 2007;357(21):2153–2165.
10. Pattishall EN, Kendig EL Jr. Sarcoidosis in children. *Pediatr Pulmonol*. 1996;22(3):195–203.
11. Milman N, Hoffmann AL. Childhood sarcoidosis: long-term follow-up. *Eur Respir J*. 2008;31(3):592–598.
12. Sharma OP. Fatigue and sarcoidosis. *Eur Respir J*. 1999;13(4):713–714.
13. Rizzato G, Palmieri G, Agrati AM, et al. The organ specific extrapulmonary presentation of sarcoidosis: a frequent occurrence but a challenge to an early diagnosis. A 3-year-long prospective observational study. *Sarcoidosis Vasc Diffuse Lung Dis*. 2004;21:119–126.
14. Rizzato G, Tinelli C. Unusual presentation of sarcoidosis. *Respiration*. 2005;72(1):3–6.
15. Baughman RP, Teirstein AS, Judson MA, et al. Clinical characteristics of patients in a case control study of sarcoidosis. *Am J Respir Crit Care Med*. 2001;164:1885–1889.
16. Adams JS, Singer FR, Gacad MA, et al. Isolation and structural identification of 1,25-dihydroxyvitamin D3 produced by cultured alveolar macrophages in sarcoidosis. *J Clin Endocrinol Metab*. 1985;60:960–966.
17. Insogna KL, Dreyer BE, Mitnick M, et al. Enhanced production rate of 1,25-dihydroxyvitamin D in sarcoidosis. *J Clin Endocrinol Metab*. 1988;66:72–75.
18. Hosking DJ, Cowley A, Bucknall CA. Rehydration in the treatment of severe hypercalcaemia. *Q J Med*. 1981;50:473–481.

19. Suki WN, Yium JJ, Von Minden M, et al. Acute treatment of hypercalcemia with furosemide. *N Engl J Med*. 1970;283(16):836–840.
20. Dahl K, Canetta PA, D'Agati VD, et al. A 56-year-old woman with sarcoidosis and acute renal failure. *Kidney Int*. 2008;74:817–821.
21. Casella FJ, Allon M. The kidney in sarcoidosis. *J Am Soc Nephrol*. 1993;3(9):1555–1562.
22. Mahévas M, Lescure FX, Boffa J-J, et al. Renal sarcoidosis: clinical, laboratory, and histologic presentation and outcome in 47 patients. *Medicine*. 2009;88:98–106.
23. Bilezikian JP. Clinical review 51: management of hypercalcemia. *J Clin Endocrinol Metab*. 1993;77(6):1445–1449.
24. Berenson JR. Treatment of hypercalcemia of malignancy with bisphosphonates. *Semin Oncol*. 2002;29:12–18.
25. Aouizerate J, Matignon M, Kamar N, et al. Renal transplantation in patients with sarcoidosis: a French multicenter study. *Clin J Am Soc Nephrol*. 2010;15(11):2101–2108.

Clinical Presentation 44

1. Magiakou MA, Smyrnaki P, Chrousos GP. Hypertension in Cushing's syndrome. *Best Pract Res Clin Endocrinol Metab*. 2006;20:467–482.
2. Cicala MV, Mantero F. Hypertension in Cushing's syndrome: from pathogenesis to treatment. *Neuroendocrinology*. 2010;92(suppl 1):44–49.
3. Kirilov G, Tomova A, Dakovska L, et al. Elevated plasma endothelin as an additional cardiovascular risk factor in patients with Cushing's syndrome. *Eur J Endocrinol*. 2003;149:549–553.
4. Mangos GJ, Whitworth JA, Williamson PM, et al. Glucocorticoids and the kidney. *Nephrology (Carlton)*. 2003;8:267–273.
5. Baid S, Nieman LK. Glucocorticoid excess and hypertension. *Curr Hypertens Rep*. 2004;6:493–499.
6. McFarlane SI, Banerji M, Sowers JR. Insulin resistance and cardiovascular disease. *J Clin Endocrinol Metab*. 2001;86:713–718.
7. Pitt B, Zannad F, Remme WJ, et al. The effect of spironolactone on morbidity and mortality in patients with severe heart failure. Randomized Aldactone Evaluation Study Investigators. *N Engl J Med*. 1999;341:709–717.
8. Weiner ID, Wingo CS. Hypokalemia–consequences, causes, and correction. *J Am Soc Nephrol*. 1997;8:1179–1188.
9. Etxabe J, Vazquez JA. Morbidity and mortality in Cushing's disease: an epidemiological approach. *Clin Endocrinol*. 1994;40:479–484.
10. Clayton RN, Raskauskiene D, Reulen RC, et al. Mortality and morbidity in Cushing's disease over 50 years in Stoke-on-Trent, UK: audit and meta-analysis of literature. *J Clin Endocrinol Metab*. 2011;96:632–642.
11. Arnardóttir S, Sigurjonsdóttir HA. The incidence and prevalence of Cushing's disease may be higher than previously thought: results from a retrospective study in Iceland 1955 through 2009. *Clin Endocrinol*. 2011;74:792–793.
12. Ragnarsson O, Olsson DS, Chantzichristos D, et al. The incidence of Cushing's disease: a nationwide Swedish study. *Pituitary*. 2019;22:179–186.
13. Bolland MJ, Holdaway IM, Berkeley JE, et al. Mortality and morbidity in Cushing's syndrome in New Zealand. *Clin Endocrinol*. 2011;75:436–442.
14. Lindholm J, Juul S, Jørgensen JO, et al. Incidence and late prognosis of Cushing's syndrome: a population-based study. *J Clin Endocrinol Metab*. 2001;86:117–123.
15. Wengander S, Trimpou P, Papakokkinou E, et al. The incidence of endogenous Cushing's syndrome in the modern era. *Clin Endocrinol*. 2019;91:263–270.
16. Sharma ST, Nieman LK, Feelders RA. Cushing's syndrome: epidemiology and developments in disease management. *Clin Epidemiol*. 2015;7:281–293.
17. Lodish MB, Keil MF, Stratakis CA. Cushing's syndrome in pediatrics: an update. *Endocrinol Metab Clin N Am*. 2018;47:451–462.
18. Stratakis CA. Cushing syndrome in pediatrics. *Endocrinol Metab Clin N Am*. 2012;41:793–803.
19. Ismail H, Broniszczak D, Markiewicz-Kijewska M, et al. Metastases of pancreatic neuroendocrine tumor to the liver as extremely rare indication for liver transplantation in children. Case report and review of the literature. *Clin Res Hepatol Gastroenterol*. 2016;40:e33–e37.

20. Rosado B, Gores GJ. Liver transplantation for neuroendocrine tumors: progress and uncertainty. *Liver Transpl.* 2004;10:712–713.
21. Navalkele P, O'Dorisio MS, O'Dorisio TM, Zamba GK, Lynch CF. Incidence, survival, and prevalence of neuroendocrine tumors versus neuroblastoma in children and young adults: nine standard SEER registries, 1975–2006. *Pediatr Blood Cancer.* 2011;56:50–57.
22. Cives M, Strosberg JR. Gastroenteropancreatic neuroendocrine tumors. *Cancer J Clin.* 2018;68:471–487.
23. Franchi G, Manzoni MF. Cytological Ki-67 in pancreatic endocrine tumors: a new "must"? *Gland Surg.* 2014;3:219–221.
24. Zimmer T, Ziegler K, Liehr RM, et al. Endosonography of neuroendocrine tumors of the stomach, duodenum, and pancreas. *Ann NY Acad Sci.* 1994;733:425–436.
25. Binstock AJ, Johnson CD, Stephens DH, et al. Carcinoid tumors of the stomach: a clinical and radiographic study. *Am J Roentgenol.* 2001;176:947–951.
26. Dolcetta-Capuzzo A, Villa V, Albarello L, et al. Gastroenteric neuroendocrine neoplasms classification: comparison of prognostic models. *Cancer.* 2013;119:36–44.
27. Gu P, Wu J, Newman E, Muggia F. Treatment of liver metastases in patients with neuroendocrine tumors of gastroesophageal and pancreatic origin. *Int J Hepatol.* 2012;2012:131659.

CHAPTER 5

Genetic Disorders

Clinical Presentation 1

A 3-year-old boy is evaluated for failure to thrive, muscle weakness, bone pain, and difficulty to walk over the past 10 months. The infant was born at term to a 28-year-old gravida 2, para 2 mother via vaginal delivery. The birth weight was 3.1 kg; length, 50 cm; and head circumference, 45 cm. The child's father had rickets as a child, which left severe deformities. He was taking vitamin D and phosphorous supplements. The patient's 6-year-old sister had a history of delayed gross motor milestones and frontal bossing. However, a workup had never been done, nor had the child been treated. A dietary history revealed that the child had been fed a soy-based formula since early infancy because he had been unable to tolerate cow's milk.

On examination, he appears as a thin male in no acute distress. Blood pressure is 96/51 mm Hg; pulse, 96 beats/min; respirations, 20/min; temperature, 37°C, weight, 11.3 kg (fifth percentile); height, 80 cm (below the third percentile); and head circumference, 49 cm (50th percentile). Heart rate is regular and there are no extra sounds or murmurs. The lungs are clear. The abdomen is soft and there are no masses. The extremities are free of rashes or edema. Neurological examination shows moderate proximal-muscle weakness with lower extremity bowing. The rest of the physical examination is uneventful. Laboratory studies reveal a hemoglobin level and a leukocyte count within reference ranges and a normal urinalysis. Serum sodium level is 137 mEq/L; potassium, 3.9 mEq/L; chloride, 100 mEq/L; bicarbonate, 28 mEq/L; blood urea nitrogen, 8 mg/dL; creatinine, 0.3 mg/ dL; albumin, 4.2 g/dL; calcium, 10.2 mg/ dL; phosphate, 1.9 mg/dL; magnesium, 1.7 mg/ dL; and alkaline phosphatase, 1829 U/L (reference range, 50-330 U/L). A random urine calcium-creatinine ratio is 0.18 (reference range, <0.22–0.26). The urine phosphate and creatinine excretion are 60 mg and 33 mg, respectively, and the iron(III) phosphate ($FEPO_4$) is 28.6% (reference range, 10–15%).

Which one the following conditions should now be considered in the differential diagnosis (select all that apply)?

A. Primary hyperparathyroidism
B. Inadequate dietary intake
C. Malabsorption of intestinal phosphate
D. Ingestion of large quantities of phosphate-binding antacids
E. Vitamin D deficiency
F. Fanconi syndrome
G. X-linked hypophosphatemic rickets
H. Oncogenic osteomalacia
I. Hyperventilation

The correct answers are E, F, and H

Comment: The elevated $FEPO_4$ signifies excessive urinary losses of phosphate. Renal phosphate wasting can result from genetic or acquired renal disorders. Acquired renal phosphate wasting syndromes can result from vitamin D deficiency, hyperparathyroidism, oncogenic osteomalacia, and Fanconi syndrome (options E, F, H).[1,2]

The genetic disorders of renal hypophosphatemic disorders generally manifest in infancy are usually transmitted as XHR.[3]

Choice A is a wrong answer, as serum calcium concentration is elevated in patients with primary hyperparathyroidism. Answers B, C, and D are also incorrect because of the inappropriately high $FEPO_4$. Choice I is the wrong answer because hyperventilation lowers serum phosphate levels by promoting a shift of phosphate into the cells, leading to respiratory alkalosis, and the $FEPO_4$ is appropriately low.

Additional laboratory studies revealed 25-hydroxyvitamin D was 71.8 ng/mL (reference range, 30–100 ng/mL); 1,25-dihydroxyvitamin D, 15 pg/dL (reference range for children, 20–70 pg/dL); and intact parathyroid hormone (PTH), 44 pg/mL (4.6 pmol/L; reference range, 10–68 pg/mL). There was no aminoaciduria or glucosuria. Radiographic studies revealed florid signs of rickets, including a rachitic rosary and cupping of the ribs, and fraying and flaying of the radius, ulna, femur, tibia, and fibula.

Clinical Presentation 2

The mother of a 16-year-old White male seeks your advice regarding prognosis and future treatment of her son, who has recently been diagnosed as having Alport syndrome.

Her husband is healthy, but her grandfather died of chronic kidney failure. Her son currently has mild sensorineural hearing impairment, lenticonus, and well-controlled hypertension (blood pressure [BP], 130/82 mm Hg) on an angiotensin-converting enzyme (ACE) inhibitor. His serum creatinine is 1.4 mg/dL, and his protein excretion is 1.0 g/day. One year ago, he underwent genetic testing as a part of a research study and was found to have a deletion mutation of the *COL4A5* gene of the X-chromosome.

Which *one* of the following choices best describes the clinical course that this patient is most likely to follow?

A. His renal failure is not likely to progress and renal transplantation will not be needed.
B. His renal failure is likely to progress, and renal transplantation is associated with a low risk (<5%) of posttransplant glomerulonephritis.
C. His renal failure is likely to progress, and renal transplantation would be associated with a moderate risk (15% or more) of posttransplant glomerulonephritis.
D. His renal failure is likely to progress, but his hearing impairment is not likely to progress.
E. His renal failure is likely to progress, and renal transplantation would be associated with a high probability of recurrent disease.

The correct answer is B

Comment: Currently, there is no specific treatment for Alport syndrome. The goal is to treat the symptoms and help slow the progression of kidney disease. This may include ACE inhibitors or angiotensin-receptor blocker medicines (medications to control high BP), diuretics, and dietary sodium restriction.

Kidney transplantation is usually very successful in patients with Alport syndrome and is considered the best treatment when kidney failure is approaching.[1]

Clinical Presentation 3

A 61-year-old female with autosomal dominant polycystic kidney disease (ADPKD) type 1 who has recently begun treatment with hemodialysis seeks your advice regarding evaluation of her 18-year-old grandson who is asymptomatic but anticipating marriage. He has recently undergone a renal ultrasound examination that disclosed no abnormalities.

What advice would you give to the grandson?

A. No further evaluation is needed because he is almost certainly unaffected.
B. Further evaluation with magnetic resonance imaging (MRI) of the kidneys is needed to determine if he is affected.
C. Further evaluation with genetic testing for mutations on chromosome 16 is needed to determine if he is affected.
D. Further evaluation with genetic testing for mutations on chromosome 4 is needed to determine if he is affected.
E. No further testing is needed because the results are likely to be inconclusive.

The correct answer is C
Comment: In the great majority of individuals with PKD, the condition is inherited in an autosomal dominant manner, known as autosomal dominant polycystic kidney disease (ARPKD). This is due to mutations in the *PKD1* gene on chromosome 16, causing type 1 disease. This accounts for more than 85% of cases.[1]

Clinical Presentation 4

An 11-year-old girl presented with short stature and was found to have chronic renal failure. The parents are cousins, but there was no family history of renal disease. There was a history of polydipsia, polyuria, and salt cravings. Her growth parameters were below the third percentile. Blood pressure is normal. Neurological examination was normal. There were no other abnormal findings. Urinalysis was negative for protein, glucose, and blood; pH was 7.0, and specific gravity was 1.008. Glomerular filtration rate (GFR) was 12 mL/min. Hemoglobin is 7.0 g/dL, white blood cells 11,500/mm^3, platelet 269,00/mm^3. Serum sodium was 130 mEq/L, potassium 4.0 mEq/L, chloride 111 mEq/L, bicarbonate 7 mEq/L, blood urea nitrogen (BUN) 80 mg/dL, creatinine 6.7 mg/dL, calcium 8.0 mg/dL, and phosphorous 6.9 mg/dL. Renal ultrasound showed bilateral small kidneys with increased echogenicity. A contrast cystogram was normal. A slit-lamp examination was normal and audiometry revealed no sensorineural loss.

What is the most likely diagnosis?

A. Cystic nephroblastoma
B. Medullary sponge kidney
C. Familial juvenile medullary cystic kidney
D. Polycystic kidney disease
E. Tuberculosis

The correct answer is C
Comment: Autosomal dominant tubulointerstitial kidney disease is caused by mutations in the genes encoding uromodulin (*UMOD*), hepatocyte nuclear factor-1β, renin, and mucin-1 (*MUC1*).

Multiple names have been proposed for these disorders, including medullary cystic kidney disease (MCKD) type 2, familial juvenile hyperuricemic nephropathy, or uromodulin-associated kidney disease for UMOD-related diseases and MCKD type 1 for the disease caused by *MUC1* mutations.

The multiplicity of these terms, as well as the fact that cysts are not pathognomonic, creates confusion.

Kidney Disease: Improving Global Outcomes proposes the adoption of a new terminology for this group of diseases using the term *autosomal dominant tubulointerstitial kidney disease* appended by a gene-based subclassification and suggests diagnostic criteria. Implementation of these recommendations is anticipated to facilitate the recognition and characterization of these monogenic diseases. A better understanding of these rare disorders may be relevant for the tubulointerstitial fibrosis component in many forms of chronic kidney disease.[1]

Clinical Presentation 5

You are asked to see a 3-year-old child who has developed growth failure, muscle weakness, and bone pain. Radiography studies indicate the presence of rickets (bow legs, thick fuzzy growth plates, and widened knee joints). Laboratory data revealed hematocrit 46%; BUN 15 mg/dL; serum creatinine 0.2 mg/dL; sodium 140 mEq/L; potassium 3.9 mEq/L; chloride 104 mEq/L; CO_2 29 mEq/L; calcium 8.1 mg/dL; phosphate 2.5 mg/dL; magnesium 1.9 mg/dL; alkaline phosphatase 3 × normal; albumin 3.9 g/dL; PTH 87 pg/mL (normal range, 10–65 pg/mL), calcidiol (25-OHD) 45 ng/mL (normal range, 10–50 ng/mL), and calcitriol [1,25 (OH)2D]. Urinalysis was within normal limits.

What is the correct diagnosis?

A. Pseudovitamin D-deficient rickets (1-alpha hydroxylase deficiency, vitamin D–dependent rickets type 1)
B. Vitamin D deficiency
C. Hypoparathyroidism
D. Pseudohypoparathyroidism
E. Hereditary vitamin D-resistant rickets

The correct answer is D

Comment: Hereditary vitamin D–resistant rickets (HVDRR) is a rare autosomal recessive disease caused by mutations in the vitamin D receptor (VDR). Patients exhibit severe rickets and hypocalcemia. Heterozygous parents and siblings appear normal and exhibit no symptoms of the disease.

HVDRR is characterized by the early onset of severe rickets, with a complete triad of clinical, biochemical, and skeletal abnormalities. Homozygous or heterozygous mutations in the *VDR* gene leading to complete or partial target organ resistance to the action of 1α, 25-dihydroxyvitamin D3, are responsible for HVDRR. Theoretically, the therapeutic goal is to overcome this tissue resistance and to normalize calcium and phosphate homeostasis. Practically, the treatment could be oriented to correct the secondary hyperparathyroidism to avoid long-term negative impact on bone health. The conventional therapeutic strategy (high-dose calcium plus active vitamin D metabolites) gives variable responses in magnitude and duration.[1]

Clinical Presentation 6

A 14-year-old male with deafness was referred for evaluation because his father had a history of deafness, branchial cysts, hypertension, and renal hypoplasia. The child was found to be deaf at the age of 18 months. Examination showed hypoplasia of the mandible, blind fistulae in the neck, preauricular sinuses, and a high arched palate. There was a narrowing of the external auditory canals, and audiometry showed a bilateral mixed hearing loss with significant conduction deficit. BP was normal. Urine test was negative for blood, and protein and culture was sterile. GFR was 115 mL/min and serum electrolytes were normal.

Renal ultrasound showed that both kidneys had dysmorphic pelvicalyceal systems, the right kidney measured 8.5 cm in length and the left kidney 10.5 cm. The voiding cystogram was normal.

Why did the father develop renal failure?

A. Alport syndrome
B. Knee-patella syndrome

C. Branchio-oto-renal syndrome
D. Reflux nephropathy

The correct answer is C

Comment: Branchiootorenal spectrum disorder is characterized by malformations of the outer, middle, and inner ear associated with conductive, sensorineural, or mixed hearing impairment, branchial fistulae and cysts, and renal malformations ranging from mild renal hypoplasia to bilateral renal agenesis.

Symptom and symptom severity can vary greatly from person to person. It can be caused by genetic changes in the *EYA1*, *SIX1*, or *SIX5* genes. It is passed through families in an autosomal dominant fashion.[1]

Conditions to consider in the differential diagnosis of the branchiootorenal spectrum disorder include Alport syndrome and thin-basement membrane disease.

Clinical Presentation 7

A 6-month-old infant was admitted for failure to thrive. She was the 2500-g product of 36-week twin pregnancy; the twin weighed 1400 g and did well. Neonatal history was unremarkable. Family history was unremarkable for hereditary diseases, seizures, or renal abnormalities. She has a mild developmental delay. Her weight was 4.9 kg and height 58 cm, both below the fifth percentile. The head circumference was 42 cm at 50th percentile. Blood pressure is elevated at 129/64 mm Hg. There was no heart murmur or cyanosis. Peripheral pulses are equal and symmetrical in both upper and lower extremities. There was no organomegaly or edema. A hypopigmented maculae was found on the left abdomen. Urinalysis was normal. Serum electrolytes including BUN and creatinine were normal. The hemoglobin was 12 g/dL. Serum aldosterone and renin levels were normal. Echocardiogram was normal. A renal ultrasound revealed markedly enlarged kidneys with cysts.

What is the most likely diagnosis?

A. Polycystic kidney disease
B. Tuberous sclerosis
C. Multicystic kidney disease
D. Juvenile medullary sponge kidney
E. Medullary cystic kidney

The correct answer is B

Comment: Tuberous sclerosis complex (TSC) is the second most common neurocutaneous disease.[1] It is inherited in an autosomal dominant pattern, although the rate of spontaneous mutation is high. Formerly characterized by the triad of mental retardation, epilepsy, and facial angiofibromas, patients with TSC may present with a broad range of clinical symptoms because of variable expressivity. TSC may affect many organs, most commonly the brain, skin, eyes, heart, kidneys, and lungs. Common features include cortical tubers, subependymal nodules, subependymal giant cell astrocytomas, facial angiofibromas, hypomelanotic spots known as Fitzpatrick patches (ash-leaf spots), cardiac rhabdomyomas, and renal angiomyolipomas. Regarding the genetic sources of epilepsy, TSC is among the most common. Epilepsy affects 90% of patients with this neurocutaneous condition, and it first becomes evident in most such individuals in the initial 2 years of life.[1] TSC provides a model for genetic epilepsy development and modification.

Anticonvulsant medication is the first treatment option for seizures, and neurosurgery is rarely required for refractory seizures. MRI, electroencephalography, and positron emission tomography scans to localize brain lesions are important before neurosurgery.

Mutations in either of two genes (*TSC1* and *TSC2*) have been determined to cause TSC; however, diagnosis continues to be based on clinical manifestations. Molecular analysis is helpful in confirming a diagnosis and genetic counseling.

This article elucidates the various neoplasms, along with their clinical significance, and suggests suitable evaluation and management strategies.

The most common and severe central nervous system manifestations of TSC include seizures, such as infantile spasms, and mental retardation.

Medical care is aimed at seizure control using various anticonvulsants. Begin treatment with monotherapy and increase the dose gradually until seizures are well controlled or the dose is limited by adverse effects.

Lymphangioleiomyomatosis may respond to therapy using progesterone and oophorectomy. Consider inotropic agents in patients with evidence of decreased contractility and cardiomyopathy resulting from rhabdomyoma. Antihypertensive medication may be required in patients with renal disease and subsequent hypertension; an ACE inhibitor may be the first drug of choice.

Kidney surgery for angiomyolipomas usually consists of enucleation or partial nephrectomy. Renal arterial embolization is an additional treatment option.

Some believe that early epilepsy surgery is associated with seizure freedom in children with TSC and intractable epilepsy.

Clinical Presentation 8

Deafness is least likely to be associated with which *one* of the following genetic disorders affecting the kidney?

A. Branchiootorenal syndrome
B. Alport syndrome
C. Alström syndrome
D. Fechtner syndrome.
E. Nail-patella syndrome.

The correct answer is E

Comment: Nail-patella syndrome, which is caused by mutations in a gene encoding for a transcription factor (*LMX1B*) expressed in the podocytes, is not associated with deafness. On the other hand, deafness is a major feature of the branchiootorenal, Alport, Alström, and Fechtner syndromes. Deafness in branchiootorenal syndrome is due to the absence or underdevelopment of the cochlea. A cochlear defect is also responsible for the hearing loss associated with Alport and Fechtner syndromes. COL4A3, AOL4A4, and COL4A5—the proteins mutated in Alport syndrome—are strongly expressed in the matrix that connects the tension fibroblast to the basilar membrane in the lateral aspect of the spiral ligament at the basal turn of the cochlea. MYHIIA—the protein mutated in Fechtner syndrome—is a nonmuscle myosin predominantly expressed in these tension fibroblasts. The structural integrity and function of the tension fibroblasts and matrix are essential to increase the tension of the basilar membrane to the degree needed for high-frequency sound reception. The pathogenesis of deafness in Alström syndrome is not understood.[1]

Clinical Presentation 9

A 13-year-old male develops right upper-quadrant pain and fever with shaking chills. An abdominal ultrasound reveals hyperechoic liver parenchyma, dilatation of several intrahepatic bile ducts, and a few bilateral renal cysts.

The defect responsible for this condition is *most* likely to be a mutation(s) in which gene?

A. *PKHD1*
B. *PKHD1*
C. *PKD2*
D. *TSC2*
E. *OFD1*

The correct answer is A
Comment: The clinical presentation and imaging studies in this patient are consistent with Caroli disease (congenital hepatic fibrosis and mild autosomal recessive polycystic kidney disease presenting with ascending cholangitis). Mutations in the recently identified *PKHD1* gene have been found in cases of congenital hepatic fibrosis and Caroli disease with minimal or mild renal involvement, as well as in patients with more typical presentations of severe ARPKD. Congenital hepatic fibrosis and dilatation of the intrahepatic bile ducts are much more rarely associated with ADPKD caused by *PKD1* or *PKD2* mutations. Mutations in *TSC2* (causing TSC) or in *PRKCSH* (causing autosomal dominant polycystic liver disease) would not be consistent with the presentation or findings in this patient.[1,2]

Clinical Presentation 10

A 9-year-old girl with sensorineural hearing loss has progressive renal insufficiency. Her father and a paternal aunt also had renal failure, and the father's renal biopsy showed features consistent with Alport syndrome.

Which *one* of the following statements is correct?

A. If mutation analysis were to be performed, it is likely that a mutation would be found in either the *COL4A3* gene or the *COL2A4* gene.
B. The risk of posttransplant antiglomerular basement membrane disease is significant and should preclude transplantation.
C. The likelihood that the children of this patient would develop evidence of syndrome is 50% of both male and female offspring.
D. A search for diffuse leiomyomatosis should be initiated.
E. Her children are at risk for the development of thin basement membrane nephropathy.

The correct answer is C
Comment: The pattern of inheritance described in this case is consistent with X-linked dominant or autosomal dominant disease. The former is more likely because autosomal dominant Alport syndrome is very rare. Although X-linked Alport syndrome is usually mild in female heterozygotes, severe disease can occur because of skewed inactivation of the X-chromosome. X-linked Alport syndrome is caused by mutations in *COL4A3* or *COL4A4*; therefore, answer A is wrong. Answer B is not correct because less than 3% of Alport patients develop anti-glomerular basement membrane (anti-GBM) disease following renal transplantation and this small risk does not preclude renal transplantation. The Alport syndrome-diffuse leiomyomatosis contiguous gene syndrome is very rare and, although it needs to be kept in mind, specific investigations for its detection (answer D) are not indicated in the absence of suggestive symptoms such as dysphagia, dyspnea, vulvovaginal leiomyomas, or juvenile cataracts. At least some cases of thin-basement membrane disease are heterozygote carriers of autosomal recessive Alport syndrome with *COL4A3* or *COL4A4* mutations. X-linked Alport syndrome is dominant, and patients with *COL4A5* mutations have Alport syndrome, not thin-basement membrane disease; therefore, answer E is wrong.[1–3]

Clinical Presentation 11

The father of a patient is being evaluated as a potential kidney donor for his 4-year-old son, who has end-stage renal disease (ESRD) secondary to focal segmental glomerulosclerosis. The potential donor undergoes a computed tomography (CT) examination of the kidneys with contrast enhancement. The CT examination reveals two cysts measuring 4 mm in diameter.

Which *one* of the following would be the best course of action?

A. Stop further evaluation as a potential donor because he meets imaging criteria for a diagnosis of ADPKD.
B. Proceed with evaluation because a diagnosis of ADPKD can be excluded by the results of CT examination.
C. Tell the patient that he probably does have ADPKD and that genetic testing on him, the recipient, and other available family members will be necessary to confirm this diagnosis.
D. Tell the patient that he probably does not have ADPKD and that genetic testing on him, the recipient, and other available family members will be necessary to confirm this diagnosis.
E. Proceed with the magnetic resonance (MR) examination of the abdomen.

The correct answer is D

Comment: The imaging criteria for the diagnosis of ADPKD in first-degree relatives of affected individuals have been based on ultrasonography. Current imaging techniques, particularly CT and MR, have a much higher resolution, and therefore the sonographic criteria developed more than a decade ago cannot be indiscriminately applied. Furthermore, although these sonographic criteria have a very high sensitivity for the diagnosis of PKD1 disease, their sensitivity for the diagnosis of PKD2 disease in individuals younger than age 30 years is very low. The presence of two cysts detected by ultrasound in a 10-year-old individual at 50% risk of ADPKD would have met the criteria for a positive diagnosis. This is not the case using CT examinations.

Therefore, answer A is wrong. Answer B is also wrong because the diagnosis of ADPKD (particularly PKD2) cannot be reliably excluded. Answers C and D could be correct, but answer D seems more likely in view of the severity of the disease in the father. Although MRI is the most sensitive technique for detecting renal cysts, it seems unlikely that many cysts detectable by MRI would have been missed by the contrast CT.[1–3]

Clinical Presentation 12

For which *one* of the following diseases is genetic testing most helpful?

A. von Hippel-Lindau disease
B. Autosomal dominant polycystic kidney disease (ADPKD)
C. TSC
D. Alport syndrome
E. Congenital hepatic fibrosis

The correct answer is A

Comment: The availability of genetic testing for von Hippel-Lindau disease has, in most cases, eliminated the need for lifelong follow-up of unaffected individuals for the early detection of the life-threatening complications of this disease. On the other hand, genetic testing for ADPKD, TSC, Alport syndrome, and congenital hepatic fibrosis is much more rarely performed because existing clinical criteria are usually adequate for the clinical management of these patients. The lack of effective therapies limits the benefits of early diagnosis, and the yield of mutation analysis is significantly less than 100%. At present, the main indication for genetic testing for ADPKD is the evaluation of living-related donors for renal transplantation when the imaging studies are inconclusive.[1–3]

Clinical Presentation 13

A 12-year-old girl is found to have a solid mass on ultrasound evaluation of the abdomen for malignant hypertension.

Which *one* of the following findings on physical examination would be most helpful in establishing the diagnosis of von Hipple-Lindau disease?

A. Fibrofolliculomas and trichodiscomas
B. Facial angiofibromas and subungual fibromas
C. Cutaneous leiomyomas
D. Retinal hemangioblastoma
E. Normal skin examination

The correct answer is D

Comment: Retinal hemangioblastomas are seen in up to 60% of the patients with von Hipple-Lindau disease, and approximately half of the cases are multifocal and bilateral. Fibrofolliculomas and trichodiscomas are characteristic of Birt-Hogg-Dube disease—an autosomal dominant syndrome associated with chromophobe and conventional renal cell carcinomas and with oncocytomas. These skin lesions typically appear as multiple, small, dome-shaped, yellowish or skin-colored papules scattered over the face, neck, scalp, and upper trunk. Facial angiofibromas or forehead plaques and periungual or subungual fibromas, along with hypomelanotic macules and shagreen patches, are major features of TSC.

Cutaneous and uterine leiomyomas, uterine leiomyosarcomas, and papillary renal cell, bladder, and breast carcinomas are part of a recently recognized syndrome caused by mutations in the gene encoding fumarate hydrate—an enzyme of the tricarboxylic acid cycle.[1]

Clinical Presentation 14

A 14-year-old male has recurrent calcium oxalate stones and excretes excessive amounts of oxalate. There is a family history of kidney stones. Glomerular filtration rate is normal, and there is no evidence of systemic oxalosis. Testing for primary hyperoxaluria reveals excessive urinary 1-glyceric acid, and genetic testing confirms a mutation in the *DGDH* gene.

What is the diagnosis?

A. The patient has primary hyperoxaluria type 1 (PH1) and will probably need liver and kidney transplantation.
B. The patient has benign dietary hyperoxaluria.
C. The patient is likely to benefit from pyridoxine therapy.
D. The patient has primary hyperoxaluria type 2 (PH2) and is unlikely to develop renal failure or systemic oxalosis.
E. The patient's children are at risk for systemic oxalosis.

The correct answer is D

Comment: Excessive urinary excretion of L-glyceric acid indicates the diagnosis of primary hyperoxaluria type 2; this is confirmed by mutations in *DGDH*. Patients with PH2 suffer from kidney stones but, in contrast to PH1, do not have systemic oxalosis, and transplantation is unnecessary. Urinary L-glyceric acid excretion is not elevated in dietary hyperoxaluria. Pyridoxine therapy is useful in some patients with PH1, but its value in PH2 has not been reported.

Because the patient does not have PH1, his children will not be at risk for systemic oxalosis.[1]

Clinical Presentation 15

An 11-year-old boy has renal Fanconi syndrome, nephrocalcinosis, and a reduced GFR.

Which *one* of the following findings would make you doubt the diagnosis of Dent disease?

A. Hypercalciuria
B. A similar syndrome in his father
C. Proteinuria
D. Rickets
E. The absence of a family history

The correct answer is B

Comment: Dent disease is inherited in an X-linked fashion, and *CLCN5* is located on chromosome X. Father-to-son inheritance is inconsistent with X-linkage. Proteinuria is a hallmark of Dent disease, and hypercalciuria is present in virtually all patients until renal function begins to decline. Rickets, although present in a minority of patients, is a well-recognized feature of the disease.

Although this is clearly a genetic disease, a family history of affected relatives may be absent, either because of incomplete information on family members or as a consequence of the highly variable severity of phenotype even within families.[1]

Clinical Presentation 16

A 6-year-old boy is being evaluated for polyuria. He is found to have nephrocalcinosis and hyperuricemia, and his physician suspects that he may have a hereditary syndrome associated with mutations in *parceling-1.*

Which *one* of the following, if observed, would be most suggestive of this diagnosis?

A. Hypokalemic metabolic alkalosis
B. Salt-wasting
C. Hypocalciuria
D. Hypomagnesemia
E. High serum levels of renin and aldosterone

The correct answer is D

Comment: Familial hypomagnesemia with hypercalciuria and nephrocalcinosis (FHHNC) is associated with mutations in paracellin-1, which is inherited in an autosomal recessive fashion. The combination of polyuria, nephrocalcinosis, and hyperuricemia in the setting of clinically significant hypomagnesemia would be strongly suggestive of this diagnosis. Unlike the Bartter or Gitelman syndromes, salt-wasting, hypokalemia, and metabolic alkalosis are not features of FHHNC.

Urinary calcium excretion is excessive in FHHNC, presumably reflecting the defect in paracellular reabsorption of divalent cations in the loop of Henle. Serum levels of renin and aldosterone are high in Bartter syndrome but normal in FHHNC.[1–3]

Clinical Presentation 17

You are asked to see a 4-year-old girl who recently developed a nephrotic syndrome. She has two siblings who developed similar problems in childhood. A renal biopsy reveals focal and segmental glomerulosclerosis.

Which *one* of the following statements is *most* likely to be correct?

A. Nephrotic syndrome will not recur after renal transplant.
B. She will likely have a mutation in the gene encoding alpha-actinin-4.
C. She should be evaluated for mitochondrial gene mutation.
D. She will likely have a mutation in the APOL 1 gene.

The correct answer is B

Comment: The history suggests a familial focal segmental glomerulosclerosis (FSGS), probably autosomal recessive. Podocin mutations have been detected in approximately one-half of these patients. The nephritic syndrome recurs in up to one-third of patients with familial FSGS following renal transplantation. In the absence of clues suggesting a mitochondrial disease, such as diabetes mellitus, hearing loss, neurological manifestations, or cardiomyopathy, evaluation for a mitochondrial gene disease is not indicated. Alpha actinin-4 mutations have been associated with a later-onset, autosomal dominant FSGS that is not consistent with the clinical presentation of this patient. Although some patients with familial FSGS can respond to combination regimens, such as methylprednisolone boluses and cyclosporine, responsiveness to glucocorticoid treatment alone is unlikely.[1]

Clinical Presentation 18

An 8-year-old hypertensive boy is referred for evaluation of hyperkalemia and metabolic acidosis and is found to have hypercalciuria and a normal serum magnesium level.

Which *one* of the following drugs is *most* likely to benefit this child?

A. Spironolactone
B. Amiloride
C. Hydralazine
D. Hydrochlorothiazide
E. Furosemide

The correct answer is D

Comment: The presence of metabolic acidosis and hyperkalemia in a child with hypertension points to a diagnosis of Gordon syndrome (familial hyperkalemic hypertension) because other familial syndromes of childhood hypertension (such as Liddle syndrome and glucocorticoid-remediable aldosteronism) are associated with hypokalemia and metabolic alkalosis. Hypercalciuria and normal serum magnesium levels are also consistent with Gordon syndrome, which in many respects represents a mirror image of Gitelman syndrome. Gordon syndrome is associated with mutations in the kinases WNK1 and WNL4 that lead to enhanced expression or function of the sodium-chloride cotransport, NCCT. Thus, therapy with thiazide diuretics corrects all of the abnormalities in Gordon syndrome. Diuretics that compete with aldosterone for binding to the receptor (spironolactone), or inhibit the epithelial sodium channel (amiloride), or the NKCC2 transporter (furosemide), have not been shown to be of benefit as the vasodilator hydralazine.[1]

Clinical Presentation 19

Mutations in the *UMOD* gene encoding the Tamm-Horsfall protein have been found in patients with which *one* of the following pairs of overlapping syndromes?

A. Bartter and Gitelman syndromes
B. Low syndrome and Dent disease
C. Familial juvenile hyperuricemic nephropathy and medullary cystic kidney disease type 2
D. Liddle syndrome and glucocorticoid-remedial aldosteronism
E. Autosomal dominant and autosomal recessive renal tubular acidosis

The correct answer is C

Comment: Familial juvenile hyperuricemic nephropathy and medullary cystic kidney disease type 2 are associated with mutations in the *UMOD* gene. It is not known why the gene encoding the Tamm-Horsfall protein should be associated with hyperuricemia, but it may be worth noting that both the Tamm-Horsfall protein and paracellin-1 are expressed in the thick ascending limb of the loop of Henle, and mutations in both are associated with hyperuricemia. The four genes mutated in Bartter syndrome are different from the *NCCT* gene that is mutated in Gitelman syndrome, and the same is true for Low syndrome and Dent disease, Liddle syndrome and glucocorticoid-remediable aldosteronism, and both the autosomal recessive and dominant forms of distal renal tubular acidosis.[1]

Clinical Presentation 20

During evaluation for growth retardation, a 5-year-old girl is found to have hyperchloremic metabolic acidosis, hypokalemia, hypercalciuria, and evidence of rickets.

Which *one* of the following statements regarding inherited distal renal tubular acidosis (RTA) is correct?

A. Mutations in sodium-bicarbonate transporter NCB1
B. Patients with distal RTA and mutations in the basolateral anion exchanger AE1 usually also have hereditary spherocytosis.
C. Mutations in the basolateral anion exchanger AE1 occur in both the dominant and recessive forms of distal RTA.
D. It goes away as the child gets older.
E. It is associated with ocular abnormalities.

The correct answer is C

Comment: The basolateral anion exchange AE1 transports bicarbonate to exit the basolateral surface of type A intercalated cells of the collecting duct and is essential to producing acidic urine. Mutations in AE1 occur in both dominant and recessive forms of distal RTA. This same gene is expressed in the erythrocyte, but the mutations associated with distal RTA are different from those associated with hereditary spherocytosis, and patients with RTA invariably do not have spherocytosis. Inherited distal RTA is not associated with ocular abnormalities, although when it occurs in association with mutations in the B1 subunit of the V-type proton ATPase, it may be associated with sensorineural deafness. The sodium-bicarbonate transporter *NBC1* is expressed in the proximal tubular cell and in the eye, and mutations in this gene are associated with inherited proximal RTA and ocular abnormalities. Inherited distal RTA does not typically improve with age.[1]

Clinical Presentation 21

A 12-year-old boy is being evaluated for progressive renal insufficiency. He has had evidence of renal Fanconi syndrome with aminoaciduria and low-molecular-weight proteinuria for the past several years. There is evidence for hypophosphatemic rickets, and he has hyperchloremic metabolic acidosis. Family history includes a maternal uncle and maternal grandfather who both reached ESRD with evidence of similar features. He has intellectual disabilities and was born with cataracts.

Which *one* of the following choices is the *most* likely diagnosis?

A. Cystinosis
B. Lowe syndrome
C. Dent disease
D. Autosomal dominant distal renal tubular acidosis
E. Primary hyperoxaluria

Correct answer is B

Comment: This boy has features of a generalized Fanconi syndrome, hypophosphatemic rickets, renal failure, and a family history consistent with X-linked inheritance. These features alone would be consistent with either Lowe or Dent disease, but several observations are valuable in distinguishing these two entities. Hyperchloremic metabolic acidosis is a common feature in Lowe syndrome but not Dent disease. Renal failure commonly occurs at an earlier age in Lowe syndrome than in Dent disease, most often not developing until the third or fourth decade in Dent disease. Intellectual disability and congenital cataracts are typical features of the oculocerebrorenal syndrome of Lowe but not of Dent disease.

Cystinosis can also be associated with Fanconi syndrome, metabolic acidosis, renal failure, and ocular and neurologic abnormalities. The eye findings in cystinosis, however, involve the retina (or, in the juvenile form, the cornea) rather than the lenses. Furthermore, cystinosis is an autosomal disease, and in this family, there is strong evidence of X-linked inheritance. Distal RTA and primary hyperoxaluria are also autosomal diseases, and neither would explain the full range of clinical abnormalities in this boy.[1]

Clinical Presentation 22

A 12-year-old girl presents with hematuria. Her past medical history is unremarkable. The family history is notable for the neonatal death of a young brother from respiratory insufficiency and renal cystic disease. An abdominal sonography reveals an enlarged liver with dilated intrahepatic bile ducts, splenomegaly, evidence of portal hypertension, and enlarged echogenic kidneys.

Which *one* of the following disorders is *most* likely present in this patient?

A. ARPKD
B. Isolated congenital hepatic fibrosis
C. Nephronophthisis from mutations in *NPHN2*
D. Isolated autosomal dominant polycystic kidney disease

The correct answer is A

Comment: In ARPKD, affected children typically present in utero with enlarged echogenic kidneys, as well as oligohydramnios secondary to poor urine output. Approximately 30% of the affected neonates die shortly after birth as a result of severe pulmonary hypoplasia and secondary respiratory insufficiency.

Among the survivors, the clinical phenotype variably includes systemic hypertension, renal insufficiency, and portal hypertension resulting from portal tract fibrosis. Marked inter-familial variation has been described in ARPKD and likely reflects the influence of modifier genes. Therefore, ARPKD (choice A) most likely fits the clinical scenario described. Isolated congenital hepatic fibrosis is by definition confined to the biliary tract. The other incorrect choices represent renal cystic diseases not typically associated with symptomatic congenital hepatic fibrosis.[1]

Clinical Presentation 23

An 18-year-old male is referred for evaluation of elevated serum creatinine (1.9 mg/dL). His maternal grandfather died of kidney failure and his mother started on dialysis when she was age 48 years. Physical examination is unremarkable except for a BP of 134/80 mm Hg. Laboratory evaluation reveals a serum creatinine of 2.0 mg/dL, uric acid 7.5 mg/dL, BUN 36 mg/dL, and bicarbonate 22 mEq/L. A 24-hour urine volume is 3600 mL and total protein excretion is 150 mg. Urine sediment is normal. Ultrasonography reveals normal-sized kidneys with increased echogenicity and a single 2-cm cyst in the right kidney. Gadolinium-enhanced MRI shows multiple small cysts ranging from 3 mm to 2 cm in diameter in the corticomedullary region.

Which *one* of the following is the *most* likely diagnosis?

A. Nephronophthisis
B. Medullary cystic kidney disease
C. Hereditary nephritis
D. ADPKD

The correct answer is B

Comment: The family history of kidney failure with an autosomal dominant pattern of inheritance and the imaging studies support a diagnosis of medullary cystic kidney disease as the cause of renal insufficiency. The diagnosis of nephronophthisis can be excluded because this is an autosomal recessive disorder that leads to end-stage renal failure in childhood or adolescence. The absence of microhematuria and proteinuria is not consistent with a diagnosis of hereditary nephritis as the cause of renal insufficiency. The development of renal insufficiency in ADPKD is always associated with marked renal enlargement. The autosomal dominant pattern of inheritance and the absence of findings consistent with congenital hepatic fibrosis rule out the diagnosis of ARPKD.[1,2]

Clinical Presentation 24

Fetal renal enlargement and increased echogenicity are noted during a routine antenatal sonogram in a 27-year-old female with a 30-week gestation. Hexadactyly is also noted. The bladder and amniotic fluid are normal. There is no history of consanguinity or inherited diseases in the family.

What is the likely diagnosis?

A. Autosomal dominant polycystic kidney disease
B. Autosomal recessive polycystic kidney disease
C. Nephronophthisis
D. Joubert syndrome
E. Bardet-Biedl syndrome

The correct answer is E

Comment: The presence of hexadactyly makes the diagnosis of Bardet-Biedl syndrome likely. Hexadactyly is not a feature of autosomal dominant polycystic kidney disease, autosomal recessive polycystic kidney disease, nephronophthisis, or Joubert syndrome.[1]

Clinical Presentation 25

A 16-year-old male presents with a 3-year history of radiographic kidney stones. His serum calcium is 12.4 mg/dL and intact PTH is 365 pg/mL. Computed tomography of the abdomen reveals a few small renal cysts and bilateral kidney stones. A Sestamibi scan reveals an enlarged parathyroid gland. His father had polycystic kidneys and died years ago from metastatic parathyroid carcinoma. No one else in the family is known to have autosomal dominant polycystic kidney disease.

Which *one* of the following choices is the *most* likely diagnosis?

A. His mother has low von Willebrand factor-cleaving protease (vWF-CP) activity.
B. He has a homozygous mutation in the *ADAMS13* gene.
C. Treatment should include plasma exchange with fresh frozen plasma.
D. He has a heterozygous mutation in the *ADAMS13* gene.

The correct answer is C

Comment: The history of recurrent episodes of microangiopathic hemolytic anemia with undetectable vWF-CP activity and absence of vWF-CP autoantibodies strongly suggest the diagnosis of inherited thrombotic thrombocytopenic purpura. Inherited thrombotic thrombocytopenic purpura is a recessive disorder caused by homozygous *ADAMTS13* mutations. Carriers of *ADAMTS13* gene mutations can have partially reduced vWF-CP activities. Transfusions of *ADAMTS13* (fresh frozen plasma or cryosupernatant) to maintain the vWF-CP activity over 3% is sufficient to prevent relapses. The only false statement is C. In the absence of *ADAMTS13* autoantibodies, plasma exchange is not necessary.[1]

Clinical Presentation 26

A 5-year-old girl presents with anasarca. Her BP is 92/60 mm Hg. The laboratory tests show serum creatinine 0.7 mg/dL, albumin 1.6 g/dL, and cholesterol 482 mg/dL. Urine protein is 6.1 g/24 hours. Oval fat bodies are found in the urine sediment.

What is the likely genetic mutation in this child?

A. Children with idiopathic nephritic syndrome benefit from genetic testing for *NPHS2* (podocin) mutations because the results will be helpful in determining whether treatment with steroids is indicated.
B. Children with steroid-resistant idiopathic nephritic syndrome benefit from genetic testing for *NPHS2* (podocin) mutations because the results will be helpful in planning for renal transplantation.
C. The majority of children with steroid-resistant idiopathic nephritic syndrome have *NPHS2* (podocin) mutations.
D. Age of onset and severity of steroid-resistant nephritic syndrome are unrelated to the type of *NPHS2* mutations.
E. *NPHS2* mutation is a good marker for the disease but is unrelated to the cause of the syndrome.

The correct answer is B

Comment: Patients with *NPHS2* mutations are less likely to have a recurrence of FSGS in the renal transplant than those without. In addition, because of the possibility that heterozygous *NPHS2* mutations could make the recipient and the donor more susceptible to the development of proteinuria and FSGS, caution has been recommended before considering transplantation from a living donor carrying an *NPHS2* mutation. Minimal change disease responsive to the administration of steroids is the most common cause of childhood nephritic syndrome. Treatment with steroids is indicated without the need of renal biopsy or genetic testing for *NPHS2*.

Choice A is therefore incorrect. *NPHS2* mutations are found in up to 30% of children with steroid-resistant idiopathic nephritic syndrome. Therefore, choice C is wrong. Choice D is also wrong because patients with mutations leading to retention of podocin in the endoplasmic reticulum have an earlier onset of the disease and a more severe phenotype than those with homozygous mutations expressed on the plasma membrane. Choice E is incorrect because disease-causing podocin mutations cause nephritic syndrome by failing to recruit nephrons into rafts either because of retention in the endoplasmic reticulum or failure to associate with rafts in the plasma membrane.[1]

Clinical Presentation 27

A 19-year-old female was found to have microscopic hematuria without proteinuria during a routine medical examination. She has been in excellent health and the remainder of her examination, including BP and general chemistries, are normal. She has a normal excretory urogram and cystoscopy. The question of hereditary nephritis is raised because her mother also has microscopic hematuria. She is concerned about being a carrier for X-linked Alport syndrome because she is planning to raise a family.

Which *one* of the following options would be *best* to evaluate the patient for carrier status of X-linked Alport syndrome?

A. Hearing test and eye examination
B. Skin biopsy
C. Kidney biopsy
D. *COL4A5* mutation analysis
E. Slit-lamp testing

The correct answer is B

Comment: The immunohistochemical study of a skin biopsy is diagnostic in approximately 80% of patients with X-linked Alport syndrome and avoids the need for a more invasive renal biopsy. Confocal microscopy of the skin with three-dimensional reconstruction of the epidermal basal membrane increases the sensitivity of the test. *COL4A5* is usually absent from epidermal and glomerular basal membranes in male patients and has a segmental distribution in female patients. Testing for *COL4A5* mutation using sequence analyses identifies more than 60% of mutations in individuals with X-linked Alport syndrome and could be considered as an alternative, but at present it is probably less sensitive than a skin biopsy. Sensorineural deafness, anterior lenticonus, pigmentary changes in the perimacular region, and corneal dystrophy (rare) or alterations in the corneal epithelial basement membrane are features of Alport syndrome. Their occurrence in females is too low to be used for diagnosis.[1,2]

Clinical Presentation 28

A 10-month-old boy presents with failure to thrive. Evaluation reveals metabolic acidosis in the context of Fanconi syndrome. His neurocognitive status is appropriate for his age, and there is no family history of a similar disorder.

Which *one* of the following genetic disorders is *most* likely present in this boy?

A. Cystinosis from *CTNS* mutations
B. Lowe syndrome from *OCRL* mutations
C. Dent disease from *CLCN5* mutations
D. Dent disease from *ORCL* mutations
E. Lowe syndrome from *CLCN5* mutations

The correct answer is A

Comment: Cystinosis is an autosomal recessive lysosomal storage disease. It is the most common inherited cause of renal Fanconi syndrome, as well as a multisystem disorder that affects the eyes, muscles, central nervous system, lungs, and various endocrine organs. These patients, however, typically do not have neurocognitive impairment. In contrast, both Lowe syndrome and Dent disease are X-linked disorders. In Lowe syndrome, full expression of Fanconi syndrome typically does not occur in infancy, whereas in Dent disease metabolic acidosis from proximal tubular dysfunction is rarely seen.[1]

Clinical Presentation 29

A 5-year-old girl presents with polyuria and failure to thrive. Diagnostic evaluation reveals that she has hypomagnesemia and hyperuricemia.

Which *one* of the following associated clinical features would *most* strongly suggest that she has defects in paracellin-1 function (*CLDN16* mutations)?

A. Autosomal recessive inheritance
B. Association of hypomagnesemia and nephrocalcinosis
C. Association of hypomagnesemia and mild hypokalemic metabolic alkalosis
D. History of neonatal seizures in a maternal cousin
E. Normal renal function

The correct answer is B

Comment: Familial hypomagnesemia with hypercalciuria and nephrocalcinosis is an autosomal recessive disorder caused by defects in paracellin-1 function. This disorder is distinguished from other magnesium-losing tubular disorders by clinical presentation during early childhood with recurrent urinary tract infections, polyuria/polydipsia, isosthenuria, and renal stones. Affected children typically have bilateral nephrocalcinosis and develop progressive renal failure. Some seek medical attention because of associated failure to thrive, vomiting, abdominal pain, titanic episodes, or generalized seizures. Besides hypomagnesemia, biochemical abnormalities include hypermagnesemia and hypercalciuria, and impaired GFR is often detected at the time of diagnosis. A substantial percentage of patients have incomplete distal renal tubular acidosis, hypocitraturia, and hyperuricemia.[1]

Clinical Presentation 30

A 4-year-old girl presents with metabolic acidosis and failure to thrive. Diagnostic evaluation reveals an isolated proximal renal tubular acidosis without associated features of renal Fanconi syndrome. She does have ocular abnormalities, including cataracts.

Which *one* of the following disorders is the *most* likely the cause of her syndrome?

A. Cystinosis from *CTNS* mutations
B. Low syndrome from *OCRL* mutations
C. Low syndrome from *CLCB5* mutations
D. Isolated proximal RTA from *SLC4A4* mutations
E. Carbonic anhydrase deficiency

The correct answer is D

Comment: RTA results from defective bicarbonate reabsorption and is commonly associated with a generalized defect in proximal tubular function (e.g., cystinosis, Lowe syndrome). However, isolated proximal RTA can occur in association with ocular abnormalities, including glaucoma, band keratopathy, and cataracts. This autosomal recessive disorder results from loss-of-function mutations in *SLC4A4*, the gene encoding the electrogenic Na+-bicarbonate exchanger, NBCe1. The clinical presentation in this patient is most consistent with isolated proximal RTA from *SLC4A4* mutations.[1]

Clinical Presentation 31

A 7-year-old boy presents with headache and severe hypertension. Diagnostic evaluation is notable for hypokalemic metabolic alkalosis, and there is no evidence of renal artery stenosis or coarctation of the aorta. His urinary 18-hydroxycortisol is within the normal range. His family history is notable for early-onset hypertension in his mother and several maternal cousins. Although his hypertension is refractory to therapy with ACE inhibitors, angiotensin-receptor blockers, and calcium channel antagonists, he responds well to amiloride therapy.

Which *one* of the following disorders is *most* likely to provide the diagnosis?

A. Liddle syndrome (or subunits of epithelial sodium channels)
B. Glucocorticoid-remediable aldosteronism
C. Gordon syndrome (mutations involving *WNK1*)
D. Gordon syndrome (mutations involving *WNK4*)
E. Autosomal dominant pseudohypoaldosteronism type 1

The correct answer is A

Comment: The constellation of clinical findings and laboratory data are most consistent with the diagnosis of Liddle syndrome. Glucocorticoid-remediable aldosteronism is typically associated with high urinary 18-hydroxy cortisol excretion, which was not observed in this patient. Hypokalemic metabolic alkalosis is inconsistent with Gordon syndrome, which is typically associated with hyperkalemic metabolic acidosis.[1]

Clinical Presentation 32

A 12-year-old boy is noted to be hypertensive during a routine medical examination. He is otherwise in excellent physical condition. Further evaluation reveals mild hyperkalemic hyperchloremic metabolic acidosis and hypercalciuria.

Which *one* of the following disorders is the *most* likely cause of this patient's syndrome?

A. Liddle syndrome
B. Gordon syndrome

C. Glucocorticoid-remediable aldosteronism
D. Activation in the mineralocorticoid receptor
E. Autosomal dominant renal tubular acidosis

The correct answer is B

Comment: Gordon syndrome or glucocorticoid-remediable aldosteronism is an autosomal dominant distal renal tubular acidosis. Among the single-gene disorders causing low-renin hypertension, Gordon syndrome is distinguished by the associated hyperkalemia and metabolic acidosis. In contrast, Liddle syndrome, glucocorticoid-remediable aldosteronism, and an activating mutation in the dominant distal RTA are not typically associated with hypertension.[1]

Clinical Presentation 33

An 11-year-old girl presented with short stature and was found to have chronic renal failure. The parents are cousins, but there was no family history of renal disease. There was a history of polydipsia, polyuria, and salt cravings. Her growth parameters were below the third percentile. BP was normal. Neurological examination was normal. There were no other abnormal findings. Urinalysis was negative for protein, glucose, and blood. The pH was 7.0, and specific gravity was 1.008. GFR was 12 mL/min. Hemoglobin is 7.0 g/dL, white blood cells 11,500/mm^3 platelet 269,000/mm^3. Serum sodium was 130 mEq/L, potassium 4.0 mEq/L, chloride 111 mEq/L, bicarbonate 7 mEq/L, BUN 80 mg/dL, creatinine 6.7 mg/dL, calcium 8.0 mg/dL, and phosphorous 6.9 mg/dL. Renal ultrasound showed bilateral small kidneys with increased echogenicity. A contrast cystogram was normal. A slit-lamp examination was normal and audiometry revealed no sensorineural loss.

What is the most likely diagnosis?

A. Cystic nephroblastoma
B. Medullary sponge kidney
C. Familial juvenile nephronophthisis
D. Polycystic kidney disease
E. Tuberosclerosis

The correct answer is C

Comment: Familial juvenile nephronophthisis and MCKD are similar diseases that develop in children and adults, respectively. NPH is an autosomal recessive disorder that is linked to mutations of genes located at least four chromosome sites. NPH may be associated with cerebroretinal degeneration and hepatic fibrosis. Familial INPH-1 has been mapped to chromosome 2 (2q12-13). The gene *NPH-1* is responsible for the synthesis of nephrocystin. These patients develop ESRD at a median age of 13 years.

Familial adolescent *NPH-3* has been mapped to chromosome 3 (3q21-22). Patients with *NPH-3* mutations develop ESRD at a median age of 19 years. *NPH-2* is the autosomal recessive form, having an infantile, perinatal, or prenatal onset. It is linked to chromosome 9q22-31. A fourth gene locus, *NPH-4*, has been postulated, accounting for rare cases. Molecular genetic diagnosis is possible. The clinical features of failure to thrive, polyuria, polydipsias, anemia, and ESRD in the presence of normal BP and normal urinalysis are most likely consistent with NPH.[1]

Clinical Presentation 34

A 3-week-old boy developed nephrotic syndrome. His mother had previously had a miscarriage at 12 weeks of gestation. His birth weight was 3.3 kg following an uneventful pregnancy, labor, and delivery. The placenta was large, but not weighed. His parents had no Finnish ancestry. Urine showed 4+ protein, 10 to 20 red blood cells, and 2 to 5 granular casts. BP was 110/49 mm Hg. Serum albumin was 1.2 g/dL and 24-hour urine contained 1.2 g of protein. Serum creatinine was 4.1 mg/dL and GFR 11 was mL/min. He died of pneumonia in the sixth week of life.

What is the most likely diagnosis?

A. Congenital syphilis
B. Diffuse mesangial glomerulosclerosis
C. Wilms tumor
D. Congenital cytomegalovirus infection
E. All of the above

The correct answer is E

Comment: The nephrotic syndrome that is present at birth or develops in the first few weeks of life may be due to several disorders including intrauterine infections (congenital syphilis, congenital cytomegalovirus disease, congenital rubella, congenital toxoplasmosis), focal and segmental glomerulosclerosis, diffuse glomerulosclerosis, and Wilms tumor, in addition to the classic Finnish type of congenital nephrotic syndrome. The Finnish type of congenital nephrotic syndrome is due to mutations of the *NPHS-1* gene located on chromosome 19 (19q13.1). This gene determines the synthesis of nephrin, which is a major constituent, of the slit pore diaphragm of the visceral glomerular epithelial cells. These mutations give rise to a nearly total deficiency of nephrin, the absence of the slit foot processes, and a marked increase in glomerular permeability to proteins. Most patients develop renal failure and die of infections or thrombosis before 5 years of age unless vigorously supported by anticoagulants, diuretics, albumin infusions, and antibiotics, as needed. Angiotensin inhibitors, nonsteroidal anti-inflammatory drugs, or glucocorticoids do not reduce proteinuria or prolong life. Renal transplantation may be life-saving, but a new disease may develop in the graft because of the formation and deposition of antinephrin antibodies.[1]

Clinical Presentation 35

A 14-month-old girl was admitted to the hospital because of respiratory distress and puffy eyes. She was one of three normal siblings. The 23-year-old mother had had three spontaneous abortions during the sixth to eighth months of pregnancy. A fetal karyotype was reported as normal. The patient did not experience any neonatal complications. She began failing to thrive at 5 months of age. Her food intake diminished and she experienced breathlessness during sleep. Medical care was not sought because of a lack of health care insurance. Physical examination revealed a protruding forehead, absent nasal bridge, and a macrocephalic head. She had a disproportional short-limbed short stature.

Her BP was 130/90 mm Hg. Eye examination was normal. Echocardiography demonstrated right ventricular hypertrophy. Urinalysis was unremarkable except for 1+ proteinuria. Hyperchloremic metabolic acidosis (pH 7.24, bicarbonate 16 mEq/L, chloride 124 mEq/L), hyperkalemia (5.5 mEq/L), and hyperphosphatemia (6.5 mg/dL) were found in association with renal insufficiency (BUN 35 mg/dL, serum creatinine 1.8 mg/dL, GFR 40 mL/min/1.73 m^2). Skeletal x-ray revealed a long, narrow, bell-shaped thorax with short horizontal ribs, short limbs, and distal phalanges. Renal sonogram showed hyperechoic cortical zones, compressed pyramids, and a mild dilatation of both pelvises. A head ultrasound demonstrated hydrocephalus. A ventriculostomy was performed to treat the hydrocephalus. She subsequently developed ESRD and underwent a successful cadaveric renal transplantation at 3 years of age.

What disorder associated with chronic renal failure can be diagnosed on the basis of the abnormalities presented in this patient?

A. Ellis-van Creveld syndrome
B. Ivemark syndrome (renal-hepatic-pancreatic dysplasia)
C. Barnes syndrome (thoracolaryngopelvic dysplasia)
D. Jeune syndrome (asphyxiating thoracic deformity)
E. Thoracopelvic dysostosis

The correct answer is D

Comment: Asphyxiating thoracic dysplasia (Jeune syndrome) is a group of autosomal recessive osteochondrodysplasias that may involve the kidneys.

Patients with Jeune syndrome typically present at birth with a small bell-shaped thoracic cage. Many experience asphyxia, with or without pulmonary infection, within the first few weeks of life. Progressive renal failure usually occurs in those who survive childhood. Histology of the kidney shows manifestations of nephronophthisis.

The nature and degree of renal involvement is variable. Tubular dilatation and atrophy, interstitial fibrosis, glomerular sclerosis, cortical cysts, cystic dysplasia, and diffuse cystic disease have been described. Early renal manifestations include proteinuria, proximal tubular dysfunction, polyuria, and hypertension. A link between Jeune syndrome and familial juvenile nephronophthisis and Laurence-Moon-Biedl syndromes has been suggested. Prenatal diagnosis of Jeune syndrome is possible.

Present knowledge suggests that the locus of the gene associated with Jeune syndrome may be situated at 12p11.2p12.2.

Because of the absence of polydactyly, nail, tooth, and heart defects, differentiation from other kinds of bone dysplasia such as Ellis-van Creveld syndrome is easy.

Ivemark syndrome can be excluded because of the absence of biliary dysgenesis and pancreatic fibrosis. Barnes syndrome and thoracopelvic dysplasia are excluded because they have an autosomal dominant mode of inheritance.

Radiologic manifestations of Jeune syndrome are variable and include a small thoracic cage with short ribs and irregular costochondral junctions. The pelvis exhibits hypoplastic iliac wings and a horizontal angle of the acetabular roof. The long bone is often short and wide.[1–3]

Clinical Presentation 36

A 22-month-old girl was admitted for failure to thrive and abnormal movements for the past few weeks. She was the 1900-g product of a 36-week twin pregnancy (the twin weighed 2500 g and did well). She had multiple upper respiratory tract infections, a history of recurrent cyanotic episodes, with upward gaze deviation and generalized floppiness. Her feeding was poor with episodes of coughing and jussive emesis for the week preceding admission. She had moderate developmental delay.

The family history was unremarkable for hereditary disorders, seizures, or renal abnormalities. Physical examination revealed an alert infant with a weight of 4.1 kg and height of 53 cm on the 25th percentile. Her BP was elevated at 129/64 mm Hg and her respiratory rate was 44/min. The heart rate was regular with a grade of 2/6 systolic ejection murmur at the left sternal border. There was no organomegaly on palpation of the abdomen. There was no cyanosis or peripheral edema. Cutaneous examination revealed a hypopigmented macula on the left abdomen, measuring 1.7 × 2.4 cm in diameter, and multiple similar lesions on the chest and lower extremities. No focal neurological signs were present.

Laboratory data revealed a serum creatinine of 0.4 mg/dL, BUN 18 mg/dL, and normal electrolytes. The hemoglobin was 12 g/dL with normal indices. Serum aldosterone and renin were normal. Urinalysis revealed a pH of 5.0, specific gravity of 1.008, and normal microscopic examination. A renal ultrasound examination revealed markedly enlarged kidneys (both kidneys measured 9.9 cm in length) with multiple noncommunicating cysts.

What is the most likely diagnosis?

A. ARPKD
B. Nephronophthisis
C. Multicystic kidney disease
D. Tuberosclerosis

The correct answer is D

Comment: The neurocutaneous syndrome tuberous sclerosis is inherited as a dominant trait, but 50% of cases appear to be new mutations. The most common skin abnormality is hypopigmented macula, usually oval- or leaf-shaped and present at birth in 80% to 90% of patients. Other cutaneous lesions include adenoma sebaceous and shagreen patches. Central nervous system disease is common and presents as convulsions in most patients. Intellectual delay is frequent. Sclerotic patches (tubers) are scattered throughout the cortical gray matter.

A CT scan of the skull is often diagnostic and reveals intracerebral calcification.

Cardiac rhabdomyomas are found in at least 50% of patients and may lead to arrhythmias.

The classic renal lesion of tuberous sclerosis is angiomyolipomas, which occur in 50% to 80% of patients and often are bilateral and multiple. Renal cysts are the second most common renal lesions and can be present with the angiomyolipomas.

Large kidney cysts can be present at birth. The radiological appearance of the kidneys is often similar to that of adult-type polycystic kidney disease. The cysts are anechoic lesions, varying in size from 2 mm to 2 cm, with thin uniform walls. Most children are asymptomatic; rarely is pain or hematuria the presenting symptom.

Proteinuria can develop. The incidence of renal carcinoma is less than 5%—surgical intervention is then indicated.

Infantile polycystic kidney disease, nephronophthisis, multicystic kidney disease, and medullary sponge kidneys are easily excluded in the absence of hypopigmented skin lesions and intracranial calcification.[1]

Clinical Presentation 37

An 18-month-old boy was hospitalized because of seizures. At birth, he was found to have male pseudohermaphrodism with hypoplastic phallus, penoscrotal hypospadias, urogenital sinus, and bilateral cryptorchidism. The karyotype was XY. On admission, BP was 130/90 mm Hg. The child had generalized edema. The child was severely oliguric. Hemoglobin was 9.5 g/dL, white blood cells 14,400/mm^3, platelet 565,000/mm^3, serum creatinine 4.8 mg/dL, BUN 53 mg/dL, serum sodium 138 mEq/L, potassium 6.5 mEq/L, calcium 8.3 mg/dL, phosphorus 6.8 mg/dL, total protein 5.6 g/dL, and albumin 1.6 g/dL. Urinalysis revealed proteinuria 4+ and microscopic hematuria. Renal ultrasound revealed a mass in the right kidney.

What was the cause of renal failure?

A. Drash syndrome
B. Congenital Torch complex
C. Hereditary nephrotic syndrome
D. Minimal change nephrotic syndrome
E. Idiopathic focal and segmental glomerulosclerosis

The correct answer is A

Comment: The mass present in the right kidney was a Wilms tumor, and renal failure was due to diffuse mesangial sclerosis (DMS). The child had all the features diagnostic of what is now well known as Drash syndrome.

This is a case of congenital nephritic syndrome with a nephritic urinary sediment and severe renal insufficiency associated with ambiguous genitalia and Wilms tumor. Most cases of congenital nephritic syndrome are of the Finnish variety. The major histological difference between diffuse mesangial and Finnish congenital nephritic syndrome is the presence of global and segmental sclerosing glomerular lesions and crescents in DMS. Both types show cystic dilatation of the proximal tubules with fetal or immature glomeruli. Progression to ESRD occurs early in DMS. It is a late or absent feature of surviving infants with DMS.[1,2]

Clinical Presentation 38

A 3-week-old male infant was referred with vomiting and renal failure. He was born following a normal pregnancy with normal antenatal ultrasound examinations.

He was delivered by emergency cesarean section for breech presentation associated with fetal distress at 42 weeks. Birth weight was 3.4 kg, and Apgar scores were 9 and 10 at 1 and 5 minutes, respectively. On examination, there was edema of the hands and feet, and he was dysmorphic with simple cup-shaped ears, short fingers with distal tapering, and flexed flexion deformity of two fingers of his hands. There was no organomegaly, and genitalia were normal.

At 3 days, he began vomiting and to lose weight. Both parents are healthy unrelated Whites. The initial investigation revealed sodium 128 mEq/L, potassium 6.3 mEq/L, BUN 65 mg/dL, creatinine 4.5 mg/dL, bicarbonate 12 mEq/L, and uric acid 16.5 mg/dL. The full blood count was normal. Cultures of blood and urine were sterile. Pyloric ultrasound examination was normal. Renal ultrasound examination demonstrated bright kidneys, both 5 cm in length. He was treated with fluids, sodium bicarbonate, and broad-spectrum antibiotics while awaiting the results of blood and urine cultures. He was discharged at 20 days, but because of persistent vomiting, he was readmitted at age 23 days. He was mildly dehydrated. BP was 95/65 mm Hg. Hemoglobin was 13.3 g/dL, white blood cell count 8900/mL, platelet 250,000/mL, sodium 131 mEq/L, potassium 4.4 mEq/L, BUN 42 mg/dL, creatinine 3.1 mg/dL, calcium 8.3 mg/dL, phosphate 7.3 mg/dL, alkaline phosphatase 420 23 IU/L, albumin 2.9 g/dL, uric acid 14.5 mg/dL, aspartate aminotransferase 55 IU/L, pH 7.23, and bicarbonate 13 mEq/L. Urinalysis revealed pH 6.0, specific gravity 1.010, sodium 44 mEq/L, and potassium 8 mEq/L. A renal ultrasound demonstrated bilateral marked echogenicity with prominent medullary pyramid. Each kidney measured 5 cm in length. A 99m diethylene-triamine-pentaacetate scan demonstrated perfusion but no function. A voiding cystoureterogram revealed bilateral grade 4 vesicoureteric reflux.

The karyotype was 46, XY. Nasogastric tube feeding was uninitiated and treatment with sodium bicarbonate and calcium carbonate supplements were commenced.

What is the most likely diagnosis?

A. Acute tubular necrosis
B. Lesch-Nyhan syndrome
C. Congenital cystic dysplasia kidney
D. Nephronophthisis

The correct answer is B

Comment: The striking ultrasonic appearance of the kidneys and the clinical recognition of gout and the very high plasma uric acid level that was disproportionately raised relative to the high serum creatinine were early clues to the presence of uric acid nephropathy and led to the appropriate diagnostic study of measuring hypoxanthine guanine phosphoribosyl-transferase (HGPRT).

Complete HGRPT deficiency is associated with presentation in infancy as Lesch-Nyhan syndrome. Uric acid overproduction is associated with developmental delay, choreoathetosis, and spasticity between 1 and 16 years. Gouty arthritis and tophi are seldom seen before puberty. Death usually occurs in the second and third decades because of renal failure or recurrent infections. Patients with a partial HGPRT deficiency often develop uric acid nephropathy and uric acid stones, but they do not develop the characteristic self-mutilation. HGPRT activity in lysed red cells is undetectable in both forms of clinical expression, but patients with partial deficiency demonstrate detectable activity in intact erythrocytes. HGPRT deficiency is X-linked, and thus both clinical syndromes occur only in males. Enzyme kinetic studies on fibroblasts of the mother were normal, implying a mutation in the case of our patient.

Although treatment with allopurinol, combined with alkalinization of the urine, may prevent the renal consequences of excess uric acid production, such therapy appears to have no effect on the distressing neurological manifestations of Lesch-Nyhan syndrome.[1]

Clinical Presentation 39

Constellation of kidney dysphasia associated with hypoplasia of cerebellar vermis, nystagmus, retinal dysplasia, ocular coloboma, mid-brain "molar sign" on the MRI of and congenital hepatic fibrosis are characteristics of which of the following abnormalities?

A. Joubert syndrome
B. Meckle-Gruber syndrome
C. Short rib syndrome
D. VACTER-L syndrome

The correct answer is A

Comment: Joubert syndrome is an uncommon autosomal recessive condition characterized by hypoplasia of the cerebellar vermis (demonstrated by MRI as the "molar tooth sign"), intellectual disability, retinal dystrophy, ocular coloboma, rotatory nystagmus, polydactyly, cystic renal dysplasia, and congenital hepatic fibrosis. Its neurologic manifestations usually come to medical attention in infancy. The syndrome was initially described in a French-Canadian family with four affected siblings by pediatric neurologists in Montreal more than 40 years ago; one of the original children had an occipital meningoencephalocele that was removed at birth.

The two different forms of renal disease that have been described in Joubert are cystic renal dysplasia and nephronophthisis (tubulointerstitial nephritis and cysts at the corticomedullary junction). Clinically, these children present with polydipsia, polyuria, anemia, growth failure, elevated creatinine, and later develop renal failure.

Recently, it has become known that Joubert syndrome is due to ciliary disorders and there is some overlap in clinical presentations with Meckel and Bardet-Biedl syndromes (e.g., occipital meningoencephalocele, congenital hepatic fibrosis, obesity, ambiguous genitalia). So far, the molecular genetics of Joubert syndrome includes eight mutations in the ciliary/basal body genes: *INPPFE*, *AH11*, *NPHP1*, *CEP290*, *TMEM67/MKS3*, *RPGR1P1L*, *ARL13B*, and *CC2D2A*. At a molecular level, it has been demonstrated that Joubert and Meckel syndromes share at least one gene mutation (*TMEM67/MKS3*) and it seems logical to infer that in the future more common mutations will be found.

Some individuals may have a mild form of the disorder with minimal motor (movement) disability and good mental development; at the other end of the spectrum is the severe motor disability with moderately impaired mental development and multiorgan impairments.

Current treatment options are symptomatic and supportive. Infant stimulation and physical, occupational, and speech therapy may benefit some children, as well as regularly monitoring symptoms. Routine screening for progressive eye, liver, and kidney complications associated with Joubert-related disorders is highly recommended.[1]

Clinical Presentation 40

Which of the following genes are implicated in the pathogenesis of dysplastic kidneys?

A. Hepatocyte nuclear factor-1 β (*HNF1β*)
B. Paired box gene 2 (*Pax2*)
C. Uromodulin (*UMOD*)
D. Eyes absent homolog 1 (*Eya1*)
E. None of the above
F. All of the above

The correct answer is F

Comment: The spectrum of congenital anomalies of the kidney and urinary tract is extremely broad and ranges from mild, asymptomatic malformations such as a double ureter or minimal ureteral pelvic obstructions to severe, life-threatening pathologies such as bilateral renal agenesis or renal dysplasia. Several of these renal abnormalities are part of a syndrome or sequence that can be confirmed and sometimes treated by a multidisciplinary approach, including fetal ultrasonography and vesicoamniotic shunt placement to relieve obstruction while in the fetal period, or by other imaging modalities, molecular analysis, and pathologic examination after birth.

Currently, it is recognized that there are two different types of renal dysplasias: obstructive and nonobstructive. In many instances of obstructive renal dysplasia, a megacystis (massively distended urinary bladder) can be observed, even by fetal ultrasound; however, there are other cases in which the obstructive component is not as obvious, and only a careful examination will detect a stenotic area, a hydroureter, or a dilated renal pelvis. Histologically, when kidneys affected by obstructive renal dysplasia have developed hydronephrosis, they usually exhibit a compressed medulla from the hydrostatic pressure produced by the accumulated urine within the pelvis. The renal cortex tends to have less fibrosis and more glomeruli, whereas the medulla is fibrotic and dysplastic; however, the histology may vary depending on the timing of the intrauterine obstruction.

To better understand the etiology and pathogenesis of renal dysplasia, many efforts have been made to further classify them as syndromic and nonsyndromic and to find the gene or genes involved in the development of the disease.

A comprehensive review article delineates evidence that 2% of the congenital anomalies of the kidney and urinary tract, even if nonsyndromic, are linked to genes. So far, the following genes have been reported: hepatocyte nuclear factor-1 β (*HNF1β*), paired box gene 2 (*Pax2*), uromodulin (*UMOD*), and eyes absent homolog 1 (*Eya1*). They have been detected in 2% of patients with nonsyndromic congenital anomalies of the kidney and urinary tract.[1]

A large study by Saisawat et al. applied massive parallel exon resequencing of 30 candidate genes in pooled DNA from 40 patients with congenital anomalies of the kidney and urinary tract and identified seven novel mutations in four genes: *RET*, *BMP4*, *FRAS1*, and *FREM2*. All of these mutations were absent in healthy controls.[2]

Clinical Presentation 41

Which of the following conditions are associated with horseshoe kidney (select all that apply)?

A. Trisomy 18
B. Turner syndrome
C. Wilms tumor
D. Cardiovascular disease

The correct answers are A, B, C, and D

Comment: Horseshoe kidney is a condition in which the kidneys are fused together at the lower end or base. By fusing, they form a "U" shape, which gives it the name "horseshoe."

Horseshoe kidney occurs during fetal development as the kidneys move into their normal position in the flank area (area around the side, just above the waist).

Horseshoe kidney occurs in about one in 500 children.

Horseshoe kidney can occur alone or in combination with other disorders. The most common disorders seen with horseshoe kidney include:

Turner syndrome: a genetic disorder seen in girls that causes them to be shorter than others and to not mature sexually as they grow into adulthood. Sixty percent of girls with Turner syndrome have horseshoe kidneys.

Trisomy 18: a serious chromosome abnormality involving defects in nearly all organ systems, including horseshoe kidney in 20% of children affected.

One-third of people with horseshoe kidneys have at least one other complication involving the cardiovascular system, the central nervous system, or the genitourinary system (which is the reproductive organs and urinary system) such as the following:

Kidney stones: crystals and proteins that form stones in the kidney that may lead to a urinary tract obstruction

Hydronephrosis: enlargement of the kidneys that is usually the result of a urinary tract obstruction

Wilms tumor: an embryonic (newly formed) tumor of the kidneys that usually occurs during early childhood renal cancer or polycystic kidney disease hydrocephaly and/or spina bifida various cardiovascular and gastrointestinal conditions, or skeletal problems.

The most common symptoms of horseshoe kidney include urinary tract infection (fever, vomiting dysfunction), kidney stones (flank pain, hematuria), and hydronephrosis.

About one-third of children with horseshoe kidney have no symptoms.

There is no known cure for a horseshoe kidney, but if patients have complications, treatment approaches may include antibiotics (to treat an underlying infection) or surgical intervention for symptomatic kidney stones.[1]

Clinical Presentation 42

A 4-year-old boy was referred for evaluation of failure to thrive. He was found to have severe intellectual delay, cataracts, areflexia, nontender joint swelling, subcutaneous nodules, and renal proximal tubular dysfunction.

What is the most likely diagnosis?

A. Zellweger syndrome (ZS)
B. Lowe syndrome
C. Smith-Lemli-Opitz syndrome
D. Dent disease
E. Cataract-dental syndrome (Nance-Horan syndrome)

The correct answer is B

Comment: Lowe syndrome (oculocerebrorenal syndrome) is characterized by congenital cataracts and glaucoma, severe intellectual disability, hypotonia with diminished to absent reflexes, and renal abnormalities. Fanconi syndrome is followed by progressive renal impairment. ESRD usually does not occur until the third to fourth decades of life.

Lowe syndrome is transmitted as an X-linked recessive trait. Despite the X-linked inheritance pattern, Lowe syndrome has occurred in a few females. The defective gene codes for inositol polyphosphate 5-phosphatase, *OCRL1*, are involved with cell trafficking and signaling.

Light microscopy of the kidney is normal early in the disorder, with endothelial cell swelling and thickening and splitting of the glomerular basement membrane seen by electron microscopy. In the proximal tubule cells, there is shortening of the brush border and enlargement of the mitochondria.

Cataracts are present at birth and kidney and brain abnormalities are associated with intellectual disabilities.

Almost all boys with Lowe syndrome have developmental and intellectual disability that can range from mild to severe. Seizures occur in approximately half of those by 6 years of age, and behavioral problems are present in some boys with Lowe syndrome. A fraction of affected males develop keloids on the corneas of one or both eyes during late childhood and adolescence. These growths are progressive and can lead to blindness.

Renal Fanconi syndrome is one of the most common kidney involvement in patients with Lowe syndrome. The GFR usually begins to fall during the second decade of life and slowly progresses to end-stage renal failure by 30 to 40 years of age.

Other signs frequent in boys with Lowe syndrome include short stature, dental cysts and abnormal dentin formation of the teeth, skin cysts, and vitamin D deficiency that can lead to soft bones, skeletal changes (rickets), bone fractures, scoliosis, and noninflammatory degenerative joint disease. Some patients have shown a delayed bleeding diathesis following surgery characterized by normal hemostasis and clot formation, only to be followed a few hours later by sudden recurrence of bleeding. This may be an important consideration with any surgery but especially both cataract surgery and glaucoma surgery in which bleeding inside the eye may have considerable consequences.

Disorders with similar symptoms to Lowe syndrome include congenital rubella, ZS, cataract-dental syndrome (Nance-Horan syndrome), Smith-Lemli-Opitz syndrome, and Dent disease.[1]

Clinical Presentation 43

A 2-month-old female infant was admitted to our hospital because of failure to thrive (FTT) associated with diarrhea and abdominal distension. She was the first child of nonconsanguineous healthy parents. Pregnancy was complicated by maternal hypertension and intrauterine growth restriction. Birth was by vaginal delivery at 38 weeks' gestation, with Apgar scores of 9 at 1 minute and 10 at 5 and 10 minutes. Her weight at birth was 2070 g (below the third percentile), length 44 cm, and head circumference 31 cm. Jaundice on the first day of life led to phototherapy for 48 hours. There was a good weight gain up to the first month of life, with regular growth below the third percentile. After the second month of life, hypotonia and poor weight gain prompted hospitalization.

On admission, the infant was severely undernourished (weighing 2940 g), with abdominal distension, intermittent stridor, and axial hypotonia. Dysmorphic features included a large anterior fontanelle and dehiscence of the interparietal space extending to the posterior fontanelle, broad nasal bridge with orbital hypertelorism, epicanthus, high-arched palate, short neck, rhizomelic shortening of proximal extremities, low-set thumb, and overlapping toes.

Transfontanel, abdominal, and renovesical ultrasounds were normal. The skeletal radiograph did not show any calcific stippling of epiphyses. A chest CT with angiography revealed two supraaortic trunks with preserved permeability (proximal stem yielding to the right brachycephalic trunk and left carotid artery, and distal stem corresponding to the left subclavian artery) and no apparent decrease in the diameter of the trachea, revealing a variant of normal cardiovascular structure. On further investigation, karyotype analysis was normal (46, XX), as were carbohydrate-deficient transferrin, phytanic and pristanic acids, and the erythrocyte plasmalogens. Brain proton MR spectroscopy revealed localized peaks at 0.9 and 1.3 ppm, possibly reflecting the presence of macromolecules and lipids/lactate, without other relevant changes in neuroimaging.

Laboratory investigations revealed increased plasma levels of very long-chain fatty acids and precursor of bile acids and deficient activity of dihydroxyacetone phosphate acyltransferase in fibroblasts. Two mutations in the *PEX1* gene were found in heterozygosity (c.2528G>A (p.G843D)/c.760dupT (p.S254fs*5)), confirmed by the patient's genetic study.

What is the likely diagnosis?

A. ZS
B. Lowe syndrome
C. Potter syndrome
D. Meckel-Joubert syndrome

The correct answer is A

Comment: This case has some particular features that are consistent with a diagnosis of ZS, based on clinical phenotype and specific laboratory and genetic abnormalities.

Zellweger spectrum disorders (ZSDs) are a group of rare, genetic, multisystem disorders that were once thought to be separate entities. These disorders are now classified as different expressions (variants) of one disease process because of their shared biochemical basis. Collectively, they form a spectrum or continuum of disease. The most severe form of these disorders was previously referred to as ZS, the intermediate form was referred to as neonatal adrenoleukodystrophy, and the milder forms were referred to as infantile Refsum disease or Heimler syndrome, depending on the clinical presentation. ZSDs can affect most organs of the body. Neurological deficits, loss of muscle tone (hypotonia), hearing loss, vision problems, liver dysfunction, and kidney abnormalities are common findings. ZSDs often result in severe, life-threatening complications early during infancy. Some individuals with milder forms have lived into adulthood. ZSDs are inherited in an autosomal recessive pattern.

ZSDs are the result of a mutation in any of the 12 *PEX* genes. Most cases of ZSD are due to a mutation in the *PEX1* gene. These genes control peroxisomes, which are needed for normal cell function. Peroxisomes break down toxins and fats. They play an important role in the development of the bones, brain, eyes, nervous system, cardiovascular and kidney.

Symptoms of ZS usually appear soon after birth. Facial abnormalities common in ZSD include broad nose bridge, epicanthal folds (skin folds at the inner corners of the eyes), flattened face, high forehead, underdeveloped eyebrow ridges, and wide-set eyes.

Other symptoms include: difficulty swallowing, hepatosplenomegaly, gastrointestinal bleeding, hearing and vision problems, jaundice, seizures, underdeveloped muscles, and movement problems.

There is no cure for ZS. Some therapies may ease symptoms, but there are not any treatments that address the cause of ZS. For example, a baby with difficulty eating may benefit from a feeding tube. But the baby won't be able to eat normally on his or her own in the future.[1]

Clinical Presentation 44

Which one of the following distinguishes autosomal recessive polycystic kidney disease (ARPKD) from autosomal dominant polycystic kidney disease (ADPKD)?

A. Bilateral enlarged kidneys
B. Hypertension
C. Abnormal renal function
D. Hepatic fibrosis
E. Polyuria

The correct answer is D

Comment: ARPKD is currently considered a primary ciliopathy that equally affects the kidneys and liver.

ARPKD has an incidence of 1:20,000 to 1:40,000 live births and a heterozygous carrier rate of 1 in 70. It occurs as a result of a mutation in a single gene named polycystic kidney and hepatic disease (*PKHD1*). Severely affected fetuses are born with oligohydramnios, Potter face, and some will develop respiratory insufficiency, but many survive the neonatal period. Of all neonatal survivors, approximately 40% have severe hepatic and renal disease. Of the remaining children, 30% present with severe renal and mild hepatobiliary disease and the other 30% with severe hepatobiliary problems and mild renal disease.

The renal pathology is extremely characteristic because it is always bilateral, the kidney is enlarged but maintains its reniform shape, and when opened it transudates a lot of urine. Histologically, the cysts are elongated and their long axis is perpendicular to the capsule. The hepatic manifestations are congenital hepatic fibrosis (CHF) that is undistinguishable from the CHF found in other ciliopathies such as Meckel, short rib, or polysplenia. Secondary to the liver fibrosis, patients develop portal hypertension, esophageal varices, hemorrhoids, upper gastrointestinal bleeding, splenomegaly, and hypersplenism.

Genetic studies have demonstrated that ARPK is associated with two genes (*PKD1* and *PKD2*). The former produces the severe form of the disease and its gene product, polycystin-1 (*PC1*), is a receptor-like integral membrane protein that seems to be involved in cell-cell matrix interactions and also plays a role in calcium homeostasis through its physical interaction with polycystin-2, the protein product of PKD2.

Parents of a child born with ARPKD who are obligate carriers may be offered preimplantation genetic diagnosis using single-cell multiple displacement amplification products for *PKHD1* haplotyping, which significantly decreases the problem of allelic dropout. This specific protocol employs whole-genome amplification of single blastomeres, multiple displacement amplification, and haplotype analysis with 20 novel polymorphic short-tandem repeat markers from the *PKHD1* gene and flanking sequences.

Once the child is born with the disease, the current treatment is symptomatic. However, in cases of severe renal and hepatobiliary disease, the combined renal-liver transplant looks promising because the outcome of liver transplant has improved recently and it has been proven that, if left unattended, CHF may lead to ascending cholangitis, sepsis, portal hypertension, and gastrointestinal bleeding. All of these complications could impact the ultimate outcome of liver transplant months or years after renal transplant. The future seems more promising for these patients because there are several preclinical trials that hopefully will discover new treatment modalities to block fluid transfer into the tubular epithelial cells and decrease or completely block cyst formation.[1,2]

Clinical Presentation 45

Which of the following therapeutic interventions is inappropriate for patient with ADPKD?

A. Administration of lipid-lowering drugs
B. Administration of ACE inhibition
C. Dietary salt and protein restrictions
D. Administration of arginine-vasopressin receptor inhibitor
E. Force fluids
F. None of the above

The correct answer is F

Comment: ADPKD is a relatively common condition that affects 1 of every 400 to 1000 live births and accounts for approximately 10% of patients with chronic renal failure requiring dialysis or transplant. ADPKD should be considered a systemic disorder that mainly affects adult patients. They also develop hepatic and pancreatic cysts, chronic hypertension, intracranial aneurysms, and cardiac valve anomalies, especially mitral valve prolapse. The likelihood of renal failure increases progressively with age after 40 years, rising to 25% by age 50, 40% at 60 years, and 75% at age 70. The kidneys of adult patients contain multiple round cysts of variable size, filled with urine and blood become extremely large extending up to 10 times their normal weight. Histology reveals completely disorganized renal parenchyma with large cystically dilated tubules and occasional glomeruli and fibrotic interstitium with chronic inflammation.

For many years, ADPKD was considered an untreatable renal disease leading to chronic renal failure and required either dialysis or transplant, but more recently there is some hope of a better treatment by early administration of an AVP (arginine-vasopressin)-V2 receptor inhibitor in individuals with subclinically detected disease. The rationale behind this therapy is that the collecting ducts and distal nephrons (that are the more severely affected by cysts in ADPKD) are sensitive to vasopressin. This receptor is the main hormonal regulator of adenyl cyclase activity in collecting ducts. To avoid dehydration, mammals live under the constant action of AVP on the distal nephron and collecting duct. When the individual drinks large volumes of water, plasma AVP levels decrease enough to make the urine more dilute than plasma; therefore, during most of the day, cyst epithelial cells undergo stimulation to secrete fluid. The circulating levels of AVP are likely elevated in patients with ADPKD to compensate for the reduced concentrating capacity of the affected kidneys and the AVP effect leads to cyst formation. The administration of an arginine-vasopressin receptor inhibitor delays the cyst formation, but does not help regenerating tubular epithelium; therefore, it is critical to start treatment as early as possible to prevent cyst formation. Other recommendations are to drink plenty of fluids, up to 3 L/day for adults and proportionately less for children, avoid caffeine, decrease salt and protein intake, add ACE inhibitors or angiotensin-receptor blockers to lower the blood pressure, decrease the amount of fat ingested, and prescribe a cholesterol-lowering agent.[1]

Clinical Presentation 46

Which of the following congenital anomalies of kidneys are associated with trisomies 13, 18, and 21 (select all that apply)?

A. Horseshoe kidney
B. Duplex kidney
C. Kidney cystic dysplasia
D. Ureteropelvic junction obstruction

The correct answers are A, B, C, and D

Comment: Trisomy 13: Numerous studies have been reported on children with trisomies 13, 18, and 21 who also have hydronephrosis, horseshoe kidney, duplex kidney/collecting system, cortical cysts and/or cystic dysplasia, glomerular microcysts, or renal hypoplasia.

Trisomy 13 (Patau syndrome) is a lethal chromosomal abnormality characterized by holoprosencephaly, arhinencephaly, macrophthalmos, cleft lip and/or palate, polydactyly, and congenital heart disease. However, associated renal anomalies can be found at autopsy. We examined a fetus that was aborted; amniocentesis demonstrated an extra chromosome. In addition to holoprosencephaly, he had polydactyly and cystic dilatation of renal tubules. The most common renal anomaly is multicystic renal cortex (34%) followed by hydronephrosis (21%).

These children are frequently born preterm and may have scalp defects, congenital heart disease, and Meckel diverticulum. A patient with trisomy 13 and bilateral renal dysplasia has been described. The patient had ectopic splenic tissue in the pancreas and a complex congenital heart disease.

Trisomy 18 primarily affects the cardiovascular system and is better known by its association to ventricular (73%) and atrial septal defects (41%), patent ductus arteriosus, and pulmonary valve anomalies. Its characteristic facial features are a prominent occiput, narrow bifrontal diameter, low-set malformed ears, small oral opening, overlapping of the fingers, and narrow pelvis. On the other hand, trisomy 18 tends to have almost the same incidence of renal anomalies as trisomy. The most common malformations are duplication of the collecting system and horseshoe kidney (25%). Less commonly identified are cortical cysts (17%) and hydronephrosis (15%). One of our patients with trisomy 18 underwent autopsy at 7 days and besides the characteristic facial features, she had agenesis of corpus callosum, overlapping of the fingers, and multicystic dysplastic kidneys.

Trisomy 21 may have renal involvement ranging from cortical microcysts, simple cysts, renal hypoplasia, and immature glomeruli deep in the cortex. These children may also develop obstructive uropathy. The largest autopsy series reported 124 fetuses and children with Down syndrome from three medical centers. These authors found renal hypoplasia in 18 cases, glomerular microcysts in 24% of children, only one of these patients had an anatomical obstruction of the urinary tract, focal tubular dilatation in 10 cases, and seven cases with simple cysts. Immature glomeruli deep into the cortex were present in 18 children (15%). There were eight patients with obstructive uropathy (6%). Four of them had cystic renal dysplasia and the other four had a combination of hydronephrosis and hydroureter.[1–3]

Clinical Presentation 47

Retinitis pigment Ida is the cardinal manifestation in which of the following syndromes?

A. Joubert syndrome
B. Short rib sundry
C. Bardet-Biedl synonym
D. Prune belly syndrome

The correct answer is C

Comment: The cardinal manifestations of Bardet-Biedl syndrome are retinitis pigmentosa, obesity, renal dysplasia, polydactyly, learning disability, and hypogenitalism. The diagnosis may be confirmed later as a young adult if the patient presents in childhood only with truncal obesity and learning disabilities but has normal vision and lacks polydactyly or syndactyly and hypogonadism. However, as patients age, visual and renal problems become more severe, and virtually 100% of individuals with Bardet-Biedl syndrome will develop poor vision. The possibility of renal insufficiency increases with age. It is inherited in an autosomal recessive manner. Interfamilial and intrafamilial phenotypic variability exists. Prenatal diagnosis in affected families can be made by fetal ultrasound examination with the detection of polydactyly and cysts in the kidneys. Once the affected gene has been detected in a family, it is possible to look for the known gene. At the present time, 18 genes have been associated with Bardet-Biedl syndrome: *BBS1*, *BBS2*, *ARL6* (*BBS3*), *BBS4*, *BBS5*, *MKKS* (*BBS6*), *BBS7*, *TTC8* (*BBS8*), *BBS9*, *BBS10*, *TRIM32* (*BBS11*), *BBS12*, *MKS1* (*BBS13*), *CEP290* (*BBS14*), *WDPCP* (*BBS15*), *SDCCAG8* (*BBS16*), *LTZFL1* (*BBS17*), and *BBIP1* (*BBS18*). Histologically, the kidneys show extensive replacement of parenchyma by round cysts lined by flat to cuboidal epithelium. The glomeruli are preserved. Persistent fetal lobulations have been described suggesting a defect in renal maturation.[1]

Clinical Presentation 48

Which of the following genetic nephrolithiasis is *not* associated with chronic kidney disease (apply all that apply)?

A. Adenine phosphoribosyltransferase deficiency
B. Dent disease
C. Cystinuria
D. FHHNC
E. Bartter syndrome
F. Primary hyperoxaluria (PH)

The correct answer is E

Comment: Several rare genetic disorders including adenine phosphoribosyltransferase deficiency, cystinuria, Dent disease, FHHNC, and PH can cause chronic kidney disease that can progress to end-stage kidney failure even during early childhood. Patients with these disorders often experience recurring stones, urinary tract infections, and upper tract obstruction requiring frequent hospitalizations that may accelerate the loss of kidney function.[1–6]

References

Clinical Presentation 1

1. Tebben PJ. Hypophosphatemia: a practical guide to evaluation and management. *Endocr Pract.* 2022;28(10):1091–1099. https://doi.org/10.1016/j.eprac.2022.07.005.
2. Smanzadeh J, Rielly RF Jr. Hypophosphatemia: an evidence-based approach to its clinical consequences and management. *Nature Clin Pract Nephrol.* 2006;2(3):136–148. https://doi.org/10.1038/ncpneph0124.
3. Assadi F. Disorder of divalent metabolism. In: Assadi F, ed. *Clinical Decisions in Pediatric Nephrology: A Problem Solving to Clinical Cases*. New York, NY: Springer; 2008:98–124.

Clinical Presentation 2

1. Rossetti S, Hopp K, Sikkink RA, et al. Identification of gene mutations in autosomal dominant polycystic kidney disease through targeted resequencing. *J Am Soc Nephrol.* 2012;23(5):915–933. https://doi.org/10.1681/ASN.2011101032.

Clinical Presentation 3

1. Rossetti S, Hopp K, Sikkink RA, et al. Identification of gene mutations in autosomal dominant polycystic kidney disease through targeted resequencing. *J Am Soc Nephrol.* 2012;23(5):915–933. https://doi.org/10.1681/ASN.2011101032.

Clinical Presentation 4

1. Eckardt KU, Alper SL, Antignac C, et al. Kidney disease: improving global outcomes. Autosomal dominant tubulointerstitial kidney disease: diagnosis, classification, and management: a KDIGO consensus report. *Kidney Int.* 2015;88(4):676–683. https://doi.org/10.1038/ki.2015.28.

Clinical Presentation 5

1. Pang Q, Qi Z, Jiang Y, et al. Clinical and genetic findings in a Chinese family with VDR-associated hereditary vitamin D-resistant rickets. *Bone Res.* 2016;4:16018. https://doi.org/10.1038/boneres.2016.18.

Clinical Presentation 6

1. Gigante M, d'Altilia M, Montemurno E, et al. Branchio-oto-renal syndrome (BOR) associated with focal glomerulosclerosis in a patient with a novel EYA1 splice site mutation. *BMC Nephrol.* 2013;14:60. https://doi.org/10.1186/1471-2369-14-60.

Clinical Presentation 7

1. Bissler JJ, Batchelor D, Kingswood JC. Progress in tuberous sclerosis complex renal disease. *Crit Rev Oncog.* 2022;27(2):35–49. https://doi.org/10.1615/CritRevOncog.2022042857.

Clinical Presentation 8

1. Richardson D, Shires M, Davidson AM. Renal diagnosis without renal biopsy. Nephritis and sensorineural deafness. *Nephrol Dial Transplant.* 2001;16:1291–1299.

Clinical Presentation 9

1. Bergmann C, Senderek J, Sedlacek B, et al. Spectrum of mutations in the genes for auto- somal recessive polycystic kidney disease (ARPKD/PKHD1). *J Am Soc Nephrol.* 2003;14:76–89.
2. Rossetti S, Torra R, Coto E, et al. A complete mutation screen of PKHD1 in autosomal recessive polycystic kidney disease pedigrees. *Kidney Int.* 2003;64:391–403.

Clinical Presentation 10

1. Badenas C, Praga M, Tazon B, et al. Mutations in the COL4A4 and COL4A3 gene cause familial benign hematuria. *J Am Soc Nephrol.* 2002;13:1248–1254.
2. Byrne MC, Budisavljevic MN, Fan Z, et al. Renal transplant in patients with Alport syndrome. *Am J Kidney Dis.* 2002;39:769–775.
3. Mothes H, Heidet L, Arrondel C, et al. Alport syndrome associated with diffuse leiomy-44 omatosis: COL4A5-COL4A6 deletion associated with a mild form of Alport nephropathy. *Nephrol Dial Transplant.* 2002;17:70–74.

Clinical Presentation 11

1. Nicolau C, Torra R, Badenas C, et al. Autosomal dominant polycystic kidney disease types 1 and 2: assessment of US sensitivity for diagnosis. *Radiology.* 1999;213:273–276.
2. Rossetti S, Chauveau D, Walker D, et al. A complete mutation screen of the ADPKD genes by DHPLC. *Kidney Int.* 2002;61:1588–1599.
3. Zand MS, Stang J, Dumalo M, et al. Screening a living donor kidney for polycystic kidney disease using heavily T2-weighted MRI. *Am J Kidney Dis.* 2001;38:612–619.

Clinical Presentation 12

1. Bergmann C, Senderek J, Selacek B, et al. Spectrum of mutations in the gene for autosomal recessive polycystic kidney disease (ARPKD/PKHD1). *J Am Soc Nephrol.* 2003;14:76–89.
2. Maranchie JK, Linehan WM. Genetic disorders and renal cell carcinoma. *Urol Clin North Am.* 2003;30:133–141.
3. Rossetti S, Torra R, Coto E, et al. A complete mutation screen of PKHD1in autosomal recessive polycystic disease (ARPKD) pedigrees. *Kidney Int.* 2003;64:391–403.

Clinical Presentation 13

1. Singh AD, Shields CL, Shields JA. von Hipple-Lindau disease. *Surv Ophthalmol.* 2001;46:117–142.

Clinical Presentation 14

1. Miliner DS, Wilson DM, Smith LH. Phenotypic expression of primary hyperoxaluria: comparative features of types I and II. *Kidney Int.* 2001;59:31–36.

Clinical Presentation 15

1. Scheinman SJ. X-linked hypercalciuric nephrolithiasis: clinical syndromes and chloride channel mutations. *Kidney Int.* 1998;53:3–17.

Clinical Presentation 16

1. Blanchard A, Jeunemaitre X, Coudol P, et al. Paracellin-1 is critical for magnesium and calcium reabsorption in the human thick ascending limb of Henle. *Kidney Int.* 2001;59:2206–2215.
2. Knrad M, Weber S. Recent advances in molecular genetics of hereditary magnesium-losing disorders. *J Am Soc Nephrol.* 2003;14:249–260.
3. Praga M, Vara J, Gonzalez-Parra E, et al. Familial hypomagnesemia with hypercalciuria and nephrocalcinosis. *Kidney Int.* 1995;47:1419–1425.

Clinical Presentation 17

1. Bertelli R, Ginevri F, Caridi G, et al. Recurrence of focal segmental glomerulosclerosis after renal transplantation in patients with mutations of podocin. *Am J Kidney Dis.* 2003;1:314–321.

Clinical Presentation 18

1. Mayan H, Vered I, Mouallem M, et al. Pseudohypoaldosteronism type II: marked sensitivity to thiazides, hypercalciuria, normomagnesemia, and low bone mineral density. *J Clin Endocrinol Metab.* 2002;87:3248–3254.

Clinical Presentation 19

1. Hart TC, Gorry MC, Hart PS, et al. Mutations of the UMOD gene are responsible for medullary cystic kidney disease Type 2 and familial juvenile hyperuricemic nephropathy. *J Med Gener.* 2002;42:882–889.

Clinical Presentation 20

1. Karet FE. Inherited distal renal tubular acidosis. *J Am Soc Nephrol.* 2002;13:2178–2184.

Clinical Presentation 21

1. Torra R, Badenas C, Perez-Oller L, et al. Increased prevalence of polycystic kidney disease type 2 among elderly polycystic patients. *Am J Kidney Dis.* 2000;36:728–734.

Clinical Presentation 22

1. Kaplan BS, Kaplan P, de Chadarevian JP, et al. Variable expression of autosomal recessive polycystic kidney disease and congenital hepatic fibrosis within a family. *Am J Med Gent.* 1988;29:639–664.

Clinical Presentation 23

1. Betz R, Rensing C, Otto E, et al. Children with nephronophthisis. *J Pediatr.* 2000;136:828–831.
2. Hildebrandt F, Jungers P, Robino C, et al. Nephronophthisis and medullary cystic kidney disease and medullary sponge kidney disease. In: Schrier R, ed. *Diseases of Kidney.* 7th ed. Philadelphia: Lippincott, Williams and Wilkins; 2001:521–528.

Clinical Presentation 24

1. Cossart M, Eurin D, Didier F, et al. Antenatal renal sonographic anomalies and postnatal follow-up of renal involvement in Bardet-Biedle syndrome. *Ultrasound Obstet Gynecol.* 2004;24:51–55.

Clinical Presentation 25

1. Koo B, Oh D, Chung SY. Deficiency of von Willebrand factor-cleaving protease activity in the plasma of malignant patients. *Thrombosis Res.* 2002;105:471–474.

Clinical Presentation 26

1. Ruf RG, Lichtenberger A, Karle SM, et al. Patients with mutations in NPHS2 (podocin) do not respond to standard steroid treatment of nephritic syndrome. *J AM Soc Nephrol.* 2004;15:722–732.

Clinical Presentation 27

1. Kashtan CE. Familial hematuria due to type IV collagen mutations: Alport syndrome and thin-basement membrane nephropathy. *Curr Opin Pediatr.* 2004;16:177–181.
2. Muda AO, Massella L, Giannakakis K, et al. Confocal microscopy of the skin biopsy in the diagnosis of X-linked Alport syndrome. *J Invest Dermatol.* 2003;121:208–211.

Clinical Presentation 28

1. Gahl W, Thoene J, Schneider J. Cystinosis. *N Engl J Med.* 2002;347:111–121.

Clinical Presentation 29

1. Konard M, Weber S. Recent advances in molecular genetics of hereditary magnesium-losing disorders. *J Am Soc Nephrol.* 2003;14:249–260.

Clinical Presentation 30

1. Igarashi T, Sekine T, Inatomi J, et al. Unraveling the molecular pathogenesis of isolated proximal renal tubular acidosis. *J Am Soc Nephrol.* 2002;13:2171–2177.

Clinical Presentation 31

1. Warnock DG. Liddle syndrome: genetics and mechanisms of Na+ channel defects. *Am J Med Sci.* 2001;322:302–307.

Clinical Presentation 32

1. O'Shaughnessy KM, Karet FE. Salt handling and hypertension. *J Clin Invest.* 2004;113:1075–1081.

Clinical Presentation 33

1. Hildebrandt F, Jungers P, Robino C, et al. Nephronophthisis and medullary cystic kidney disease and medullary sponge kidney disease. In: Schrier R, ed. *Diseases of Kidney.* 7th ed. Philadelphia: Lippincott, Williams and Wilkins; 2019:521–528.

Clinical Presentation 34

1. Hamed RMA, Shomaf M. Congenital nephritic syndrome: a clinicopathological study of thirty children. *J Neprol.* 2001;14:104–109.

Clinical Presentation 35

1. Donaldson MCD, Warner AA, Trompeter RS, et al. Familial juvenile nephronophthisis, Jeune's syndrome and associated disorders. *Arch Dis Child.* 1985;60:426–434.
2. Gruskin AB, Baluarte HJ, Cote ML, et al. The renal disease of thoracic asphyxiate dystrophy. *Birth Defects.* 1974;10:44–50.
3. Nagai T, Nishimura G, Kato R, et al. Del (12) (p11.21p12.2) associated with an asphyxiating thoracic dystrophy or chondroectodermal dysplasia-like syndrome. *Am J Med Genet.* 1995;55:8–16.

Clinical Presentation 36

1. Stapleton FB, Johnson D, Kaplan GE, et al. The cystic renal lesion in tuberculosis. *J Pediatr.* 1980; 97:574–579.

Clinical Presentation 37

1. Drash A, Sherman F, Hartmann WH, et al. A syndrome of pseudo-hermaphroidism, Wilm's tumor, hypertension, and degenerative renal disease. *J Pediatr.* 1970;76:585–593.
2. Hamed RMA, Shomaf M. Congenital nephritic syndrome: a clinico-pathological study of thirty children. *J Nephrol.* 2001;14:194–199.

Clinical Presentation 38

1. Holland PC, Dillon JM, Pincott J, et al. hypoxanthine guanine phosphoribosyl-transferase deficiency presenting with gout and renal failure in infancy. *Arch Dis Child.* 1983;58:831–833.

Clinical Presentation 39

1. Joubert M, Jean-Jacques E, Robb JP, et al. Familial agenesis of the cerebellar vermis. A syndrome of episodic apnea, abnormal eye movements, ataxia, and retardation. *Neurology.* 1969;19:813–825.

Clinical Presentation 40

1. Yosypiv IV. Congenital anomalies of the kidney and urinary tract: a genetic disorder? *Int J Nephrol.* 2012;2012:909083.
2. Saisawat P, Tasic V, Vega-Warner V, et al. Identification of two novel CAKUT-causing genes by massively parallel exon resequencing of candidate genes in patients with unilateral renal agenesis. *Kidney Int.* 2012;81:196–200.

Clinical Presentation 41

1. Kang M, Kim YC, Lee H, et al. Renal outcomes in adult patients with horseshoe kidney. *Nephrol Dial Transplant.* 2021;36(3):498–503. https://doi.org/10.1093/ndt/gfz217.

Clinical Presentation 42

1. Bökenkamp A, Ludwig M. The oculocerebrorenal syndrome of Lowe: an update. *Pediatr Nephrol.* 2016;31:2201–2212. https://doi.org/10.1007/s00467-016-3343-3.

Clinical Presentation 43

1. Schutgens RBH, Wanders RJA, Heymans HSA, et al. Zellweger syndrome: biochemical procedures in diagnosis, prevention and treatment. *J Inherit Metab Dis.* 1987;10(Suppl 1):33–45. https://doi.org/10.1007/BF01812845.

Clinical Presentation 44

1. Tobin JL, Beales PL. The nonmotile ciliopathies. *Genet Med.* 2009;11:386–402.
2. Sweeney WE, Avner ED. Pathophysiology of childhood polycystic kidney diseases: new insights into disease-specific therapy. *Pediatr Res.* 2014;75:148–157.

Clinical Presentation 45

1. Torres VE. Vasopressin antagonists in polycystic kidney disease. *Semin Nephrol.* 2008;28:306–317.

Clinical Presentation 46

1. Uehling DT, Gilbert E, Chesney R. Urologic implications of the VATER association. *J Urol.* 1983; 129:352–354.
2. Egli F, Stalder G. Malformations of kidney and urinary tract in common chromosomal aberrations. *Humangenetik.* 1973;18:16–32.
3. Balci S, Güçer S, Orhan D, Karagöz T. A well-documented trisomy 13 case presenting with a number of common and uncommon features of the syndrome. *Turkish J Pediatr.* 2008;50:595–599.

Clinical Presentation 47

1. Green JS, Parfrey PS, Harnett JD, et al. The cardinal manifestations of Bardet–Biedl syndrome, a form of Laurence–Moon–Biedl syndrome. *N Eng J Med.* 1989;321:1002–1009.

Clinical Presentation 48

1. Blanchard A, Jeunemaitre X, Coudol P, et al. Paracellin-1 is critical for magnesium and calcium reabsorption in the human thick ascending limb of Henle. *Kidney Int.* 2001;59:2206–2215.
2. Knrad M, Weber S. Recent advances in molecular genetics of hereditary magnesium-losing disorders. *J Am Soc Nephrol.* 2003;14:249–260.
3. Praga M, Vara J, Gonzalez-Parra E, et al. Familial hypomagnesemia with hypercalciuria and nephrocalcinosis. *Kidney Int.* 1995;47:1419–1425.
4. Gahl W, Thoene J, Schneider J. Cystinosis. *N Engl J Med.* 2002;347:111–121.
5. Vezzoli G, Arcidiacono T, Citterio L. Classical and modern genetic approach to kidney stone disease. *Kidney Int Rep.* 2019;4(4):507–509. https://doi.org/10.1016/j.ekir.2019.01.006.
6. Gefen AM, Sethna CB, Cil O, et al. Genetic testing in children with nephrolithiasis and nephrocalcinosis. *Pediatr Nephrol.* 2023;38(8):2615–2622. https://doi.org/10.1007/s00467-023-05879-0.

CHAPTER 6

Glomerulonephritis

Clinical Presentation 1

A 17-year-old pregnant woman was referred for evaluation of chronic constipation, dehydration, decreased muscle tone, polyuria, and polydipsia.

Her last menstrual period was 7 weeks ago. She has been on no medications.

Her past medical history and family history are unremarkable. The parents are unrelated.

Physical examination revealed a fair-complexioned female in no acute distress. Her weight was 59 kg and height was 160 cm. Blood pressure was 120/76 mm Hg, pulse rate 78 beats/min, and temperature 37°C. She appeared pale and had mild dehydration.

Abdomen was distended. Liver was 3 cm below the right costal margin. There was no splenomegaly. Rectal examination revealed a large amount of firm stool requiring manual removal. The stool was heme negative. Muscle tone was decreased and deep tendon reflexes were present and symmetric throughout.

Urinalysis revealed a specific gravity of 1.009, pH 6.0, trace glucose, and 1+ protein but no blood. Hemoglobin was 9.6 g/dL, hematocrit 31%, white blood cells (WBC) 10,000/mm^3 with a normal differential, and platelets 419,000/mm^3.

Serum electrolytes were: sodium 133 mmol /L, potassium 3.8 mmol/L, chloride 98 mmol/L, and bicarbonate 18 mEq/L. Blood urea nitrogen was 27 mg/dL, serum creatinine 1.0 mg/dL, glucose 91 mg/dL, calcium 9.7 mg/dL, magnesium 3.9 mg/dL, phosphorus 3.0 mg/dL, alkaline phosphatase 132 U/L; total protein 6.8 g/dL, and albumin 3.8 g/dL.

A spot urine protein-to-creatinine ratio was 0.32. Urine osmolality was 300 mOsm/kg H_2O.

Further laboratory studies showed generalized aminoaciduria, increased fractional excretion of beta 2-microglobulin and low tubular phosphate.

Which diagnoses should receive further consideration (select all that apply)?

A. Diabetes insipidus
B. Wilson disease
C. Cystinosis
D. Galactosemia

Correct answers are A, B, C, and D

If we proceed in a stepwise fashion, which of the following would be the best initial laboratory test for the correct diagnosis of this patient (select all may apply)?

A. Slit-lamp eye examination
B. Blood ceruloplasmin level
C. Vasopressin following water deprivation test
D. Blood galactose-1-phosphate uridylyltransferase

The correct answer is A

If this patient happens to have cystinosis, would you start therapy with cysteamine?

A. Yes
B. No

The correct answer is B

Comment: Constellation of polyuria, polydipsia, generalized aminoaciduria, hyponatremia, hypokalemia, and non-gap metabolic acidosis is consistent with the diagnosis of renal Fanconi syndrome.[1]

Constipation secondary to dehydration has also been described both in the infantile and juvenile forms of cystinosis.[2]

Although cystinosis is the most common identifiable cause of the inherited renal Fanconi syndrome in children, other metabolic diseases (tyrosinemia, galactosemia, glycogen storage diseases), Wilson disease, Dent disease, and Lowe syndrome should also be considered in the differential diagnosis of the renal Fanconi syndrome. Some cystinosis patients with atypical presentations may also be initially diagnosed as nephrogenic diabetes insipidus.

Three clinical forms of cystinosis have been described on the basis of severity of symptoms and age of onset: infantile cystinosis, characterized by renal proximal tubulopathy and progression to end-stage renal disease before 12 years of age; juvenile form, with a markedly slower rate of progression; and adult form, with only ocular abnormalities. Slit-lamp examination of the cornea showing cysteine crystal deposits is considered the best initial test to confirm the diagnosis of cystinosis.

Complete Fanconi syndrome often does not develop in late-onset cystinosis, but renal function deteriorates as in infantile nephropathic cystinosis, and patients often experience end-stage renal failure within a few years of diagnosis.

Pregnant women with cystinosis should not be treated with cysteamine because of its teratogenic effects on developing fetus, particularly in the first trimester.[3,4]

Studies in animals have shown reproductive toxicity, including teratogenesis and fetotoxicity, at doses less than the recommended human maintenance dose. Observed teratogenic findings were cleft palate, kyphosis, heart ventricular septal defects, microcephaly, and exencephaly. No study has been performed during pregnancy or breast-feeding, so it should not be used by pregnant or breast-feeding women (option A).[2–4]

Clinical Presentation 2

A 10-year-old asymptotic male with new onset of nephrotic range proteinuria (2 g/m^2/day), with no edema and low normal serum albumin (3.7 g/dL). No edema, normal blood pressure (BP), normal urine sediment, and normal creatinine, normal ultrasound, normal complement, and no evidence of positive glomerulonephritis (GN) markers including negative PLA2R, and normal hepatitis/HIV serology. Growth and development are also normal. Family history is unremarkable.

Biopsy showed minimal change, 20 glomeruli in the sample, and no fibrosis or scarring. Electron microscopy (EM) is pending.

Which of the following do you recommend (choose all that apply)?

A. Start immunosuppressive as usual with minimal change disease.
B. Order nephrotic syndrome gene panel.
C. Watch and wait.

D. Start angiotensin-converting enzyme (ACE) inhibitor.
E. Other

The correct answers are A, C, D, and E

Would your answer change if focal segmental glomerulosclerosis (FSGS) were found on biopsy?

A. Yes, it would.
B. No, it would not.

The correct answer is A

Comment: This patient is not presenting with full-blown nephrotic syndrome. Mildly low serum albumin and heavy proteinuria are concerning for a primary podocytopathy, especially focal segmental glomerulosclerosis (FSGS).

It is recommended to wait for EM findings to look for the extent of foot process effacement and the appearance of glomerular basement membrane (GBM) on EM (option C).[1–4]

For now, we should start ACE inhibitors/angiotensin receptor blockers and (option D) and would not do steroids or any other immunosuppression at this stage.

We also should consider doing genetic testing including *NPH2*, *WT1*, and *CLCN5* (option B)[3,4] and ask for evaluation of hypercalciuria and low-molecular-weight proteinuria such as beta-2 microalbuminuria to rule out Dent disease (option E).

In Dent disease, the EM shows no or minimal podocyte effacement with FSGS histopathology.

Should EM reveal minimal change disease (MCD) or primary FSGS (negative genetic results), we should start steroids alone, and if the steroids fail to achieve remission following 6 weeks of therapy, we should then consider this case as steroid-resistant nephrotic syndrome (SRNS) and begin treatment with rituximab (RTX; induction therapy) plus mycophenolate mofetil (MMF; maintenance therapy).

In a recent randomized controlled trial, Assadi et al.[2] compared the efficacy and safety of RTX-cyclosporine A (CsA) MMF (n = 32) vs. RTX-CsA (n = 34) in 66 children with SRNS (MC, n = 15; FSGS, n = 47; and diffuse mesangial hyperplasia (DMH), n = 4) between the ages 2 and 6 years and found RTX-MMF was superior to RTX-CsA both in maintaining the remission and causing fewer adverse events in all cases of renal histology lesions.[1–4]

Clinical Presentation 3

The mother of an 8-year-old boy with steroid-sensitive idiopathic nephrotic syndrome seeks advice regarding future therapy for her son. He has had four relapses of nephrotic syndrome in the last year, each time responding rapidly to oral prednisone. Relapses have occurred when prednisone was tapered to <20 mg every other day.

He now has reduced stature for his age and developed behavioral disorder believed to be due to excess glucocorticoids.

Another physician has advised the mother that a 10-week course of oral cyclophosphamide is essential to control her son's disease and prevent further relapses. However, the mother is very fearful of the adverse side effects of cyclophosphamide.

Which *one* of the following statements is correct?

A. Alternate drugs, other than cyclophosphamide, are available to control the disease at an acceptable level of side effect.
B. Continuation of glucocorticoid therapy is the best option.
C. A course of cyclophosphamide is indicated and is preferable to all other options.

D. All therapy should be stopped while awaiting a spontaneous remission.
E. No treatment advice can be given unless a renal biopsy is performed.

The correct answer is E

Comment: Guidelines from the International Study of Kidney Disease in Children, Kidney Disease: Improving Global Outcomes (KDIGO) and, more recently, from the International Pediatric Nephrology Association have been modified and adopted across the world, depending on the availability of medications and preferences by parents and physicians. A review of country-specific guidelines shows that despite minor differences, there is reasonable consensus on the management of both steroid-sensitive and steroid-resistant nephrotic syndrome in children. Harmonizing guidelines and considering region-specific preferences will be useful for uniform guidance for physicians, parents, and patient groups, as well as for allowing comparisons of outcome.[1]

Several randomized controlled trials (RCTs) have investigated the duration and dose of corticosteroid therapy for the initial episode of nephrotic syndrome. Findings from four multicenter trials on more than 800 patients that compared standard (8–12 weeks) to prolonged (16–26 weeks) initial prednisone therapy consistently favor limiting initial therapy to 8 to 12 weeks.

An updated meta-analysis comparing 2 months versus 3 months or longer was not associated with increased risk of relapse.

Individual patient data analyses of two European studies suggest that initial therapy for 12 weeks was better than 8 weeks in terms of delaying the time to first relapse and fewer relapses on short-term follow-up. Furthermore, prolonged therapy in young children might reduce the risk of first relapse but not frequent relapses. Similar findings were reported in a recent RCT on patients with onset of disease before age 4 years, which showed that extending the duration of initial therapy beyond 12 weeks postponed the time to first relapse without altering the risk of frequent relapses.

Based on the results of these trials, the International Pediatric Nephrology Association recommends that initial therapy should comprise 6 weeks each of daily and alternate-day prednisone therapy. KDIGO guidelines recommend that physicians could either follow 8 weeks or 12 weeks of initial treatment, with empiric advice to prefer the former in patients with rapid (<7 days) remission or comorbidities such as obesity or hypertension, and consider prolonged (26–24 weeks) therapy in young patients with delayed remission.

Clinical Presentation 4

A 10-year-old boy develops idiopathic nephrotic syndrome. His BP is 138/74 mm Hg and he has massive anasarca. His serum creatinine is 0.8 mg/dL, urine protein excretion is 12 g/day, serum albumin is 1.8 g/dL, and serum cholesterol is 480 mg/dL. Serum C3 and C4 concentrations are normal. Urinalysis reveals 10 to 15 erythrocytes per high-power field (HPF), numerous hyaline and granular and fatty acid casts, and oval fat bodies. The patient's mother refuses to permit a renal biopsy.

What would be the most appropriate initial therapy for this patient?

A. 40 mg/m^2 prednisone daily for 2 weeks, then 20 mg/m^2 every other day for an additional 2 weeks
B. 60 mg/m^2 prednisone daily for 4 weeks, then 40 mg/m^2 for an additional 4 weeks, 500 mg of intravenous methylprednisolone daily for three doses; repeat monthly for 6 months
C. 5 mg/kg cyclosporin per day and 20 mg/m^2 of prednisone every other day for 4 months
D. 2.5 mg/kg levamisole three times weekly for 6 months

The correct answer is C

Comment: We recommend kidney biopsy be obtained at the onset of nephrotic syndrome to establish a histological diagnosis to determine the treatment plan in patients (1) whose age is younger than 1 year or older than 6 years, (2) with persistent hematuria and frank hematuria, (3) with hypertension and renal dysfunction, (4) with hypocomplementemia, and (5) with extrarenal symptoms (e.g., rash, purpura) because these patients are likely to have other histological types than minimal-change disease.[1,2]

Kidney biopsy is also recommended in patients showing steroid resistance and in patients given long-term calcineurin inhibitor therapy, even without renal dysfunction at 2 to 3 years into the therapy to assess for any nephrotoxicity.

Clinical Presentation 5

A 15-year-old boy is referred for a second opinion regarding his diagnosis of focal and segmental glomerulosclerosis documented by renal biopsy 3 months ago. The patient's proteinuria was first noted 6 months ago on a routine check-up. He is moderately obese. Physical examination shows a weight of 86 kg, height 160 cm, BP 148/92 mm Hg, and no edema is present. He has 2.6 g of proteinuria daily, serum albumin is 4.2 g/dL, serum cholesterol is 232 mg/dL, blood urea nitrogen (BUN) is 18 mg/dL, and creatinine is 1.2 mg/dL. A review of his renal biopsy shows 10 glomeruli, of which two show segmental sclerosis; the other eight were markedly hypertrophied. There is 40% effacement of foot processes on electron microscopy, but no electron-dense deposits or tubuloreticular inclusions are found.

Along with counseling about weight reduction, initial appropriate treatment for this patient would be which *one* of the following?

A. Use of an ACE inhibitor or an angiotensin II receptor antagonist.
B. Start 4 to 6 mg/kg cyclosporin per day for 4 to 6 months.
C. Start 2.0 g of mycophenolate mofetil daily for 6 months.
D. Intravenous cyclophosphamide at 1 g/m^2 monthly for 6 months.
E. Prednisone 40 mg daily or every other day for a 6-month course.

The correct answer is A

Comment: FSGS is a histological pattern of glomerular injury, rather than a single disease, that is caused by diverse clinicopathological entities with different mechanisms of injury with the podocyte as the principal target of lesion. It is considered the most common glomerular cause leading to end-stage renal disease (ESRD).

Primary FSGS, which usually presents with nephrotic syndrome, is thought to be caused by circulating permeability factors that have a main role in podocyte foot process effacement.

Secondary forms of FSGS include maladaptive FSGS secondary to glomerular hyperfiltration such as in obesity or in cases of loss in nephron mass, virus-associated FSGS, and drug-associated FSGS that can result in direct podocyte injury.

Genetic FSGS has increasingly been recognized and a careful evaluation of patients with atypical primary or secondary FSGS should be performed to exclude genetic causes.

Unlike primary FSGS, secondary and genetic forms of FSGS do not respond to immunosuppression and tend not to recur after kidney transplantation.

Distinguishing primary FSGS from secondary and genetic causes has a prognostic significance and is crucial for an appropriate management. In this review, we examine the pathogenesis, clinical approach to distinguish between the different causes, and current recommendations in the management of FSGS.[1,2]

Clinical Presentation 6

A 16-year-old girl with idiopathic focal and segmental glomerulosclerosis and 8 g of proteinuria daily has been treated with an ACE inhibitor and prednisone for 4 months without reduction in her proteinuria. Her serum creatinine is 1.4 mg/dL.

Which *one* of the following therapies should be offered to her at this point?

A. Continue prednisone in a tapering dose to complete a full year of treatment 2 to 3 mg/kg.
B. Start oral cyclophosphamide per day for 2 to 4 months.
C. Start 1.0 g of oral mycophenolate mofetil twice daily for 6 months.
D. Start 3 to 5 mg/kg oral cyclosporine per day for 6 months.
E. Start induction therapy with rituximab followed by maintenance mycophenolate mofetil for 12 months.

The correct answer is E

Comment: In a recent RCT, Assadi et al. compared the efficacy and safety of maintenance mycophenolate versus cyclosporine following rituximab in children with steroid-resistant nephrotic syndrome with FSGS and found that a combination of rituximab plus mycophenolate in maintaining remission was superior to rituximab plus cyclosporine with fewer adverse effect in 12 months of follow-up.[1]

Clinical Presentation 7

A 14-year-old girl is found to have proteinuria on a urinalysis done for a school sports team physical examination. Her blood pressure is 118/70 mm Hg and she has no edema.

Laboratory data show normal BUN and creatinine; urinalysis shows trace protein with 20 to 15 erythrocytes per HPF. Serum albumin is 3.2 g/dL, cholesterol 272 mg/dL, and 24-hour urinary protein excretion 4.2. Serologic tests include antinuclear antibodies (ANA), hepatitis B and C, and serum complement; all are negative or normal. A renal biopsy reveals membranous nephropathy with well-defined spike formation and no mesangial deposits.

The best treatment for this patient includes which *one* of the following?

A. An ACE inhibitor, a low-cholesterol diet, and the use of a statin
B. 2.0 g of oral mycophenolate mofetil daily for 6 months
C. 60 mg of prednisone daily in a tapering dose for at least 6 months
D. 3 to 4 mg/kg cyclosporine per day for 4 to 6 months
E. Intravenous methylprednisolone "pulse" of 1000 mg daily for 3 days followed by oral steroids alternating with monthly with oral cyclophosphamide

The correct answer is A

Comment: In a large prospective study of 1205 renal biopsies reviewed at The Hospital for Sick Children, Toronto, 14 patients had a clinicopathologic diagnosis of idiopathic membranous glomerulopathy. Typical thickening of glomerular capillary basement membranes, a spike-and-dome pattern, and subepithelial electron-dense deposits were noted. Strong deposits of immunoglobulin G (IgG) and weaker deposits of C3, IgM, and IgA were present in glomeruli. Stages of membranous glomerulopathy on EM were I in one biopsy, II in nine biopsies, and III in four biopsies.

At presentation, 11 patients had nephrotic syndrome, 7 had hypertension, and 8 had hematuria. Now four are in remission, seven have active disease with normal renal function, and three have renal failure.

Patients with hypertension, presence of nephrotic syndrome, hematuria, and being younger than age 6 years at the onset tended to do worse. Administration of steroids or immunosuppressive drugs did not adversely affect outcome. Furthermore, clinical outcome did not correlate with stage of disease. Hence, pathologic and most clinical features do not predict long-term prognosis in children with membranous glomerulopathy. Based on these observations, a conservative and less aggressive therapeutic approach is recommended for children with normal renal function and normal BP.[1,2]

Clinical Presentation 8

A 17-year-old woman with a 2-year history of well-documented systemic lupus erythematosus but without known prior renal disease develops fever, increased joint pains, and worsening facial rash. On physical examination, her BP is 140/90 mm Hg and she has a molar rash and multiple erythematous lesions on her arms and torso and pitting ankle edema.

Her laboratory evaluation shows an elevated anti-double-stranded DNA antibody titer, a low total hemolytic complement (CH50), and a low C3 level. The WBC count is 3600/mm^3, hematocrit is 22%, and platelet count is 95,000/mm^3. BUN is 23 mg/dL and creatinine is 1.6 mg/dL. The urinalysis shows 4+ proteinuria and many erythrocytes and red blood cell casts. A 24-hour urinary protein excretion is 4.5 g. A renal biopsy is performed and shows World Health Organization class IV diffuse proliferative lupus nephritis.

Which of the following treatment regimens has been shown to give the best long-term efficacy with the fewest side effects for the patient described here?

A. 750 to 1000 mg of mycophenolate mofetil twice daily for at least 6 months
B. 2 mg/kg oral cyclophosphamide per day combined with alternate-day prednisone with conversion of the cyclophosphamide to 2 mg/kg oral azathioprine per day at 6 months
C. Intravenous monthly "pulse" cyclophosphamide for 6 months with follow-up mycophenolate mofetil (MMF) or azathioprine for 2 years
D. Intravenous "pulse" cyclophosphamide and intravenous "pulse" methylprednisolone for 6 months with follow-up doses every third month
E. 4 to 5 mg/kg cyclosporine per day and prednisone starting at 60 mg/day and then tapering the dose for a minimum treatment duration of 6 months

The correct answer is C

Comment: Despite the continuing development of immunomodulatory agents and supportive care, the prognosis associated with lupus nephritis (LN) has not improved substantially in the past decade, with end-stage kidney disease still developing in 5% to 30% of patients within 10 years of LN diagnosis.

Modalities that better preserve kidney function and reduce the toxicities of concomitant glucocorticoids are needed in the development of therapeutics for LN. In addition to the conventional recommended therapies for LN, there are newly approved treatments as well as investigational drugs in the pipeline, including the newer generation of calcineurin inhibitors and biologic agents. In view of the heterogeneity of LN in terms of clinical presentation and prognosis, the choice of therapies depends on a number of clinical considerations. Molecular profiling, gene-signature fingerprints, and urine proteomic panels might enhance the accuracy of patient stratification for treatment personalization in the future.

Immunosuppressive therapy in patients with class I/II LN should be guided by extrarenal disease manifestations unless the patients have nephrotic syndrome resulting from lupus podocytopathy, which is managed as a minimal change disease.

The initial treatment of active proliferative (± membranous) LN is glucocorticoids plus either MMF or low-dose (Euro-Lupus) intravenous cyclophosphamide.

Although glucocorticoids have generally been given in high doses for LN, emerging data suggest that lower doses may be equally effective but with fewer short- and long-term toxicities.

Following initial therapy of proliferative LN, mycophenolate mofetil is the preferred immunosuppressive and should be continued for at least 36 months.

Class V lupus nephritis is managed with RAS blockade, BP optimization, hydroxychloroquine, and the addition of immunosuppression in patients who develop nephrotic range proteinuria.[1,2]

Clinical Presentation 9

A 12-year-old White girl presents with recurrent episodes of gross hematuria in the previous 1 year. Her blood pressure is 150/95 mm Hg. No edema is present. A urinalysis reveals 50 to 100 erythrocytes per HPF (50% dysmorphic), several erythrocyte casts, and 4+ proteinuria. Six months ago, her serum creatinine was 0.9 mg/dL. Her serum creatinine is now 1.9 mg/dL and a random urine protein/creatinine ratio is 2.0. A renal biopsy reveals that 30% of the glomeruli are involved, with focal and segmental or circumferential cellular crescents. The remaining glomeruli show mesangial proliferation and focal and segmental glomerulosclerosis. The immunofluorescence study shows 3+ IgA, 2+ IgG, 1+ IgM, 3+ C3, negative C1q, and 3+ fibrin/fibrinogen.

In addition to blood pressure control with an ACE inhibitor, which *one* of the following therapies would you add to her regimen as initial therapy?

A. Omega-3 fatty acid (fish oils) 6 g daily
B. Oral prednisone at 60 mg daily
C. Cyclosporine at 5 mg/kg daily
D. Oral cyclosporine at 60 mg daily plus cyclophosphamide at 1.5 mg/kg daily
E. Oral mycophenolate mofetil (Cellcept) at 500 mg twice daily

The correct answer is A

Comment: At this stage of kidney tissue involvement, not only will immunosuppression be ineffective, but its use may be associated with serious adverse effects and high risk of morbidity and mortality.[1,2]

Clinical Presentation 10

A 14-year-old girl is discovered to have microscopic hematuria during a routine examination. Her physical examination, including BP, is normal. You see her for further investigation. History reveals that her younger sister, age 6 years, also has persistent microscopic hematuria. There is no family history of deafness. The patient denies flank pain, fever, urinary tract symptoms, or episodes of gross hematuria. Laboratory values include a serum creatinine of 0.6 mg/dL, and the urine shows 30 to 50 erythrocytes and 1 to 2 leukocytes per HPF. No casts are seen.

A 24-hour urine reveals 18 mg of protein and a creatinine clearance of 110 mL/min.

Which of the following tests is most likely to reveal the correct diagnosis (select all that apply)?

A. Renal biopsy
B. Urinary beta-2 microglobulin
C. Audiogram
D. Computed tomography (CT) scan of the abdomen with contrast
E. Cystoscopy

The correct answers are A and B

Comment: Microscopic hematuria without proteinuria is a common clinical finding. When urological causes are excluded, usual findings on renal biopsy are IgA nephropathy, Alport syndrome, or thin basement membrane nephropathy (which has an excellent prognosis).

Urinary microalbumin is a sensitive and noninvasive biomarker to discriminate between the IgA and thin basement membrane disease.[1]

Urinary microalbumin excretion was assessed in 76 children with asymptomatic microscopic hematuria in whom the presence of proteinuria, hypertension, reduced renal function, hypercalciuria, urinary tract infection, or structural abnormality of the urinary tract had been excluded. MA/Cr μg/mg was <4. Twenty-two (29%) patients had microalbuminuria (MA/Cr >30 μg/mg) and 54 (71%) had normal albumin excretion. Of those with normoalbuminuria, 38 (70%) had normal renal tissue, 15 (28%) thin glomerular basement membrane (TGBM) disease, and 1 (2%) IgA nephropathy. In contrast, 20 (91%) of those with microalbuminuria had IgA nephropathy and 2 (9%) had TGBM disease.

Statistical analysis showed no significant differences between the mean MA/Cr ratio for children with TGBM disease and those with normal glomerular findings. Fourteen of the 20 children with IgA nephropathy who also had microalbuminuria were treated with an ACE inhibitor. Over a mean follow-up of 51 months, none developed overt proteinuria; hematuria resolved and microalbuminuria returned to normal in eight (57%) during therapy with the ACE inhibitor. In contrast, hematuria persisted and proteinuria developed in the other untreated children. None of the children with TGBM disease developed overt proteinuria after a mean of 51 months. Hematuria was persistent in children with TGBM disease, but often resolved in those whose biopsies were completely normal.

These data suggest that determination of urinary microalbumin excretion is warranted in the routine examination of children with isolated microscopic hematuria. Routine screening for microalbuminuria may help identify a subgroup of patients with IgA nephropathy who are at high risk for progressive kidney disease and need more intensive therapy and closer follow-up.[1]

Clinical Presentation 11

An 18-year-old man, who is HIV seropositive, presents with generalized edema. He is found to have nephrotic syndrome with 2.1 g proteinuria daily and serum creatinine of 2.1 mg/d. Large echogenic kidneys are seen by ultrasonography. The serum complement is normal and the ANA is negative. He has no active infections.

Which *one* of the following statements is most correct concerning a renal biopsy in this patient?

A. Renal biopsy would be of little value because he has classic HIV-associated nephropathy.
B. Renal biopsy is indicated to differentiate HIV-associated nephritis from other causes of glomerular diseases to direct therapy.
C. Renal biopsy is contraindicated because of the risks of bleeding or infection.
D. Renal biopsy is not indicated because he has a severely elevated serum creatinine level.

The correct answer is A

Comment: Histological features of HIV-associated nephritis (HIVAN) include collapsing FSGS as a result of podocyte proliferation and tubular dilatation with atrophy and flattening of tubular epithelial cells. Interstitial edema and lymphocyte infiltration often accompany interstitial fibrosis in patients with HIVAN.[1]

Kidney biopsy is contraindicated in HIV patients with small and contracted kidneys, single kidney, polycystic kidney disease, hydronephrosis, and presence of urinary tract infection.[1,2]

To distinguish HIVAN from other forms of renal disease (e.g., immune complex glomerulonephritis, IgA nephropathy), patients who are seropositive for HIV require a kidney biopsy. The typical practice is to obtain a biopsy specimen if the patient's daily protein excretion is greater than 1 g.[1,2]

Clinical Presentation 12

A 16-year-old boy is discovered to have idiopathic nephrotic syndrome and a reduced serum C3 level. His BP is 147/90 mm Hg. Urine protein excretion is 3.8 g/day and serum creatinine 1.5 mg/d/L. Lupus, hepatitis B, and hepatitis C serologies are negative. Cryoglobulins are not found on repeated examinations.

A renal biopsy shows the lesion of diffuse proliferative glomerulonephritis by light microscopy. Electron microscopy shows both subepithelial and subendothelial electron-dense deposits. The basement membrane is reduplicated, multilayered, and fenestrated.

In addition to control of BP with an ACE inhibitor, what would you recommend next?

A. 2.0 mg/kg cyclophosphamide per day and 20 mg of prednisone every other day for 6 months
B. 4.0 mg/kg cyclosporine per day and 20 mg of prednisone every other day for 6 months
C. 40 mg of prednisone every other day for 6 months, then 20 mg every other day for an additional 6 months
D. No additional therapy is advisable.
E. 500 mg mycophenolate mofetil twice daily for 6 months

The correct answer is C

Comment: Approaches to treatment of idiopathic membranoproliferative glomerulonephritis (MPGN) have included immunosuppression, inhibiting platelet-induced injury with aspirin and dipyridamole, minimizing glomerular fibrin deposition with anticoagulants, and use of steroidal and nonsteroidal anti-inflammatory agents.[1,2]

Only a handful of RCTs have been published with sufficient power to determine the benefits of therapy for MPGN. The use of variable end points (e.g., reduction in proteinuria, renal function measured using variable techniques) further confounds the data.

Thus, the optimal treatment of idiopathic MPGN is not clearly defined. Specific therapies should be reserved for patients with MPGN who have one or more of the following indications:

Proteinuria exceeding 3 g/d, active interstitial or glomerular disease (crescents) on biopsy, impaired renal function at presentation, and a progressive decline in renal function.[1,2]

Clinical Presentation 13

A 15-year-old boy was admitted with a 2-week history of abdominal fullness and pain. Physical examination revealed a lethargic but alert male. Vital signs were blood pressure 130/45 mm Hg, pulse 116/min, respiratory rate 24/min, temperature 98.6°F. There was a palpable left supraclavicular node and firm, nontender hepatosplenomegaly. Laboratory studies showed hematocrit 34%, WBC 11,600/mm^3, BUN 36 mg/dL, serum creatinine 2.9 mg/dL, sodium 136 mEq/L, chloride 97 mEq/L, potassium 5.6 mEq/L, CO_2 20 mEq/L, calcium 6.9 mg/dL, phosphate 7.0 mg/dL, uric acid 20 mg/dL, and albumin 3.7 g/dL. Urinalysis showed pH 5.0, no protein, no casts or red blood cells (RBCs) but many uric acid crystals.

Which diagnoses should receive most consideration in this case (select all that apply)?

A. Acute interstitial nephritis
B. Tumor lysis syndrome
C. Urinary tract obstruction
D. Rhabdomyolysis
E. Acute glomerulonephritis

The correct answers are B and D

Comment: Tumor lysis syndrome occurs when tumor cells release their contents into the bloodstream, either spontaneously or in response to therapy, leading to the characteristic findings of hyperuricemia, hyperkalemia, hyperphosphatemia, and hypocalcemia.[1]

Tumor lysis syndrome is a metabolic and oncologic emergency frequently encountered in clinical practice. This condition is prevalent in both adult and pediatric patients undergoing chemotherapy. Most of the symptoms seen in patients with tumor lysis syndrome are related to the release of intracellular chemical substances that cause impairment in the functions of target organs. This can lead to acute kidney injury, fatal arrhythmias, and even death.

Because this condition is so lethal, it is imperative to identify patients at high risk for developing tumor lysis syndrome and start early preventive therapy. Quick and early recognition of the renal and metabolic derangement associated with tumor lysis syndrome and initiation of treatment can save the patient's life.[1]

Rhabdomyolysis is a complex process associated with morbidity and mortality. Although the condition is often caused by direct traumatic injury, other potential etiologies are drugs, toxins, infections, muscle ischemia, electrolyte and metabolic disorders, genetic disorders, exertion or prolonged bed rest, and temperature-induced states such as neurologic malignant syndrome (NMS) and malignant hyperthermia. Rhabdomyolysis is exhibited by a triad of symptoms including myalgia, weakness, and myoglobinuria, with an elevation in creatinine kinase level being the most sensitive test for muscle injury–induced rhabdomyolysis. All clinicians should be aware of common causes, diagnosis, and treatment options.[2]

Clinical Presentation 14

A 19-year-old female patient has been treated with hemodialysis for the past 14 years after rejection of a cadaver transplant. Her original disease was Henoch-Schoenlein purpura (HSP). She now presents with ascending pain and weakness in her hands and feet. There are prominent contractures of her extremities that have caused her to become bedridden over the past 4 months. Her major problems associated with hemodialysis have been hyperphosphatemia (7–8.5 mg/dL) and hypercalcemia (10–11 mg/dL) after vitamin D therapy. Her parathyroid hormone (PTH) levels are mildly elevated at 56 pg/mL, although they have been substantially higher in the past. A workup for collagen vascular disease, including vasculitis, has been negative, as have Lyme titer and thyroid function tests. Blood glucose has never been elevated. Electromyography and nerve conduction studies are normal. Muscle biopsy shows atrophy and intramuscular calcification.

What is the most likely cause of this condition?

A. Uremic myopathy
B. Mitochondrial myopathy
C. Scleroderma
D. Calcific uremic arteriopathy
E. Recurrent HSP

The correct answer is D

Comment: In its most florid form, calcific vasculopathy may be manifested as calciphylaxis. A small fraction of patients with ESRD, particularly those treated with dialysis, develop deep skin ulcerations in association with calcification of subcutaneous arterioles. Uremic peripheral neuropathy is a distal, symmetrical, mixed sensorimotor. It occurs more commonly in men and is independent of the underlying disease. There is no specific myopathy associated with uremia.

Arthralgia and myalgias characterize diffuse scleroderma. Early diffuse cutaneous systemic sclerosis includes arthritic symptoms. A specific myopathy is not seen.[1]

Recurrent HSP does not manifest a specific myopathic picture, as seen in this case.

Clinical Presentation 15

A 14-year-old male patient begins hemodialysis treatments under your care. His original disease was FSGS. Physical examination is unremarkable. His serum calcium is 9.7 mg/dL, phosphate 6.1 mg/dL, and PTH 340 pg/mL. To optimize his management, you initiate therapy with sevelamer hydrochloride to maintain his serum phosphate level within an acceptable range.

Which of the following statements *best* describes the likely response of this patient to sevelamer hydrochloride in comparison with calcium acetate?

A. Sevelamer hydrochloride will be more effective in reducing serum phosphate levels.
B. Calcium acetate will be more effective in reducing serum phosphate level.
C. Sevelamer hydrochloride will be effective at reducing PTH levels.
D. Sevelamer hydrochloride use will result in less hyperchloremia as a late complications.

The correct answer is D

Comment: Sevelamer hydrochloride (Renagel) significantly lowers serum phosphorous in hemodialysis patients but with minimal effects on serum calcium in comparison to treatment with standard calcium-based phosphate binders. Patients with the highest PTH levels (>300 pg/mL) experienced the greatest reduction in PTH. The effect on PTH levels, however, may be inconsistent.[1]

Clinical Presentation 16

An 18-year-old woman maintained on hemodialysis for the past 6 years because of congenital kidney dysplasia presents with a large necrotic lesion of the skin of her upper thigh. She is obese, has mild glucose intolerance and poorly controlled hypertension, and has been receiving large doses of iron dextran and erythropoietin for resistant anemia as well as enalapril for hypertension. Her serum phosphate level has ranged from 6 to 9 mg/dL, serum albumin from 2.2 to 2.9 g/dL, and serum calcium from 8.8 to 9.0 mg/dL. Serum magnesium is 2.6 mg/dL, alkaline phosphatase 165 IU/L, and serum PTH 450 pg/mL. A biopsy of her skin lesion reveals medial calcification and intimal hyperplasia of small arteries and fat necrosis.

Which of her clinical characteristics is a key risk factor for this condition?

A. Iron dextrin therapy
B. Hypertension
C. Hypomagnesemia
D. Hyperphosphatemia
E. Erythropoietin therapy

The correct answer is D

Comment: Hyperphosphatemia is the strongest predictor of calciphylaxis in patients receiving hemodialysis treatment. There is a 3.5-fold increase in the risk of calciphylaxis associated with each 1-mg/dL increase in the serum phosphate concentrations. Body mass index, diabetes, hypertension, hypomagnesemia, aluminum, and higher dosages of erythropoietin and iron dextran are not independent predictors of calciphylaxis.[1]

Clinical Presentation 17

A 9-year-old patient with a 5-year history of chronic hemodialysis for the treatment of FSGS begins to complain of bone pain and muscle weakness. The workup of the patient revealed the following: serum calcium 9.2 mg/dL, PO_4 5.2 mg/dL, intact PTH level 250 pg/mL, and plasma aluminum 433 g/dL. Bone mineral density was reduced with a total *Z* score (SD from the mean of a healthy, age- and gender-matched reference population) of −1.25.

Which of the following should be done now?

A. Bone biopsy
B. 1,25 (OH)2 vitamin D measurement
C. Bone-specific alkaline phosphatase measurement
D. Procollagen-icarbixy-terminal propeptide level
E. 2-microglobulin level

The correct answer is A

Comment: This patient's clinical picture is consistent with low turnover bone disease; therefore, aluminum toxicity must be considered. In the presence of significant aluminum exposure, bone biopsy seems indicated in the following cases: before parathyroidectomy and before starting long desferrioxamine treatment, given the risks of deafness and fatal mucormycosis as complications of treatment. Bone alkaline phosphatase is not sensitive enough to distinguish between low and normal turnover. Procollagen-icarboxy-terminal propeptide is not a specific indicator of bone disease because it is not well controlled with bone histology.[1]

Clinical Presentation 18

A 12-year-old male patient on maintenance hemodialysis is referred to you from an outside hospital for help with treating his renal osteodystrophy. The patient has been poorly compliant with his phosphate binders and has multiple PTH measurements in the 1400 pg/mL range. He has also had a fractured fibula after minor trauma. The referring nephrologist has tried to suppress the patient's PTH levels with intravenous calcitriol but has produced hypercalcemia to 12.5 mg/dL on several occasions.

In reviewing a number of treatment options, which would you recommend to the patient?

A. 22-oxacalcitriol because it will likely prove more beneficial than calcitriol
B. Paricalcitol because it will likely prove more beneficial than calciferol
C. Parathyroidectomy
D. 1-Alfa-hydroxyvitamin D2 because it will likely prove more beneficial than calcitriol
E. 1-Alfa hydroxyvitamin D3 because it will likely prove more beneficial than calcitriol

The correct answer is C

Comment: The indications for parathyroidectomy, two of which apply to this patient, have classically included: (1) hypercalcemia and hyperphosphatemia in the presence of very high PTH levels

(>800 pg/mL), as in this patient, with concurrent resistance to pharmacologic control; (2) fractures and tendon avulsions; (3) when the estimated weight of a parathyroid gland exceeds 1 g; and (4) calcific arteriolopathy, which some experts have considered to be an absolute indication.[1]

Clinical Presentation 19

A 10-year-old boy was referred to you for evaluation and treatment of persistent post-renal transplant hypophosphatemia. He has been treated with cyclosporine and prednisone but has complained of some persistent muscle aches. Physical examination was unremarkable except for mild proximal muscle weakness in the lower extremities. He is on no medications except for his immunosuppressive agents. Laboratory values revealed the following: creatinine 1.2 mg/dL, calcium 9.6 mg/dL, phosphate 2.1 mg/dL, intact PTH 38 pg/mL, and fractional excretion of phosphate 28%.

Which of the following is the most likely cause of his renal phosphate wasting?

A. PTH
B. Cyclosporine
C. Phosphatonin
D. 1,25 (OH)2 vitamin D3
E. Glucocorticoids

The correct answer is C

Comment: Green et al. studied the mechanism of posttransplant hypophosphatemia and found that sera from hypophosphatemic posttransplant patients inhibited PO_4 transport in vitro in a PTH-independent mechanism. This finding is consistent with the concept that there are PTH-independent humoral agents (phosphating) that dramatically reduce PO_4 reabsorption, and they may underline disorders of phosphate transport, as seen in oncogenic osteomalacia.

Cyclosporine does not produce phosphate wasting, nor does 1,25 (OH)2 D3. Glucocorticoids are phosphaturic but do not produce the severe degree of phosphate wasting seen in this case.[1]

Clinical Presentation 20

Which *one* of the following statements is *true* regarding the effective prevention of hyperphosphatemia in patients receiving adequate dialysis therapy?

A. Calcitriol administration does not alter dietary phosphate absorption.
B. Avoiding processed foods will reduce phosphate absorption.
C. Avoiding meat-derived phosphate will be more beneficial than avoiding plant-derived phosphate.
D. $CaCO_3$ is less effective than sevelamer hydrochloride for the control of serum phosphorus.

The correct answer is C

Comment: Any evaluation of dietary phosphorus adequacy should consider not only the content of phosphorus in food but also the bioavailability of phosphorus because most phosphorus in plants is in the form of phytate. Because humans do not have the phytase enzyme that is required to degrade phytate and to release phosphorus, phytate is poorly digested in the human gastrointestinal tract and therefore limits phosphorus absorption from plant sources. Phosphorus in meat is well absorbed because it is found mostly as intracellular organic compounds that are easily hydrolyzed in the gastrointestinal tract, releasing inorganic phosphorus for absorption.[1]

Clinical Presentation 21

A 15-year-old boy is evaluated for muscle weakness and bone pain over the past 5 months. Physical examination reveals marked proximal myopathy but no other abnormalities. Laboratory studies reveal the following: calcium 10.2 mg/dL, phosphorous 1.2 mg/dL, immunoreactive PTH 23 pg/mL (normal, 10–65 pg/mL), 1,25 (OH)2 vitamin D 8 pg/mL (normal, 10–55 pg/mL), and tubular reabsorption of phosphate 75% (normal, 90%). A CT scan shows a 3 × 4-cm tumor of the right thigh. The tumor is removed and the patient fully recovers.

Which *one* of the following is responsible for phosphoric action of the tumor?

A. PTH-related protein
B. 25 (OH) vitamin D fibroblast growth factor 23
C. Stanniocalcin
D. Calcitonin
E. 25 (OH) vitamin D

Comment: Recent evidence suggests that the tumor product responsible for the phosphaturic action is fibroblast growth factor 23 (FGF-23), a member of a large family of proteins involved in regulating fibroblast function. In the oncogenic osteomalacia, there is overproduction of FGF-23. In hereditary X-linked hypophosphatemic rickets there is mutation in an endopeptidase that normally inactivates FGF-23 and prevents high levels of the cytokine from migrating from bone to act systemically and in the kidney. In autosomal dominant hypophosphatemic rickets, there are mutations in the gene encoding FGF-23, so that it is functional.[1]

Clinical Presentation 22

A 15-year-old girl on maintenance hemodialysis for 8 years is transferred to your clinic and found to have severe refractory hyperparathyroidism (PTH 1400 pg/mL), serum calcium 10.6 mg/dL, and phosphorus 6.9 mg/dL. The patient has mild bone pain, and radiologic studies show moderate signs of hyperparathyroidism.

The increased level of PTH is confirmed on three separate occasions. Ultrasound revealed a single parathyroid mass with a long axis of 6 mm. The other three glands were enlarged, but each was less than 5 mm in length.

Which *one* of the following therapies should the patient receive?

A. Total parathyroidectomy with autotransplantation of parathyroid tissue
B. Two 6-week trials of high-dose calcitriol
C. Increase in bath calcium level to 3.0 mEq/L
D. Calcimimetic therapy

The correct answer is A

Comment: The indications for percutaneous ethanol injection include serum PTH >800 pg/mL, symptoms such as severe itching or bone pain, evidence of high-turnover bone disease, exclusion of aluminum bone disease by desferrioxamine, resistance to medical therapy including calcitriol pulse therapy, and the long axis of the target parathyroid gland detected by ultrasonography exceeding 5 mm and shown to have a positive blood flow by power-Doppler ultrasonography. Patients failing to have adequately sized glands will likely require surgical removal. Increasing calcium in the dialysate or increasing vitamin D intake would be inappropriate in this hypercalcemic patient. Calcimimetic agents would be ineffective in this patient with the enlarged parathyroid mass greater than 5 mm in length.[1]

Clinical Presentation 23

A 17-year-old male presents with two large areas of skin necrosis on his left thigh. He has been treated with hemodialysis for the past 6 years for chronic kidney disease. He has received intermittent small doses of calcitriol but has developed hypercalcemia to 12.0 mg/dL. His physical examination is unremarkable except for moderate obesity and intact pulses throughout his lower extremities. The necrotic areas of skin are superficial, but they measure 4 × 5 cm each. Laboratory studies revealed calcium 9.6 mg/dL, phosphate 5.6 mg/dL, and immunoreactive PTH 180 pg/mL.

Which *one* of the following choices *best* explains this clinical condition?

A. Calciphylaxis associated with adynamic bone disease
B. Calciphylaxis with intermittent hyperphosphatemia
C. Calciphylaxis secondary to intermittent hyperparathyroidism
D. Vasculitis
E. Occult atheroembolic disease

The correct answer is A

Comment: This patient has developed skin necrosis associated with calcific vasculopathy. This syndrome is called calciphylaxis. Because he demonstrates hypercalcemia with therapeutic doses of vitamin D, he likely has adynamic bone disease as well. The association of the two conditions has been reported and is linked by the role of recurrent episodes of hypercalcemia. Hyperphosphatemia does play a role, but the elevation of serum phosphate is typically persistent. Hyperparathyroidism is frequently found associated with calciphylaxis, but in this case the iPTH level is below that associated with the full picture of symptomatic hyperparathyroidism including accelerated bone turnover and hypercalcemia with small doses of vitamin D. Vasculitis and atheroembolic disease are important entities in the differential diagnosis of calciphylaxis but are not associated with the tendency to hypercalcemia found in this patient.[1]

Clinical Presentation 24

A 6-year-old girl has undergone renal transplantation as therapy for ESRD resulting from FSGS. She has received a living related kidney from her father. She has done well postoperatively. Her therapy includes a regimen of low-dose prednisone, cyclosporine, and mycophenolate mofetil. At 6 months after transplantation, a dual-energy x-ray absorptiometric scan demonstrates a 10% loss of bone mass compared with her pretransplantation study.

Which *one* of the following maneuvers would have likely prevented this bone loss?

A. Low protein intake
B. Elimination of mycophenolate mofetil
C. Use of vitamin D and calcium therapy
D. Use of vitamin D and calcium therapy

The correct answer is D

Comment: Low doses of active vitamin D and calcium partially prevent bone loss at the lumbar spine and proximal femur during the first 6 months after renal transplantation. Recently, prophylactic bisphosphonate treatment has shown promise, but the exact indications for its use in this setting remain to be determined. Steroid therapy contributes to bone loss, but not cyclosporine or mycophenolate.[1]

Clinical Presentation 25

Calcimimetics are thought to decrease both serum calcium and PTH levels through which of the following mechanisms of action (select all that apply)?

A. Activation of PTH receptors in bone
B. Enhanced excretion of PTH in the kidney
C. Enhanced metabolism of PTH to inactive fragments
D. Activation of the calcium-sensing receptor (CaSR) on chief cells of the parathyroid to suppress PTH secretion

The correct answers are B and D

Comment: Calcimimetics are calcium receptor agonists that act on the parathyroid gland by increasing the sensitivity of the receptor to calcium. Treatment with cinacalcet HCl causes significant decreases in PTH without elevating serum calcium or phosphate levels.[1]

Clinical Presentation 26

A 12-year-old boy treated with hemodialysis presents with a serum calcium level of 10.7 mg/dL, phosphate of 5.9 mg/dL, iPTH level of 1065 pg/mL, and a parathyroid gland weight of 5.0 g as determined by ultrasonography. Previous attempts with oral calcitriol therapy to suppress PTH had produced a 15% fall in PTH levels.

Which of the following treatments should be ordered next?

A. Aggressive use of sevelamer to lower serum phosphate level
B. Intravenous calcitriol (1.0 μg) at the time of dialysis treatment
C. Intravenous 25 (OH) vitamin D
D. Parathyroidectomy

The correct answer is D

Comment: The indications for parathyroidectomy include (1) hypercalcemia and hyperphosphatemia in the presence of very high PTH level (>800 pg/mL) with failure to lower PTH levels after 6 to 8 weeks of vitamin D analog and/or calcimimetics therapy; (2) fractures and tendon avulsions; (3) calcific arteriolopathy; and (4) hypertrophied gland and weight >4.0 g as determined by ultrasonography.[1]

Clinical Presentation 27

A 7-year-old boy with dialysis-dependent ESRD and chronic hip pain had a magnetic resonance imaging (MRI) scan that revealed aseptic necrosis that was attributed to previous glucocorticoid therapy for asthma. Two hours after the MRI, he had his scheduled hemodialysis treatment. His predialysis serum calcium was 5.4 mg/dL, phosphorus 5.6 mg/dL, and albumin 3.6 g/dL. He has been closely followed for moderate secondary hyperparathyroidism and has received vitamin D supplementation.

Which is the *most* likely explanation for these findings?

A. Gadodiamide (Omniscan)-induced spurious hypocalcemia
B. Parathyroid infarction
C. Gadopentetate (Magnevist)-induced spurious hypocalcemia
D. Inadvertent barium administration

The correct answer is A

Comment: Gadodiamide binds with colorimetric agents used in assaying serum calcium and produces a spurious hypocalcemia. Parathyroid infarct is a rare event. Gadopentetate does not produce the same effect. Barium administration is associated with hypokalemia, and barium sulfate used in radiologic studies does not enter the circulation. A defective laboratory instrument is always possible, but gadodiamide predictably produces this artificial finding.[1]

Clinical Presentation 28

A 10-year-old boy was referred to you for evaluation and treatment of persistent postrenal transplant hypophosphatemia. He has been treated with cyclosporine and prednisone but has complained of some persistent muscle aches. Physical examination was unremarkable except for mild proximal muscle weakness in the lower extremities. He is on no medications except for his immunosuppressive agents. Laboratory values revealed the following: creatinine 1.2 mg/dL, calcium 9.6 mg/dL, phosphate 2.1 mg/dL, intact PTH 38 pg/mL, and fractional excretion of phosphate 28%.

Which of the following is the most likely cause of his renal phosphate wasting?

A. PTH
B. Cyclosporine
C. Phosphatonin
D. 1,25 (OH)2 D3
E. Glucocorticoids

The correct answer is C

Comment: Green et al. studied the mechanism of posttransplant hypophosphatemia and found that sera from hypophosphatemic posttransplant patients inhibited PO_4 transport in vitro in a PTH-independent mechanism. This finding is consistent with the concept that there are PTH-independent humoral agents (phosphating) that dramatically reduce PO_4 reabsorption, and they may underline disorders of phosphate transport, as seen in oncogenic osteomalacia.

Cyclosporine does not produce phosphate wasting, nor does 1,25 (OH)2 D3. Glucocorticoids are phosphaturic but do not produce the severe degree of phosphate wasting seen in this case.[1]

Clinical Presentation 29

A 15-year-old male is found to have an antineutrophil cytoplasmic antibody (ANCA) associated with microscopic polyangiitis with both renal and pulmonary involvement. He is treated with oral prednisone and cyclophosphamide.

The prednisone is tapered and discontinued after 4 months; azathioprine is substituted for cyclophosphamide at 6 months. His initial serum creatinine was 2.1 mg/dL, and it decreased to a nadir of 1.7 mg/dL after 6 months of therapy. He is now seen for a follow-up examination 1 year after the initial diagnosis. He is asymptomatic. Therapy consists of 100 mg of azathioprine daily and 10 mg of enalapril daily. His blood pressure is 130/80 mm Hg. Physical examination is normal. Urinalysis reveals 1 to 2 erythrocytes and 1 WBC per HPF, occasional granular casts, and 2+ proteinuria. The serum creatinine is now 1.8 mg/dL. The sedimentation rate is 20 mm/h. An ANCA test performed 1 week ago was positive with a titer of 1:128. Previous values have been intermittently positive at low titer.

What would you do next?

A. Reinstitute cyclophosphamide at 2.0 mg/kg/day; stop azathioprine.
B. Reinstate cyclophosphamide at 1.0 mg/kg/day; stop azathioprine.
C. Continue azathioprine; observe carefully.
D. Start prophylactic trimethoprim-sulfamethoxazole.
E. Discontinue azathioprine; begin mycophenolate mofetil at 1.0 mg twice daily.

The correct answer is C

Comment: Pauci-immune necrotizing and crescentic GN is a frequent component of ANCA vasculitis. ANCA vasculitis is associated with ANCA specific for myeloperoxidase (MPO-ANCA) or proteinase 3 (PR3-ANCA). A diagnosis of ANCA vasculitis should always specify the serotype as MPO-ANCA positive, PR3-ANCA positive, or ANCA-negative. To fully characterize a patient, the serotype also should be accompanied by the clinicopathologic variant if this can be determined: microscopic polyangiitis, granulomatosis with polyangiitis (Wegener), eosinophilic granulomatosis with polyangiitis (Churg-Strauss), or renal-limited vasculitis.

Immunomodulatory and immunosuppressive therapies are used to induce remission, maintain remission, and treat relapses. Over recent years, there have been major advances in optimizing treatment by minimizing toxic therapy and using more targeted therapy.[1]

In the present case study, patient's renal function and laboratory findings have substantially improved after switching to cyclophosphamide to azathioprine. The best approach at this point is to continue azathioprine with close follow-up (option C).

Clinical Presentation 30

A 12-year-old girl was referred for a new onset of diffuse arthralgias involving fingers, toes, shoulders, knees, and temporomandibular joints. She denied hematuria, abdominal pain, or hematochezia. The arthralgias were worse in the morning with severe intensity. She was taking ibuprofen 800 mg three times daily. The patient had no past medical history of known renal, gastrointestinal, or cardiorespiratory disease.

On examination she had polyarticular arthritis and palpable purpura involving the buttocks area with the upper and lower extremities. She was afebrile. Her blood pressure was 145/89 mm Hg. Examination of heart, lungs, and abdomen was normal. She had anemia with a of hematocrit 22.4%. Her urinalysis was positive for microhematuria and 3+ proteinuria. Her creatinine and BUN were 45 and 2.1 mg/dL, respectively. Her serum complement and ANA were also normal.

ANCA testing was performed and she tested positive for IgG C-ANCA (anti-proteinase 3) and negative for myeloperoxidase antibodies. A percutaneous kidney biopsy showed pauci-immune necrotizing and crescentic glomerulonephritis with global glomerulosclerosis, interstitial fibrosis, and tubular atrophy. The glomerulonephritis demonstrated mild activity and moderate chronicity. There was no evidence of immune complex–mediated disease.

What is (are) the likely diagnosis(es)?

A. HSP
B. Pauci-immune vasculitis
C. Wegener's granulomatosis
D. Microscopic polyangiitis
E. Churg Strauss (eosinophilic granulomatosis with polyangiitis)

The correct answers are A, B, and C

Comment: The finding of a positive ANCA in association with HSP has been described in both pediatric and adult cases.[1,2] The presence of IgA ANCA has been found in anywhere between 28% and 79% of patients with HSP,[3] and it has been suggested to be able to help confirm the diagnosis of childhood HSP.[2] Also, the presence of ANCA in HSP has been associated with a more severe course in adults.[3] On the other hand, the presence of IgG ANCA in HSP is still unclear and of unknown significance.

The positive IgG anti-proteinase 3 C-ANCA (PR3-ANCA) in our patient allowed for a working diagnosis of HSP but brought further consideration of ANCA-associated vasculitis. ANCA-associated vasculitis includes Churg-Strauss (eosinophilic granulomatosis with polyangiitis), Wegener granulomatosis (granulomatosis with polyangiitis), and microscopic polyangiitis, among others.[4]

Because of the consideration of other etiologies, a renal biopsy was performed, which showed pauci-immune necrotizing and crescentic glomerulonephritis with global glomerulosclerosis, interstitial fibrosis, and tubular atrophy. The glomerulonephritis demonstrated mild activity and moderate chronicity. There was no evidence of immune complex–mediated disease, and it represented an ANCA-mediated glomerulonephritis.

Based on renal biopsy and being ANCA positive, the patient was given pulse methylprednisolone, mycophenolate mofetil, and rituximab.

Clinical Presentation 31

A 7-year-old girl with lupus nephritis with kidney biopsy revealing diffuse proliferative lesion (type IV) was admitted because of persistent abdominal pain, nausea, and vomiting for the last 2 weeks. Her medications, including pulse methyl prednisolone (1000 mg/m^2/d for 3 days and then monthly for 24 months), oral prednisolone (1 mg/kg/day), and cyclophosphamide (750 mg/m^2 first 6 months and then every 3 months), had been started and continued at least for 2 years. Treatment with ramipril and losartan for hypertension and proteinuria also had been started and continued. The titers of ANA and anti-dsDNA have decreased and serum C3 and C4 levels increased during the follow-up.

Physical examination revealed abdominal distension with dilated veins over the anterior abdominal wall, massive ascites, and marked edema. Abdominal palpation showed hepatomegaly and splenomegaly each 5 cm below the costal margin. Her weight and height were within normal ranges. Her body temperature, respiratory rate, heart rate, and blood pressure were 36.7°C, 22 breaths/min, 65 beats/min, and 115/65 mm Hg, respectively. There were no cutaneous vasculitis or abnormal neurologic signs.

On initial laboratory evaluation, WBC count was 14.000/mm^3 (80% neutrophils and 20% lymphocytes); hemoglobin was 17.4 g/dL, and platelet count was 23.000/mm^3 with prolonged prothrombin time (41.2 seconds). Peripheral blood smear demonstrated no abnormal cells. Serum studies included a blood urea nitrogen of 21.41 mg/ dL, serum creatinine 1.14 mg/dL, uric acid 10.22 mg/dL, sodium 135 mmol/L, potassium 5.07 mmol/L, calcium 8.2 mmol/L, phosphorus 2.9 mg/dL, chloride 108 mmol/L, magnesium 2.06 mmol/L, total protein 6.0 g/dL, albumin 2.8 g/dL, aspartate aminotransferase 6267 U/L, alanine amino-transferase 2454 U/L, alkaline phosphatase 168 U/L, gamma-glutamyl transferase 259 U/L, total bilirubin 9.1 mg/dL, direct bilirubin 1.4 mg/dL, lactic dehydrogenase 5384 U/L, creatine phosphokinase 113 U/L, and creatine phosphokinase-MB fraction 145.4 U/L.

Erythrocyte sedimentation rate was 18 mm/h (normal range, 1–15 mm/h); and C-reactive protein was 0.64 mg/dL (normal range, up to 0.35 mg/dL). Urinalysis showed a specific gravity of 1030, pH of 6.0, proteinuria of 3+, two erythrocytes, and one leukocyte/HPF. Protein excretion was determined as 68 mg/m^2/h in 24-hour urine sample. Urine and blood cultures were negative for any evidence of infection. Serum viral markers including Epstein-Barr virus, hepatitis A, B, and C virus, cytomegalovirus, human immunodeficiency virus, and herpes simplex virus were negative.

Additional parameters were as follows: lactate 39.7 mmol/L (4.5–19.8), NH3 243 μmol/L (normal range, <109 μmol/L), and pro-brain-type natriuretic peptide (pro-BNP) 598 pg/mL (normal range, <110 pg/mL). Contrast-enhanced axial CT images showed mottled appearance of the liver, perihepatic ascites, pleural effusion of the left hemithorax, thrombosed hepatic veins, narrowed intrahepatic inferior vena cava, and sparring of the caudate lobe.

What is your diagnosis?

A. Renal vein thrombosis
B. Budd-Chiari syndrome secondary
C. Cirrhosis of the liver
D. Hepatitis

The correct answer is A

Comment: Systemic lupus erythematosus is a typical autoimmune disease characterized by multiple system involvement and is associated with anti-phospholipid antibody syndrome in approximately 36% of patients.[1] Anti-phospholipid antibody syndrome is associated with recurrent arterial and venous thrombosis, fetal loss, and thrombocytopenia. Thrombosis resulting in various clinical manifestations can occur in any small or large vessel in the body. The thrombosis of the intrahepatic proportion of the inferior vena cava, called Budd-Chiari syndrome, secondary to anti-phospholipid antibody syndrome has been noted in previous reports.[2] A previous study of 43 patients with anti-phospholipid antibody syndrome-associated Budd-Chiari syndrome showed that two-thirds of these patients were girls, and the first clinical appearance of anti-phospholipid antibody syndrome, despite the absence of the other clinical systemic lupus erythematosus findings, was Budd-Chiari syndrome.[2]

In anti-phospholipid antibody syndrome, thrombosis can develop anywhere in the body or in any organ, ranging from 29% to 69%[2] and results in different clinical manifestations depending on the organ involved and the location/degree of the involvement.[2]

Similarly, the liver dysfunction that occurs in Budd-Chiari syndrome varies according to the rate and degree of venous hepatic occlusion and ranges from an asymptomatic state to fulminant hepatic failure.[3]

Many studies have shown that anti-phospholipid antibodies, including lupus anticoagulant and anti-cardiolipin antibodies, positive patients are prone to recurrent thrombosis and spontaneous fetal loss episodes, which is termed *anti-phospholipid antibody syndrome*, classified as either primary or secondary.[2]

Budd-Chiari syndrome can develop in the clinical course of systemic lupus erythematosus and should be considered in the differential diagnosis when such a patient develops abdominal pain, nausea, vomiting, hepatomegaly, ascites, and massive lower extremities edema. Systemic lupus erythematosus patients should be screened for anti-phospholipid antibody syndrome, even if there is not any clinical sign of thrombosis.

Clinical Presentation 32

A 3-year-old girl was admitted for evaluation of generalized edema. She was born prematurely at 25th gestational week with a birth weight of 875 g and was hospitalized in the neonatal intensive care unit for 4 months. Her parents were first cousins once removed and had a healthy 6-year-old daughter.

On physical examination, she had a weight of 6400 g (<third percentile), height of 65 cm (<third percentile), and head circumference of 42 cm (<third percentile). The patient had a pulse rate 83/min, respiratory rate 18/min, and blood pressure of 123/76 mm Hg (>95th + 12 mm Hg) appropriate for stage 2 hypertension. She had generalized edema, disproportionate short stature, short neck and trunk, frontal bossing, broad and depressed nasal bridge and bulbous nasal tip, thick frenulum, fine and sparse hair, high-pitched voice, tapering fingers/toes, lumbar lordosis and protruding abdomen, and waddling gait.

Laboratory tests revealed mild iron-deficiency anemia (hemoglobin 10.1 g/dL, hematocrit 31%, iron 35 μg/dL [normal, 50–350], ferritin 15 ng/mL [normal, 30–300]), leukopenia (2.7 103/μL), lymphopenia (0.970 103/μL), hypoalbuminemia (albumin 1.7 g/dL), and high total cholesterol level (269 mg/dL). Urinalysis demonstrated 2+ proteinuria. Spot urine protein was 129.2 mg/dL, urine creatinine 11.28 mg/dL, and the urine protein/creatinine ratio of 11.45 mg/mg creatinine. Serum complement C3 (105 mg/dL) and C4 (22 mg/dL) were within normal limits. She was diagnosed with nephrotic syndrome based on clinical and laboratory findings.

Decreased total CD3+ (32% [normal, 50–75%]), CD4+ (13% [normal, 25–55%]), and T cells were observed. Serum IgG was decreased (659 mg/dL [normal, 700–1600]), whereas IgA and IgM levels were in the normal range. Thyroid hormone panel revealed elevated thyroid-stimulating hormone (6.55 mIU/L [normal, 0.54–4.53]) and normal free T4 levels (14.7 mIU/L [normal, 11–22.5]). There were no mucopolysaccharides in the urine, and urinary oligosaccharides level was normal for age. Eye examination revealed hypermetropia and astigmatism. Cardiac echocardiography was normal.

Radiological examination demonstrated spondylometaphyseal dysplasia, platyspondyly, metaphyseal irregularities of long bones, increased concavity of forearm bones, metacarpals and phalanges, irregular and horizontal acetabular roofs, and unossified proximal femoral epiphyses.

Enalapril was administered for hypertension and proteinuria. Growth hormone therapy was initiated and renal biopsy was performed. Histopathology of the renal biopsy specimen demonstrated 2/36 global sclerosis, 3/36 segmental sclerosis, and minimal focal atrophy, with the remaining glomeruli apparently normal. Immunofluorescence evaluation was negative for IgG, IgM, IgA, C3, fibrinogen, C1q, kappa, and lambda. A diagnosis of FSGS was made based on renal histopathology. Because hypertension was severe, hydrochlorothiazide and atenolol were added to the hypertension regimen.

What is your diagnosis?

A. Osteochondrodysplasias
B. Mainzer-Saldino syndrome
C. Nail-patella syndrome
D. Schimke immunoosseous dysplasia
E. Ellis-van Creveld syndrome

The correct answer is D

Comment: Schimke immunoosseous dysplasia (SIOD) is characterized by short stature, spondyloepiphyseal dysplasia, nephropathy, and T-cell immune deficiency. The diagnosis of SIOD is usually based on clinical findings, especially in patients with nephrotic syndrome.[1] Genetic analysis can confirm the diagnosis and lead to early interventions that may prevent the fatal outcome of SIOD patients.

SIOD is a rare autosomal recessive disorder that manifests as disproportionate short stature, facial dysmorphic features, spondyloepiphyseal dysplasia, SRNS progressing to ESRD, and T-cell deficiency.

Additionally, lymphopenia, anemia, thrombocytopenia, neutropenia, cerebrovascular events (transient ischemic attack, stroke, headache), hyperpigmented macules, hypothyroidism, developmental delay, and occasionally non-Hodgkin lymphoma have been reported.[1,2] In the case presented here, clinical findings were suggestive for the diagnosis, which was ascertained at the initial evaluation. The present patient had homozygote c.1606_1701delinsTTCCC mutations at exon 10 of the *SMARCAL1* gene. Treatment is symptomatic. Nephropathy has been reported as steroid resistant, and although transient partial response to calcineurin inhibitors has been reported, renal pathology has always progressed to ESRD. Renal transplantation when possible has been effective for the ESRD.[2] Growth hormone therapy for short stature has been reported as ineffective.[2]

Clinical Presentation 33

A 13-year-old boy was referred for high creatinine (serum creatinine 2.1 mg/dL) detected on a routine checkup. There was no history of abdomen pain, hematuria, recurrent urinary tract infections, reduced urine output, rashes, or edema. However, he had complaints of polyuria and polydipsia over the past 5 to 6 months. He was on no medications. He was the product of nonconsanguineous marriage. He developed severe myopia at 4 years of age and has been using glasses for the same since then; however, there was no visual loss. On examination, the child was obese. His weight was 58 kg, height 140 cm, and BMI 33.5 kg/m^2. There was no edema, rashes, or pallor. BP was 110/76 mm Hg (normal) and other vitals were within normal ranges for his age. There were no dysmorphic features. Eye examination revealed normal anterior segment but high myopia. His vision was 6/12 bilaterally with corrective glasses (right: 14.0 D/left: 14.50 D). No pigment deposits were present on the retina. There were no other abdominal, cardiac, respiratory, or neurological findings on examination.

Laboratory investigations showed hemoglobulin 10.1 g/dL, serum sodium 139 mEq/L, potassium 4.2 mEq/L, chloride 99 mEq/L, BUN 70 mg/dL, and creatinine 2.0 mg/dL. Estimated glomerular filtration rate (GFR) was 31.5 mL/min/1.73 m^2, serum calcium, phosphorus, and vitamin D3 levels were normal but serum magnesium was low 1.1 mg/dL. Serum intact PTH was 152 pg/mL and uric acid 7.2 mg/dL. Capillary blood pH was 7.30. Urinalysis showed pH 7.3, specific gravity 1.020, and 1+ albumin. A 24-hour urine protein was 550 mg, calcium was 3.2 mg/kg, creatinine 8.5 mg/kg, urine calcium to creatinine ratio 0.4, phosphorus 530 mg/1.73 m^2, oxalate 16 mg, sodium 88 mEq, and uric acid 285 mg,

Abdominal ultrasound was suggestive of bilateral nephrocalcinosis which appeared as dense calcific deposits on x-ray of the kidneys, ureters, and bladder.

What is your diagnosis?

A. Dent disease
B. Familial hypomagnesemia with hypercalciuria and nephrocalcinosis (FHHNC)
C. Cystinuria
D. Primary hyperoxaluria

The correct answer is B

Comment: There are many disorders that may present with nephrocalcinosis, including Bartter syndrome, disorders of calcium sensing receptors, idiopathic calcium and kidney stone diseases, disorders of vitamin D metabolism resulting from *CYP24A1* mutations presenting as idiopathic infantile hypercalcemia type 1 (HCINF1) or type 2 because of mutations of sodium, phosphate co-transporter (NaPi 2a) (SLC34A1), hypervitaminosis D, and primary distal renal tubular acidosis. However, chronic kidney disease (CKD) is not seen in these disorders.

Our patient had anemia, elevated urea, and creatinine with an eGFR of 31 mL/min/1.73 m^2 (CKD stage 3) with hyperparathyroidism, and normal calcium and vitamin D levels and hypomagnesemia with hypercalciuria and hyperuricemia and subnephrotic proteinuria, which rule out calcium-sensing receptor and vitamin D metabolism defects.

Clinical disorders associated with nephrocalcinosis that lead to CKD at an early age are Dent disease, cystinosis, FHHNC, cystinuria, and primary hyperoxaluria.

The presence of low-molecular-weight proteinuria, hypercalciuria, and kidney stones or nephrocalcinosis with stage 5 CKD should raise the suspicion of Dent disease. In these disorders, the proximal tubular dysfunction may also cause phosphaturia, glycosuria, and metabolic acidosis (Fanconi-Bickel syndrome). The progression to CKD occurs by age 30 to 50 years, and sometimes even later.[1] The diagnosis of Dent disease may be confirmed on genetic analysis by looking for the presence of *OCRL1* or *CLCN5* mutations.[1] In the given case, however, no metabolic acidosis was present and features of proximal tubular dysfunction such as phosphaturia and glycosuria were absent. The screen for β_2-microglobulin was negative. Slit-lamp examination ruled out deposits of cysteine in the cornea, and the absence of Fanconi-Bickel syndrome completely ruled out cystinosis.[1–3]

FHHNC is a rare autosomal recessive disorder that presents with loss of magnesium and calcium, thereby causing magnesium wasting, hypercalciuria, nephrocalcinosis, and kidney failure. There may not be significant protein excretion, but early presentation with loss of magnesium in urine and hypomagnesemia is characteristic of the disease. Most children would develop kidney failure in adolescence or early adulthood resulting from a progressive CKD setting from early in life. A defect in claudins that are present at the tight junctions of the thick ascending limb of the loop of Henle (encoded by *CLDN16* or *CLDN19*) is implicated in the development of FHHNC.

The kidney manifestations resulting from both mutations are identical, but with *CLDN19* there is severe ocular involvement, which may present with myopia, pigment retinitis, macular coloboma, strabismus, astigmatism, nystagmus, macular scars, macular degeneration, anisocoria, and retinochoroiditis.[2] The clinical features in the current context make the diagnosis of FHHNC type 2 highly likely.[3] This was confirmed by next-generation sequencing. An autosomal recessive homozygous missense mutation in exon 4 of the *CLDN19* gene transcript was detected, which was a novel pathogenic variant.

This child was initiated on hydrochlorothiazide, magnesium supplements, and potassium citrate (to combat hypercalciuria and repress crystallization) and advised large-volume fluid intake.

The presence of dense unilateral or bilateral radiopaque stones like those from calcium oxalate should also raise the suspicion of primary hyperoxaluria. This is highly likely if the child presents early in life and has persistent nausea and vomiting, leading to failure to thrive or progressive CKD even without a history of passing stones. They may present with reduced kidney function over a period of time, and more than 65% present before the age of 10 years with stone disease.[3]

Children with cystinuria will present with recurrent urinary tract stones in childhood. The individuals may be hypotonic at birth, presenting with delayed growth early in life, and may have hyperphagia and excessive weight gain later on. The average age at stone detection is early teenage years. A significant proportion of adults may develop CKD later in life.[1] The diagnosis may be confirmed by detecting cysteine, ornithine, lysine, and arginine in a urine sample.

Clinical Presentation 34

A 15-year-old girl presented with 2 weeks' history of arthritis involving the right ankle, knee, and hip joints. Her medical history was unremarkable.

Physical examination was normal. There was no swelling, tenderness, or warmth in any of her joints. Her weight was 57 kg (<third percentile) and height was 162 cm (<third percentile). She had a pulse rate of 78/min and respiratory rate of 16/min, axillary temperature of 36.5°C, and blood pressure of 110/70 mm Hg (<95th percentile).

Laboratory findings at admission were as follows: WBC count 6590/mm^3, hemoglobin 12.5 g/dL, platelets 26,1000/mm^3, C-reactive protein 0.3 (N < 0.2) mg/dL, erythrocyte sedimentation rate 10 mm/h, BUN 40 mg/dL, creatinine 1.4 mg/dL, total protein 6.2 g/dL, albumin 3.5 g/dL, total cholesterol 160 mg/dL, and triglyceride 86 mg/dL. Parathyroid hormone level was

68 pg/mL (18.5–88.0 pg/mL). Estimated GFR was calculated as 65 mL/min/1.73 m^2. Urinalysis revealed proteinuria 3+, and 12 erythrocytes/HPF and 9 leukocytes/HPF were demonstrated in urine microscopy. Spot urine protein/creatinine ratio was calculated as 2.9 mg/mg creatinine. Protein excretion was 70 mg/m^2/h according to 24-hour timed collected urine.

Serum complement levels of C3 (92 mg/dL) and C4 (24.8 mg/dL) were normal, ANA was positive at 1/160 titer (with granular pattern), whereas anti-dsDNA, anti-SSA, anti-SSB, anti-Sm, anti-Sm/anti-ribonucleoprotein (RNP), anti-Scl 70, anti-Jo1, anti-Ssa/52, anti-ribosomal P protein, anti-histone antibody, cytoplasmic ANCA (cANCA/PR3), perinuclear ANCA (pANCA/MPO), and rheumatoid factor were all negative. ACE level (23.4 U/L) was normal. Ultrasonography showed increased renal parenchymal echogenicity in both kidneys. MRI of the sacroiliac joint was normal. Kidney biopsy was performed according to clinical and laboratory findings.

Histopathology of the kidney biopsy specimen indicated 36/46 global sclerosis (78%) and 3/46 focal segmental sclerosis (6%). Fibrocellular crescent was observed in one glomerulus and cellular crescent in two. Most of the glomeruli had narrowing, synechiae, mesangial enlargement, and mesangial cell increase in the Bowman space in nonsclerotic glomeruli. Mesangial cell increase was accompanied by lymphocytes. Significant thickening, rigidity, and occasional double contours were present in the capillary basement membranes. Signs of moderate tubular atrophy and injury to the tubular epithelium were observed. Mild to moderate lymphocyte cell infiltration with interstitial fibrosis was observed in the interstitium. Immunofluorescence microscopy showed accumulation in the mesangium and periphery of the glomerular capillary basement membranes (thin granular form) for IgG, C3, C1q, kappa, and lambda. Congo red and crystal violet dye stains were negative. In EM, glomerular basement membrane borders were irregular and thickened because of prominent, subepithelial, and subendothelial-located electron-dense deposits suggesting the diagnosis of MPGN.

Which diseases should be considered on the differential diagnosis list?

A. Systemic lupus erythematosus (SLE)
B. Sjögren syndrome (SS)
C. Rheumatoid arthritis (RA)
D. Monoclonal gammopathies

The correct answers are A, B, and C

Comment: Immune complex-mediated membranoproliferative glomerulonephritis (IC-MPGN) was diagnosed in the kidney biopsy of the patient who presented with arthralgia, microscopic hematuria, severe proteinuria, high serum creatinine level, and positive ANA in the granular pattern.

IC-MPGN has been accompanied with many infections such as hepatitis B, hepatitis C,[1] autoimmune diseases,[2,3] and monoclonal gammopathies.[4] Some of these diseases are extremely rare in childhood, such as SS.[5]

Because our patient had arthralgia, positive ANA (with granular pattern), and IC-MPGN on kidney biopsy, we considered systemic autoimmune diseases including SLE, SS, and RA in the differential diagnosis.

For the differential diagnosis of associated diseases: hepatitis B surface antigen, hepatitis C antibody, and HIV screens were found to be negative. The presence of a monoclonal gammopathy was excluded with normal serum and urine protein electrophoresis. Lymphoma and leukemia were not considered in the patient because she had a normal physical examination. Also, no atypical cells were found in her peripheral blood smear.

Our patient did not have any of the clinical findings suggestive of SLE. Serum complement levels of C3 and C4 were normal, anti-dsDNA was negative, and therefore she did not fulfill the diagnostic criteria of SLE.[6] RA was not considered because the duration of her complaint was as short as 2 weeks and rheumatoid factor (RF) was in the normal range.

An extremely rare cause of IC-MPGN in children is SS. Although our patient did not complain about dry mouth and/or eyes, the ophthalmological evaluation revealed she suffered from dry eyes. Schirmer test showed decreased tear secretion (≤5 mm in 5 minutes). Although she had no history of swelling in the salivary glands, the biopsy showed focal lymphocytic sialoadenitis, with a focus score of 5 per 4 mm^2 of glandular tissue.

Primary SS (pSS) is diagnosed using the American College of Rheumatology/European League Against Rheumatism[7] criteria in adults. There are no criteria established for children and adolescents.

Ocular dryness was present in her examination, although she did not complain about it at admission. Moreover, her Schirmer test was ≤5 mm/5 minutes (decreased tear secretion) and her focus score was 5 foci/4 mm^2 on minor salivary gland biopsy. The complaint of ocular dryness appeared 2 weeks later. Therefore, she fulfilled the criteria of SS according to American College of Rheumatology/European League Against Rheumatism criteria. Additionally, the presence of granular pattern ANA positivity supported the diagnosis of pSS because this type of positivity is seen when the target antigens are nRNP/Sm, SS-A, and SS-B in the cell nucleus. The diagnosis was accepted as pSS.

Clinical Presentation 35

A 16-year-old male patient admitted because of fatigue, severe right flank pain, and rectal bleeding and elevated serum creatinine (1.4 mg/dL), bilateral hydroureteronephrosis, and bilateral echogenic kidneys 3 weeks ago. Micturating cystourethrography revealed grade 2 vesicoureteral reflux (VUR) on the right. Scintigraphy revealed 66% functioning right kidney with a nonobstructive stasis and 34% functioning left kidney with poor perfusion and concentrating ability. With these findings, a diagnosis of CKD secondary to VUR was made. He had no previous urinary tract infection or symptoms of dysfunctional bladder. He had a laboratory examination 2 years ago that revealed normal urea (21 mg/dL) and creatinine (0.5 mg/dL) levels. He had no abdominal imaging before 3 months ago. In his family history, he had a cousin with a diagnosis of infantile myxoid mesenchymal tumor.

His body weight was 53 kg (third percentile); his height was 175 cm (45th percentile). Abdominal examination revealed a nontender, distended abdomen with grade 2 ascites. Organomegaly was not detected.

Laboratory examination revealed the following values: WBC 9.570/mm^3, hemoglobin 12/dL, platelet 450,103 μL, glucose 97 mg/dL, urea 56 mg/dL, creatinine 2.2 mg/dL, aspartate aminotransferase (AST) 66 U/L, alanine aminotransferase (ALT) 103 U/L, amylase 97 U/L, lipase 7 U/L, albumin 3.6 g/dL, sodium 137 mEq/L, potassium 3.9 mEq/L, magnesium 1.7 mg/dL, chloride 99 mEq/L, calcium 8.8 mg/dL, and phosphorus 3.9 mg/dL. Alpha-fetoprotein and βHCG values were normal, and hepatitis markers were negative. Ascites sample was transudate. No atypical cells were detected in the ascites sample. Serum ascites albumin gradient was 1.1 g/dL. Abdominal ultrasonographic examination revealed mild dilatation in intrahepatic bile ducts, grade 2 dilatation in both kidney pelvicalyceal structures, widespread free fluid in peritoneal compartments, and increased wall thickness in the rectosigmoid region. Hydroureteronephrosis was more severe compared with previous ultrasonography (pelvis anteroposterior diameter from 28 to 35 mm on the left, 16 mm to 20 mm on the right).

MRI of the abdomen revealed dilatation in the intrahepatic biliary tract, which is thought to be secondary to external compression, dilatation compatible with grade 2 hydroureteronephrosis in both kidneys, constriction secondary to external pressure or tumoral infiltration at the level of the ureter pelvis, a luminal mass lesion that holds the lumen in a 10-cm segment proximal to the rectum, and invasion of the mass lesion into the bladder posterior wall and distal segment of both ureters. Sigmoidoscopy revealed a malignant tumor occupying the lumen of the distal sigmoid colon.

What is the likely cause of hydronephrosis?

A. VUR
B. External pressure secondary to intraabdominal tumor
C. Ureteropelvic junction obstruction
D. Posterior ureteral valves

The correct answer is B

Comment: Hydroureteronephrosis is classified based on the presence or absence of reflux and obstruction. The variant with reflux but no obstruction is high-grade vesicoureteral reflux with a dilated ureter. In primary VUR, there is a failure of this anti-reflux mechanism because of a congenitally short intravesical ureter. Secondary VUR is frequently associated with an anatomic obstruction (for example, posterior urethral valves) or a functional bladder obstruction (for example, bladder bowel dysfunction and neurogenic bladder). The severity of VUR can be influenced by the degree and chronicity of obstruction.[1]

If progression in hydronephrosis is observed in patients with hydroureteronephrosis for a known cause such as VUR, intra-abdominal tumors should be kept in mind, including signet ring cell carcinoma (SRCC), a rare and rapidly progressing tumor in this age group capable of compressing the ureter.

After a histopathologic diagnosis of SRCC, chemotherapy was started as a modified FOLFOX 6 regimen that includes oxaliplatin 85 mg/m^2 day 1, leucovorin 400 mg total dose over 2 hours day 1, fluorouracil 400 mg/m^2 bolus day 1, followed by 2400 mg/m^2 over 46 hours, and panitumumab 6 mg/kg every 2 weeks, was started. The patient is well after 3 months of follow-up. After chemotherapy, the creatinine level decreased to 0.7 mg/dL and hydroureteronephrosis of the right kidney regressed, whereas hydroureteronephrosis in the left kidney persisted.

Clinical Presentation 36

A 10-year-old boy was admitted for evaluation of recurrent painless episodes macroscopic hematuria over the previous 2 weeks. He reported three episodes of passage of red-colored urine, occurring immediately after exercise and lasting for two or three urinations. No fever or other symptoms were reported. The family history was negative for kidney disease and hematological disorders, apart from nephrolithiasis in the father.

On admission, the boy was hemodynamically stable. His blood pressure was 116/78 mm Hg (95th percentile for his height), and physical examination was normal. His body mass index was 21.5.

The hemoglobin level, WBC, and platelet counts, levels of serum electrolytes and creatinine, and liver function tests were all within the normal range. The fractions of serum complement C3 and C4 were in the lower normal range (C3 84 mg/dL, normal range, 83–177 mg/dL; and C4 15 mg/dL, normal range, 15–45 mg/dL). The antistreptolysin O antibodies titer was 613 IU/mL (normal <200 IU/mL), and throat swab culture was positive for group A β-hemolytic *Streptococcus*, although no clinical symptoms of streptococcal tonsillitis or skin infection were reported.

Urinalysis revealed a specific gravity of 1.016, pH 7, negative albumin, hemoglobin 4+, and erythrocytes 80 to 100 cells/HPF. A 24-hour urine collection revealed calcium excretion 2.6 mg/kg and total protein excretion 84 mg/m^2. Urine culture was negative. Urinary tract ultrasound was normal, and abdominal x-ray showed no calculi.

What is the most likely diagnosis?

A. Postinfectious glomerulonephritis
B. Alport syndrome
C. Nephrolithiasis
D. Hypercalciuria
E. Nutcracker syndrome

The correct answer is E

Comment: The pattern of gross hematuria, painless episodes of gross hematuria after exercise without persistent microscopic hematuria, and the finding of normal C3 complement fraction exclude poststreptococcal glomerulonephritis from the differential diagnosis. The normal calcium excretion in the 24-hour urine collection rules out hypercalciuria. Nephrolithiasis was excluded from the differential diagnosis, based on absence of pain and normal ultrasound and abdominal x-ray, which failed to show a stone in the urinary tract. Other causes of macroscopic hematuria were excluded, including urinary tract infection (negative urine culture) and coagulation disorders (normal blood coagulation tests).

The onset of macroscopic hematuria after exercise with resolution at rest, and the exclusion of other, more common causes of hematuria, led to the most likely diagnosis of nutcracker syndrome (NCS). To confirm the diagnosis of NCS, Doppler ultrasonography and magnetic resonance angiography were performed.

Doppler ultrasonography revealed a reduced angle between the superior mesenteric artery and the abdominal aorta and a sharp change in the width of the left renal vein by 0.2 between the above vessels to 0.62 at the left kidney portal, findings compatible with nutcracker syndrome. Magnetic resonance angiography revealed a very acute angle between the superior mesenteric artery and the aorta (about 25 degrees, with an acceptable value of 38 degrees) and dilatation of the left renal vein at about 8 mm before its intersection with the upper mesenteric artery, whereas after the intersection, the diameter was estimated at about 2.5 mm. These findings and the patient's clinical presentation were consistent with the diagnosis of NCS.[1,2]

Clinical Presentation 37

A 14-year-old girl with Wilson disease (WD) was referred because of proteinuria. WD was diagnosed 4 months prior by liver biopsy, which was performed because of persistently high transaminase levels, low serum ceruloplasmin, and high 24-hour urine copper levels. She was treated with penicillamine and zinc and had a well-controlled serum copper level. Urine analysis revealed proteinuria at the sixth month of the penicillamine treatment, which was negative before.

On admission to our nephrology department, her weight was 43 kg (–1.93 standard deviation), height was 158 cm (–0.46 standard deviation), and blood pressure was 105/60 mm Hg. She was a thin girl, and physical examination was unremarkable. Laboratory findings were as follows: hemoglobin 14.1 g/dL, total leukocyte count 5.960/mm^3, platelet count 199,000/mm^3, serum urea 14 mg/dL, creatinine 0.2 mg/dL, albumin 3.5 g/dL, aspartate aminotransferase 30 U/L, and alanine aminotransferase 35 U/L. C-reactive protein and erythrocyte sedimentation rate were also normal. Urinalysis showed a specific gravity of 1.005 and pH of 6.0, proteinuria (++), and glucose (-). Microscopic examination of urine revealed a red blood cell count of 3 and a WBC count of 4/HPF. Spot urine protein-to-creatinine ratio was 2.4 mg/mg in random urine and 1 mg/mg in the first-morning urine samples. Daily urinary protein excretion was 2291 mg (1648 mg/m^2/day) and albumin excretion was 1202 mg/day. Urinary β2-microglobulin was 0.19 mg/L (normal range, 0–0.2 mg/L). Serum complement C3 (1.18 g/L) and C4 (0.17 g/L) levels were within the normal range. Viral serology was unremarkable. In addition, ANA, anti-double-stranded DNA, and anti-neutrophil cytoplasmic antibodies (proteinase 3 and myeloperoxidase) were negative. Kidney ultrasonography findings were as follows: right kidney size 100 × 45 mm, parenchymal thickness 13 mm, left kidney size 114 × 54 mm, parenchymal thickness 16 mm, and renal echogenicity was normal. A simple cyst of 13 mm in size was observed in the upper pole of the left kidney.

Because of nephrotic range proteinuria and decreased serum albumin level, kidney biopsy was performed.

The light and immunofluorescence microscopy demonstrated diffuse thickening and granular IgG staining of the glomerular basement membrane. EM demonstrated subepithelial electron-dense deposits.

What is your diagnosis based on the kidney biopsy findings?

A. Membranous nephropathy
B. Membranoproliferative glomerulonephritis
C. Focal segmental glomerulosclerosis
D. Minimal change mesangial hypercellularity

The correct answer is A

Comment: The histological findings on the kidney biopsy are consistent with membranous glomerulonephritis. The cause of membranous nephropathy in this case was penicillamine treatment, which was confirmed with the resolution of proteinuria after switching the penicillamine treatment to trientine hydrochloride.

Membranous nephropathy is a rare cause of proteinuria in the pediatric age group (about 5%), and secondary causes such as infections (hepatitis B virus, hepatitis C virus, syphilis) and drugs are more common in children compared with adults.[1] Routine urine analysis during follow-up of children with WD is essential for the diagnosis of kidney involvement because of the disease itself or as a side effect of penicillamine treatment. In children, who develop proteinuria under penicillamine treatment, membranous nephropathy must be kept in mind, and switching of penicillamine to trientine hydrochloride should be preferred.

Kidney involvement in WD mainly manifests as tubulopathy with findings of renal tubular acidosis, glucosuria, phosphaturia, aminoaciduria, proteinuria (i.e., low molecular weight), hypercalciuria, and nephrolithiasis.[2] Copper is mainly deposited in the epithelium of proximal and distal convoluted tubules in the kidney, which induces cell swelling and degeneration. Acute kidney injury resulting from acute hemolytic anemia at the first presentation has also been reported.[3]

Glomerular involvement as microscopic hematuria (11%) and microalbuminuria (34%) has been reported in pediatric WD cases, which were resolved after penicillamine treatment.[4] In the same report, transient microscopic hematuria and microalbuminuria have also been reported during penicillamine treatment. Glomerulonephritis in patients with WD (without penicillamine treatment) is rarely reported. Immunoglobulin A nephropathy (IgAN) was reported in a patient with a known WD.[3] Inversely, it is also reported that patients whose first presentation was immunoglobulin A nephropathy were diagnosed as having WD concomitantly or during follow-up[5] with WD.

Clinical Presentation 38

A 10-year-old girl, born of a nonconsanguineous marriage, presented with history of poor urinary stream, continuous dribbling, and primary enuresis. She had history of recurrent febrile urinary tract infections and constipation since birth. She had been prescribed antibiotics and laxatives intermittently by her primary care physician. At the age of 8 years, she was seen in a urology clinic and was found to have a solitary right kidney with hydroureteronephrosis and urinary bladder wall diverticuli on ultrasonography. She was managed as a case of dysfunctional voiding with an oral alpha adrenoceptor antagonist, tamsulosin, and clean intermittent catheterization, which she discontinued after a few months. There was no history of maternal diabetes or any antenatal infection, and the parents were not informed of any abnormalities on antenatal ultrasound. Her birth and family history were noncontributory. She had age-appropriate mental, social, and motor milestones.

On examination, her height was 120 cm and weight was 19 kg (both less than third percentile), and she was stage 1 on Tanner's sexual maturity scale. She had mild pallor and stage 1 hypertension (BP 122/80 mm Hg). She had no edema, breathlessness, or bony deformities. Her spine was normal with normal-appearing external genitalia. There was hypoplasia of the left thenar eminence compared with the right hand with no restriction in the movements of left thumb at the first metacarpophalangeal and interphalangeal joints. There were no palpable lumps in the abdomen or in the inguinal region. She did not have anosmia, and hearing assessment was normal. Neurological examination was unremarkable except for weak anal tone. Perineal sensation was preserved.

Her laboratory parameters showed anemia, elevated serum creatinine, low serum bicarbonate, low vitamin D, and elevated parathormone level. Urine microscopy showed abundant WBCs, and culture grew a significant colony count of *Escherichia coli*. There was no proteinuria or hematuria. Serum electrolytes were sodium 139 mEq/L, potassium 3.5 mEq/L, chloride 90 mEq/L, bicarbonate 14 mEq/L, BUN 22 mg/dL, creatinine 2.2 mg/dL, calcium 9.2 mg/dL, phosphorous 5.3 mg/dL, alkaline phosphatase 431 IU/L, vitamin D3 11.0 ng/mL, and intact PTH 180 pg/mL. Venous blood gas showed pH was 7.32, PCO_2 17 mm Hg, and bicarbonate 13 mEq/L.

The abdominal ultrasonography confirmed the presence of solitary right kidney (8.8 × 4.1 cm, at 50th percentile in kidney length chart) with hydroureteronephrosis, poor corticomedullary differentiation, and irregular thickening of bladder wall. The uterus and ovaries were absent. She underwent urinary catheterization, and urinary tract infection was treated with intravenous ceftriaxone. For constipation, she received daily enemas and later maintenance therapy with oral lactulose. After confirming a normal urine analysis, a micturating cystourethrogram was performed. Micturating cystourethrogram showed an elongated bladder outline with sacculations giving a "Christmas tree" appearance. Later, MRI of the pelvis and lumbosacral spine was done, which showed a neurogenic bladder with irregular walls and sacculations, solitary right hydroureter, and solitary right gross hydronephrosis. The sagittal T2 image revealed a neurogenic bladder and dilated rectum with an absent müllerian structure between the two organs. There is an absent coccyx and lower sacral segments (block arrow). Coronal T2 image showed partial agenesis of the sacrum with absent lower sacral segments and coccyx. The solitary right kidney had hydronephrosis.

What is your diagnosis?

A. Neurogenic bladder
B. Ureterocele
C. Ureteropelvic junction obstruction
D. Bladder neck obstruction

The correct answer is A

Comment: This girl with a solitary kidney had urinary incontinence and constipation since birth along with recurrent urinary tract infections, resulting in the development of CKD stage IV (eGFR 22 mL/min/1.73 m^2 by modified Schwartz formula). She was underweight with short stature and had hypertension, anemia, metabolic acidosis, vitamin D deficiency, and hyperparathyroidism, which are manifestations of CKD. The solitary right kidney did not show compensatory hypertrophy and had loss of poor corticomedullary differentiation with hydroureteronephrosis in the absence of vesicoureteric reflux. These findings and increased bladder wall thickness on ultrasound suggested presence of concomitant bladder dysfunction probably from anatomical or functional obstruction. A patulous anus and characteristic "Christmas tree" appearance of urinary bladder with irregular contours were suggestive of a neurogenic bladder. Both ovaries and uterus were absent. As the patient was phenotypically female, this prompted us to consider 46, XY disorders of sexual development like androgen insensitivity syndrome (OMIM 300068). She was in her early adolescence; hence, we could not comment on the development of secondary sexual characteristics. Patients with androgen insensitivity syndrome usually do not have extragenital anomalies.[1] The presence of genitourinary abnormalities, abnormal thumb of the left hand with loss of thenar prominence, and probable neurogenic bladder raised the suspicion of multisystem structural involvement. Patients with Kallmann syndrome may rarely have solitary kidney with genital and skeletal abnormalities, but they have associated anosmia and a family history of delayed or absent puberty.[2] Hence, we revisited our differential diagnosis to a syndrome that involved müllerian duct agenesis, congenital anomalies of kidney and urinary tract, and the skeletal system. We further evaluated the patient for Mayer-Rokitansky-Küster-Hauser syndrome.

Clinical Presentation 39

A 14 year-old girl was the only child born to nonconsanguineous parents. She was admitted for evaluation of right first-finger pain, weakness, and lack of appetite of 10-day duration. The patient's medical and family histories were not significant for a systemic disease.

On physical examination, she appeared pale. Her weight was 40 kg (fifth percentile) and height 151 cm (<10th percentile). Blood pressure was 111/73 mm Hg. There was no evidence of arthritis. The remaining physical examination was unremarkable.

Admission laboratory test values were: WBCs 14,300/μL, hemoglobin 7.5 g/dL, hematocrit 22%, and platelets 245,000/μL. Urea, creatinine, and uric acid levels were 119 mg/dL, 1.3 mg/dL, and 12 mg/dL, respectively, and measured creatinine clearance was 42 mL/min per 1.73 m^2. Daily urine output was normal (1.9–2.3 mL/kg per hour), with a urine osmolarity of 357 mOsm/L. Tubular reabsorption of phosphate was 80% (normal range ≥85%), and fractional excretion of uric acid was 2.5% (normal range >14 ± 5.3%). Urine analysis did not show glycosuria, proteinuria, aminoaciduria, or hypercalciuria. There were no red or WBCs. Urine culture showed no growth. Renal ultrasound demonstrated bilateral renal parenchymal hyperechogenicity with normal dimensions and without ureteral dilatation or renal cysts.

Voiding cystourethrography was normal. Dimercaptosuccinate renal scintigraphy demonstrated a low renal uptake and a high background activity. A renal biopsy was performed and 68 glomeruli were sampled; 50% were globally sclerosed. The remaining glomeruli were unremarkable, and no deposition of crystalloid was observed. The biopsy revealed chronic interstitial nephritis and moderate-to-severe tubular atrophy and interstitial fibrosis, especially in the neighboring sclerosed glomerulus. The blood vessels were unremarkable. Direct immunofluorescence studies showed no significant immunoglobulin or complement deposition.

Which diseases(s) should be considered in the differential diagnosis of this clinical picture?

A. Hypoxanthine-guanine phosphoribosyltransferase deficiency
B. Medullary cystic kidney disease type 2
C. Familial juvenile hyperuricemic nephropathy
D. Medullary sponge kidney

The correct answer is C

Comment: Hypoxanthine-guanine phosphoribosyl-transferase deficiency is an X-linked disorder that results in the overproduction of uric acid. The patient's female gender and the absence of neurological symptoms, history of nephrolithiasis, or urate granulomas on renal biopsy argued against partial hypoxanthine-guanine phosphoribosyltransferase deficiency. On the other hand, renal ultrasound did not demonstrate renal cysts; therefore, the diagnosis of medullary cystic kidney disease type 2 was ruled out. The most likely etiology of the hyperuricemic chronic renal disease could be familial juvenile hyperuricemic nephropathy. This clinical picture is an autosomal dominant disorder characterized by hyperuricemia, low fractional renal urate excretion, progressive chronic interstitial nephritis, and chronic renal failure. Renal impairment usually appears between 15 and 40 years of age, leading to ESRD within 10 to 20 years.[1–4]

Familial juvenile hyperuricemic nephropathy is caused by mutations in the uromodulin gene (*UMOD*) located at 16p11.2-12 that encodes for uromodulin or Tamm-Horsfall glycoprotein, the most abundant protein in normal urine. Several mutations in the *UMOD* gene have been identified in some families. Thus, to achieve exact diagnosis, the patient was tested for *UMOD* mutations by polymerase chain reaction (PCR) amplification of genomic DNA and bidirectional automated DNA sequencing of all exons in the coding region of the *UMOD* gene.

Clinical Presentation 40

A 6-year-old girl was admitted to the emergency department with diffuse edema on the eyelids and lower extremities and decreased urinary output. On physical examination, bibasilar crackles and distended abdomen with mild ascites were evident. Her height (100 cm) was below the 3rd percentile, weight (16 kg) was between the 10th and 25th percentiles, and BP was 125/80 mm Hg. Her medical history was unremarkable, except for night blindness, which developed in early childhood. There was no history of kidney disease in her family and her parents were nonconsanguineous.

Laboratory tests at admission revealed a normal complete blood count. Dipstick urinalysis revealed a pH of 6, specific gravity of 1015, 3+ red blood cells (+3), and trace proteinuria. Other laboratory findings were as follows: blood pH 7.30, PCO_2 30 mm Hg, bicarbonate 19.8 mmol/L, urea 164 mg/dL, serum creatinine 6.3 mg/dL, albumin 4.1 g/dL, sodium 131 mmol/L, potassium 3.6 mmol/L, uric acid 8.3 mg/dL, magnesium 1.3 mg/dL, calcium 8.1 mg/dL, phosphorus 5.8 mg/dL, alkaline phosphatase 111 U/L, and PTH 228.5 pg/mL (normal, 15–65 pg/mL). Tubular reabsorption of phosphate was 63.41% (normal, >85%), fractional sodium excretion was 4.1% (normal, <1%), and fractional potassium excretion was 22.8% (normal, <15%). Urinary protein/creatinine ratio was 2.2. The GFR calculated using the Schwartz formula was 8.59 mL/min/1.73 m^2, and creatinine clearance calculated on 24-hour collected urine was 14.6 mL/min/1.73 m^2. The ultrasound showed bilateral small kidneys (length, left kidney 69 mm and right kidney 67 mm) and increased renal echogenicity. Thus, renal biopsy was not planned for the patient. Ophthalmological examination revealed bilateral diffuse choroidal and retinal atrophy, retinitis pigmentosa sine pigmento-retinal arteriolar attenuation, and peripapillary atrophy.

During follow-up, an irregular appearance in her fingers drew special attention. Radiographs of the upper and lower extremities revealed symmetrical shortening of the ulna in both forearms, shortening of all the phalanges, and widening of the proximal metaphyseal joints. On an x-ray of the coxofemoral joints, epiphyseal surface irregularities, especially those on the left, were observed.

Because the patient was accepted as having stage 5 chronic kidney disease, she was involved in a peritoneal dialysis program. Investigations for vesicoureteral reflux and other urological pathological conditions were normal. Following the peritoneal dialysis period for 3 months, she underwent renal transplantation from her mother.

What is the most likely diagnosis for this patient?

A. Mainzer-Saldino (conorenal) syndrome
B. Jeune syndrome

C. Senior-Loken syndrome
D. Familial brachydactyly

The correct answer is A

Comment: Taking into account the end-stage CKD, retinitis pigmentosa (RP), cone-shaped epiphyses (CSE), and coxofemoral findings, the most likely diagnosis is Mainzer-Saldino (conorenal) syndrome in our patient.[1,2] Genetic analysis to demonstrate an IFT140 or IFT172 mutation would be the next step to confirm the diagnosis.

Mainzer-Saldino syndrome (MSS) or conorenal syndrome is a rare autosomal recessive ciliopathy that is characterized by CSE, CKD, RP, and radiographic abnormalities of the proximal femur.[1–4] The clinical entity was first described in two siblings (a 14-year-old girl and a 10-year-old boy) in the same family. Both patients had nephropathy characterized by failure to concentrate and acidify the urine, suggesting a dysfunction in distal tubules and collecting ducts along with RP, CSE, and cerebellar ataxia. The younger patient had femoral neck abnormalities as well.[1,2]

In our patient, we have observed all of the four components. However, she never showed any sign of cerebral ataxia, and head circumference was normal. The most striking finding in MSS is the CSE, which is described as a projection of the distal surface of an epiphysis beyond the proximal border of its diaphysis.[2] The CSE in the feet, at the distal phalanx of the thumb or middle phalanx of the fifth finger of the hand is usually seen as variants of normal.[2] However, CSE located at the proximal phalanges or at the middle phalanges of fingers 3 and 4 of the hands are more likely to be associated with a malformation syndrome.[2] In our patient, CSE was observed in all phalanges of the hands. The CSE may be associated with many syndromes including trichorhinophalangeal syndrome, metaphyseal chondrodysplasias, and familial brachydactyly subtypes.[2] In combination with nephronophthisis, the CSE has been reported in asphyxiating thoracic dystrophy, also known as Jeune syndrome.[5] At the first admission of our patient, exclusion of urological problems, prominent short stature, and retinal findings were suggestive of Senior-Loken syndrome. However, because of end-stage kidney disease and renal atrophy, kidney biopsy could not be performed to show the findings of nephronophthisis. In addition, genetic analyses have not been conducted. When the CSE in the hands was realized in the follow-up, genetic testing was performed for MSS. Mutations in genes encoding intraflagellar transport complexes A (IFT-A) and B (IFT-B) proteins lead to ciliopathies, which are defined as a collection of complex developmental disorders of multiple organs and/or systems.[6] Skeletal ciliopathies were found to be associated with mutations in genes mostly encoding IFT-A, and rarely in those encoding IFT-B complexes.[6,7] MSS has been suggestive of a ciliopathy with regard to retinal dystrophy, nephronophthisis, and skeletal findings, and because of the transmission profile, an autosomal recessive inheritance was assumed. Initially, candidate genes for IFT-A and IFT-B complexes were defined and mutations in *IFT140* and *IFT172* were found in patients with MSS.[6,7] IFT140 is an IFT-A protein that regulates retrograde protein transport in ciliated cells.[7] IFT172 was found to be the only IFT-B protein shown to interact with IFT140 in mice[8] and is involved in an interaction between IFT-A and IFT-B subcomplexes.[6]

Clinical Presentation 41

A 10-year-old male child was referred by his primary care physician to the pediatric rheumatology clinic with long-standing albuminuria and a weakly positive ANA (enzyme-linked immunosorbent assay [ELISA]) as a suspected case of lupus nephritis. A brief febrile illness 3 years earlier had prompted a urine analysis, which documented moderate albuminuria (2+). Subsequently, his renal biochemistry was found to be normal and sonography revealed bilateral bulky kidneys. Varying but persistent albuminuria (2+ to 4+) was documented on subsequent urine examinations. He had received periodic high doses of steroids to no effect.

He was born to a nonconsanguineous marriage and had lost his mother when she was 33 years of age to an undiagnosed medical renal disease. His father had remarried, and his 2-year-old half-brother was well. His weight was 25.48 kg and his height was 134 cm. There was no edema, hypertension, clinical stigmata of lupus, or any syndromic features. Urine examination showed albuminuria (4+) devoid of RBCs or casts. Twenty-four-hour urinary protein was 4.6 g and the urinary protein electrophoresis showed a selective albumin band. BUN and creatinine were 8.8 and 0.4 mg/dL, respectively. Serum albumin and cholesterol were normal. Repeat ANA testing immunofluorescent (IF) was negative, and C3 and C4 were normal.

In view of the long-standing steroid-resistant proteinuria and family history of renal disease, a kidney biopsy was performed. Light microscopy revealed normocellular glomeruli showing mild mesangial widening and focal mild basement membrane thickening; on PAS stains Congo red stains were negative. Nonspecific, faint deposits of IgG, IgM, IgA, C3, and C1q were seen along the capillary loops, not conforming to any diagnostic pattern. Ultrastructure revealed bundles of banded collagen in the focally vacuolated lamina densa as has been described in nail-patella syndrome (NPS). The foot processes were focally obliterated. No electron-dense deposits were seen.

What is your diagnosis?

A. NPS
B. Alport syndrome
C. Congenital ectodermal defects
D. Pachyonychia congenital

The correct answer is A

Comment: In view of the findings of the kidney biopsy, the patient was clinically and radiologically reassessed for all the features of NPS. Nails were unremarkable; the patient had normal patellae, and no pelvic horns were seen radiologically. Other than mild pectus excavatum and bilateral in-turned fifth toes, there were no remarkable stigmata. Joint examination, especially of the elbows, was normal.

The normal glomerular basement membrane is composed of a triple helical molecule of type IV collagen showing sieve-like arrangements.[1] In NPS, abnormal banded collagen (type III) is detected in the lamina densa of the basement membranes.

Hereditary osteo-onycho-dysplasia or NPS is an autosomal dominant entity (OMIM 161200) characterized by absence of the patella, nail dystrophy, and renal abnormalities.[2] The renal abnormality is seen in 35% to 45% of cases. It may be a late manifestation and is responsible for the morbidity and mortality of this condition. The diagnostic morphologic features are noted only using EM.[3,4]

A few reported cases have renal features typical of this syndrome in isolation, without the nail and skeletal anomalies.[5] This entity has been called the nail-patella-like glomerulopathy (OMIM 256020).

The typical clinical presentation of nail-patella-like glomerulopathy is steroid-resistant proteinuria; hypertension is rarely associated with hematuria. Few patients present in renal failure and some progress to chronicity, suggesting a poorer prognosis. Light microscopy reveals nonspecific changes of focal and diffuse basement membrane thickening with mesangial widening. Immunofluorescence studies may be negative or show nonspecific deposits of granular IgM and C3. Both of these show no specific morphological changes, which may help establish the diagnosis. The diagnostic features are seen only with EM. These consist of lucent areas in the basement membrane with intramembranous inclusions of fibrillary collagen. The collagen may also be seen in the mesangium. The lamina densa is devoid of the basket-weave pattern or splitting or large vacuoles like those seen in Alport syndrome.

The only two conditions showing banded collagen in the basement membrane are NPS and nail-patella-like glomerulopathy. Banded collagen may be found in the other regions of the glomerulus (other than the basement membrane) in collagen fibrotic glomerulopathy. In fact, the lamina densa in cases of collagenofibrotic glomerulopathy are free of any collagen fibers. Rarely, very focal deposition of intramembranous collagen may be noted in advanced chronic glomerulopathies.

No specific treatment is available for NPS and nail-nail-patella-like glomerulopathy. The patients are managed only symptomatically. Patients of NPS treated with renal transplantation have not shown any recurrence of the disease.[5]

Clinical Presentation 42

A 2-day-old male neonate was born at 36 weeks' gestation. He was the second child of parents who reported no consanguinity. His twin sibling had died at 10 weeks of gestation. Weight, length, and head circumference at birth were 2090 g (<third percentile), 43 cm (<third percentile), and 31 cm (<third percentile), respectively. The Apgar score was 6, 8, 9 at 1, 5, and 10 minutes, respectively. Because of respiratory distress, the newborn was transferred to the neonatal intensive care unit.

On examinations, he had multiple petechiae, inverted nipples, and scrotal and penile edema. Facial dysmorphisms, such as a broad nasal bridge and distinctly low-set ears, as well as small eyes with pronounced hypertelorism, were present. The right foot presented as pes supinatus with digitus quintus subductus.

The patient suffered from congenital nephrotic syndrome (CNS) with generalized edema, severe proteinuria (645 mg/dL), hypoalbuminemia (20.6 g/L), and low serum IgG (on day 27: <40 mg/dL [normal range, 660–1750 mg/dL]). He was treated with daily protein substitutions (6 mL/kg human albumin 20%) and IgG substitutions. High blood pressure developed. Attempts to treat the CNS with corticoids were unsuccessful. Levels of thyroid hormones were normal at 14 days of age, but subsequently decreased: thyroid-stimulating hormone 0.44 (reference, 0.72–11.00) μU/mL, free T4 0.52 (reference, 0.89–2.20) ng/dL, and free T3 1.05 (reference, 1.95–6.04) pg/mL. Thrombocytes were low (70,000/μL). Seizures started at 52 days of age, and electroencephalography revealed a burst suppression pattern in the frontocentral region of the right hemisphere. Because of muscular hypotonia, a biopsy of the quadriceps femoris was performed, showing a predominance of type 2 muscle fibers (approximately 75% of all fibers) and relatively small type 1 muscle fibers (about 30% smaller than type 2 fibers). At 6 weeks of age, the patient developed pneumonia and sepsis. Anuria occurred, and the boy died from kidney and respiratory failure a week later.

What is your diagnosis?

A. *ALG1* gene mutation
B. *WT1* gene mutation
C. *PLCE1* gene mutation
D. *LAMB2* gene mutation
E. *NPHS2* gene mutation

The correct answer is A

Comment: CNS is usually caused by genetic defects affecting the glomerular filter. The most common defects are nephrin mutations, whereas defective *WT1*, *PLCE1*, *LAMB2*, or *NPHS2* gene products are less common.[1,2] Additionally, CNS has been described in association with metabolic diseases, such as respiratory chain deficiency.[3] Variants in integrin α3 (ITGA3) are known to cause lung disease in combination with nephrotic syndrome.[4] The most common nongenetic causes are infectious diseases, such as cytomegalovirus infection[5,6] and congenital syphilis.[7]

CNS can also occur in congenital disorders of glycosylation (CDG). So far, it has been described in the subtypes PMM2-CDG, ALG1-CDG, and various cases of CDG-x (i.e., cases in which the subtype has not been identified).

Taking the dysmorphic and multiorgan presentation of the described patient into account, the differential diagnosis in the presented case consists of mitochondrial cytopathy, CDG, and ITGA3 disease. The most likely option with regard to the typical dysmorphic presentation (i.e., inverted nipples and facial dysmorphisms) is CDG.

The analysis of serum transferrin is the primary diagnostic tool for cases with suspicion of CDG. This group of diseases affects the glycosylation process and is known to cause a great variety of symptoms in almost all organ systems. There are two distinct pathologic patterns: the type 1 pattern with a decreased tetrasialo-fraction and increased di- and asialo-transferrin fractions; and the type 2 pattern, which shows an additional increase in the mono- and/or trisialo-transferrin bands.[8]

Having obtained a pathological transferrin test, genetic analysis of the genes associated with CNS in CDG should be initiated. If this leads to no result, whole-exome sequencing is another option, which may facilitate the identification of the causative gene. However, this method has limitations, especially in consanguineous families where a vast number of variants and mutations is not unusual.

In the majority of cases, CNS is caused by underlying genetic defects leading to disruption of the glomerular filtration barrier resulting in proteinuria, hypoproteinemia, and generalized edema.[1,9,10] In the described patient, CNS was caused by a metabolic disease affecting the glycosylation of glycoproteins (ALG1-CDG). Sanger sequencing of the *ALG1* gene was performed and the patient was found to be homozygous for the mutation c.773C>T [S258L] in the *ALG1* gene (rs28939378),[11] which results in a defect of β1,4-mannosyltransferase. The parents were heterozygous for this mutation. Renal manifestations of CDG other than CNS are rare.

Clinical Presentation 43

A 17-year-old girl was referred for evaluation of proteinuria. A diagnosis of diabetes had been made 2 years earlier after a short history of polyuria, polydipsia, weight loss, and tiredness. A presumptive diagnosis of type 1 diabetes was made based on the short history, blood glucose concentration of 14.9 mmol/L, and significant ketosis at presentation. Diabetic control had been excellent, and in fact, the insulin dose had required reduction.

Six months after the diagnosis of diabetes, her urine was tested for protein as part of routine diabetes monitoring. Glycated hemoglobin (HbA1C) levels were low at 4.8% (29 mmol/mol). Early morning urine protein/creatinine ratios were 282, 268, and 170 mg/mmol. Plasma electrolytes, urea, creatinine, calcium, phosphate, and PTH levels were all normal, as were plasma complement C3 and C4 concentrations.

The past medical history was notable for poor stamina that had forced her to give up playing soccer several years previously. Since the onset of diabetes, she had begun to suffer from pain in the lower abdomen and knees. The symptoms were very distressing and interfered with sleep and socializing. She was seen by multiple specialists and had undergone numerous tests, including knee radiographs, abdominal magnetic resonance scans, and numerous blood tests. No diagnosis was made.

The patient was the younger of two children born to healthy, unrelated parents. There was no family history of diabetes, deafness, or renal disease. Her height was 145.3 cm (*Z* score −3.01) and her weight was 42.4 kg (*Z* score −2.25). There was no edema. Her systolic/diastolic BP was 98/68 mm Hg. Her abdomen was not distended and soft to palpation. There was generalized tenderness but no masses or peritonism. The rest of the examination was unremarkable.

Laboratory tests showed a normal full blood count and a slightly raised erythrocyte sedimentation rate of 28 mm/h, but a normal C-reactive protein concentration of <1 mg/L. The plasma creatinine was 0.9 mg/dL giving an estimated GFR of 86 mL/min/1.73 m^2. The urine protein/creatinine ratio was markedly elevated at 483 mg/mmol (normal, <23 mg/mmol; nephrotic range, >200 mg/ mmol), and the plasma albumin concentration was slightly reduced at 31 g/L. The HbA1C level was low at 34 mmol/mol and the C-peptide level was 1046 pmol/L. Tests for islet cell and glutamic acid decarboxylase antibodies were negative. Audiometry showed that the patient had normal hearing. The renal biopsy showed 40 glomeruli, of which 13 were globally sclerosed and five had segmental sclerosis. There was no nodular glomerulosclerosis and immunostaining was negative.

What is the diagnosis?

A. Analgesic nephropathy
B. Diabetic nephropathy
C. Alport syndrome
D. Hereditary nephrotic syndrome (NPHS) 1

The correct answer is D

Comment: In a patient with diabetes and proteinuria, the initial thought is often diabetic nephropathy. However, patients with diabetes are more likely to have conditions other than diabetic nephropathy.[1] This is particularly true in patients with short duration of diabetes and good metabolic control. Our patient has diabetes, which is somewhat atypical for type 1 diabetes with negative autoantibodies and an unusually very low HbA1C levels.[2] The renal biopsy showed FSGS, and she has other clinical features, including short stature, poor effort tolerance, and abdominal pain.

The patient had received large doses of analgesics, but the renal disease is unusual for analgesic nephropathy, which typically presents with papillary necrosis and reduced GFR. The association with drugs other than phenacetin remains speculative.[3] Finally, the patient could have two or more unrelated conditions. Therefore, it is appropriate to consider genetic causes of diabetes that may account for some or all of these features.

Genetic testing revealed a mutation in mitochondrial DNA, m.3243A>G, which is the most common cause of maternally inherited diabetes and deafness (MIDD), a mitochondrial disorder characterized by maternally transmitted diabetes and sensorineural deafness. She was also found to be heterozygous for a missense variant of NPHS1, c.2746G>T; p (Ala916Ser). The patient therefore has MIDD, and the renal disease may be aggravated by the *NPHS1* variant.

Maternally inherited diabetes and deafness has been previously reported.[4] It is caused in the great majority of cases by an adenine to guanine substitution at position 3243 of the mitochondrial DNA (m.3243A>G) encoding the gene for leucine transfer RNA. MIDD is frequently misdiagnosed as type 1 or type 2 diabetes, depending on the age of the patient and mode of presentation. Approximately 1% of cases of diabetes are thought to be caused by mutations in mitochondrial DNA, and the m.3243A>G mutation accounts for about 85% of these.[5] The key clinical features are diabetes and deafness and their presence in maternal relatives. As the case of our patient demonstrates, these are not always present. The diabetes usually presents insidiously, but in 20% of cases it presents acutely, with ketoacidosis present in 8% of the latter cases.[6] Approximately 75% of diabetic patients with the m.3243A>G mutation have deafness, which is sensorineural and the result of cochlear disease.[7] Renal disease is common in patients with MIDD, especially females. In one series of 74 patients with MIDD, proteinuria was greater in these patients than in control diabetic patients, and CKD stage 3 or greater was 4- to 6-fold higher despite lower HbA1C, lower blood pressure and a 3.7-fold lower incidence of diabetic retinopathy than controls.[8] The most common histological pattern in patients undergoing renal biopsy is FSGS, but tubulointerstitial disease and renal cysts have also been described. The combination of nephropathy and deafness may lead to a mistaken diagnosis of Alport syndrome.[9] Several other features present in this patient are also explained by the m.3243A>G mutation, including short stature, which is common and caused by a deficiency of growth hormone–releasing hormone.[10,11] Gastrointestinal complaints are also common, especially constipation and pseudoobstruction.[5] The inability to play competitive soccer likely reflects impaired energy utilization and skeletal myopathy. Cardiomyopathy, retinal macular dystrophy, and stroke, features not present in our patient, are also described. Our patient had early onset of several features. This is likely to reflect high levels of heteroplasmy for the mutant mitochondrial DNA. The severity and early onset of renal disease may also be due to the presence of a heterozygous mutation in *NPHS1*. This gene codes for nephrin, an important component of the glomerular slit diaphragm, and homozygous mutations cause Finnish type congenital nephrotic syndrome. A diagnosis of MIDD has several important implications for treatment. Metformin should not be used for treating the diabetes because of the increased risk of lactic acidosis. Antibiotics such as tetracyclines and chloramphenicol, which interfere with mitochondrial function, should also be avoided. Coenzyme Q10 has been shown to be beneficial in preventing hearing loss and delaying progression of diabetes.[12] In patients who progress to end-stage renal failure, great caution should be exercised in using maternal relatives as kidney donors.

Clinical Presentation 44

A 6-year-old boy was admitted to our clinic with a suspected diagnosis of an inborn error of metabolism (IEM). He was born at term with a birth weight of 3620 g with an uneventful delivery. He was the first child of nonconsanguineous parents, and his sibling was healthy. He presented with fever and proteinuria 9 months ago; hepatosplenomegaly and lymphocyte vacuolation on peripheral blood smear had been noticed incidentally. His motor and cognitive development was normal. He was investigated for a suspected metabolic disorder, mainly mucopolysaccharidosis and mucolipidosis. However, urine glycosaminoglycan level and enzyme screening for mucopolysaccharidosis and mucolipidosis were normal.

On admission, his weight was 17 kg (10th–25th percentile) and his height 106 cm (3rd–10th percentile). He had a mildly coarse face. The liver was 8 cm, and the spleen was 4 cm below the costal margin. Routine laboratory investigations showed mild anemia, elevated urea levels, and proteinuria. Results were as follows: WBCs 10,400/mm^3, hemoglobin 5.8 g/dL (11–14.5), mean corpuscular volume 71.9 fL (76.5–90.6), platelets 164,000/mm^3 (150–450), urea 45 mg/dL (11– 39), creatinine 1.32 mg/dL (0.5–1.2), iron 52 μg/dL (50–120), total iron binding capacity 274 ng/mL (110–370), AST 27 U/L (0–50), ALT 10 U/L (0–50), gamma glutamyl transferase 19 U/L (3–22), alkaline phosphatase 154 U/L (93–300), uric acid 2.1 mg/dL (3.5–7.2), total protein 5.6 g/dL (5.7–8), albumin 3.1 g/dL (3.8–5.4), and urinary protein 3+. Arterial BP results were normal.

Abdomen ultrasonography showed upper limit of normal liver size, splenomegaly, bilateral nephromegaly, and bilateral increased renal parenchyma echogenicity. Skeletal imaging revealed dysostosis multiplex. Ophthalmologic examination revealed cherry-red spot. Chitotriosidase level was found highly elevated at the 5731 nmol/h/mL (0–90) level. Bone marrow aspiration showed foamy cells indicating a storage disease. Leukocyte cystine content, glucocerebrosidase, and sphingomyelinase enzyme levels were normal. Twenty-four-hour urine protein level was 203 mg/m^2/h and exhibited nephrotic range proteinuria. Erythropoietin and calcitriol treatments were commenced.

Kidney biopsy showed diffuse cytoplasmic vacuolization of tubular epithelial cells and glomerular sclerosis and segmental and global sclerosis.

What is your diagnosis?

A. Nephrosialidosis
B. Hurler syndrome
C. Tyrosinosis
D. Cystinuria
E. Sialidosis

The correct answer is E

Comment: Sialidosis is a rare lysosomal storage disorder characterized by neuraminidase deficiency leading to proteinuria and kidney failure.[1] Sialidosis may involve almost all organs and systems, either as a part of a systemic clinical picture or individually. The kidney is one of the target organs for inherited metabolic disorders, and a variety of IEMs present with different types of kidney disorders. Fanconi syndrome, proteinuria, renal tubular acidosis, nephrolithiasis, kidney cysts, acute kidney injury, and chronic kidney disease can be clinical manifestations of IEMs. Specific patterns of kidney involvement could be indicative of an underlying IEM. Kidney failure is a well-defined severe morbidity in Fabry disease, primary hyperoxaluria, cystinosis, and methylmalonic acidemia. Nephrosialidosis is a very rare subgroup of the lysosomal storage disorders leading to proteinuria and kidney failure.[1] The patient has a life-limiting inherited metabolic disease and kidney failure because of this disorder. Genetic counseling and information about the condition should be given to the parents. To date, the age of symptom onset in all cases is before 2 years of age, and most patients have died before age 10 years. Our patient became dialysis-dependent at 8 years of age. In comparison with other cases reported before, the mild clinical phenotype in our patient may be associated with compound heterozygosity. It is difficult to say anything definite about the prognosis in this case.

It is caused by mutations in the *NEU1* gene on chromosome 6p21.[2] Neuraminidase deficiency affects glycoprotein degradation and leads to abnormal accumulation of sialyl oligosaccharides and glycoproteins. Sialidosis is divided into two groups: type 1 and type 2. Clinical severity is heterogeneous depending on the residual enzyme activity. Type 1 sialidosis is the milder form and usually presents in the second decade with neurological findings. Type 2 presents with earlier onset and mucopolysaccharide-like phenotype with dysostosis multiplex and organomegaly. Rarely, type 2 may affect the kidneys and lead to proteinuria progressing to nephrotic syndrome and chronic kidney disease.

Clinical Presentation 45

A 4-year-old healthy girl presented with anasarca of 2 days and a sudden onset of abdominal pain. Vital signs including BP at admission were normal. Abdominal tenderness and moderate edema of the eyelids and legs were revealed on physical examination. Her medical history did not include arthralgia or exanthema including purpura. Laboratory tests following admission were WBCs 10,500/mm^3, hemoglobin 13.4 g/dL, platelets 104,000/mm^3, serum total protein 4.3 g/dL, albumin 0.9 g/ dL, creatinine (Cr) 0.24 mg/dL, and IgG 733 mg/dL. C3 (145 mg/dL), C4 (41 mg/dL), and CH50 (40.7 U/mL) were all in the normal range. The urine protein to Cr ratio (Up/Cr) was 19.40 g/gCr, and the urine sediment revealed more than 100 red blood cells per HPF. The antinuclear antibodies (ANA: 1>1:160), anti-double-stranded DNA antibodies (19 IU/mL), and anti-SSA antibodies (64 times) were positive, but anti-SSB antibodies and rheumatoid factor were negative. Other serological markers including the hepatitis B and C antibodies, antineutrophil cytoplasmic antibodies, anti-glomerular basement membrane antibodies, anti-cardiolipin beta-2-glycoprotein 1 antibodies, anti-phospholipid antibodies, and lupus anticoagulant were negative. The abdominal ultrasonography findings were also normal.

A kidney biopsy was performed. Light microscopy revealed thickening of the glomerular capillary loops and mild mesangial proliferation. The tubulointerstitium was infiltrated by lymphocytes and plasma cells. Immunofluorescence examinations revealed IgG (2+), IgA (2+), C4d (2+), and C3 (1+) deposits along the capillary wall and IgM (1+) and C1q (1+) deposits in the mesangial region. EM revealed diffuse epithelial foot process effacement and electron dense deposits in the subepithelial and mesangial regions. Continuous administration of albumin improved abdominal manifestation. A dose of 60 mg/m^2 body surface area per day of prednisolone (PSL) was initiated after the pathological findings were revealed, making it possible to discontinue administration of albumin. However, nephrotic range proteinuria and hypoalbuminemia persisted even after 4 weeks of PSL administration. Cyclosporine A (CsA) and lisinopril were simultaneously instituted, and the urinary protein gradually decreased with these treatments. Sudden onset of mild intermittent back pain was observed 2 weeks after concomitant administration of immunosuppressive drugs, and close monitoring revealed tachycardia at standing or sitting in the morning. Her vital signs were body temperature, 36.8°C; oxygen saturation, 96% (room air); respiratory rate, 20 breaths/min; BP, 105/72 mm Hg; and heart rate, 110 beats/min at rest and 160 beats/min at waking up.

The laboratory tests at this point were WBCs $11.6 \times 10^3/\mu L$; hemoglobin 14.6 g/dL; platelets $117 \times 10^3/\mu L$; CRP 0.08 mg/dL; albumin 1.5 g/dL; Cr 0.14 mg/dL; total cholesterol 469 mg/dL; amylase 66 U/L; IgG 388 mg/dL; and Up/Cr 5.25 g/gCr.

What is the likely diagnosis of the kidney disease?

A. Sjögren syndrome
B. Hepatitis C
C. Lupus nephritis
D. Malignancy

The correct answer is C

Comment: The pathological features of the glomerular capillary loop thickening and subepithelial deposits of immune complexes typically indicate membranous nephropathy (MN). Inflammatory cell infiltration into the interstitium and mesangial deposits on EM are suggestive of secondary MN. IgG subclass staining revealed codominance of IgG1 and IgG2, and the M-type phospholipase A2 receptor staining was negative in her glomeruli, which also supported the diagnosis of secondary MN. The positive findings of ANA and anti-double-stranded DNA antibodies and the nephritis on kidney biopsy were consistent with SLE, according to the criteria of the Systemic Lupus International Collaborating Clinics,[1] despite the patient being very young to be diagnosed with SLE and demonstrated no physical findings of SLE except for nephritis. No symptoms associated with lacrimal gland or salivary gland, suggestive of Sjögren syndrome, were found. No other cause of secondary MN was obvious during the follow-up.

Patients with nephrotic syndrome (NS) are at an increased risk of various complications including infections, kidney dysfunction, and thromboembolism (TE).[2] Our patient was afebrile, and no inflammatory reaction or kidney dysfunction was observed on laboratory examinations. TE in patients with NS can occur in the renal vein or pulmonary artery, which can cause back and chest pain. Coagulation investigations and imaging findings such as ultrasonography (US) and contrast-enhanced CT are useful in the evaluation of thrombus formation. Lung perfusion scintigraphy could reveal the presence of pulmonary embolism (PE). The coagulation tests performed in this case were prothrombin time-international normalized ratio (PT-INR), 0.86; D-dimer, 11.8 μg/mL; fibrinogen, 233 mg/dL; and antithrombin III, 124.6%. Her activated protein C and protein S were normal. Her US and contrast-enhanced CT revealed a thrombus extending from the bilateral renal vein branch to the vicinity of the right atrium, and blood flow in the inferior vena cava (IVC) could not be confirmed using color Doppler US. Lung perfusion scintigraphy revealed decreased perfusion segmentally in the pleural lobes of both lungs, indicating multiple bilateral microemboli. The PE and TE in the renal vein and IVC were responsible for the tachycardia and back pain, respectively; decline of the venous return caused by IVC thrombus could have induced tachycardia during standing or sitting in the morning.

Heparin was administered as anticoagulant therapy with activated partial thromboplastin time to 60 to 80 seconds and was subsequently replaced by warfarin. The dose of warfarin was adjusted with PT-INR value between 2.0 and 3.0. After the initiation of the anticoagulant therapy, US revealed shrinking of the thrombi in the IVC and renal vein over time, followed by a dramatic improvement in tachycardia and back pain. Two months after the anticoagulant therapy, US and contrast-enhanced CT demonstrated the IVC and renal vein without evidence of residual thrombus, and lung perfusion scintigraphy showed normal findings. Complete remission was achieved 4 months after the initiation of CyA and lisinopril. The remission was maintained with the administration of CyA, lisinopril, and PSL (15 mg/m^2 BSA) every other day. No recurrence of thrombosis was observed, continuing warfarin with PT-INR value between 1.5 and 2.0.

Patients with NS can have various complications, of which TE is one of the most serious severe.[3] The development of NS-related TE has been attributed to the urinary loss of fibrinolytic and anticoagulant proteins, such as antithrombin III and protein S, and increased platelet aggregation and fibrinogen levels.[4,5] Other intrinsic and extrinsic factors including hemoconcentration, hyperlipidemia, dehydration, immobilization, intravascular catheter placement, and medications such as corticosteroids and diuretics have also been indirectly associated with thrombus formation in NS.[3,6,7] The incidence of TE in adults with NS is reported as approximately 25%.[8,9] Therefore, TE can always be assumed as a possible complication in adult patients with NS. In contrast, the incidence of TE in childhood NS has been reported as 2% to 9.2%,[6,8,9] which is less frequent than in adults. Age older than 12 years at onset has been a significant independent predictor of TE in children,[8] suggesting that younger children are at a much lower risk of TE. These differences have been proposed to be attributed to several protective mechanisms against TE in children, including a reduced capacity to produce thrombin, an increased capacity of alpha-2 macroglobulin to inhibit thrombin, and enhanced antithrombotic capacity by the vessel wall.[10] Membranous histology of MN and SLE class V is the greatest risk for TE in both adults and children,[8,11] although the mechanism is not yet clear. MN is a rare underlying cause of NS in children,[12] which may contribute to the low frequency of TE. Responsiveness to steroids has also been implicated in the risk of developing NS-associated TE, with steroid-resistant NS being of a higher risk than steroid-sensitive NS.[13] Consequently, although there are few reports of TE in younger children, our patient would have been at a relatively high risk of TE, considering the features of histology and steroid responsiveness. In cases with a higher risk of TE resulting from NS, the disease is most frequently seen in the veins of the lower extremities[8] but is also common in the renal veins and pulmonary arteries,[14,15] of which PE can be the most potentially life-threatening. Accordingly, back pain, gross hematuria, impaired kidney function, chest pain, hypoxia, and dyspnea are well known as the main symptoms of TE. However, it is often overlooked that these symptoms are usually too subtle to trigger a diagnosis of TE, and occasionally the patients are even asymptomatic. In a review of 74 cases with renal vein thrombosis in adults with NS, asymptomatic patients outnumbered the symptomatic patients.[16] Another report indicated that 84% of NS patients with PE were asymptomatic.[17] Similarly, in our case, despite the large thrombi in the IVC and renal veins and multiple PE, the symptoms suggestive of TE or PE were mild during the course of the disease. TE may not be uncommon in childhood NS because it has simply been previously undetected. Thus, in pediatric patients as well as adults with NS, the development of NS-related TE should be carefully considered, regardless of the underlying disease.

Contrast-enhanced CT and scintigraphy, which can reliably detect TE, cannot be routinely performed in children because of the need for sedation, radiological exposure, and cost effectiveness. It is essential to identify children with NS at higher risk for TE and then proceed with more sensitive imaging studies in them. A previous report showed that as many as 30% of childhood NS patients with hemoglobin >16 g/dL, fibrinogen >400 mg/L, and serum total cholesterol >10 mmol/L had PE and TE in renal veins,[18] indicating that a severe hypercoagulable state can be a risk. Additionally, an albumin level <2.8 g/dL, and severity of proteinuria were also suggested as risk factors for TE[9,19] in addition to age, histology, and steroid responsiveness as mentioned before. The close association between NS-related PE and D-dimer has been demonstrated, with a cumulative probability of PE in patients with NS of approximately 90% when D-dimer >8.9 mg/L was reached.[20] US has also yielded promising results in the diagnosis of renal vein thrombosis.[21] In our case, coagulation tests and abdominal US without overlooking mild symptoms led to more sensitive imaging studies of contrast-enhanced CT and lung perfusion scintigraphy, resulting in TE and PE detection.

Prophylactic anticoagulant therapy to prevent NS-related thrombosis in childhood NS has not been clearly established because of the lack of large and prospective RCTs to confirm the safety and efficacy of the therapy. International guidelines suggest NS patients with prominent hypoalbuminemia (<2.5 g/dL) and additional risks for TE should be considered for prophylactic anticoagulation with warfarin.[22] However, prophylactic anticoagulation may be associated with an increased risk of bleeding events,[23,24] and warfarin can also be associated with kidney injury.[25,26] The timing of initiation or resumption of prophylactic anticoagulation would be hesitant in view of a kidney biopsy. Considering the underlying disease in our case, it would also be possible that we could have considered ways to introduce immunosuppressive agents other than steroids at an earlier stage for faster remission. Prophylactic anticoagulation could have been initiated, given the risk of TE in our case. However, the decision of prophylactic anticoagulation is always challenging because the expected benefits and adverse events must be carefully examined, considering the backgrounds of each patient, including the age and activity level, as well as the risk of developing TE. In the future, large and prospective randomized control trials on prophylactic anticoagulation for NS-related TE in children are expected to be conducted.

TE in pediatric NS is truly an "old and new" complication, although TE is a well-known complication of NS, the evidence on its prevention and treatment is sparse, especially in children. It should always be kept in mind that patients with NS can develop TE and PE, even younger children, and that the symptoms of NS-related TE are mild or often asymptomatic. Even for asymptomatic patients, routine noninvasive tests such as US and coagulation tests can lead to the detection of TE and PE. The treatment strategy for prophylactic anticoagulation in patients with NS should be determined by carefully examining each case for the risk of developing TE and the expected benefits and adverse events of this treatment.

Clinical Presentation 46

A previously healthy 13-year-old girl was admitted with 1 day of fever; temperature maximum 105°F (40°C); vomiting; pain in the ankles, wrists, and proximal right metacarpophalangeal joints; and a rash on the palms, soles, and distal legs. She did not give a history of sore throat, headache, visual changes, vaginal discharge, dysuria, urinary urgency or frequency, or any drug intake. She had unprotected sex with two male partners 1 month prior.

At admission, she had a temperature of 102.5°F (39.1°C), heart rate 110 beats/min, BP 95/65 mm Hg, capillary refill <2 seconds. She had painful petechiae over the palms, soles, and lower legs, moderate swelling of both ankle joints, and erythema and tenderness of the dorsum of the right foot attributed to acute tenosynovitis. She had no periorbital or pedal edema, no pharyngitis, no cervical lymphadenopathy, and no perianal or genital lesions.

Initial laboratory tests included hematocrit 31%, WBC 30,000/mm^3, with 65% neutrophils and 24% immature neutrophils, C-reactive protein 180 mg/L, erythrocyte sedimentation rate 64 mm/hour. Urinalysis showed protein 100 mg/dL, 41 red blood cells/HPF, >182 WBC/HPF, and 4+ WBC clumps. Blood chemistries showed serum creatinine 2.9 mg/dL, BUN 39 mg/dL, serum albumin 3.5 g/dL, normal electrolytes and liver enzymes, complement C3 12 (70–225) mg/dL, C4 14 (14–55) mg/dL, anti-nuclear antibody positive 1:320 titer with homogenous pattern; and negative antimyeloperoxidase, antiproteinase-3, and anti-DNA antibodies. A rapid streptococcal antigen test from a throat swab was negative.

She was started on vancomycin and ceftriaxone for presumed bacterial sepsis and doxycycline for possible tickborne infection.

On hospital day 2, she became hypotensive with oliguria and required vasopressor support with dopamine despite infusion of 4 L of normal saline (0.9%). Urine PCR was positive for

Neisseria gonorrhoeae DNA. Testing for other sexually transmitted infections was done and was unremarkable for syphilis, hepatitis C, or HIV. She was immune to hepatitis B with presence of hepatitis B surface antibody. There was no growth of bacteria on blood or urine culture. An echocardiogram was normal with no evidence of vegetations.

On hospital day 3, her blood pressure stabilized, fever defervesced, ankle pain improved, and serum creatinine decreased to 1.2 mg/dL, but she manifested fluid overload with anasarca and dyspnea requiring supplemental oxygen. The latter resolved with diuretic therapy. The renal and pelvic US examination showed no evidence of pelvic inflammatory disease or abscess.

On day 5, serum creatinine increased to 2.3 mg/dL despite normal BP and perfusion. Urinalysis showed protein 300 mg/dL and several RBCs, and mixed cellular casts and urine protein/creatinine ratio was 1.1 mg/mg (normal, <0.2). Antistreptolysin titer was 860 Todd units/mL (<330) and anti-DNAse B was <250 U/mL (<310 U/mL). Serum complement levels were as follows: C3 6 mg/dL (83–177), C4 9 mg/dL (15–45), CH50 10 (40–62) U/mL, C5 3 (7–20) mg/dL, C6 36.3 (28–69) μg/mL, C7 56.4 (35.3–96.5) μg/mL, C8 43 (49–106) μg/mL, and C9 71.3 (33–95) μg/mL. Serum parvovirus IgM was not sent because the rash was petechial and purpuric rather than typical malar or reticulated erythema seen with parvovirus. Also, given the abrupt onset of clinical symptomatology and absence of any identifiable chronic infection or chronic autoimmune condition, the index of suspicion for cryoglobulinemia was low, and cryoglobulin testing was not done.

On day 6, serum creatinine was 2.7 mg/dL, serum albumin 2.6 g/dL, and cholesterol 116 mg/dL. She never manifested nephrotic range proteinuria, and thus the low serum albumin was attributed to hemodilution associated with fluid retention and protein catabolism.

A renal biopsy was performed. All 19 glomeruli sampled for light microscopy showed diffuse and global severe endocapillary proliferative and exudative glomerulonephritis with many infiltrating neutrophils. Patchy interstitial inflammation and oedema occupied 15% to 20% of the cortical parenchyma. Focal RBC and WBC casts were seen. Immunofluorescence microscopy of 5 glomeruli showed dominant 2 to 3+ granular deposits of C3 involving the glomerular capillary walls and mesangium in a "starry sky" pattern with 1 to 2+ IgG, negative IgM, trace to 1+ IgA, and trace sparse C1q. Electron microscopy performed on five glomeruli showed marked diffuse and global proliferation of mesangial and endothelial cells, numerous infiltrating neutrophils, abundant subepithelial hump-shaped electron-dense deposits without spike formation, and scattered small segmental mesangial and subendothelial electron-dense deposits.

She received intravenous ceftriaxone for 10 days, oral doxycycline for 7 days, amlodipine 5 mg daily for 3 weeks for hypertension, and enalapril 10 mg daily for 16 months. Serum C4 normalized 10 days after admission and C3, C5, and C8 values returned to normal 5 weeks after admission. Serum creatinine improved to 0.7 mg/dL 6 weeks after admission. The urine protein/creatinine ratio was 0.3 to 0.36 for the next 6 months and has been stable around 0.22 g thereafter. Urinalysis 16 months after disease onset showed 100 mg/dL protein and 1 to 3 RBC/HPF.

What is your diagnosis?

A. Postinfectious GN
B. Membranoproliferative GN
C. Lupus nephritis
D. Cryoglobulinemia

The correct answer is A

Comment: Our patient presented with hypocomplementemic acute nephritic syndrome including reduced GFR, fluid overload, hematuria, leukocyturia, and proteinuria. Although the serum creatinine improved transiently with hemodynamic support, she subsequently manifested significant but nonnephrotic range proteinuria, further decrease in GFR, and anasarca from fluid retention, reflecting an evolving glomerulonephritis temporally associated with active systemic infection. The kidney biopsy findings of diffuse proliferative glomerulonephritis with many infiltrating neutrophils and hump-shaped subepithelial immune complex deposits of IgG and C3 resemble the changes seen in acute poststreptococcal glomerulonephritis. The patient, however, did not have any preceding sore throat or impetigo. A rapid streptococcal antigen test was negative at presentation; therefore, no throat culture was obtained. An elevated streptolysin titer together with a normal anti-DNase B level is a discordant antibody response. This serology in the setting of lack of preceding or current pharyngitis or skin infection provides evidence against a bona fide streptococcal infection.

Our patient presented with signs and symptoms consistent with disseminated gonococcal infection including fever, vasculitic petechia, tenosynovitis, arthralgias, and arthritis.[1–3] Gonococcal DNA was detected in urine by PCR.

The most common presentation of sexually transmitted *N. gonorrhoeae* infection is cervicitis in women and urethritis in men.[4] A history of recent symptomatic genital infection is uncommon in patients with disseminated gonococcal infection. The latter condition generally presents with abrupt onset of malaise, tenosynovitis, skin lesions of hemorrhagic macules, pustules or vesicles, polyarthralgia, and asymmetric polyarthritis. The skin lesions generally involve distal extremities and are often transient, as in our case.[5] The risk of dissemination probably depends on microbial virulence as well as host immune factors.

In disseminated gonococcal infection, the blood culture is positive in fewer than half of cases and the skin culture is positive in 10% to 15% of cases. This is due to the fastidious nature of *N. gonorrhoeae,* as its viability is dependent on proper transport in a humid and carbon dioxide–rich atmosphere, as well as the proper use of chocolate blood agar for culture. By contrast, *N. gonorrhoeae* can be isolated from a mucosal site in about 80% of cases, as occurred in our patient.[6]

Deficiencies in the complement system have been associated with disseminated disease.[7,8] Our patient had low C3, C4, C5, and C8 levels during the acute illness, but they normalized within 5 weeks, providing evidence against congenital complement deficiency and supporting active complement consumption associated with acute nephritis.

Most patients with poststreptococcal glomerulonephritis show only low serum C3, reflecting activation of the alternative complement pathway, whereas only a minority of patients also have low C4. Our patient had decreases in both C3 and C4. The C4 value returned to normal within 10 days, whereas the C3 value normalized later at 5 weeks, suggesting possible involvement of both the classical and alternative pathways of complement. In a recent study of acute infection-related glomerulonephritis, one-third of patients showed both low C3 and C4 levels[7] similar to the findings in our patient.

Clinical Presentation 47

A 4-month-old male infant was born to healthy, unrelated parents, at 39 weeks of gestation, weighing 4160 g. The pregnancy was uneventful. His 3.5-year-old sister had a history of allergy to eggs and had been treated for many otitis media infections. The mother's second pregnancy ended with spontaneous abortion in the first trimester. The mother had a microhematuria of unknown cause.

The infant was evaluated at the age of 6 weeks because of a rash and suspected allergy to milk. The rash subsided when the mother, who was breastfeeding him, went on a milk-free diet. He was otherwise healthy until the day after his first vaccination against diphtheria, tetanus, pertussis, poliomyelitis, *Hemophilus influenza* type B, and *Pneumococcus* when he was 3 months old.

The infant became febrile for 3 days starting from the day after vaccination, was well again for another 14 days, and then suddenly presented with macrohematuria and mild periorbital edema. He was sent for evaluation to our department. The physician did not see him when he was febrile, so there were no firm data regarding the cause of the fever. Theoretically, this may have been the case of infection or nonspecific fever after vaccination.

At admission, he looked well although somewhat irritable with no signs of respiratory tract infection, no skin rash, and with mild periorbital edema. He was very well grown, with weight of 7900 g (81st percentile) and height of 68 cm (95th percentile). BP was normal at 82/55 mm Hg, with pulse around 138/min. Physical examination of his heart, lung, abdomen, and extremities showed normal results. Peripheral pulses were palpable.

At admission, laboratory studies revealed macrohematuria and nephrotic range proteinuria (protein/creatinine was 4104 g/mol), mild hypoalbuminemia 3.0 g/dL, and elevated serum urea 34 mg/dL and creatinine 0.9 mg/dL with estimated GFR 31 mL/min/1.73 m^2). Immunoglobulin levels were as follows: IgE 13 kU/L (reference range, 0–13 kU/L), IgG 5.72, IgA 0.52, and IgM 2.0 g/L (reference range for IgG, 2.41–6.13, IgA 0.1–0.46, IgM 0.26–0.6 g/L), whereas antistreptolysin 0 level was 54 IU/mL (reference range, 0–170 IU/mL). Kidneys were of normal shape and size but hyperechoic on ultrasound. Total hemolytic complement activity was very low (alternative pathway 40 IU, reference range, 40–120 IU; classical pathway 9%, reference range, 72–128%). C3 component was only mildly decreased (851 mg/L; reference range, 970–1576 mg/L), whereas concentrations of all other complement components were within the reference range, except for C2 component, which was extremely low (1.72 mg/L; reference range, 14–25 mg/L). C5-9 lytic complex was elevated in urine (424 µg/L; reference value, <30 µg/L) and in plasma it was within the reference range (303 µg/L; reference range, 300–350 µg/L). Antiextractable nuclear antigen, antinuclear antibodies, anti-double-stranded DNA antibodies, anticardiolipin antibodies, anti-beta2-glycoprotein I antibodies, antibodies against C1q, and antineutrophil cytoplasmic antibodies were negative.

On the basis of physical examination and the results of basic laboratory tests, the diagnosis of nephritic syndrome, postvaccination, was suspected, despite very low C2 complement. A renal biopsy was performed, which showed a diffuse, nonuniform endoproliferative (20/25, 80%), mesangioproliferative (5/25, 20%), and extracapillary crescentic (6/25, 24%) glomerulonephritis. Extensive focal (40–50%) active mixcellular tubulointerstitial nephritis was also found. Immunofluorescence analysis showed IgA stained ++, IgG+, IgM+, kappa and lambda+, C3++, C1q+, and fibrin/fibrinogen+. Deposits, mostly IgA and C3, were located in the glomerular capillary wall and in the mesangium. Electron microscopy showed that deposits were mesangial and subepithelial in cases when they did not form characteristic humps. It was concluded that this was an immune complex–mediated GN, most probably an atypical postinfectious GN (postvaccine GN) with predominant IgA and C3 deposits in immune-complexes and no humps on electron microscopy. The composition of immune deposits described in our patient could also be found in IgA GN or HSP, but the clinical course of our patient excluded these two conditions with great probability.

The patient was treated with three pulses of methylprednisolone (10 mg/kg) for 3 consecutive days, followed by 1 mg/kg of methylprednisolone daily for 6 weeks. Thereafter, the steroids were tapered gradually and withdrawn completely in a 4-month period. He went into complete remission after 6 weeks of treatment and, at the moment of writing of this report, had been off all treatment for 4 months and was doing fine. He had normal renal function, normal BP, no proteinuria or hematuria, normal kidney US, but had persistently decreased total hemolytic complement activity (alternative pathway 41 IU, reference range, 40–120 IU; classical pathway 7%; reference range, 72–128%). C3 component and C5-9 lytic complex in urine normalized, whereas C2 component stayed low (3.16 mg/L; reference range, 14–25 mg/L).

What is your diagnosis?

A. IgA nephropathy
B. Hereditary C2 complement deficiency GN
C. HSP
D. Membranoproliferative GN

The correct answer is B

Comment: Our patient was simultaneously vaccinated against diphtheria, tetanus, pertussis, polio, *Hemophilus influenza* type B, and *Pneumococcus*. Eighteen days after vaccination, he presented with clinical and laboratory signs of nephritic syndrome. Immune complex–mediated GN was histologically confirmed with predominant IgA and C3 deposits in immune complexes and no humps on electron microscopy. Specific antigens in glomerular immune complexes in glomerular immune complexes proved that the boy had formed specific antibodies in protective titers against all the received vaccines.

Genetic testing revealed two heterozygous mutations on gene for C2 component. The first one was 28-base pair deletion of genomic DNA, which results in a premature termination of transcription. The second was a missense mutation that changes glutamate into aspartate at position 298. The same mutations were found also in his older sister, whereas the parents refused to be tested, establishing the diagnosis of hereditary C2 complement GN.

Genetically determined C2 deficiency is the most common of inherited complement deficiencies. Homozygous or complete C2 deficiency can present with a variety of symptoms, from asymptomatic state to systemic lupus erythematosus-like illness, polymyositis, glomerulonephritis, Hodgkin lymphoma, vasculitis, HSP, and recurrent pyogenic infections with encapsulated bacteria, such as *Streptococcus pneumoniae*, *Haemophilus influenza* type b, and *Neisseria meningitides*. Patients may also have a combination of multiple autoimmune phenomena, especially various cutaneous manifestations and pyogenic infections.[1–3] On the other hand, in most individuals, partial C2 deficiency has no clinical importance.[2,4,5]

Development of GN after vaccination has been reported earlier but as a very rare event and never in a patient with C2 deficiency. Postvaccine GN can present with a variety of clinical and histological pictures. It has been described after hyperimmunization with pertussis vaccine as a diffuse vasculitis and death,[6] after influenza H1N1 vaccination as a membranous GN,[7] after hepatitis B vaccine as a vaccine-related SLE,[8] and after pneumococcal vaccination as a crescentic GN from anti-glomerular basement membrane disease.[9] Nephrotic syndrome has been described after measles vaccination[10] and after antirabies vaccine.[5]

There was a question about the patient's further vaccination. Because approximately 50% of C2-deficient patients have an increased susceptibility to bloodborne infections caused by encapsulated organisms (e.g., pneumococcus, *H. influenza*, and meningococcus), vaccination represents a treatment of choice against sepsis, meningitis, arthritis, and osteomyelitis.[7–9] On the other hand, they are at increased risk of developing SLE, glomerulonephritis, inflammatory bowel disease, dermatomyositis, anaphylactoid purpura, and vasculitis,[7–9] with all these conditions being possibly triggered by environmental factors like infection or vaccination.

Clinical Presentation 48

A 19-year-old girl presented with generalized weakness, loss of appetite, frothy urine, gradual decrease in urine output followed by facial puffiness, and bipedal edema for the past 1 month. She was having pain in the epigastric region and recurrent vomiting for the past 1 week. The patient had no history of significant medical or surgical illness except hypothyroidism, for which she was on thyroxine supplementation (levothyroxine 150 μg/day) for the past 12 months. On systemic evaluation, she was found to have hypertension, anemia, and bipedal edema. Initial laboratory evaluations revealed BUN 265 mg/dL, serum creatinine 11.4 mg/dL, and hemoglobin (Hb) 9 g/dL. Urinalysis showed 2+ proteinuria and 10 to 15 RBCs per HPF. Urinary albumin creatinine ratio was 5.8. She was managed with hemodialysis and blood transfusions. As the presentation was suggestive of rapidly progressive glomerulonephritis (RPGN), serological tests including ANA, antistreptolysin O, serum complements C3 and C4, antineutrophilic cytoplasmic antibodies (ANCA), extractable nuclear antibody (ENA), hepatitis C, hepatitis B, HIV, anti-GBM antibody, and cryoglobulins were done and found to be negative. Renal US evaluation revealed a slightly larger kidney size with increased echogenicity and no evidence of renal artery stenosis on the Doppler study. Kidney biopsy was done and the tissue sample was sent for light microscopy, immunofluorescence, and electron microscopic study. Light microscopy revealed cellular crescents in all nine glomeruli. The underlying tufts were markedly compressed and exhibited an irregular increase in mesangial matrix and cellularity with focal neutrophil infiltration, whereas there was no evidence of tuft necrosis. The mesangial areas were periodic acid–Schiff positive. Tubular atrophy and interstitial fibrosis involved about 40% of sampled cortical parenchyma. Tubules showed cytoplasmic vacuolar changes and severe acute tubular injury. Immunofluorescence (IF) showed confluent staining along mesangial and capillary walls of IgG (3+) and C3 (2+), whereas IgA, IgM, and C1q were negative. Staining for lambda was 3+, whereas kappa (k) was negative. Electron microscopy showed widespread foot process effacement. There was the expansion of mesangial and few subendothelial regions, which were occupied by aggregates of nonbranching, randomly oriented fibrillary structures measuring from 13.1 to 29.6 nm (mean fibril diameter, 21.3 nm). Conventional immune complex type electron-dense deposits were not identified. Tubuloreticular inclusions were not seen in the endothelial cell cytoplasm of glomerular or peritubular capillaries. Because the patient's age and presentations were not typical of fibrillary glomerulonephritis (FGN), serum protein electrophoresis and serum-free light chain assay were done to evaluate monoclonal gammopathy; both were negative. Further immunohistochemical staining with DNAJB9 was done, which showed intense (3+) positivity along the glomerular mesangial areas and capillaries. Thus, renal biopsy finding was consistent with the diagnosis of crescentic fibrillary glomerulonephritis (CFGN) showing monotypic IgG lambda type deposits.

After initial reporting of crescentic GN in biopsy, intravenous methylprednisolone 500 mg was given for 3 days followed by oral prednisolone 1 mg/kg/day and oral cyclophosphamide with dose adjustment. After confirmation of diagnosis as crescentic CFGN, we continued the same immunosuppressive treatment. As patient remained oliguric and continued to be dialysis-dependent even after 2 months of treatment, immunosuppressive drugs were withdrawn and supportive treatment was continued as for ESRD.

How do you treat this patient?

A. Steroid alone
B. Combination of steroid and cyclophosphamide
C. Combination of steroid and rituximab
D. There is no consensus on the optimal treatment of CFGN because of the paucity of clinical data.

The correct answer is D

Comment: CFGN is uncommon and carries the worst prognosis among FGN.[1] Without electron microscopic study, CFGN is likely to remain undiagnosed. Electron microscopy and special immunohistochemical stains play a significant role in the diagnosis of rare glomerular diseases, especially deposition diseases. CFGN usually does not respond to available therapy and mostly progresses to ERSD. There is no consensus on the optimal treatment of fibrillary glomerulonephritis because of the paucity of clinical data.

FGN presents most commonly in five patterns in light microscopic evaluation. These are membranoproliferative, mesangial proliferative, membranous, diffuse proliferative, and diffuse global sclerosis pattern. Although uncommon, CFGN may present as crescentic GN as in this case. Prognosis is directly related to the histological pattern of the disease. The mesangial proliferative and membranous patterns have a milder course, whereas membranoproliferative and diffuse proliferative have poorer prognosis.[2] FGN is considered primarily idiopathic, but infections, malignancies (particularly lymphoproliferative diseases), and autoimmune disorders are seen in up to one-third of cases.[3]

Crescentic GN as defined by the presence of crescents in >50% of glomeruli has rarely been reported in FGN and has the worst prognosis, with the majority leading to ESRD within the next few months. The IF findings in FGN usually show intense staining for IgG usually accompanied by C3, kappa, and lambda, and sometimes also staining for IgM, C1q, and/or IgA. In 5% of cases of FGN, the IF shows monotypic pattern staining with IgG with for kappa or lambda light chain with or without circulating monoclonal protein, as in our patient.[3]

After initial reporting of crescentic GN in biopsy, intravenous methylprednisolone 500 mg was given for 3 days followed by oral prednisolone 1 mg/kg/day and oral cyclophosphamide with dose adjustment. After confirmation of diagnosis as crescentic CFGN, we continued the same immunosuppressive treatment.[3] Because the patient remained oliguric and continued to be dialysis-dependent even after 2 months of treatment, immunosuppressive drugs were withdrawn and supportive treatment was continued as for ESRD.

CFGN responds poorly to the treatment and optimum treatment remains largely unknown. The scarcity of clinical data makes it more difficult to make a guideline for the treatment. Most of the series used steroids with or without either cyclophosphamide or rituximab with variable success. The University of North Carolina (UNC) series[1] showed one in nine patients treated with rituximab had a response, whereas Javaugue et al.[3] reported partial remission in five of seven patients treated with rituximab. Hogan et al.[4] treated 12 FGN patients with rituximab of which 5 reached ESRD. Those who responded to the treatment were having lower serum creatinine levels at presentation (three having baseline serum creatinine <1.2 mg/dL). Although adequate data are not available regarding posttransplant recurrence of FGN, Nasr et al.[5] reported recurrence of FGN in 33% of 14 cases who underwent renal transplantation. Recent data by Mallett et al.,[6] exploring ANZDATA registry, reported outcomes similar to the overall transplant population and recurrence in one of 13 transplant patients who received renal allografts because of FGN-related ESRD.

Clinical Presentation 49

A 15-year-old male with history of hypertension, interstitial lung disease of unclear etiology, and recurrent right pleural effusion was admitted for further evaluation. His outpatient medications were esomeprazole, hydrochlorothiazide plus valsartan, fluticasone, and salmeterol.

He was admitted at the emergency department with anorexia, asthenia, and right pleuritic thoracalgia lasting for 2 weeks. There was no history of new medications. He mentioned an episode of polyarthralgia and edema of lower extremities 1 year before, which had a spontaneous resolution. On admission, he was afebrile and his blood pressure was 170/91 mm Hg. He had diminished pulmonary sounds on the inferior lobes. The presence of puffy hands was notorious. The rest of his physical examination was unremarkable.

Initial investigation revealed a normocytic and normochromic anemia (hemoglobin 11 g/dL), C-reactive protein of 0.84 mg/dL, erythrocyte sedimentation rate of 89 mm/h, BUN 114 mg/dL, and serum creatinine of 3.5 mg/dL. Urinalysis presented with hematuria and proteinuria and an urinary sediment with numerous RBCs (10–30 per HPF) and rare leukocytes (<5 per HPF). Chest radiography showed bilateral pleural effusion. Mild increased parenchymal echogenicity was found in the renal ultrasound with no dilation of the urinary system. Normocytic and normochromic anemia (Hb 11 g/dL), normal serum creatinine of 0.98 mg/dL, and a normal urinalysis were present in laboratory analysis 2 years before.

An RPGN was suspected, and an extended investigation showed a 24-hour urinary protein excretion of 5.9 g, hypoalbuminemia of 2.8 g/dL, hypercholesterolemia (total cholesterol 228 mg/dL and low-density lipoprotein 153 mg/dL), and hypertriglyceridemia (298 mg/dL). A strongly positive ANA (1/1280) with speckled pattern and positive anti-RNP antibodies was apparent, but the remaining immunologic studies were negative, including ANCA, anti-glomerular basement membrane antibodies, anti-dsDNA, anti-La, anti-Ro, and anti-Sm. The complement levels (C3 and C4) were within the normal range, and serum electrophoresis excluded a monoclonal gammopathy. Peripheral blood cultures were sterile. Tests for HIV, hepatitis C virus, and hepatitis B virus were negative.

Renal biopsy revealed 10 of 11 glomeruli with cellular crescents, some with fibrinoid necrosis and rupture of Bowman capsule. There was periglomerular fibroedema, also involving 30% of the cortex. Severe inflammatory infiltrate, mainly mononuclear, was present in the interstitium. There were spots of acute tubular necrosis, but most of the tubules were preserved. Immunofluorescence was negative. Electron microscopy was not performed. These changes were compatible with pauci-immune crescentic glomerulonephritis (CrGN). Steroid therapy was initiated with a favorable response, but given the severity of the biopsy findings, cyclophosphamide was added. As a complication of immunosuppressive therapy, bacterial pneumonia was successfully treated. For better characterization of the severity of the respiratory disease, a chest CT scan showed lung cavities with destruction of the lung parenchyma in both inferior lobes and a right pleural effusion. A pulmonary CT scan performed 2 years before already showed these cavities, which were stable in size. A bronchoscopy showed ulcerative lesions in the superior lobar bronchus that may be suggestive of vasculitis, diffuse inflammatory signs, as well as abundant secretions. Bronchoalveolar lavage was negative for *Mycobacterium tuberculosis* and other agents. At this point, a systemic disease with renal and respiratory involvement, previously present but undiagnosed, was considered, which led to a capillaroscopy revealing a secondary Raynaud phenomenon and a late scleroderma pattern.

Echocardiography excluded pulmonary hypertension. Spirometry results disclosed a normal forced vital capacity (4.43 L, 99% of predicted), normal static volumes (total lung capacity of 6.61 L, 93% of predicted), normal airway resistance, and a reduced diffusing capacity (4.03 mmol/min/kPa, 40.7% of predicted).

What is your diagnosis?

A. ANCA-negative CrGN associated with a mixed connective tissue disease (MCTD)
B. Wegener granulomatosis
C. Eosinophilic polyangiitis
D. Microscopic polyangiitis

The correct answer is A

Comment: Our patient presented with RPGN. His clinical presentation and findings on kidney biopsy were compatible with the diagnosis of MCTD. After induction therapy with cyclophosphamide, the patient started on azathioprine (2 mg/kg/day). He showed a significant improvement with serum creatinine decreasing to 1.2 mg/dL. Three months after the initial episode, the patient was asymptomatic. A continuous renal function improvement was evident (serum creatinine, 0.97 mg/dL; proteinuria, 335 mg/24 hours, with a normal urinary sediment), as well as an improvement in the respiratory symptoms and in the pulmonary function tests.

One of the most common causes of RPGN is pauci-immune CrGN.[1,2] In the majority of cases, this condition has a positive serologic marker, the ANCAs, but in approximately 10% there are no circulating ANCAs, and this subgroup has been known as the ANCA-negative pauci-immune CrGN.

In majority of cases, pauci-immune CrGN is associated with systemic small-vessel vasculitis, such as granulomatosis with polyangiitis, microscopic polyangiitis, and eosinophilic granulomatosis with polyangiitis, but also with renal limited vasculitis in a small number of cases. CrGN and RPGN share a common serologic hallmark, defined by the presence of ANCAs, and for this reason it is known as ANCA-associated vasculitis.

However, there is a small group of pauciimmune CrGN without ANCA positivity, representing about 10% of cases.[1–3] Most of these cases are idiopathic and not associated with connective tissue diseases (MCTD).[3] MCTD is defined as a syndrome that shares features of systemic sclerosis, polymyositis, and SLE. A laboratory characteristic of this syndrome is a high titer of anti-RNP antibodies and positive ANAs with a high-titer speckled pattern.

The antibodies to double-stranded DNA (dsDNA) Sm, Ro, and La might also be present, although not dominant or persistent. Renal involvement in MCTD is less common than in typical SLE. It occurs either as a membranous nephropathy or, less frequently, as mesangioproliferative glomerulonephritis or renal vasculopathy of scleroderma.[4] Pauci-immune CrGN is a rare form of renal involvement in MCTD and is sparsely reported. The authors aim to describe a case of a pauci-immune CrGN, with negative ANCA, which was associated with MCTD.

MCTD is a rare syndrome with overlap features of rheumatic disorders, such as SLE, systemic sclerosis, and polymyositis with the serologic marker of high titers of anti-RNP antibodies. The Alarcon-Segovia and Kahn diagnostic criteria are the most used algorithms for establishing the diagnosis of MCTD.[5] Both classifications include serological (high titers of anti-RNP antibodies) and clinical (swollen hands, synovitis, myositis, and Raynaud phenomenon) criteria.[6] This patient presented with a higher titer of anti-RNP antibodies, swollen hands, synovitis, and Raynaud phenomenon, fulfilling the diagnosis criteria for MCTD. Although almost any organ can be involved in MCTD, severe renal involvement is infrequent, and it is hypothesized that high titers of anti-RNP antibodies may protect against the development of diffuse proliferative glomerulonephritis.[7–11] The most common presentations of renal disease in MCTD are membranous nephropathy and mesangioproliferative glomerulonephritis. Interstitial nephropathy and renal vasculopathy are less frequent and could lead to malignant hypertension as observed in scleroderma renal crisis.[9–11]

Specific therapeutic protocols for patients with CrGN and MCTD are not available because of the rarity of this association. The treatment for MCTD should be individualized depending on organ involvement and severity.[6] In this case report, the therapeutic approach was based on the most commonly accepted strategy for pauci-immune CrGN because of the magnitude of the renal involvement and included cyclophosphamide in combination with high-dose steroids, followed by azathioprine. Successful use of azathioprine as maintenance therapy was reported in one case of pauci-immune CrGN associated with MCTD.[12] Azathioprine has also been used on MCTD with good results, especially when there is pulmonary, articular, or neurologic involvement.[6] As expected, the renal outcomes would have been better if the treatment started in the early stages of the disease.[5] A favorable clinical outcome was observed, with renal function recovery, normalization of urinary sediment, significant proteinuria reduction, and substantial improvement in pulmonary function tests. This multiorgan improvement after immunosuppression consolidated the hypothesis of a common immune origin in both renal and pulmonary dysfunctions.

Clinical Presentation 50

A 17-year-old previously healthy woman without significant past medical history presented feeling generally unwell and fatigued over the preceding 2 months. The patient did not usually take any regular medications. She reported a recent history of intermittent joint pains in her hands, which had become more severe over the past week despite a short course of nonsteroidal anti-inflammatory medications (naproxen). Active urinary sediment had been noted elsewhere in the 1-month period before attendance to nephrology clinic when the patient visited the emergency department of her local district general hospital, though urine microscopic analysis was otherwise unremarkable. The patient did not report any ocular or nasal symptoms, rash, or hemoptysis. She was hypertensive with a BP of 200/118, whereas the remainder of the clinical examination was unremarkable. Urine microscopic analysis was positive for protein (0.8 g proteinuria) and blood (<50 RBCs/HPF). Blood tests showed evidence of acute kidney injury with serum creatinine

2.8 mg/dL and moderately raised inflammatory markers, with C-reactive protein being 102 mg/L, and anemia (hemoglobin 8.5 g/dL; liver function tests and coagulation studies were all normal). Immunology screening identified serum positivity to ANCA and abnormal levels of the myeloperoxidase (MPO) ELISA, with MPO ELISA titer being 55 IU/mL (normal range, <20 IU/mL). Immunology tests including complement C3 and C4, ANAs, anti-glomerular basement membrane antibodies, and free light chains, were all unremarkable. Chest x-ray and CT of the chest and abdomen were not suggestive of any systemic pathology, including lymphadenopathy.

A tentative diagnosis of MPO ANCA-associated small vessel vasculitis with renal involvement was suspected. An urgent renal biopsy was scheduled. The ANCA MPO titer was only mildly raised above the normal reference range, and the patient was well with stable kidney function; hence, oral steroid therapy (prednisolone 30 mg once daily) was initiated 3 days before kidney biopsy. The kidney biopsy showed cellular and fibrous crescents with negative immunohistochemistry, in keeping with pauci-immune glomerulonephritis. There was moderate tubulointerstitial fibrosis. Surprisingly, significant tubulointerstitial inflammation was also seen with a predominance of plasma cells. These were later confirmed to be IgG4-producing plasma cells on immunohistochemistry, with the presence of IgG4 deposits confirmed following immune deposit staining, and the infiltration of 10 IgG4 cells per HPF in keeping with IgG4-related disease. Further serum samples were sent to determine serum IgG4 levels, which were found to be raised at 1.94 g/L (reference range, ≤1.35 g/L).

The patient was commenced on cyclophosphamide 1 g intravenously with further doses of cyclophosphamide scheduled, whereas her daily prednisolone dose continued. The patient's BP control was also optimized during this time with amlodipine 5 mg once daily, and she was commenced on atorvastatin 20 mg daily. Oral co-trimoxazole and fluconazole were started for prophylaxis of infection. The patient was discharged in good health. We discussed further immunosuppression for this unusual presentation and decided to switch her immunosuppressive regime to rituximab because of its presumed ability to effectively treat both IgG4-related disease and ANCA-associated vasculitis with a milder side effect profile compared with cyclophosphamide. Rituximab was initiated with single-dose intravenous methylprednisolone 250 mg, and oral prednisolone was reduced to 15 mg daily. When last seen in the clinic after one dose of rituximab, the patient appeared well with her kidney and inflammatory parameters much improved (serum creatinine 159 μmol/L and C-reactive protein <1.0 mg/L) and serum IgG4 levels falling back to within normal ranges (0.52 g/L). No active urinary sediment was detected. The patient also reported settling of her joint pain symptoms in this clinic appointment following the multiple immunosuppressive treatments administered. She was scheduled for her second dose of rituximab treatment 2 weeks following this appointment.

What is the likely diagnosis?

A. Churg-Strauss syndrome
B. Microscopic polyangiitis
C. ANCA-associated vasculitis with IgG4 tubulointerstitial nephritis
D. Wegener granulomatosis disease

The correct diagnosis is C

Comment: Our patient presented with a 2-month history of malaise and joint pain and was found to have acute kidney injury, hematuria, and proteinuria. Initial immunological tests revealed positive anti-neutrophil cytoplasmic antibodies with a peri-nuclear pattern (pANCA). An ELISA for anti-MPO antibodies was also positive, leading to a tentative diagnosis of ANCA-associated small vessel vasculitis with renal involvement. Steroid treatment was commenced and an urgent kidney biopsy was performed. This showed crescentic glomerulonephritis but also demonstrated concurrent tubulointerstitial nephritis with a dominance of IgG4-producing plasma cells. Serum

IgG4 levels were also elevated. The patient was initially treated with intravenous cyclophosphamide and steroids and then switched to rituximab. When last seen, she was well after one dose of rituximab, with kidney function, inflammatory parameters, and serum IgG4 levels returning to normal levels. The concurrent presentation of ANCA-associated vasculitis and IgG4 renal disease is rare, with only a few cases reported in the literature.

Histological identification of IgG4-producing plasma cells with concurrent crescentic glomerulonephritis in the presence of positive ANCA ELISA testing led to the diagnosis in the case presented here.[1] Serum IgG4 is a sensitive marker for IgG4-related disease but is currently considered to lack diagnostic specificity.[2] It is also worth considering the fact that both IgG4 immunohistochemistry in renal biopsies and serum IgG4 measurements are not easily accessible worldwide. The latter is certainly not currently part of routine blood tests in patients with unexplained renal impairment. Of note, elevated serum IgG4 levels are somewhat nonspecific and also seen in chronic inflammatory conditions (e.g., inflammatory bowel disease) and malignancies (e.g., lymphoma).[3] It is therefore possible that some cases of this unusual presentation are not diagnosed and reported. Clinicians should be aware of the association, and use of IgG4 immunohistochemistry in renal biopsies and measurement of serum IgG4 should be employed in unusual cases of ANCA-associated vasculitis, for example when there is tubulointerstitial nephritis or fibrotic extrarenal disease. In summary, a high degree of suspicion is required to validate this unusual combination of diagnoses.

IgG4-related disease is a recently recognized syndrome that affects multiple organs through inflammation, fibrosis, or both.[4] The concept of IgG4-related disease was initially described in 2001 by Hamano et al.,[2] who reported raised serum IgG4 levels in a subgroup of patients diagnosed with autoimmune pancreatitis. Since then, IgG4-related disease has been observed in the pancreas and biliary tract, salivary glands, lung, aorta and retroperitoneum, endocrine glands, and the kidney.[5] The most common form of kidney involvement in IgG4-related disease is tubulointerstitial nephritis with both acute and chronic disease manifestations.[6] IgG4-related membranous nephropathy is also seen.[6] Concurrent IgG4-related disease and ANCA-associated vasculitis is very uncommon, and a distinct new syndrome has been proposed.[7] We report a case of concurrent IgG4-related tubulointerstitial nephritis and ANCA MPO crescentic glomerulonephritis. We describe our case and provide a brief review of the literature in terms of pathophysiology, diagnostic recommendations, and management options based on current evidence.

Concurrent subacute presentation of IgG4-related kidney disease with ANCA-associated MPO crescentic glomerulonephritis is uncommon.[8]

The evidence for treatment of this unusual presentation is weak simply because of the rarity of this presentation, and larger studies seem unlikely at present. Anecdotal reports consider cyclophosphamide combined with steroid therapy as a potentially effective treatment option for concurrent IgG4-related kidney disease and ANCA-associated vasculitis.[9] Rituximab use has been described in the treatment of IgG4-related kidney disease because of its ability to deplete B cells and have a better side effect profile compared to cyclophosphamide combined with steroid therapy.[10] It is tempting to think of rituximab as a potentially ideal drug in treating the concurrent presentation of IgG4 disease and ANCA-associated vasculitis, but this assumption will require further exploration.[11]

Clinical Presentation 51

A 19-year-old male with a history of hepatitis B and C infections presented with acute kidney injury (serum creatinine, 5.6 mg/dL) and *Enterococcus faecalis*–infective endocarditis (IE). He denied any current or previous recreational drug use, including cocaine, and sexual activity.

Blood cultures returned positive for *E. faecalis* that was treated with ampicillin and ceftriaxone, the latter for a synergistic activity for the treatment of possible IE pending results of an echocardiogram. Initial transthoracic echocardiogram revealed a 1.5 × 1-cm mass on the anterior tricuspid valve leaflet along with a 1 × 0.5-cm echo-dense mobile mass on the implantable cardioverter-defibrillator (ICD) wire of the right atrial side of his tricuspid valve. The ICD was later extracted, and the left ventricle lead was tunneled to the right side.

The patient's creatinine continued to rise during his admission (peak, 9.2 mg/dL) and was accompanied by microscopic hematuria and proteinuria on urinalysis. Consequently, the possibility of GN was entertained. A low C3 (0.5 g/L) and C4 (0.07 g/L) and strongly positive PR3-ANCA (>8.0 AI) with a negative p-ANCA prompted a renal biopsy, which revealed focal segmental proliferative and necrotizing glomerulonephritis affecting >50% of glomeruli with cellular and fibrocellular crescents and some segmental sclerosis, indicative of chronicity. Immunofluorescence and electron microscopy demonstrated a paucity of any significant immune complexes, and, given the severity and extent of necrotizing lesions, a diagnosis of pauci-immune GN consistent with ANCA vasculitis was made.

The rheumatology service advised initiation of immunosuppression for possible salvage of renal function given that the patient's creatinine had plateaued at 8.6 mg/dL; he became anuric and was initiated on intermittent hemodialysis 1 month following his admission to hospital. However, there are few data on the management of chronic inactive hepatitis B infection in patients who are on dialysis, limiting the provision of induction therapy with rituximab or cyclophosphamide in our patient. He was initiated on intravenous methylprednisolone 250 mg daily for 3 days, followed by an oral prednisone taper starting at 60 mg daily. This decision was made in conjunction with the infectious diseases service, given that he had sterilized his blood cultures roughly 1.5 weeks before steroid provision. The patient's clinical course became complicated by development of pneumonia and candidemia, and he did not recover his renal function. The cardiovascular surgery team advised against surgery given the patient's complex medical status and comorbidities, and he died 3 months into his admission.

How would you manage infective endocarditis-associated ANCA vasculitis in this patient?

A. Combination of steroids and cyclophosphamide
B. Steroids and antibiotics alone
C. Induction therapy with either cyclophosphamide or rituximab
D. Insufficient data to recommend any specific treatment

The correct answer is D

Comment: Our patient with a history of chronic hepatitis B and C infections presented with acute kidney injury and *E. faecalis* IE. An elevated proteinase-3 (PR3)-ANCA and pauci-immune GN on renal biopsy were discovered, corresponding to ANCA-mediated GN.

Of the five cases of ANCA GN in the setting of IE reported in the literature, all had markedly elevated levels of PR3-ANCA, with either a subacute or chronic course of infection. Patients were treated with a combination of steroids and cyclophosphamide (2/5), steroids and antibiotics alone (1/5), or with valvular replacement (2/5). Renal function was recovered in 4/5 patients. Infection is a major etiologic player in the formation of ANCA; however, the role of PR3-ANCA in IE remains unclear. The development of GN during infection is associated with significant morbidity and mortality, and diagnosis requires a high index of clinical suspicion. Although antibiotics hasten renal recovery in immune-complex-mediated GN in IE, ANCA-associated renal vasculitis often requires treatment with immunosuppression through induction with either cyclophosphamide or rituximab.[1]

Kidney biopsy is essential in differentiating IE-related GN resulting from infection and immune complex deposition versus ANCA-associated vasculitis. A paucity of reports on the development of GN in IE-associated ANCA vasculitis exists, highlighting the rarity of our case and lack of clear therapeutic strategies in a patient with active infection requiring immunosuppression. In this case, the patient's chronic hepatitis B and C coinfection presented a unique challenge.

Various patterns of kidney injury have been described during the course of IE, including renal cortical necrosis in the event of septic emboli or thrombotic microangiopathy, acute interstitial nephritis, and tubular necrosis as a consequence of drugs, bacterial toxins, or intravascular volume depletion.[1] GN represents a unique form of renal injury that might also complicate the course of SLE,[2,3] typically through circulating immune complex deposition within glomeruli.

Subacute and chronic inflammatory states including infection may also induce the formation of ANCAs[4,5] that may subsequently result in blood vessel damage leading to manifestations of vasculitis.[6,7] Unlike immune complex–mediated GN in which renal recovery parallels the resolution of infection,[8] pauci-immune GN requires immunosuppression, posing a therapeutic challenge in the setting of bacterial sepsis.

Clinical Presentation 52

A 16-year-old male was admitted with a 5-year history of proteinuria and hypertension. He started to have a complaint of headache 1 year ago and was found to have malignant hypertension (204/151 mm Hg), and the funduscopic examination revealed flame hemorrhages and exudates. Urinalysis revealed proteinuria (3+) and dysmorphic red blood cells (5–8/HPF). The 24-hour proteinuria excretion was 3.76 g, and the serum creatinine value was 1.04 mg/dL (normal range, 0.50–1.50 mg/dL). He was treated with ramipril (5 mg/d) and nifedipine (30 mg/d). His BP was well controlled (110–120/70–80 mm Hg), his serum creatinine value was stable, and the amount of proteinuria decreased to 2.94 g/24 hours.

On admission, his BP was 110/70 mm Hg, temperature 36.3°C, heart rate 80 beats/min, and respiratory rate 20 breaths/min. The patient had mild bilateral symmetrical lower extremity edema. The remaining of examinations were unremarkable.

Laboratory data revealed proteinuria of 0.93 to 1.72 g/24 hours, serum creatinine of 1.36 mg/dL, and serum albumin of 3.2 g/dL. Hemoglobin level was 13.4 g/dL and the platelet count was 252 × 10^9 cells/L. Plasma C3 was 0.165 g/L and C4 was 0.177 g/L. Complement alternative pathway was overactivated with decreased plasma C3 and elevated plasma Bb, C3a, C5am, and sMAC levels. Serum IgG level was 8.05 g/L, IgA 1.01 g/L, and IgM 0.93 g/L. C-reactive protein was <1.0 mg/L. Anti-streptolysin O, antineutrophil cytoplasmic antibodies, anti-glomerular basement membrane antibodies, and anti-nuclear antibodies were all negative. HBsAg, anti-HCV, anti-HIV, and TP-Ab were also negative. Chest x-ray and abdominal ultrasound were normal.

A renal biopsy was performed. Light microscopic examination exhibited that 5/32 glomeruli were globally sclerosed. Other glomeruli showed moderate to severe mesangial expansion with a lobular appearance, and segmental thickening of the glomerular basement membrane with double contours. Immunofluorescence examination revealed strong granular staining for C3c (+++), weak staining for IgA (+), IgM (+), and trace C1q along the glomerular capillary wall and in the mesangium, but negative staining for IgG. Electron microscopy showed subendothelial and mesangial electron-dense deposits, with extensive effacement of the foot processes of podocytes.

What is your diagnosis?

A. IgA nephropathy
B. Dense deposit disease

C. C1q nephropathy
D. C3 glomerulonephritis

The correct answer is D

Comment: Our patient's renal biopsy demonstrated C3c-dominant deposition on immunofluorescence. The complement alternative pathway was overactivated with decreased plasma C3 and elevated plasma Bb, C3a, C5a, and sMAC levels. Thus, a diagnosis of C3 glomerulonephritis (C3G) was suspected. The electron microscopy further excluded the subtype of dense deposit disease (DDD), confirming the diagnosis of C3GN with an MPGN pattern.[1]

The alternative pathway activation in C3GN was driven by either inherited or acquired defects. Acquired causes included C3Nef, anti-CFH autoantibodies, anti-C3b autoantibodies, or anti-CFB antibodies. Genetic factors included *CFH*, complement factor I (*CFI*), membrane cofactor protein (*MCP*), complement factor B (*CFB*), and *C3* as well as CFH-related protein 5 (*CFHR5*) internal duplication, *CFHR1-3* hybrid, *CFHR1* duplication, and *CFHR2-5* hybrid.[2] Genetic testing in our patient showed variants of *CFH, THBD*, and *MBL2* and a novel variant of *C2* mutant genes.

CFH is one of the key inhibitors of the alternative pathway. The *CFH* Val62Ile variant (rs800292) and Tyr402His variant (rs1061170), which locate within regions that bind C3b, heparin, and C-reactive protein, have been shown to confer susceptibility to DDD patients.[3] Meanwhile, the Tyr402His variant had significant association with an increased risk of developing age-related macular degeneration, another complement-associated disease.[4] Furthermore, the two variants have been reported in the postpartum atypical hemolytic uremic syndrome, which was also the result of inappropriate activation of the complement alternative pathway.[5] Thus, we inferred that these two variants might result in a mutant CFH protein with reduced regulatory capacity to prevent complement overactivation. Thrombomodulin is an endothelial anticoagulant glycoprotein that can regulate the complement alternative pathway by enhancing factor I–mediated C3b inactivation after binding C3b and CFH. Based on a study in a large cohort demonstrating that the *THBD* Ala473Val variant could increase the probability of developing C3G,[6] it was speculated that the mutant protein might reduce the binding capacity of C3b and CFH to inactive C3b, although the functional studies on *THBD* Ala473Val were lacking. In general, the common variants *CFH* Val62Ile, *CFH* Tyr402His, and *THBD* Ala473Val found in our patient might cause the dysregulation of the complement alternative pathway and increase susceptibility to C3GN.

Another *CFH* variant Glu936Asp (rs1065489) was previously demonstrated to be associated with host susceptibility to meningococcal disease in genome-wide association studies.[7] CFH has been shown to be exploited by *Neisseria meningitidis* to escape host immune control.[8] Binding of *N. meningitidis* to CFH would protect the bacterium from complement-mediated damage. Thus, we thought that this variant would increase the binding ability between CFH and *N. meningitidis* and then facilitate the escape of the bacteria from host immune responses. The *MBL2* Gly54Asp variant (rs1800450) was found to decrease MBL2 protein stability and expression,[9] which was supported by the lower plasma MBL level (342.89 ng/mL) in our patient that could be defined as partial MBL deficiency (50–1000 ng/mL).[10] MBL is a soluble pattern recognition receptor that initiates the activation of the complement MBL pathway after binding to carbohydrate, and its deficiency was reported to increase the risk of various infections such as sepsis.[11] Therefore, the common variants *CFH* Glu936Asp and *MBL2* Gly54Asp might help explain our patient's history of meningitis.

The renal prognosis of C3G is poor, and previous reports showed that approximately 50% of DDD patients progressed to ESRD in 10 years.[12] C3GN had a better prognosis than DDD, although the latest study by Bomback et al. showed that there was no significant difference in renal prognosis between DDD and C3GN.[8] Unfortunately, there were still no high-level randomized trials for the treatment of C3GN, and the therapy for the disease was mainly based on low-quality evidence consisting of case series, case reports, retrospective cohort studies, and expert opinion.[13] General treatments include antihypertensive therapy and lipid-lowering therapy. Specific interventions include plasma infusion or exchange, immunosuppressive therapy, and eculizumab. Because our patient had genetic defects of circulating proteins without acquired autoantibodies, he received fresh frozen plasma infusion, and immunosuppressants were not initiated. He responded well with an elevated plasma C3 level, well-controlled proteinuria, and stable renal function. Moreover, anti-complement therapy (eculizumab) has been a novel and pathogenesis-based treatment method for the disease in recent years. C3G patients with deteriorating renal function, severe nephrotic syndrome, elevated sMAC levels, and active renal biopsy changes, might be more likely to benefit from this therapy based on previous studies.[14]

Clinical Presentation 53

A 17-year-old woman was referred for evaluation of persistent hematuria and proteinuria. She had a history of fever and sore throat lasting 1 week that occurred 6 months earlier and were associated with abdominal pain and dark urine. She did not receive any antimicrobial agents. Significant findings on physical examination at that time included a BP of 140/90 mm Hg and 2+ edema. Laboratory evaluation showed a serum creatinine value of 1.4 mg/dL, urinalysis with 2+ protein and 3+ blood, and a 24-hour urinary protein excretion of 680 mg. The C3 level was 46 mg/dL (reference range, 75–175 mg/dL) and the C4 level was 23 mg/dL (reference range, 14–40 mg/dL). A throat culture was negative for β-hemolytic streptococci, and an antistreptolysin O titer was 200 IU/mL (upper limit of normal, 200 IU/mL). The serum albumin concentration was 3.6 g/dL.

A renal biopsy was performed and showed a pattern of membranoproliferative GN on light microscopy. No crescents were observed. Immunofluorescence microscopy showed bright (3+) mesangial and capillary wall C3 staining. Electron microscopy showed mesangial, intramembranous, and subendothelial deposits, as well as a few subepithelial hump-like deposits. Postinfectious GN and type III membranoproliferative GN were diagnosed. The patient was treated symptomatically, but proteinuria and hematuria persisted. The current evaluation shows a hemoglobin level of 11.8 g/dL, a serum creatinine concentration of 1.3 mg/dL, urinalysis with 3+ blood and 3+ protein, quantitative proteinuria of 2.2 g/24 hours, C3 concentration of 44 mg/dL, and C4 concentration of 22 mg/dL.

To further evaluate this patient, which test you would now order?

A. Antinuclear antibodies
B. Hepatitis B and C serology
C. Anti-deoxyribonuclease (DNase) antibody titers
D. Serum C1q level
E. Antibodies to complement-regulating proteins

The correct answer is E

Comment: Postinfectious GN is a form of GN that develops after an infection; it is especially common in children and in the elderly.[1–4] Often the infection is minor (e.g., pharyngitis) and has usually resolved by the time clinical evidence of an ongoing GN is manifested. The lag time between the start of the infection and the clinical manifestations can vary from a few days to weeks, and disease severity ranges from asymptomatic hematuria to an acute nephritic syndrome, renal failure, and fluid overload. On renal biopsy, postinfectious GN is characterized by proliferative GN on light microscopy, mesangial and/or capillary wall bright C3 staining with or without immunoglobulin on immunofluorescence microscopy, and subepithelial hump-like deposits on electron microscopy.[4,5] In some cases, there is no clinical or serologic evidence of a preceding infection, and the diagnosis of postinfectious GN is based solely on these renal biopsy findings. It should be also recognized that over the past 30 years, an important shift in epidemiology, bacteriology, and outcome of GN related to infection has occurred.[5] A substantial number of cases now occur in adults, particularly the elderly, alcoholic persons, and patients who are immunocompromised. Because the presence of an infection is often ongoing at the time of renal biopsy, the term *infection-related GN* has been suggested as more appropriately describing this condition.[6] In contrast to children, adults are more likely to have infection-related GN secondary to nonstreptococcal infections, particularly staphylococcal infection, and the overall prognosis in terms of renal and patient survival is poor.

The pathogenesis of acute postinfectious GN has been the subject of recent reviews.[7,8] It is important to recognize that no animal model can reproduce the classic findings of abundant neutrophil infiltration and subepithelial humps characteristic of human postinfectious GN.[8] Nevertheless, it has been proposed that the initial phase of the process is characterized by deposition of bacterial antigens (e.g., streptococcal) in the glomeruli (planted). This phase is followed by production of antibodies that interact in situ with the planted antigens.[2,9] Antigens that enter the circulation after the antibody response is fully under way form immune complexes in circulation. Most of these immune complexes are cleared from the circulation by the liver and spleen, but those that escape the phagocytic system may deposit in the glomeruli and thus induce immune complex–mediated GN.[7] Reduction in serum C3 complement levels is a constant feature during the initial phase of postinfectious GN.[10,11] The hypocomplementemia is due to activation of the alternative pathway (AP) of complement, whereas C1q, C2, and C4 complement levels (classic pathway) are usually normal. In some patients with poststreptococcal GN, low C3 levels have been associated with the transient expression of circulating autoantibodies against the C3 convertase complex (i.e., C3 nephritic factors).[12] These antibodies result in stabilization of the enzyme, increase in convertase activity, and enhanced C3 cleavage by the AP of complement.[13]

In most cases, GN resolves in a matter of weeks without specific treatment. Similarly, hypocomplementemia usually resolves within 8 weeks. However, in a minority of cases, urinary and complement abnormalities may persist or take longer to resolve, with some patients even progressing to ESRD.[1,2,4,14–17] These cases have been labeled as "atypical," "persistent," or "chronic" postinfectious GN. Until recently, the cause of these atypical cases was unknown. A recent study postulates that cases of atypical postinfectious GN are due to a defect in the regulating mechanisms of the AP of complement that prevent downregulation of complement activation after resolution of the infection.[18] As a consequence, there is excessive deposition of complement proteins and breakdown products in the glomeruli, resulting in persistence of the inflammatory response.

That study included 11 patients (5 women and 6 men; mean age, 35.1 years [range, 2–71 years]) who fulfilled the diagnostic criteria of atypical postinfectious GN, defined as (1) persistent hematuria and proteinuria, with or without history of preceding infection; (2) renal biopsy showing features of postinfectious GN; and (3) abnormalities of the complement AP. Five of the 11 patients had a history of upper respiratory tract infection or impetigo. In the remaining six, no antecedent illness was documented. Serum creatinine at presentation ranged from 0.5 to 3.1 mg/dL (mean, 1.4 mg/dL), with mean proteinuria of 5139 mg/24 hours (range, 500–15,760 mg/24 hours). C3 levels were low in seven patients, and C4 levels were normal in all patients. All biopsies showed proliferative GN; the most common pattern was diffuse endocapillary proliferative GN, followed by mesangial proliferative and membranoproliferative GN on light microscopy. On immunofluorescence microscopy, bright (3+) mesangial and capillary wall C3 staining was seen in all but one case, which showed mild (1+) C3 staining. Two cases also showed mild mesangial and capillary wall staining for IgG (1–2+). Electron microscopy showed the hallmark of postinfectious GN in all cases: hump-like subepithelial deposits, which were numerous in six patients. Ten of 11 patients also had mesangial and subendothelial deposits. Functional and genetic studies of the AP identified autoantibodies or mutations in complement genes in 10 of 11 patients. Seven patients were positive for C3 nephritic factors, which were associated with other functional abnormalities of the AP in six patients. Four patients had mutations of complement genes, including three patients with mutations in CFH and one patient with a mutation in CFHR5.

The study shows that patients with atypical postinfectious GN have an underlying defect in the complement AP. Results of the study are supported by recent case reports of patients initially diagnosed as having a postinfectious GN who subsequently were found to have a proliferative form of GN called C3GN.[19,20] Thus, it can be postulated that under normal circumstances, the activation of the AP by an infection is quickly brought under control once the infection abates. However, in patients with a defect in AP regulation, there is continual AP activation with deposition of complement proteins and their breakdown products in the glomeruli, even after resolution of the infection, leading to the development of atypical proliferative GN. If the defect is mild, AP control eventually occurs with resolution of the GN. If the defect in AP regulation is more severe, hematuria and proteinuria persist, often exacerbated by recurrent bouts of infection. Recent studies have shown that dysregulation of the AP also results in C3GN. C3GN is characterized by glomerular C3 deposition and the presence of numerous deposits in the mesangium and capillary walls, including subepithelial deposits.[21–24] Thus, there is considerable overlap in the biopsy findings of patients with atypical postinfectious GN and those with C3GN.[25] This overlap is not surprising because both types are due to abnormalities of complement AP. Indeed, review of previous reports on prolonged hypocomplementemia in patients with poststreptococcal GN show kidney biopsy findings compatible with the diagnosis of C3GN.[15] It is also likely that many cases of familial poststreptococcal GN represent undiagnosed C3 glomerulopathy.[26] Therefore, atypical postinfectious GN should be considered a C3 glomerulopathy, and testing for abnormalities in the AP of complement in all patients with atypical postinfectious GN is recommended (option E).

The clinical presentation, laboratory evaluation, and renal biopsy findings of this case are not compatible with the diagnosis of systemic lupus erythematosus (option A) or cryoglobulinemic GN (option B). In lupus nephritis, immunofluorescence microscopy usually shows a "full house," meaning that all or almost all immunoreactants (IgG, IgA, IgM, κ and λ light chains, C1q, C3) are present. This is unusual in other forms of GN. On electron microscopy evaluation, in addition to immune complex deposits (discrete electron dense immune-type deposits), a very common ultrastructural finding is the presence of tubuloreticular inclusions. On the other hand, in cryoglobulinemic GN, immunofluorescence microscopy typically shows diffuse, pseudo-linear peripheral capillary wall and mesangial staining for IgM, IgG, and C3, with a relatively stronger staining for IgM and κ (compared with λ) light chain, which reflects the typical clonal restriction of type II cryoglobulins. On electron microscopy, cryoglobulin deposits often display an organized substructure: short, curved, thick-walled tubular structures with a diameter of about 30 nm that appear annular on cross-sections.

Anti-DNase antibody testing (option C) detects antigens produced by group A streptococcus and is elevated in most patients with rheumatic fever and poststreptococcal GN. This test is often done concurrently with the antistreptolysin O titer, and subsequent testing is usually performed to detect differences in the acute and convalescent blood samples. Anti-DNase testing was not performed at presentation and will probably have negative results at this time. The first component of complement (C1) is composed of three subunits, designated as C1q, C1r, and C1s. C1q recognizes and binds to immunoglobulin complexed to antigen and initiates activation of the classic pathway of complement. Serum C1q levels (option D) are usually normal in conditions associated with abnormalities of the AP of complement (e.g., C3GN), although they may be mildly decreased early in the course of postinfectious GN.

Clinical Presentation 54

A 38-year-old man has a history of apparently idiopathic membranous nephropathy diagnosed 3 years ago. Proteinuria at diagnosis was 15 g/24 hours, and the serum creatinine level was 1.4 mg/dL. Anti–phospholipase 2 receptor antibodies (PLA2R) on ELISA were 7350 U/mL (negative <40 U/mL) measured on a stored serum sample 1 year later. He was treated with angiotensin II blockade for 4 months, but proteinuria persisted at >10 g/24 hours. He was then treated with a combination of methylprednisolone, 1 g intravenously, at the start of months 1, 3, and 5; oral prednisone, 0.5 mg/kg per day, on months 1, 3, and 5; and oral cyclophosphamide, 2.0 mg/kg per day, on months 2, 4, and 6. His proteinuria declined to 9 g/24 hours and 4 g/24 hours at 6 and 12 months, respectively, after the end of the treatment but has increased to 5.5 g/24 hours over the past 3 months. He is now asking you about further therapy. Current medications are lisinopril, 20 mg orally each day, and atorvastatin, 10 mg daily.

Pertinent findings on physical examination include BP of 110/75 mm Hg, pulse of 72 beats/min, and trace edema of the ankles. Laboratory tests show a hemoglobin concentration of 12.8 g/dL, serum creatinine concentration of 1.3 mg/dL, serum albumin level of 3.4 g/dL, urinalysis showing heme 1+, and proteinuria of 5.4 g/24 hours. The serum C3 level is 110 mg/dL (reference range, 75–175 mg/dL).

In this patient, you would now recommend which of the following?

A. Urinary IgG and β2-microglobulin excretion
B. Serum IgG4 level
C. Repeat anti-PLA2R antibody level
D. Renal US with Doppler examination of renal veins
E. Repeat renal biopsy

The correct answer is E

Comment: Idiopathic MN is a common immune-mediated glomerular disease and remains the leading cause of nephrotic syndrome in White adults.[1] Although in most patients the disease progresses relatively slowly, approximately 40% of patients eventually develop ESRD.[2] Because of its frequency, it remains the second or third most common cause of primary glomerulopathy leading to ESRD.[3] Patients with MN who remain nephrotic are at an increased risk for thromboembolic[4] and cardiovascular[5–7] events. Available immunosuppressive therapies include the use of corticosteroids combined with cytotoxic agents, as well as calcineurin inhibitors. These therapies are at least partially successful in reducing proteinuria, but their use is controversial, is associated with significant adverse effects, and carries a high rate of relapse.[7] To date, the best proven long-term therapy for patients with MN consists of the combined use of corticosteroids and cyclophosphamide—the Ponticelli protocol—and it was used in this patient. Proteinuria decreased substantially, but it never decreased to <4 g/24 hours and more recently has increased to 5.5 g/24 hours. The question to answer is: Does proteinuria in this patient reflect active immunologic disease or is it a consequence of renal damage? This question is clinically relevant and introduces the concept that immunologic remission should be added to clinical remission (based on proteinuria) and that both be used in judging treatment (conservative versus immunosuppressive) in MN.

Some qualitative aspects of proteinuria, such as urinary excretion of α1-microglobulin, β2-microglobulin, IgG, and IgM (option A), have been reported as strong predictors for renal disease progression.[8–11] However, little is known regarding factors that may predict response to therapy, and the only studies that have evaluated the use of urinary markers for this purpose concluded that neither absolute levels of urinary IgG, β2-microglobulin, or α1-microglobulin at baseline or 12 months nor the percentage of reduction between baseline and 12 months clearly predicted the occurrence of a remission, a relapse to nephrotic range proteinuria, or longer-term outcomes.[12,13] It is unknown whether the use of these markers could predict active immunologic disease.

IgG4-related disease represents a recently recognized group of multiorgan diseases characterized by hypergammaglobulinemia with elevated serum total IgG and/or IgG4 levels, a high level of serum IgG4, and dense infiltration of IgG4-positive cells into multiple organs.[14,15] The term *IgG4-related sclerosing disease* is also used for this entity because it results in a sclerosing lesion of multiple organs, including the kidney, with formation of pseudotumors.[16,17] Patients with renal involvement are often elderly men presenting with progressive renal failure. There are several other characteristics. Patients often have elevated serum total IgG and/or IgG4 levels or hypergammaglobulinemia. Kidney biopsy usually shows a tubulointerstitial nephritis (TIN) with moderate to marked increase in IgG4-positive plasma cells, with or without tubular basement membrane deposits. The term IgG4-related TIN has been proposed to describe this entity.[15] A paucity of cases of IgG4-related TIN with MN has also been described (option B).[18,19] The absence of systemic organ involvement and TIN in this case make the diagnosis of an IgG4-related MN unlikely.

Renal ultrasonography with Doppler examination of renal veins (option D) is indicated to rule out renal vein thrombosis. Acute renal vein thrombosis is usually characterized by a recent episode of acute flank pain, macroscopic hematuria, flank tenderness at percussion, worsening proteinuria, and deterioration of renal function.[20] Hypoalbuminemia, particularly a serum albumin concentration <2.8 g/dL, is the most significant independent predictor of venous thrombotic risk in patients with MN.[21] In view of this, it is unlikely that our patient has developed acute renal vein thrombosis, although asymptomatic chronic renal vein thrombosis cannot be ruled out. However, there is no convincing evidence that chronic renal vein thrombosis is associated with worsening renal function or proteinuria.[20]

Anti-PLA2R antibodies (option C) are present in 70% to 82% of patients with idiopathic MN but are not present in the serum of healthy controls or patients with other glomerular and autoimmune diseases.[22,23] Levels of anti-PLA2R correlate strongly correlated with disease activity and response to therapy: Disappearance of the antibody is associated with remission of proteinuria and reappearance of the antibody heralds a relapse of nephrotic syndrome.[24,25] Taken together, these observations suggest that detection and quantification of circulating anti-PLA2R levels may provide a tool for monitoring disease activity and treatment efficacy in patients with MN.[26] On the other hand, low titers of anti-PLA2R have been detected in patients in remission, whereas the presence of high titers of anti-PLA2R antibodies did not preclude the development of spontaneous remission.[27] Similarly, discrepancies between circulating anti-PLA2R antibodies and detectable PLA2R in glomerular deposits have been reported in a study of 42 consecutive patients with primary MN.[26–27] In 21 patients, anti-PLA2R antibodies were present in circulation and PLA2R was seen in glomerular deposits. However, three patients with high levels of circulating anti-PLA2R antibodies did not have detectable PLA2R in glomerular deposits, suggesting that antibodies were not nephritogenic or that epitopes were poorly accessible at the time of kidney biopsy; among the 18 patients with no detectable circulating anti-PLA2R antibodies, 10 had positive PLA2R glomerular staining. Debiec and Ronco suggest that these apparently discordant findings might be due to the rapid clearance of antibodies from the circulation and deposition in glomeruli or to patients with persistent proteinuria resulting from glomerular ultrastructural damage but immunologically inactive disease. Therefore, the persistence of proteinuria in some cases may be the consequence of an altered architecture of the filtration barrier because of long-standing disease and remodeling process in the glomerular basement membrane.

In the present case, serial anti-PLA2R testing was not available, and although a current negative test result would probably reflect immunologic remission, a single positive anti-PLA2R test result would not necessarily correlate with immunologic activity. As such, we believe the only way to accurately establish disease activity in this patient is to perform renal biopsy (option E).

References

Clinical Presentation 1

1. Servais A, Morinière V, Grünfeld JP, et al. Late-onset nephropathic cystinosis: clinical presentation, outcome, and genotyping. *Clin J Am Nephrol.* 2008;3(1):27–35. https://doi.org/10.2215/CJN.01740407.
2. Assadi FK, Sandler RH, Wong PW, et al. Infantile cystinosis presenting as chronic constipation. *Am J Kidney Dis.* 2002;39(6):E24. https://doi.org/10.1053/ajkd.2002.33415.
3. Beckman DA, Mullin JJ, Assadi FK. Developmental toxicity of cysteamine in the rat: effects on embryo-fetal development. *Teratology.* 1998;58(3–4):96–102. https://doi.org/10.1002/(SICI)1096-9926(199809/10)58:3/4<96AID-TERA53.0.CO;2-7.
4. Assadi FK, Mullin JJ, Beckman DA. Evaluation of the reproductive and developmental safety of cysteamine in the rat: effects on female reproduction and early embryonic development. *Teratology.* 1998;58(3–4):88–95. https://doi.org/10.1002/(SICI)1096-9926(199809/10)58:3/4<88::AID-TERA43.0.CO;2-5.

Clinical Presentation 2

1. Sethi SK, Otto EA, Ma S, Duggal R, Vega-Warner V, Kher V. A boy with proteinuria and focal global glomerulosclerosis: question and answers. *Pediatr Nephrol.* 2015;30(11):1945–1949. https://doi.org/10.1007/s00467-014-2959-4.
2. Assadi F, Mazaheri M, Sadeghi-Bodj S. Randomized controlled trial to compare safety and efficacy of mycophenolate vs. cyclosporine after rituximab in children with steroid-resistant nephrotic syndrome. *Pharmacotherapy.* 2022;42(9):690–696. https://doi.org/10.1002/phar.2721.
3. Bitsori M, Vergadi E, Galanakis E. A novel CLCN5 splice site mutation in a boy with incomplete phenotype of Dent disease. *J Pediatr Genet.* 2019;8(4):235–239. https://doi.org/10.1055/s-0039-1692172.
4. Solanki AK, Arif E, Morinelli T, et al. A novel CLCN5 mutation associated with focal segmental glomerulosclerosis and podocyte injury. *Kidney Int Rep.* 2018;3(6):1443–1453. https://doi.org/10.1016/j.ekir.2018.06.003.

Clinical Presentation 3

1. Sinha A, Bagga A. Clinical practice guidelines for nephrotic syndrome: consensus is emerging. *Pediatr Nephrol.* 2022;37:2975–2984. https://doi.org/10.1007/s00467-022-05639-6.

Clinical Presentation 4

1. Sinha A, Bagga A. Clinical practice guidelines for nephrotic syndrome: consensus is emerging. *Pediatr Nephrol.* 2022;37:2975–2984. https://doi.org/10.1007/s00467-022-05639-6.
2. Ishikura K, Matsumoto S, Sako M, et al. Clinical practice guideline for pediatric idiopathic nephrotic syndrome 2013: medical therapy. *Clin Exp Nephrol.* 2015;19:6–33. https://doi.org/10.1007/s10157-014-1030-x.

Clinical Presentation 5

1. Salvatore SP, Chevalier JM, Kuo SF, et al. Kidney disease in patients with obesity: it is not always obesity-related glomerulopathy alone. *Obes Res Clin Pract.* 2017;11(5):597–606. https://doi.org/10.1016/j.orcp.2017.04.003.
2. Shabaka A, Tato Ribera A, Fernández-Juárez G. Focal segmental glomerulosclerosis: state-of-the-art and clinical perspective. *Nephron.* 2020;144(9):413–427. https://doi.org/10.1159/000508099.

Clinical Presentation 6

1. Assadi F, Mazaheri M, Sadeghi-Bodj S. Randomized controlled trial to compare safety and efficacy of mycophenolate vs. cyclosporine after rituximab in children with steroid-resistant nephrotic syndrome. *Pharmacotherapy.* 2022;42(9):690–696. https://doi.org/10.1002/phar.2721.

Clinical Presentation 7

1. Rovin BH, Adler SG, Barratt J, et al. Executive summary of the KDIGO 2021 guideline for the management of glomerular diseases. *Kidney Int.* 2021;100(4):753–779. https://doi.org/10.1016/j.kint.2021.05.015.
2. Chen A, Frank R, Vento S, et al. Idiopathic membranous nephropathy in pediatric patients: presentation, response to therapy, and long-term outcome. *BMC Nephrol.* 2007;8;11. https://doi.org/10.1186/1471-2369-8-11.

Clinical Presentation 8

1. Mok CC, Teng YKO, Saxena R, et al. Treatment of lupus nephritis: consensus, evidence and perspectives. *Nat Rev Rheumatol.* 2023;19:227–238. https://doi.org/10.1038/s41584-023-00925-5.

2. Robin BH, Adler SG, Sharon G, et al. Executive summary of the KDIGO 2021 guideline for the management of glomerular diseases. *Kidney Int.* 2021;100:753–779.

Clinical Presentation 9

1. Prakash S, Gharavi AG. Assessing genetic risk for IgA nephropathy: state of the art. *Clin J Am Soc Nephrol.* 2021;16(2):182–184. https://doi.org/10.2215/CJN.19491220.
2. Chadban SJ, Ahn C, Axelrod DA, et al. KDIGO clinical practice guideline on the evaluation and management of candidates for kidney transplantation. *Transplantation.* 2020;104(4S1 Suppl 1):S11–S103. https://doi.org/10.1097/TP.0000000000003136.

Clinical Presentation 10

1. Assadi FK. Value of urinary excretion of microalbumin in predicting glomerular lesions in children with isolated microscopic hematuria. *Pediatr Nephrol.* 2005;20(8):1131–1135. https://doi.org/10.1007/s00467-005-1928-3.

Clinical Presentation 11

1. Wyatt CM. Kidney disease and HIV infection. *Top Antivir Med.* 2017;25(1):13–16.
2. Rivera FB, Ansay MFM, Golbin JM, et al. HIV-associated nephropathy in 2022. *Glomerular Dis.* 2022;3(1):1–11. https://doi.org/10.1159/000526868.

Clinical Presentation 12

1. Kovala M, Seppälä M, Räisänen-Sokolowski A, Meri S, Honkanen E, Kaartinen K. Diagnostic and prognostic comparison of immune-complex-mediated membranoproliferative glomerulonephritis and C3 glomerulopathy. *Cells.* 2023;12(5):712. https://doi.org/10.3390/cells12050712.
2. Gan G, Michel M, Max A, et al. Membranoproliferative glomerulonephritis after intravitreal vascular growth factor inhibitor injections: a case report and review of the literature. *Br J Clin Pharmacol.* 2023;89(1):401–409. https://doi.org/10.1111/bcp.15558.

Clinical Presentation 13

1. Adeyinka A, Bashir K. Tumor lysis syndrome. In: Treasure Island (FL): StatPearls Publishing; 2023.
2. Torres PA, Helmstetter JA, Kay AM, Kay AD. Rhabdomyolysis: pathogenesis, diagnosis, and treatment. *Ochsner J.* 2015;15(1):58–69.

Clinical Presentation 14

1. Kunis CL, Markowitz GS, Liu-Jarin X, et al. Painful myopathy and end-stage renal disease. *Am J Kidney Dis.* 2001;37:1098–1104.

Clinical Presentation 15

1. Bleyer AJ, Burke SK, Dillon M, et al. A comparison of the calcium-free phosphate binder Sevelamer hydrochloride with calcium acetate in the treatment of treatment of hyperphosphatemia in dialysis patients. *Am J Kidney Dis.* 1999;33:694–701.

Clinical Presentation 16

1. Mazhar AR, Johnson RJ, Gillen D, et al. Risk factors and mortality associated with calciphylaxis in end-stage renal disease. *Kidney Int.* 2001;60:324–332.

Clinical Presentation 17

1. Ferreria MA. Diagnosis of renal osteodystrophy: when and how to use biochemical markers and non-invasive methods; when bone biopsy is needed. *Nephrol Dial Transplant.* 2000;5:S8–S14.

Clinical Presentation 18

1. Schomig M, Ritz E. Management of disturbed calcium metabolism in uremic patients: 2. Indications for parathyroidectomy. *Nephrol Dial Transpl.* 2000;5:25–29.

Clinical Presentation 19

1. Green J, Debby H, Lederer E, et al. Evidence for a PTH-independent humeral mechanism in post-transplant hypophosphatemia and phosphaturia. *Kidney Int.* 2000;60:1182–1196.

Clinical Presentation 20

1. Uribarri J, Calvo MS. Hidden sources of phosphorus in the typical American diet: does it matter in nephrology? *Semin Dial.* 2003;16:186–188.

Clinical Presentation 21

1. Jonsson KB, Zahradnik R, Larsson T, et al. Fibroblast growth factor 23 in oncogenic osteomalacia and x-linked hypophosphatemia. *N Engl J Med.* 2003;348:1656–1663.

Clinical Presentation 22

1. Tanaka R, Kakuta T, Fujisaki T, et al. Long-term (3-years) prognosis of parathyroid function in chronic dialysis patients after percutaneous ethanol injection therapy guided by color Doppler ultrasonography. *Nephrol Dial Transept.* 2003;18(suppl 3):S58–S61.

Clinical Presentation 23

1. Wilmer WA, Magro CM. Calciphylaxis: emerging concept in prevention, diagnosis, and treatment. *Semin Dial.* 2002;15:172–186.

Clinical Presentation 24

1. DeSevaux RG, Hoitsma AJ, Corstens FH, et al. Treatment with vitamin D and calcium reduces bone loss after renal transplantation: a randomized study. *J Am Soc Nephrol.* 2002;13:1608–1614.

Clinical Presentation 25

1. Rodriguez M, Nemeth E, Martin D. The calcium-sensing receptor: a key factor in the pathogenesis of secondary hyperparathyroidism. *Am J Physiol Renal Physiol.* 2005;288:F253–F264.

Clinical Presentation 26

1. Ritz E. Which is the preferred treatment of advanced hyperparathyroidism in a renal patient? II. Early parathyroidectomy should be considered as the first choice. *Nephrol Dial Transplant.* 1994;9:1819–1821.

Clinical Presentation 27

1. Choyke PL, Knopp MV. Pseudohypocalcemia with MR imaging contrast agents: a cautionary tale. *Radiology.* 2003;227:627–628.

Clinical Presentation 28

1. Green J, Debby H, Lederer E, et al. Evidence for a PTH-independent humeral mechanism in post-transplant hypophosphatemia and phosphaturia. *Kidney Int.* 2000;60:1182–1196.

Clinical Presentation 29

1. Jennette JC, Nachman PH. ANCA glomerulonephritis and vasculitis. *Clin J Am Soc Nephrol.* 2017;12(10):1680–1691. https://doi.org/10.2215/CJN.02500317.

Clinical Presentation 30

1. Zhang Y, Wu YK, Ciorba MA, Ouyang Q. Significance of antineutrophil cytoplasmic antibody in adult patients with Henoch-Schönlein purpura presenting mainly with gastrointestinal symptoms. *World J Gastroenterol.* 2008;14:622–626.
2. Pohl M. Henoch–Schönlein purpura nephritis. *Pediatr Nephrol.* 2015;30:245–252.
3. Boulis E, Majithia V, Mcmurray R. Adult-onset Henoch–Schonlein purpura with positive c-ANCA (anti-proteinase 3): case report and review of literature. *Rheumatol Int.* 2013;33:493–496.
4. Calatroni M, Oliva E, Gianfreda D, et al. ANCA-associated vasculitis in childhood: recent advances. *Ital J Pediatr.* 2017;43:46.

Clinical Presentation 31

1. Love PE, Santoro SA. Antiphospholipid antibodies: anticardiolipin and the lupus anticoagulant in systemic lupus erythematosus (SLE) and in non-SLE disorders: prevalence and clinical significance. *Ann Intern Med.* 1990;112:682–698.
2. Espinosa G, Font J, García-Pagan JC, et al. Budd-Chiari syndrome secondary to antiphospholipid syndrome: clinical and immunologic characteristics of 43 patients. *Medicine (Baltimore).* 2001;80:345–354.
3. Sciascia S, Mario F, Bertero MT. Chronic Budd-Chiari syndrome, abdominal varices, and caput medusae in 2 patients with antiphospholipid syndrome. *J Clin Rheumatol Pract Rep Rheum Musculoskelet Dis.* 2010;16:302.

Clinical Presentation 32

1. Morimoto M, Lewis DB, Lücke T, et al. Schimke immunoosseous dysplasia. In: Adam MP, Ardinger HH, Pagon RA, et al., eds. *GeneReviews® [Internet].* Seattle (WA): University of Washington; 1993–2018. https://www.ncbi.nlm.nih.gov/books/NBK1376/.

2. Lipska-Ziętkiewicz BS, Gellermann J, Boyer O, et al. Low renal but high extrarenal phenotype variability in Schimke immuno-osseous dysplasia. *PLoS One*. 2017;12:e0180926. https://doi.org/10.1371/journal.pone.0180926.

Clinical Presentation 33

1. Lloyd SE, Gunther W, Pearce SH, et al. Characterization of renal chloride channel, CLCN5, mutations in hypercalciuric nephrolithiasis (kidney stones) disorders. *Hum Mol Genet*. 1997;6:1233–1239.
2. Edvardsson VO, Goldfarb DS, Lieske JC, et al. Hereditary causes of kidney stones and chronic kidney disease. *Pediatr Nephrol*. 2013;28:1923–1942.
3. Rule AD, Krambeck AE, Lieske JC. Chronic kidney diseases in kidney stone formers. *Clin J Am Soc Nephrol*. 2011;6:2069–2075.

Clinical Presentation 34

1. Doutrelepont JM, Adler M, Willems M, et al. Hepatitis C infection and membranoproliferative glomerulonephritis. *Lancet*. 1993;341:317.
2. Bishof NA, Welch TR, Beischel LS, et al. DP polymorphism in HLA-A1, -B8, -DR3 extended haplotypes associated with membranoproliferative glomerulonephritis and systemic lupus erythematosus. *Pediatr Nephrol*. 1993;7(3):243–246.
3. Sun IO, Hong YA, Park HS, et al. Type III membranoproliferative glomerulonephritis in a patient with primary Sjögren's syndrome. *Clin Nephrol*. 2013;79:171–174.
4. Sethi S, Zand L, Leung N, et al. Membranoproliferative glomerulonephritis secondary to monoclonal gammopathy. *Clin J Am Soc Nephrol*. 2010;5:770–782.
5. Anaya JM, Ogawa N, Talal N. Sjögren's syndrome in childhood. *J Rheumatol*. 1995;22:1152–1158.
6. Aringer M, Costenbader K, Daikh D, et al. 2019 European League Against Rheumatism/American College of Rheumatology classification criteria for systemic lupus erythematosus. *Arthritis Rheumatol*. 2019;71(9):1400–1412.
7. Shiboski CH, Shiboski SC, Seror R, et al. 2016 American College of Rheumatology/European League Against Rheumatism classification criteria for primary Sjögren's syndrome: a consensus and data-driven method- ology involving three international patient cohorts. *Arthritis Rheum*. 2017;69:35–45.

Clinical Presentation 35

1. Heikkilä J, Rintala R, Taskinen S. Vesicoureteral reflux in conjunction with posterior urethral valves. *J Urol*. 2009;182:1555–1560. https://doi.org/10.1016/j.juro.2009.06.057.

Clinical Presentation 36

1. Alaygut D, Bayram M, Soylu A, Cakmakcı H, Türkmen M, Kavukcu S. Clinical course of children with nutcracker syndrome. *Urology*. 2013;82:686–690. https://doi.org/10.1016/j.urology.2013.03.048.
2. Shin JI, Park JM, Lee SM, et al. Factors affecting spontaneous resolution of hematuria in childhood nutcracker syndrome. *Pediatr Nephrol*. 2005;20:609–613. https://doi.org/10.1007/s00467-004-1799-z.

Clinical Presentation 37

1. Menon S, Valentini RP. Membranous nephropathy in children: clinical presentation and therapeutic approach. *Pediatr Nephrol*. 2010;25:1419–1428. https://doi.org/10.1007/s00467-009-1324-5.
2. Di Stefano V, Lionetti E, Rotolo N, La Rosa M, Leonardi S. Hypercalciuria and nephrocalcinosis as early feature of Wilson disease onset: description of a pediatric case and literature review. *Hepat Mon*. 2012;12:e6233. https://doi.org/10.5812/hepatmon.6233.
3. Zhuang XH, Mo Y, Jiang XY, Chen SM. Analysis of renal impairment in children with Wilson's disease. *World J Pediatr*. 2018;4:102–105. https://doi.org/10.1007/s12519-008-0019-5.
4. Helmy H, Fahmy M, Abdel Aziz H, Ghobrial C, Abdel Hameed N, El-Karaksy H. Urinary abnormalities in children and adolescents with Wilson disease before and during treatment with d-penicillamine. *J Gastroenterol Hepatol*. 2019;34:1824–1828. https://doi.org/10.1111/jgh.14653.
5. Shimamura Y, Maeda T, Gocho Y, Ogawa Y, Tsuji K, Takizawa H. Immunoglobulin A nephropathy secondary to Wilson's disease: a case report and literature review. *CEN Case Rep*. 2019;8:61–66. https://doi.org/10.1007/s13730-018-0365-7.

Clinical Presentation 38

1. Hughes IA, Davies JD, Bunch TI, et al. Androgen insensitivity syndrome. *Lancet*. 2012;380:1419–1428. https://doi.org/10.1016/S0140-6736(12)60071-3.

2. Kim S-H, Hu Y, Cadman S, Bouloux P. Diversity in fibroblast growth factor receptor 1 regulation: learning from the investigation of Kallmann syndrome: diversity in fibroblast growth factor receptor 1 regulation. *J Neuroendocrinol.* 2007;20:141–163. https://doi.org/10.1111/j.1365-2826.2007.01627.x.

Clinical Presentation 39

1. Puig JG, Miranda ME, Mateos FA, et al. Hereditary nephropathy associated with hyperuricemia and gout. *Arch Intern Med.* 1993;153:357–365.
2. Tinschert S, Ruf N, Bernascone I, et al. Functional consequences of a novel uromodulin mutation in a family with familial juvenile hyperuricaemic nephropathy. *Nephrol Dial Transplant.* 2004;19:3150–3154.
3. Nasr SH, Lucia JP, Galgano SJ, et al. Uromodulin storage disease. *Kidney Int.* 2008;73:971–976.
4. Scolari F, Caridi G, Rampoldi L, et al. Uromodulin storage diseases: clinical aspects and mechanisms. *Am J Kidney Dis.* 2004;44:987–999.

Clinical Presentation 40

1. Mainzer F, Saldino RM, Ozonoff MB, et al. Familial nephropathy associated with retinitis pigmentosa, cerebellar ataxia and skeletal abnormalities. *Am J Med.* 1970;49:556–562.
2. Saldino RM, Mainzer F. Cone-shaped epiphyses (CSE) in siblings with hereditary renal disease and retinitis pigmentosa. *Radiology.* 1971;98:39–45.
3. Giedion A. Phalangeal cone shaped epiphysis of the hands (PhCSEH) and chronic renal disease the conorenal syndromes. *Pediatr Radiol.* 1979;8:32–38.
4. Beals RK, Weleber RG. Conorenal dysplasia: a syndrome of cone-shaped epiphysis, renal disease in childhood, retinitis pigmentosa and abnormality of the proximal femur. *Am J Med Genet.* 2007;143A:2444–2447.
5. Jeune M, Beraud C, Carron R. Dystrophie thoracique asphyxiante de caractere familial. *Arch Pediatr.* 1955;12:886–891.
6. Bizet AA, Schmidts M, Porath JD, et al. Defects in the IFT-B component IFT172 cause Jeune and Mainzer Saldino syndromes in humans. *Am J Hum Genet.* 2013;93:915–925.
7. Perrault I, Saunier S, Hanein S, et al. Mainzer-Saldino syndrome is a ciliopathy caused by IFT140 mutations. *Am J Hum Genet.* 2012;9:864–870.
8. Follit JA, Xu F, Keady BT, et al. Characterization of mouse IFT complex B. *Cell Motil Cytoskeleton.* 2009;66:457–468.

Clinical Presentation 41

1. Gubler MC. Inherited diseases of the glomerular basement membrane. *Nat Clin Pract Nephrol.* 2008;4:24–37.
2. Sweeney E, Fryer A, Mountford R, et al. Nail–patella syndrome: a review of the phenotype aided by developmental biology. *J Med Genet.* 2003;40:153–162.
3. Hoyer JR, Michael AF, Vernier RL, et al. Renal disease in nail-patella syndrome: clinical and morphologic studies. *Kidney Int.* 1972;2:231–238.
4. Morita T, Laughlin LO, Kawano K, et al. Nail–patella syndrome. *Arch Intern Med.* 1973;131:271–277.
5. Zuppan CW, Weeks DA, Cutler D. Nail patella glomerulopathy without associated constitutional abnormalities. *Ultrastruct Pathol.* 2003;27:357–361.

Clinical Presentation 42

1. Kari JA, Montini G, Bockenhauer D, et al. Clinico-pathological correlations of congenital and infantile nephrotic syndrome over twenty years. *Pediatr Nephrol.* 2014;29(11):2173–2180.
2. Lionel AP, Joseph LK Simon A. Pierson syndrome—a rare cause of congenital nephrotic syndrome. *Indian J Pediatr.* 2014;81:1416–1417.
3. Goldenberg A, Ngoc LH, Thouret MC, et al. Respiratory chain deficiency presenting as congenital nephrotic syndrome. *Pediatr Nephrol.* 2005;20:465–469.
4. Nicolaou N, Margadant C, Kevelam SH, et al. Gain of glycosylation in integrin alpha3 causes lung disease and nephrotic syndrome. *J Clin Invest.* 2012;122:4375–4387.
5. Guo AH, Lu M. Two cases of congenital nephrotic syndrome resulting from cytomegalovirus infection. *Zhonghua Er Ke Za Zhi.* 2005;45:872–873.
6. Rahman H, Begum A, Jahan S, et al. Congenital nephrotic syndrome, an uncommon presentation of cytomegalovirus infection. *Mymensingh Med.* 2008;17:210–213.
7. Xiao HJ, Liu JC, Zhong XH. Congenital syphilis presenting congenital nephrotic syndrome in two children and related data review. *Beijing Da Xue Xue Bao.* 2011;43:911–913.

8. Marquardt T, Denecke J. Congenital disorders of glycosylation: review of their molecular bases, clinical presentations and specific therapies. *Eur J Pediatr.* 2003;162:359–379.
9. Jalanko H. Congenital nephrotic syndrome. *Pediatr Nephrol.* 2009;24:2121–2128.
10. Avni EF, Vandenhoute K, Devriendt A, et al. Update on congenital nephrotic syndromes and the contribution of US. *Pediatr Radiol.* 2011;41:76–81.
11. Kranz C, Denecke J, Lehle L, et al. Congenital disorder of glycosylation type Ik (CDG-Ik): a defect of mannosyltransferase I. *Am J Hum Genet.* 2004;74:545–551.

Clinical Presentation 43

1. Sharma SG, Bomback AS, Radhakrshnan J, et al. The modern spectrum of renal biopsy findings in patients with diabetes. *Clin J Am Soc Nephrol.* 2013;8:1718–1724.
2. Lombardo F, Valenzise M, Wasniewska M, et al. Two-year prospective evaluation of the factors affecting honeymoon frequency and duration in children with insulin dependent diabetes mellitus: the key role of age at diagnosis. *Diabetes Nutr Metab.* 2002;15:246–251.
3. Yaxley J, Litfin T. Non-steroidal anti-inflammatories and the development of analgesic nephropathy: a systematic review. *Renal Fail.* 2016;5:1–7.
4. van den Ouweland JM, Lemkes HH, Ruitenbeek W, et al. Mutation in mitochondrial tRNA Leu(UUR) gene in a large pedigree with maternally transmitted type 2 diabetes and deafness. *Nat Genet.* 1992;1:368–371.
5. Murphy R, Turnbull TM, Walker M, Hattersley AT. Clinical features, diagnosis and management of maternally inherited diabetes and deafness (MIDD) associated with the 3243A>G mitochondrial point mutation. *Diabetic Med.* 2008;25(4):383–399.
6. Guillausseau PJ, Dubois-Laforge D, Massin P, et al. Heterogeneity of diabetes phenotype in patients with 3243-bp mutation of mitochondrial DNA (maternally inherited diabetes and deafness or MIDD). *Diabetes Metab.* 2004;30:181–186.
7. Yamasoba T, Oka T, Tsukuda K, et al. Auditory findings in patients with maternally inherited diabetes and deafness harboring a point mutation in the mitochondrial transfer RNA Leu(UUR) gene. *Laryngoscope.* 1996;106:49–53.
8. Massin P, Dubois-Laforgue D, Meas T, et al. Retinal and renal complications in patients with a mutation of mitochondrial DNA at position 3,243 (maternally inherited diabetes and deafness). A case–control study. *Diabetologica.* 2008;51(9):1664–1670.
9. Jansen JJ, Maassen JA, van der Woude FJ, et al. Mutation in mitochondrial tRNALeu(UUR) gene associated with progressive kidney disease. *J Am Soc Nephrol.* 1997;8:118–1124.
10. Ohkubo K, Yamano A, Nagashima M, et al. Mitochondrial gene mutations in the tRNA (Leu(UUR)) region and diabetes: prevalence and clinical phenotypes in Japan. *Clin Chem.* 2001;47:1641–1648.
11. Koga Y, Akita Y, Takane N, et al. Heterogeneous presentation in A3243G mutation in the mitochondrial tRNA(Leu(UUR)) gene. *Arch Dis Child.* 2000;82:407–411.
12. Suzuki S, Hinokio Y, Ohtomo M, et al. The effects of coenzyme Q10 treatment on maternally inherited diabetes and deafness, and mitochondrial DNA 3243 (A to G) mutation. *Diabetologia.* 1998;41:584–588.

Clinical Presentation 44

1. Maroofian R, Schuele I, Najafi M, et al. Parental whole exome sequencing enables sialidosis type II diagnosis due to an NEU missense mutation as an underlying cause of nephrotic syndrome in the child. *Kidney Int Rep.* 2018;3:1454–1463.
2. Khan A, Sergi C. Sialidosis: a review of morphology and molecular biology of a rare pediatric disorder. *Diagnostics (Basel).* 2018;8:E29.

Clinical Presentation 45

1. Petri M, Orbai AM, Alarcón GS, et al. Derivation and validation of the systemic lupus international collaborating clinics classification criteria for systemic lupus erythematosus. *Arthritis Rheum.* 2012;64:2677–2686.
2. Andolino TP, Reid-Adam J. Nephrotic syndrome. *Pediatr Rev.* 2003;36:117–125.
3. Orth SR, Ritz E. The nephrotic syndrome. *N Engl J Med.* 1998;338:1202–1211.
4. Zaffanello M, Franchini M. Thromboembolism in childhood nephrotic syndrome: a rare but serious complication. *Hematology.* 2007;12:69–73.
5. Lau SO, Tkachuck JY, Hasegawa DK, et al. Plasminogen and anti-thrombin III deficiencies in the childhood nephrotic syndrome associated with plasminogenuria and antithrombinuria. *J Pediatr.* 1980;96:390–392.

6. Lilova MI, Velkovski IG, Topalov IB. Thromboembolic complications in children with nephrotic syndrome in Bulgaria (1974–1996). *Pediatr Nephrol.* 2000;15:74–78.
7. Citak A, Emre S, Sâirin A, et al. Hemostatic problems and thromboembolic complications in nephrotic children. *Pediatr Nephrol.* 2000;14:138–142.
8. Kerlin BA, Blatt NB, Fuh B, et al. Epidemiology and risk factors for thromboembolic complications of childhood nephrotic syndrome: a Midwest Pediatric Nephrology Consortium (MWPNC) study. *J Pediatr.* 2009;155:105–110.
9. Kerlin BA, Ayoob R, Smoyer WE. Epidemiology and pathophysiology of nephrotic syndrome-associated thromboembolic disease. *Clin J Am Soc Nephrol.* 2012;7:513–520.
10. Babyn PS, Gahunia HK, Massicotte P. Pulmonary thromboembolism in children. *Pediatr Radiol.* 2005;35:258–274.
11. Glassock RJ. Prophylactic anticoagulation in nephrotic syndrome: a clinical conundrum. *J Am Soc Nephrol.* 2007;18:2221–2225.
12. Yokoyama H, Taguchi T, Sugiyama H, Sato H. Committee for the Standardization of Renal Pathological Diagnosis and for Renal Biopsy and Disease Registry in the Japanese Society of Nephrology. Membranous nephropathy in Japan: analysis of the Japan Renal Biopsy Registry (J-RBR). *Clin Exp Nephrol.* 2012;16:557–563.
13. Andrew M, Brooker LA. Hemostatic complications in renal disorder of the young. *Pediatr Nephrol.* 1996;10:88–99.
14. Singhal R, Brimble KS. Thromboembolic complications in the nephrotic syndrome: pathophysiology and clinical management. *Thromb Res.* 2006;118:397–407.
15. Barbano B, Gigante A, Amoroso A, et al. Thrombosis in nephrotic syndrome. *Semin Thromb Hemost.* 2013;39:469–476.
16. Llach F, Koffler A, Finck E. On the incidence of renal vein thrombosis in the nephrotic syndrome. *Arch Intern Med.* 1977;137:333–336.
17. Zhang LJ, Zhang Z, Li SJ, et al. Pulmonary embolism and renal vein thrombosis in patients with nephrotic syndrome: prospective evaluation of prevalence and risk factors with CT. *Radiology.* 2014;273:897–906.
18. Zhang LJ, Wang ZJ, Zhou CS, et al. Evaluation of pulmonary embolism in pediatric patients with nephrotic syndrome with dual energy CT pulmonary angiography. *Acad Radiol.* 2012;19:341–348.
19. Lionaki S, Derebail VK, Hogan SL, et al. Venous thromboembolism in patients with membranous nephropathy. *Clin J Am Soc Nephrol.* 2012;7:43–51.
20. Yang Y, Lv J, Zhou F, et al. Risk factors of pulmonary thrombosis/embolism in nephrotic syndrome. *Am J Med Sci.* 2014;348:394–398.
21. Braun B, Weilemann LS, Weigand W. Ultrasonic demonstration of renal vein thrombosis. *Radiology.* 1981;138:157–158.
22. Beck L, Bomback AS, Choi MJ, et al. KDOQI US commentary on the 2012 KDIGO clinical practice guideline for glomerulonephritis. *Am J Kidney Dis.* 2013;62:403–441.
23. Medjeral-Thomas N, Ziaj S, Condon M, et al. Retrospective analysis of a novel regimen for the prevention of venous thromboembolism in nephrotic syndrome. *Clin J Am Soc Nephrol.* 2014;9:478–483.
24. Kelddal S, Nykjær KM, Gregersen JW, et al. Prophylactic anticoagulation in nephrotic syndrome prevents thromboembolic complications. *BMC Nephrol.* 2019;20:139.
25. Brodsky SV, Satoskar A, Chen J, et al. Acute kidney injury during warfarin therapy associated with obstructive tubular red blood cell casts: a report of 9 cases. *Am J Kidney Dis.* 2009;54:1121–1126.
26. Brodsky SV, Nadasdy T, Rovin BH, et al. Warfarin-related nephropathy occurs in patients with and without chronic kidney disease and is associated with an increased mortality rate. *Kidney Int.* 2011;80:181–189.

Clinical Presentation 46

1. Ebright JR, Komorowski R. Gonococcal endocarditis associated with immune complex glomerulonephritis. *Am J Med.* 1980;68(5):793–796.
2. Charles RW. Gonococcal infections. *In: Feigin and Cherry's Textbook of Pediatric Infectious Diseases.* 2014:1271–1301. Elsevier, United States.
3. Rice PA, Lieberman JM. Neisseria gonorrhoeae. *Princ Pract Pediatr Infect Dis.* 2012;126:741–748.
4. Dagan R, Cleper R, Davidovits M, et al. Post-infectious glomerulonephritis in pediatric patients over two decades: severity-associated features. *Isr Med Assoc J.* 2016;18:336–340.
5. Rompalo AM, Hook EW, Roberts PL, et al. The acute arthritis-dermatitis syndrome. The changing importance of Neisseria gonorrhoeae and Neisseria meningitidis. *Arch Intern Med.* 1987;147:281.

6. O'Brien JP, Goldenberg DL, Rice PA. Disseminated gonococcal infection: a prospective analysis of 49 patients and a review of pathophysiology and immune mechanisms. *Medicine*. 1983;1983:395.
7. Nasr SH, Radhakrishnan J, D'agati VD. Bacterial infection-related glomerulonephritis in adults. *Kidney Int*. 2013;83(5):792–803.
8. Rodríguez-Iturbe B, Rubio L, García R. Attack rate of poststreptococcal nephritis in families. A prospective study. *Lancet*. 1981;1(8217):401–403.

Clinical Presentation 47

1. Pickering MC, Botto M, Taylor PR, et al. Systemic lupus erythematosus, complement deficiency, and apoptosis. *Adv Immunol*. 2000;76:227–324.
2. Jönsson G, Truedsson L, Sturfelt G, et al. C2 deficiency in Sweden: frequent occurrence of invasive infection, atherosclerosis, and rheumatic disease. *Medicine (Baltimore)*. 2005;84:23–34. https://doi.org/10.1097/01.md.0000152371.22747.1e.
3. Hauck F, Lee-Kirsch Ma, Aust D, et al. Complement C2 deficiency disarranging innate and adaptive humoral immune responses in a pediatric patient: treatment with rituximab. *Arthritis Care Res (Hoboken)*. 2011;63:454–459.
4. Wen L, Atkinson JP, Giclas PC. Clinical and laboratory evaluation of complement deficiency. *J Allergy Clin Immunol*. 2004;113:585–593. https://doi.org/10.1016/j.jaci.2004.02.003.
5. Glass D, Raum D, Gibson D, et al. Inherited deficiency of the second component of complement. rheumatic disease associations. *J Clin Invest*. 1976;58:853–861. https://doi.org/10.1172/JCi108538.
6. Bishop WB, Carlton RF, Sanders LL. Diffuse vasculitis and death after hyperimmunization with pertussis vaccine. Report of a case. *N Engl J Med*. 1966;274:616–619. https://doi.org/10.1056/neJM196603172741107.
7. Kutlucan A, Gonen I, Yildizhan E, et al. Can influenza H1n1 vaccination lead to the membranous glomerulonephritis? *Indian J Pathol Microbiol*. 2012;55:239–241. https://doi.org/10.4103/0377-4929.97893.
8. Santoro D, Vita G, Vita R, et al. HLA haplotype in a patient with systemic lupus erythematosus triggered by hepatitis B vaccine. *Clin Nephrol*. 2010;74:150–153. https://doi.org/10.5414/Cnp74150 Medline:20630136.
9. Tan SY, Cumming AD. Vaccine related glomerulonephritis. *BMJ*. 1993;306:248. https://doi.org/10.1136/bmj.306.6872.248-b.
10. Kuzemko JA. Measles vaccination and the nephrotic syndrome. *BMJ*. 1972;4:665–666. https://doi.org/10.1136/bmj.4.5841.5865.

Clinical Presentation 48

1. Schober FP, Jobson MA, Poulton CJ, et al. Clinical features and outcomes of a racially diverse population with fibrillary glomerulonephritis. *Am J Nephrol*. 2017;45(3):248–256. https://doi.org/10.1159/000455390.
2. Rosenstock JL, Markowitz GS. Fibrillary glomerulonephritis: an update. *Kidney Int Rep*. 2019;4:917–922. https://doi.org/10.1016/j.ekir.2019.04.013.
3. Javaugue V, Karras A, Glowacki F, et al. Long-term kidney disease outcomes in fibrillary glomerulonephritis: a case series of 27 patients. *Am J Kidney Dis*. 2013;62:679–690. https://doi.org/10.1053/j.ajkd.2013.03.031.
4. Hogan J, Restivo M, Canetta PA, et al. Rituximab treatment for fibrillary glomerulonephritis. *Nephrol Dial Transplant*. 2014;29:1925–1931. https://doi.org/10.1093/ndt/gfu189.
5. Nasr SH, Valeri AM, Cornell LD, et al. Fibrillary glomerulonephritis: a report of 66 cases from a single institution. *Clin J Am Soc Nephrol*. 2011;6:775–784. https://doi.org/10.2215/CJN.08300910.
6. Mallett A, Tang W, Hart G, et al. End-stage kidney disease due to fibrillary glomerulonephritis and immunotactoid glomerulopathy—outcomes in 66 consecutive ANZDATA registry cases. *Am J Nephrol*. 2015;42:177–184. https://doi.org/10.1159/000440815.

Clinical Presentation 49

1. Chen M, Kallenberg CG, Zhao MH. ANCA-negative pauci-immune crescentic glomerulonephritis. *Nat Rev Nephrol*. 2009;5:313–318.
2. Sampathkumar K, Ramakrishnan M, Sah AK, et al. ANCA negative pauci-immune glomerulonephritis with systemic involvement. *Indian J Nephrol*. 2010;20:43–47.
3. Chen M, Yu F, Wang SX, et al. Antineutrophil cytoplasmic autoantibody-negative pauci-immune crescentic glomerulonephritis. *J Am Soc Nephrol*. 2007;18:599–605.
4. Tewari R, Badwal S, Kumar A, et al. Anti-neutrophil cytoplasmic antibody negative crescentic paucimmune glomerulonephritis in a case of scleroderma with systemic lupus erythematosus overlap. *Saudi J Kidney Dis Transpl*. 2016;27:602–605.

5. Alarcón-Segovia D, Cardiel MH. Comparison between 3 diagnostic criteria for mixed connective tissue disease. Study of 593 patients. *J Rheumatol.* 1989;16:328–334.
6. Ortega-Hernandez OD, Shoenfeld Y. Mixed connective tissue disease: an overview of clinical manifestations, diagnosis and treatment. *Best Pract Res Clin Rheumatol.* 2012;26:61–72.
7. Farhey Y, Hess EV. Mixed connective tissue disease. *Arthritis Rheum.* 2005;10:333–342. https://doi.org/10.1002/art.1790100508.
8. Bennett RM, O'Connell DJ. Mixed connective tissue disease: a clinicopathologic study of 20 cases. *Semin Arthritis Rheum.* 1980;10:25–51.
9. Kobayashi S, Nagase M, Kimura M, et al. Renal involvement in mixed connective tissue disease. Report of 5 cases. *Am J Nephrol.* 1985;5:282–289.
10. Kitridou RC, Akmal M, Turkel SB, et al. Renal involvement in mixed connective tissue disease: a longitudinal clinicopathologic study. *Semin Arthritis Rheum.* 1986;16:135–145.
11. Bennett RM, Spargo BH. Immune complex nephropathy in mixed connective tissue disease. *Am J Med.* 1977;63(4):534–541.
12. Mampilly N, Mathew M. A case of ANCA negative pauci-immune crescentic glomerulonephritis in mixed connective tissue disease. *BMH Med J.* 2015;2:47–52.

Clinical Presentation 50

1. Jackson DA, Elsawa SF. Factors regulating immunoglobulin production by normal and disease-associated plasma cells. *Biomolecules.* 2015;5:20–40.
2. Jeong HJ, Shin SJ, Lim BJ. Overview of IgG4-related tubulointerstitial nephritis and its mimickers. *J Pathol Transl Med.* 2016;50:26–36.
3. Wang Z, Zhu M, Luo C, et al. High level of IgG4 as a biomarker for a new subset of inflammatory bowel disease. *Sci Rep.* 2018;8(1):10018.
4. Stone JH, Zen Y, Deshpande V. IgG4-related disease. *N Engl J Med.* 2012;366:539–551.
5. Narayan AK, Baer A, Fradin J. Sonographic findings of IgG4-related disease of the salivary glands: case report and review of the literature. *J Clin Ultrasound.* 2018;46:73–77.
6. Saeki T, Kawano M. IgG4-related kidney disease. *Kidney Int.* 2014;85:251–257.
7. Danlos FX, Rossi GM, Blockmans D, et al. Antineutrophil cytoplasmic antibody-associated vasculitides and IgG4-relat- ed disease: a new overlap syndrome. *Autoimmun Rev.* 2017;16:1036–1043.
8. Galante JR, Daruwalla CP, Roberts ISD, et al. An unusual presentation of propylthiouracil-induced anti-MPO and PR3 positive ANCA vasculitis with associated anti- GBM antibodies, IgA nephropathy and an IgG4 interstitial infiltrate: a case report. *BMC Nephrol.* 2020;21:295.
9. Zhang P, Yin Q, Wang W, et al. Clinicopathological features of IgG4-related kidney disease. *Clin Nephrol.* 2020;94:135–141.
10. Quattrocchio G, Barreca A, Demarchi A, et al. IgG4-related kidney disease: the effects of a Rituximab-based immunosuppressive therapy. *Oncotarget.* 2018;9:21337–21347.
11. Pendergraft 3rd WF, Cortazar FB, Wenger J, et al. Long-term maintenance therapy using rituximab-induced continuous B-cell depletion in patients with ANCA vasculitis. *Clin J Am Soc Nephrol.* 2014;9(4):736–744.

Clinical Presentation 51

1. Beck L, Bomback AS, Choi MJ, et al. KDOQI US commentary on the 2012 KDIGO clinical practice guideline for glomerulonephritis. *Am J Kidney Dis.* 2013;62:403–441.
2. Nasr SH, Radhakrishnan J, D'Agati VD. Bacterial infection-related glomerulonephritis in adults. *Kidney Int.* 2013;83:792–803.
3. Boils CL, Nasr SH, Walker PD, et al. Update on endocarditis-associated glomerulonephritis. *Kidney Int.* 2015;87:1241–1249.
4. Konstantinov KN, Ulff-Møller CJ, Tzamaloukas AH. Infections and antineutrophil cytoplasmic antibodies: triggering mechanisms. *Autoimmun Rev.* 2015;14:201–203.
5. Ying C-M, Yao D-T, Ding H-H, et al. Infective endocarditis with antineutrophil cytoplasmic antibody: report of 13 cases and literature review. *PLoS One.* 2014;9:e89777.
6. Chirinos JA, Corrales-Medina VF, Garcia S, et al. Endocarditis associated with antineutrophil cytoplasmic antibodies: a case report and review of the literature. *Clin Rheumatol.* 2007;26:590–595.
7. Konstantinov KN, Harris AA, Hartshorne MF, et al. Symptomatic anti-neutrophil cytoplasmic antibody-positive disease complicating subacute bacterial endocarditis: to treat or not to treat? *Case Rep Nephrol Urol.* 2012;2:25–32.

8. Sexton DJ, Spelman D. Current best practices and guidelines. Assessment and management of complications in infective endocarditis. *Cardiol Clin.* 2003;21:273–282.

Clinical Presentation 52

1. Pickering MC, D'Agati VD, Nester CM, et al. C3 glomerulopathy: consensus report. *Kidney Int.* 2013;84:1079–1089.
2. Chauvet S, Roumenina LT, Bruneau S, et al. A familial C3GN secondary to defective C3 regulation by complement receptor 1 and complement factor H. *J Am Soc Nephrol.* 2016;27:1665–1677.
3. Iatropoulos P, Noris M, Mele C, et al. Complement gene variants determine the risk of immunoglobulin-associated MPGN and C3 glomerulopathy and predict long-term renal outcome. *Mol Immunol.* 2016;71:131–142.
4. Hageman GS, Anderson DH, Johnson LV, et al. A common haplotype in the complement regulatory gene factor H (HF1/CFH) predisposes individuals to age-related macular degeneration. *Proc Natl Acad Sci U S A.* 2005;102:7227–7232.
5. Song D, Yu XJ, Wang FM, et al. Overactivation of complement alternative pathway in postpartum atypical hemolytic uremic syndrome patients with renal involvement. *Am J Reprod Immunol.* 2015;74:345–356.
6. Fakhouri F, Jablonski M, Lepercq J, et al. Membrane cofactor protein, and factor I mutations in patients with hemolysis, elevated liver enzymes, and low platelet count syndrome. *Blood.* 2008;112:4542–4545.
7. Davila S, Wright VJ, Khor CC, et al. Genome-wide association study identifies variants in the CFH region associated with host susceptibility to meningococcal disease. *Nat Genet.* 2010;42:772–776.
8. Schneider MC, Prosser BE, Caesar JJ, et al. Neisseria meningitidis recruits factor H using protein mimicry of host carbohydrates. *Nature.* 2009;458:890–893.
9. Kalia N, Sharma A, Kaur M, et al. A comprehensive in silico analysis of non-synonymous and regulatory SNPs of human MBL2 gene. *Springerplus.* 2016;5(1):811.
10. Hoeflich C, Unterwalder N, Schuett S, et al. Clinical manifestation of mannose-binding lectin deficiency in adults independent of concomitant immunodeficiency. *Hum Immunol.* 2009;70:809–912.
11. Liu L, Ning B. The role of MBL2 gene polymorphism in sepsis incidence. *Int J Clin Exp Pathol.* 2015;8:15123–15127.
12. Smith RJ, Alexander J, Barlow PN, et al. New approaches to the treatment of dense deposit disease. *J Am Soc Nephrol.* 2007;18(9):2447–2456.
13. Goodship TH, Cook HT, Fakhouri F, et al. Atypical hemolytic uremic syndrome and C3 glomerulopathy: conclusions from a "Kidney Disease: Improving Global Outcomes" (KDIGO) Controversies Conference. *Kidney Int.* 2017;91:539–551.
14. Bomback AS, Smith RJ, Barile GR, et al. Eculizumab for dense deposit disease and C3 glomerulonephritis. *Clin J Am Soc Nephrol.* 2012;7:748–756.

Clinical Presentation 53

1. Rodriguez-Iturbe B, Musser JM. The current state of poststreptococcal glomerulonephritis. *J Am Soc Nephrol.* 2008;19:1855–1864.
2. Eison TM, Ault BH, Jones DP, et al. Post-streptococcal acute glomerulonephritis in children: clinical features and pathogenesis. *Pediatr Nephrol.* 2011;26:165–180.
3. Nasr SH, Fidler ME, Valeri AM, et al. Postinfectious glomerulonephritis in the elderly. *J Am Soc Nephrol.* 2011;22:187–195.
4. Nasr SH, Markowitz GS, Stokes MB, et al. Acute postinfectious glomerulonephritis in the modern era: experience with 86 adults and review of the literature. *Medicine (Baltimore).* 2008;87:21–32.
5. Montseny JJ, Meyrier A, Kleinknecht D, et al. The current spectrum of infectious glomerulonephritis. Experience with 76 patients and review of the literature. *Medicine (Baltimore).* 1995;74:63–73.
6. Nasr SH, Radhakrishnan J, D'Agati VD. Bacterial infection-related glomerulonephritis in adults. *Kidney Int.* 2013;85(5):792–803. https://doi.org/10.1038/ki.2012.407.
7. Nadasdy T, Hebert LA. Infection-related glomerulonephritis: understanding mechanisms. *Semin Nephrol.* 2011;31:369–375.
8. Yousif Y, Okada K, Batsford S, et al. Induction of glomerulonephritis in rats with staphylococcal phosphatase: new aspects in post-infectious ICGN. *Kidney Int.* 1996;50:290–297.
9. Rodríguez-Iturbe B, Batsford S. Pathogenesis of poststreptococcal glomerulonephritis a century after Clemens von Pirquet. *Kidney Int.* 2007;71:1094–1104.

10. Madaio MP, Harrington JT. Current concepts. The diagnosis of acute glomerulonephritis. *N Engl J Med.* 1983;309:1299–1302.
11. Rodríguez-Iturbe B. Epidemic poststreptococcal glomerulonephritis. *Kidney Int.* 1984;25:129–136.
12. Fremeaux-Bacchi V, Weiss L, Demouchy C, et al. Hypocomplementaemia of poststreptococcal acute glomerulonephritis is associated with C3 nephritic factor (C3NeF) IgG autoantibody activity. *Nephrol Dial Transplant.* 1994;9:1747–1750.
13. Daha MR, Austen KF, Fearon DT. Heterogeneity, polypeptide chain composition and antigenic reactivity of C3 nephritic factor. *J Immunol.* 1978;120:1389–1394.
14. Hoy WE, White AV, Dowling A, et al. Post-streptococcal glomerulonephritis is a strong risk factor for chronic kidney disease in later life. *Kidney Int.* 2012;81:1026–1032.
15. Dedeoglu IO, Springate JE, Waz WR, et al. Prolonged hypocomplementemia in poststreptococcal acute glomerulonephritis. *Clin Nephrol.* 1996;46:302–305.
16. Baldwin DS, Gluck MC, Schacht RG, et al. The long-term course of poststreptococcal glomerulonephritis. *Ann Intern Med.* 1974;80:342–358.
17. Popovic-Rolovic M. Serum C3 levels in acute glomerulonephritis and postnephritic children. *Arch Dis Child.* 1973;48:622–626.
18. Sethi S, Fervenza FC, Zhang Y, et al. Atypical postinfectious glomerulonephritis is associated with abnormalities in the alternative pathway of complement. *Kidney Int.* 2013;83:293–299.
19. Sandhu G, Bansal A, Ranade A, et al. C3 glomerulopathy masquerading as acute postinfectious glomerulonephritis. *Am J Kidney Dis.* 2012;60:1039–1043.
20. Vernon KA, Goicoechea de Jorge E, Hall AE, et al. Acute presentation and persistent glomerulonephritis following streptococcal infection in a patient with heterozygous complement factor H-related protein 5 deficiency. *Am J Kidney Dis.* 2012;60:121–125.
21. Sethi S, Fervenza FC, Zhang Y, et al. C3 glomerulonephritis: clinicopathological findings, complement abnormalities, glomerular proteomic profile, treatment, and follow-up. *Kidney Int.* 2012;82:465–473.
22. Servais A, Frémeaux-Bacchi V, Lequintrec M, et al. Primary glomerulonephritis with isolated C3 deposits: a new entity which shares common genetic risk factors with haemolytic uraemic syndrome. *J Med Genet.* 2007;44:193–199.
23. Sethi S, Fervenza FC. Membranoproliferative glomerulonephritis—a new look at an old entity. *N Engl J Med.* 2012;366:1119–1131.
24. Sethi S, Fervenza FC, Zhang Y, et al. Proliferative glomerulonephritis secondary to dysfunction of the alternative pathway of complement. *Clin J Am Soc Nephrol.* 2011;6:1009–1017.
25. Sethi S, Nester CM, Smith RJ. Membranoproliferative glomerulonephritis and C3 glomerulopathy: resolving the confusion. *Kidney Int.* 2012;81:434–441.
26. Rodríguez-Iturbe B, Rubio L, García R. Attack rate of poststreptococcal nephritis in families. A prospective study. *Lancet.* 1981;1:401–403.

Clinical Presentation 54

1. Medawar W, Green A, Campbell E, et al. Clinical and histopathologic findings in adults with the nephrotic syndrome. *Ir J Med Sci.* 1990;159:137–140.
2. Ruggenenti P, Chiurchiu C, Brusegan V, et al. Rituximab in idiopathic membranous nephropathy: a one-year prospective study. *J Am Soc Nephrol.* 2003;14:1851–1857.
3. Cattran DC. Idiopathic membranous glomerulonephritis. *Kidney Int.* 1994;59:1983–1994.
4. Wagoner RD, Stanson AW, Holley KE, et al. Renal vein thrombosis in idiopathic membranous glomerulopathy and nephrotic syndrome: incidence and significance. *Kidney Int.* 1983;23:368–374.
5. Ordoñez JD, Hiatt RA, Killebrew EJ, et al. The increased risk of coronary heart disease associated with nephrotic syndrome. *Kidney Int.* 1993;44:638–642.
6. Wheeler DC, Bernard DB. Lipid abnormalities in the nephrotic syndrome: causes, consequences, and treatment. *Am J Kidney Dis.* 1994;23:331–346.
7. Fervenza FC, Sethi S, Specks U. Idiopathic membranous nephropathy: diagnosis and treatment. *Clin J Am Soc Nephrol.* 2008;3:905–919.
8. Bazzi C, Petrini C, Rizza V, et al. Urinary N-acetyl-beta-glucosaminidase excretion is a marker of tubular cell dysfunction and a predictor of outcome in primary glomerulonephritis. *Nephrol Dial Transplant.* 2002;17:1890–1896.
9. Branten AJ, du Buf-Vereijken PW, Klasen IS, et al. Urinary excretion of beta2-microglobulin and IgG predict prognosis in idiopathic membranous nephropathy: a validation study. *J Am Soc Nephrol.* 2005;16:169–174.

10. Hofstra JM, Deegens JK, Willems HL, et al. Beta-2-microglobulin is superior to N-acetyl-beta-glucosaminidase in predicting prognosis in idiopathic membranous nephropathy. *Nephrol Dial Transplant.* 2008;23:2546–2551.
11. du Buf-Vereijken PW, Wetzels JF. Treatment-related changes in urinary excretion of high and low molecular weight proteins in patients with idiopathic membranous nephropathy and renal insufficiency. *Nephrol Dial Transplant.* 2006;21:389–396.
12. Irazabal MV, Eirin A, Lieske J, et al. Low- and high-molecular-weight urinary proteins as predictors of response to rituximab in patients with membranous nephropathy: a prospective study. *Nephrol Dial Transplant.* 2013;28:137–146.
13. Saeki T, Nishi S, Imai N, et al. Clinicopathological characteristics of patients with IgG4-related tubulointerstitial nephritis. *Kidney Int.* 2010;78:1016–1023.
14. Stone JH, Zen Y, Deshpande V. IgG4-related disease. *N Engl J Med.* 2012;366:539–551.
15. Cornell LD, Chicano SL, Deshpande V, et al. Pseudotumors due to IgG4 immune-complex tubulointerstitial nephritis associated with autoimmune pancreatocentric disease. *Am J Surg Pathol.* 2007;31:1586–1597.
16. Kamisawa T, Okamoto A. IgG4-related sclerosing disease. *World J Gastroenterol.* 2008;14:3948–3955.
17. Cravedi P, Abbate M, Gagliardini E, et al. Membranous nephropathy associated with IgG4-related disease. *Am J Kidney Dis.* 2011;58:272–275.
18. Fervenza FC, Downer G, Beck LH, et al. IgG4-related tubulointerstitial nephritis with membranous nephropathy. *Am J Kidney Dis.* 2011;58:320–324.
19. Llach F. Hypercoagulability, renal vein thrombosis, and other thrombotic complications of nephrotic syndrome. *Kidney Int.* 1985;28:429–439.
20. Lionaki S, Derebail VK, Hogan SL, et al. Venous thromboembolism in patients with membranous nephropathy. *Clin J Am Soc Nephrol.* 2012;7:43–51.
21. Beck LH Jr, Bonegio RG, Lambeau G, et al. M-type phospholipase A2 receptor as target antigen in idiopathic membranous nephropathy. *N Engl J Med.* 2009;361:11–21.
22. Qin W, Beck LH Jr, Zeng C, et al. Anti-phospholipase A2 receptor antibody in membranous nephropathy. *J Am Soc Nephrol.* 2011;22:1137–1143.
23. Beck LH Jr, Fervenza FC, Beck DM, et al. Rituximab-induced depletion of anti-PLA2R autoantibodies predicts response in membranous nephropathy. *J Am Soc Nephrol.* 2011;22:1543–1550.
24. Hofstra JM, Beck LH Jr, Beck DM, et al. Anti-phospholipase A_2 receptor antibodies correlate with clinical status in idiopathic membranous nephropathy. *Clin J Am Soc Nephrol.* 2011;6:1286–1291.
25. Herrmann SM, Sethi S, Fervenza FC. Membranous nephropathy: the start of a paradigm shift. *Curr Opin Nephrol Hypertens.* 2012;21:203–210.
26. Hofstra JM, Debiec H, Short CD, et al. Antiphospholipase A2 receptor antibody titer and subclass in idiopathic membranous nephropathy. *J Am Soc Nephrol.* 2012;23:1735–1743.
27. Debiec H, Ronco P. PLA2R autoantibodies and PLA2R glomerular deposits in membranous nephropathy. *N Engl J Med.* 2011;364:689–690.

CHAPTER 7

Hypertension

Clinical Presentation 1

An asymptomatic 10-year-old boy is evaluated for hypertension (HTN) diagnosed during a recent physical examination. He does not remember being told about hypertension in the past, and he has no family history of hypertension. He is not taking any medications.

On physical examination, his blood pressure (BP) is 170/60 mm Hg in both upper extremities. The heart rate is 65/min and regular. Carotid examination is normal; estimated central venous pressure is not elevated. The apical impulse is displaced and sustained. An ejection click is noted at the apex and left sternal border. There is a grade 2/6 early systolic murmur noted at the second right intercostal space. No diastolic murmur is noted over the anterior precordium. Systolic and diastolic murmurs are noted over the patient's back. There is no bruit noted over the abdomen. The lower extremity pulses are reduced and delayed.

Which of the following is the most likely diagnosis in this patient?

A. Coarctation of the aorta
B. Essential HTN
C. Pheochromocytoma
D. Renal vascular disease

The correct answer is A

Comment: This patient has classic features of aortic coarctation.[1] He has a pulse delay between the upper and lower extremities (radial artery to femoral artery delay). The BP in the lower extremities, when measured, will be lower than the BP noted in the upper extremities. The patient also has an ejection click and an early systolic murmur consistent with a bicuspid aortic valve, which is present in more than 50% of patients with aortic coarctation. The systolic and diastolic murmurs noted over the back are related to collateral vessels, which also cause the sign of rib notching, seen on this patient's chest radiograph on the inferior surface of the posterior upper thoracic ribs bilaterally.

Essential HTN is a common cause of systemic HTN, but the physical examination features of this patient are not explained by this diagnosis. In addition, a family history of HTN is common in patients with essential HTN.

Pheochromocytoma causes paroxysmal HTN in about half of affected patients; other pheochromocytomas present similar to patients with essential HTN. The signs and symptoms of pheochromocytoma are variable. The classic triad of sudden severe headaches, diaphoresis, and palpitations carries a high degree of specificity (94%) and sensitivity (91%) for pheochromocytoma in hypertensive patients. The absence of all three symptoms reliably excludes the condition. Finally, the physical examination features in this patient do not reflect this diagnosis.

Renovascular HTN resulting from fibromuscular disease of the renal arteries usually presents in patients younger than 35 years of age. Atherosclerotic renovascular disease is more common in older patients and is frequently associated with vascular disease in other vessels (carotid or coronary arteries and peripheral vessels). Azotemia is often observed in patients with atherosclerotic renovascular HTN. Renal artery stenosis cannot explain this patient's cardiac and peripheral vascular examination findings.[1]

Clinical Presentation 2

Which nonpharmacological intervention has the greatest approximate impact on systolic BP among patients with HTN?

A. Following a DASH dietary pattern
B. Performing aerobic physical activity for 90 to 150 minutes per week
C. Losing weight to reach an ideal body weight
D. Reducing intake of dietary sodium

The correct answer is A

Comment: Nonpharmacological interventions are effective in lowering BP and may aid patients with HTN in achieving their target BP. The 2019 American College of Cardiology/American Heart Association Guideline on the Primary Prevention of Cardiovascular Disease Studies suggests that the DASH diet had the greatest impact on lowering systolic BP compared with physical activity, salt restriction, and weight loss.[1] The DASH diet reduced systolic BP levels within 2 weeks of starting the plan. Not only was BP reduced, but total cholesterol and low-density lipoprotein were lower, too.[2]

Clinical Presentation 3

Which of the following risk factors is *not* commonly associated with pheochromocytoma?

A. Neurofibromatosis-1 (NF1)
B. von Hippel-Lindau (VHL) syndrome
C. Multiple endocrine neoplasia (MEN) type 1
D. Elevated succinyl dehydrogenase levels
E. Elevated RET

The correct answer is D

Comment: VHL disease is an autosomal dominant disorder with variable penetrance.[1] The *VHL* protein gene is on chromosome 3p25 and functions normally as a tumor suppressor by inhibiting transcription elongation. Missense mutations outside the elongation binding domain can cause the VHL disease. Affected persons can develop cerebellar and retinal hemangiomas, pheochromocytoma, renal cell carcinoma, pancreatic cysts, and endolymphatic inner ear tumors. Although some VHL families present with MEN-2, others may present only with pheochromocytoma. Thus, patients presenting with apparently isolated pheochromocytoma should be evaluated for VHL disease and MEN-2.[1]

Clinical Presentation 4

In a 17-year-old woman with no known established cardiovascular disease, a mean BP is 142/78 mm Hg and a glomerular filtration rate (GFR) is 56 mL/min/1.73 m^2 despite the use of enalapril 10 mg twice daily, amlodipine 5 mg twice daily, and atenolol 25 mg daily.

Which of the following would be the best first step in terms of pharmacological therapy?

A. Add spironolactone, 25 mg daily
B. Add terazosin, 1 mg twice daily
C. Increase atenolol to 50 mg daily.
D. Change enalapril to losartan HCT, 100/12.5 mg daily, and stop atenolol.

Correct answer is A

Comment: Spironolactone is the most effective fourth medication for treating HTN in patients already on treatment with triple regimens that include an angiotensin-converting enzyme (ACE) inhibitor or angiotensin receptor blocker (ARB), amlodipine, and a thiazide-like diuretic.[1]

Clinical Presentation 5

An 18-year-old female who is a devoted singer has hypertension, which has been well controlled with enalapril for the past month. She calls to report a new, intolerable side effect, and she requests to be switched to a different drug.

Which of the following adverse effects is most likely to be intolerable to this patient?

A. Frequent urination
B. Dysgeusia
C. Dry cough
D. Headache

The correct answer is C

Comment: Dry cough, which is the most common side effect reported with ACE inhibitors, would be intolerable to a singer, and develops in approximately 10% of patients treated with ACE inhibitors. In half of these patients, the ACE inhibitor has to be discontinued.[1]

Clinical Presentation 6

A 16-year-old male presented for evaluation of treatment-resistant HTN. He recalled being told that his systolic BP was high when he was in elementary school; however, he did not begin taking antihypertensive medications until age 10 years. Despite multiple antihypertensive regimens, his HTN has been difficult to control and is consistently above his BP target (<140/90 mm Hg) in multiple settings, including the physician's office and at home. His current regimen consists of 320 mg of valsartan, 200 mg/d of extended-release metoprolol, and 10 mg/d of amlodipine, which were his only medications. He had previously taken 25 mg/d of hydrochlorothiazide (in combination with valsartan and metoprolol); however, this was discontinued because of the inability to reach his BP target and the development of hypokalemia (potassium level, 2.8 mmol/L). The patient reported that he adhered strictly to a low-sodium diet, rarely drank alcohol, never smoked, and rode a stationary bicycle for 60 minutes every day. He had intentionally lost about 11.4 kg in the past 4 years. His medical history included obesity, hyperlipidemia, impaired fasting glucose levels, hypothyroidism treated with thyroid hormone replacement therapy, gout, and obstructive sleep apnea treated with continuous positive airway pressure (CPAP). He was recently evaluated in the sleep clinic, and his obstructive sleep apnea was being adequately treated with his current CPAP settings. The patient reported adherence to his antihypertensive medication regimen and CPAP use. He denied using nonsteroidal antiinflammatory drugs or stimulant medications. He also denied headaches, palpitations, and diaphoresis.

Findings on physical examination were as follows: BP, 158/88 mm Hg (average of six readings in the left arm sitting); pulse, 51 beats/min and regular; and body mass index (BMI) 47 (weight in kg/kg/height in m^2).

Other than an obese appearance, his physical examination was unremarkable.

Laboratory testing yielded the following results (reference ranges provided parenthetically): sodium level, 140 mEq/L (135–145 mEq/L); potassium level, 3.3 mmol/L (3.6–5.2 mmol/L); and creatinine level, 0.8 mg/dL (0.8–1.3 mg/dL). Electrocardiography revealed sinus bradycardia with borderline left ventricular hypertrophy. Renal ultrasonography revealed normal kidney size with no evidence of renal artery stenosis. Echocardiography revealed a mild increase in left ventricular thickness, normal function, and no valvular abnormalities.

In addition to advising continued efforts toward weight loss, which one of the following is the most appropriate next step in the management of this patient's HTN?

A. Advise follow-up blood pressure check in 3 months.
B. Increase extended-release metoprolol to 300 mg/day.
C. Evaluate for identifiable (secondary) causes of hypertension.
D. Refer the patient to a cardiologist.
E. Add clonidine.

Correct answer is C

Comment: This patient has medically complicated obesity, as evidenced by his body weight and multiple weight-related comorbid conditions (HTN, hyperlipidemia, impaired fasting glucose level, and obstructive sleep apnea). Additional weight loss, including consideration of bariatric surgery, will be paramount to improving BP control and lowering his overall cardiovascular risk. However, in the meantime, maintaining his current drug regimen is not appropriate. Further titration of his beta-blocker dose is unlikely to provide additional BP lowering and would likely induce symptomatic bradycardia given his current resting heart rate. His HTN was considered to be resistant because he had been unable to reach his BP goal despite taking three appropriate medications.

After completing a thorough review of adherence to lifestyle decisions and medications, the most appropriate next step in management would be to evaluate for identifiable secondary causes of HTN such as sleep apnea, renovascular disease, primary aldosteronism, Cushing syndrome, pheochromocytoma, and thyroid disease. This patient's history of developing HTN at a young age (<10 years) and hypokalemia with diuretic use are additional factors that suggest the need to evaluate for other contributors to his HTN.

Clonidine can be used as therapy for essential HTN and would be a reasonable agent to add; however, at this point, it is important to pursue other etiologies.

Further laboratory tests revealed: a thyroid-stimulating hormone level of 3.14 mIU/mL (0.30–5.0 mIU/mL); 24-hour urinary free cortisol level, 17 μg (3.5–45 μg/24 h); plasma free metanephrine level, <0.20 nmol/L (<0.50 nmol/L); plasma free normetanephrine level, 0.24 nmol/L (<0.90 nmol/L); plasma aldosterone concentration (PAC), 16 ng/dL (1–21 ng/dL); plasma renin activity (PRA) level, <0.6 ng/mL/h (0.6–3.0 ng/mL/h); and PAC:PRA ratio, 27 (<20).[1–3]

Clinical Presentation 7

Which one of the following best explains this patient's very low plasma renin level?

A. Hypoaldosteronism
B. Primary hyperaldosteronism
C. Restriction of dietary sodium
D. Pheochromocytoma

The correct answer is B

Comment: In the setting of a normally responsive renin-angiotensin-aldosterone (RAA) axis, hypoaldosteronism (e.g., primary adrenal insufficiency) would cause an elevated PRA, not a suppressed one as in this patient. In contrast, primary aldosteronism promotes negative feedback on the RAA axis, resulting in a low PRA level, making this the correct answer. Concomitant antihypertensive drug therapy is important to consider when interpreting the results of renin and aldosterone levels. ACE inhibitors (ACEIs) block conversion of angiotensin I to angiotensin II, which in turn decreases aldosterone levels. This inhibition actually causes elevated renin secretion through the RAA axis feedback. As a result, a low PRA level in a patient taking an ACEI or ARB should increase clinical suspicion for primary aldosteronism, as in this case. Restriction of dietary sodium results in increased aldosterone production via increased renin secretion. In pheochromocytoma, catecholamines are released that increase sympathetic neural tone and increase renin levels.[1–3]

Clinical Presentation 8

Which one of the following is the most appropriate next test to confirm the diagnosis?

A. Sodium-loading test with measurement of 24-hour urine aldosterone excretion
B. Computed tomography (CT) of the adrenal glands
C. Adrenal venous sampling (AVS)
D. BP response to a trial of a mineralocorticoid antagonist
E. Fine-needle aspiration biopsy of the adrenal glands

The correct answer is A

Comment: An increased PAC/PRA ratio alone is not diagnostic for primary aldosteronism. Primary aldosteronism must be confirmed by demonstrating inappropriate aldosterone secretion. Confirmatory testing can be done by evaluating 24-hour urine aldosterone levels after a sodium load, making this the correct answer. This functions to maximally suppress intrinsic aldosterone secretion. CT of the adrenal glands is not a good confirmatory study because it does not provide information regarding the functional status of any potentially visualized abnormalities. Surgical removal of an adenoma, which has not been proven to be functional, would be premature, so this would not contribute to the patient's current management. Adrenal venous sampling is useful to distinguish between subtypes of primary aldosteronism but is only indicated after confirmatory blood testing is complete. Empirical treatment with a mineralocorticoid antagonist would be premature because some patients may benefit from surgical intervention. Fine-needle aspiration biopsy of the adrenal glands has no role in the workup of primary aldosteronism. Occasionally, fine-needle aspiration biopsy is useful in the investigation of an adrenal mass suspected to be metastatic disease in the setting of a known malignancy.

However, it has no role in an isolated adrenal mass workup because cytology cannot distinguish a benign adrenal mass from adrenal carcinoma.

The patient was referred for a sodium-loading test with measurement of 24-hour urine aldosterone excretion. The patient consumed a 6000-mg sodium diet for 3 days. His 24-hour urine collection revealed the following results: urine volume, 3008 mL; creatinine concentration, 0.8 mg/dL (0.8–1.3 mg/dL); 24-hour urine sodium level, 343 mmol/24 h (40–217 mmol/24 h); sodium concentration, 114 mmol/L (135–145 mmol/L); and aldosterone, 17 μg/24 h (<12 μg/24 h if 24-hour urine sodium level is >200 mmol).

Because the urine aldosterone level was well above the 12 μg/24 h cutoff, the diagnosis of primary aldosteronism, resulting from either adrenal adenoma or idiopathic adrenal hyperplasia, was entertained. CT of the abdomen with 3-mm cuts through the adrenal glands did not demonstrate adrenal masses.[1–3]

Clinical Presentation 9

Which one of the following is the most appropriate next step in management?

A. Radionuclide scintigraphy of the adrenal glands
B. Magnetic resonance imaging (MRI) of the adrenal glands
C. Follow-up CT of the adrenal glands in 6 months
D. Proceed directly to surgery
E. Adrenal venous sampling

The correct answer is E

Comment: Radionuclide scintigraphy with iodocholesterol was formerly used to correlate adrenal function with visualized anatomic lesions to help clarify a target for possible surgical resection. However, this patient has no clear radiographic evidence of an adrenal adenoma. An MRI of the adrenal glands cannot rule out unilateral aldosterone-producing disease and would not contribute any additional information for this patient. Although serial CT imaging, like MRI, may reveal a new adrenal lesion, nonfunctioning adrenal incidentalomas are relatively common in patients older than age 40 years, and this would not provide any information regarding whether the lesion was hormonally functional. Moreover, aldosterone-producing adenomas can be very small, so CT imaging may not universally exclude this disorder. Adrenal venous sampling performed by an experienced interventional radiologist is the only means of detecting laterality of disease. Even though AVS is not available at all medical centers, it should be considered in all patients willing to pursue surgical management. If not initially pursued, it should be reconsidered in patients who either do not tolerate or do not benefit from medical management. Proceeding directly to adrenalectomy without prior AVS in this case would not be indicated because the disease could be bilateral. AVS was offered, but the patient did not wish to pursue surgical treatment. In the absence of an obvious adrenal carcinoma or adrenal adenoma, he was thought most likely to have the idiopathic bilateral hyperplasia subtype of primary aldosteronism.[1–3]

Clinical Presentation 10

Which one of the following is the most appropriate empirical treatment option for this patient?

A. Low-dose glucocorticoid
B. Mineralocorticoid antagonist
C. Triamterene
D. More aggressive salt restriction
E. Percutaneous radiofrequency ablation

The correct answer is B

Comment: Low-dose glucocorticoid is only used as first-line therapy in the subtype of primary aldosteronism known as glucocorticoid-remediable aldosteronism, which is a very rare genetic condition that needs to be confirmed with specific genetic testing before initiating treatment. The best treatment option for this patient with bilateral disease is medical treatment with a mineralocorticoid receptor antagonist such as spironolactone or eplerenone. Triamterene is a potassium-sparing diuretic agent that also targets the distal renal tubule; however, unlike spironolactone and eplerenone, it is not an aldosterone antagonist and is therefore not the preferred agent. A low-salt diet is a reasonable recommendation for all patients with HTN but would not be sufficient for this patient. Percutaneous radiofrequency ablation is occasionally used to treat unilateral adrenal lesions but would clearly not be useful in this scenario.

The patient began a therapeutic trial of an aldosterone antagonist, eplerenone, at a dose of 50 mg by mouth twice daily. After 2 months of therapy, his valsartan and metoprolol doses were decreased by 50%, with systolic BP maintained in the range of 135 to 145 mm Hg.[1–3]

Clinical Presentation 11

Which of the following patient vignettes is most consistent with true resistant HTN in a 19-year-old patient without established cardiovascular or chronic kidney disease?

A. Office BP (mean of repeated measurements) 146/96 mm Hg on losartan 100 mg daily, and amlodipine 5 mg daily
B. Office BP (mean of repeated measurements) 136/86 mm Hg on losartan 100 mg daily, amlodipine 5 mg daily, and hydrochlorothiazide 25 mg daily, with a mean home BP readings of 132/82 mm Hg
C. Office BP (mean of repeated measurements) 146/90 mm Hg on losartan 100 mg daily, amlodipine 5 mg daily, and hydrochlorothiazide 25 mg daily, with a mean home BP readings of 126/76 mm Hg

The correct answer is C
Comment: Resistant HTN is defined as HTN that is poorly responsive to treatment and requires the use of multiple medications to achieve acceptable BP ranges.[1]

Clinical Presentation 12

A 19-year-old male reports to the emergency room after being seen at his primary care physician's clinic. His BP on entering the emergency room is 171/100 mm Hg and he has shortness of breath with a headache. He has a past medical history of hypertension for 3 years. He denies smoking and illicit drug use. He rarely drinks alcohol. His medications are the following: lisinopril 20 mg once per day and hydrochlorothiazide 25 mg once per day. His laboratory tests are all within normal limits.

Which of the following is appropriate for this patient?

A. Check medication adherence.
B. Emphasize restriction of sodium in diet.
C. Potentially increase the current dose of hydrochlorothiazide to 50 mg daily.
D. Reevaluate in a week.
E. All of the above.

The correct answer is E
Comment: The following can all contribute to the development of both hypertension and resistant hypertension: obesity, physical inactivity, a diet high in salt, heavy alcohol drinking, and poor adherence to medication.[1]

Clinical Presentation 13

Which of the following hypertensive scenarios requires immediate treatment?

A. A 3-year-old boy with a history of renal disease and stage I HTN, now with systolic BP (SBP) >the 99th percentile

B. A 2-month-old girl admitted for labial abscess with SBP >the 99th percentile and tachycardia
C. A 10-year-old girl admitted for asthma with SBP at the 98th percentile with tachypnea
D. A 4-year-old boy admitted for bronchiolitis with SBP >the 99th percentile with lethargy

The correct answer is D

Comment: The most likely of these to need immediate treatment is the child with bronchiolitis who has a hypertensive emergency; the elevation of the BP combined with the end-organ symptom of lethargy is highly concerning, especially in a setting of few other causes.[1] Though option B could be considered hypertensive urgency, the BP is likely increased by the pain associated with the abscess, and therefore pain medications could be tried first. The asthmatic only has stage I HTN, which is most likely influenced by the steroid treatment of asthma, and his tachypnea is likely from the asthma. Finally, the patient with a history of HTN and renal failure would be considered a chronic patient, and though oral medications could be used, a conversation with the nephrologist should occur.

Clinical Presentation 14

A 17-year-old woman with long-standing lupus nephritis presents to her physician for her biannual checkup. She is currently taking no medication and she feels generally well.

On physical examination, her BP is 160/98 mm Hg. Pressures were equal in both arms. Previous BP readings have been in the range of 130/70 mm Hg.

Her physician asks her to return a week later for a recheck of the pressure. At that time, repeat blood pressure was 158/100 mm Hg. The remainder of the physical examination was normal.

Laboratory studies were serum creatinine 4.3 mg/dL, urea nitrogen 38 mg/dL, and potassium 5.1 mEq/L. A 24-hour urine protein was 1.2 g. These laboratory results were only slightly higher than those taken 6 months earlier. This patient is presumed to have HTN as the result of her lupus nephritis.

What is the first-line antihypertensive agent for this patient?

A. Thiazide diuretic
B. ACEI
C. Sympathetic blocker such as Aldomet
D. Beta-blocker

The correct answer is B

Comment: In chronic kidney disease (CKD) with proteinuria, either ACEIs or ARBs reduce urinary protein and slow the progression of renal failure.

Hypertension is present in approximately 80% to 85% of patients with CKD and is thought to be multifactorial (sodium retention, increased activity of the renin-angiotensin system, and enhanced activity of the sympathetic nervous system).

In patients with proteinuria (defined as protein excretion above 500–1000 mg/day) CKD, first-line therapy consists of an ACEI or ARB as first-line therapy for the treatment of HTN.[1,2] ACEIs, in addition to reducing intraglomerular pressure, reduce the excretion of urinary protein (both of which delay the progression of renal failure). ARBs have a similar effect.[1,2] Aside from BP control, the aim is to reach less than 1000 mg/day of protein spilling into the urine.

In patients with edema, a thiazide diuretic can be added as a second-line drug; chlorthalidone is preferred over hydrochlorothiazide because of its longer duration of action. A dihydropyridine calcium channel blocker (CCB) is appropriate as a second-line drug for patients without fluid retention. Neither a beta-blocker nor a sympathetic, such as Aldactone, demonstrate the protective effect of ACEIs or ARBs.

Clinical Presentation 15

A 12-year-old girl with CKD stage III (GFR 34 mL/min/2.73 m^2) is hypertensive and her BP is not controlled on a regimen of hydralazine 20 mg three times a day, atenolol 50 mg daily, and 12.5 mg of hydrochlorothiazide daily.

Which of the following is (are) *most* appropriate to choose (select all that apply)?

A. Switch diuretic to chlorthalidone.
B. Consider other medications in lieu of hydralazine and atenolol.
C. Add clonidine.
D. Increase hydrochlorothiazide to 25 mg.

The correct answers are A and B

Comment: Evidence suggests greater cardiovascular protection with other classes of antihypertensive agents (ACEIs/CCBs) versus beta-blockers (atenolol). Hydrochlorothiazide is not as effective a diuretic agent as chlorthalidone.

To initiate therapy to lower this patient's BP, hydrochlorothiazide should be changed to chlorthalidone, and next, a substitute should be found for hydralazine (either amlodipine or combination ACEI/ARB, preferably in a combination tablet).[1]

Three maneuvers can lead to better BP control over shorter periods. First, use combination antihypertensive agents earlier and more often, especially in HTN stage II or higher; second, identify resistant HTN earlier and use spironolactone when possible. Third, avoid less efficacious medications (hydralazine and clonidine) from days gone by.

Clinical Presentation 16

You evaluate a 15-year-old girl with chronic HTN whose BP remains above target despite a daily regimen of benazepril 20 mg, chlorthalidone 25 mg, and amlodipine 10 mg.

What is next on your therapeutic plan?

A. Add an agent from another class, such as hydralazine or clonidine.
B. Characterize the patient as having resistant HTN and initiate therapy with 25 mg of spironolactone (potassium levels permitting).
C. Add an ARB.
D. Switch from amlodipine to verapamil.

Correct answer is B

Comment: Resistant HTN is defined as BP not controlled on a complementary three-drug regimen with a diuretic as one of the agents. Spironolactone has become a "go-to" agent for treating resistant HTN.[1,2] If it works, it may allow the patient to discontinue other antihypertensive agents. It is a pharmaceutical backbone for resistant HTN treatment.

Clinical Presentation 17

You are seeing a 15-year-old male for the first time. He has untreated HTN (168/106 mm Hg and BP has been elevated on at least three occasions). There is currently no evidence of target organ dysfunction (heart, neurological, or eyegrounds).

From a therapeutic perspective, what is the best initial approach?

A. Initiate treatment with 25 mg of hydrochlorothiazide.

B. Consider initiating treatment with a two-agent combination pill.
C. Delay pharmacologic intervention and treat with salt restriction.
D. Consider initiating treatment with triple drugs including an ACEI, a CCB, and a thiazide diuretic.

The correct answer is B

Comment: The patient qualifies for a diagnosis of stage II HTN (BP >160/>100 mm Hg). A single agent will not suffice to lower the patient's BP to target level. Many studies have also demonstrated that combination therapy reduces the risk of cardiac events, is more efficacious, and improves adherence, BP control, and time-to-target BP. Combination therapy with appropriately chosen agents (such as amlodipine and an ARB) augments effects of either agent taken alone. The days of "maxing out" monotherapy before initiating combinations are over.[1]

Clinical Presentation 18

A 15-year-old male presents to your office for a follow-up of his BP medication. He is currently taking amlodipine 10 mg/d along with lisinopril 20 mg/day. He has been doing well and has had no adverse effects from this regimen. His BP readings at home and in the office average about 130/80 mm Hg. He has no history of cardiovascular disease. Nevertheless, he asks you if any simple changes can be made to decrease his cardiovascular risks.

Based on current literature, what intervention may decrease his cardiovascular-related morbidity and mortality?

A. Adding hydrochlorothiazide to the regimen
B. Taking his BP medication at bedtime
C. Adding a beta-blocker to the regimen
D. No change is needed; his BP is well controlled.

The correct answer is A

Comment: When two or more drugs are used, they should be from different antihypertensive drug classes. In most patients, the drugs should be selected from among the three preferred classes (i.e., ACEIs [or ARBs], CCBs, and thiazide diuretics).

Evidence suggests treating with the combination of an ACEI (or ARB) and a CCB, preferably a dihydropyridine calcium blocker. In addition, it is also recommended to prescribe these two agents as a single-pill combination, if feasible. Single-pill combinations lead to greater BP reduction, increased attainment of BP goals, and better medication adherence as compared with free equivalents, in which the two drugs are prescribed separately.

The combination of an ACEI (or ARB), a CCB with a thiazide diuretic is a reasonable alternative, particularly in patients who have conditions that can benefit from a thiazide diuretic (e.g., edema, osteoporosis, calcium nephrolithiasis with hypercalciuria).[1]

Initially, serum electrolytes and serum creatinine should be monitored 1 to 3 weeks after initiation or titration of ACEIs, ARBs, mineralocorticoid receptor antagonists, and diuretics. In patients on stable doses of medications, electrolytes and creatinine are typically monitored annually.

If BP is uncontrolled, it is typically recommended to escalate doses of individual antihypertensive drugs to at least half the maximum recommended dose (i.e., to a moderate or high dose) before adding additional therapy. After goal BP is attained, patients should be followed every 3 to 6 months.

Clinical Presentation 19

A 17-year-old woman has been on antihypertensive drug therapy for the past 3 months. During her most recent visit, her fasting blood glucose level was found to be 243 mg/dL.

Which agent in an antihypertensive drug regimen would be most likely to have caused her glucose intolerance?

A. Diltiazem
B. Lisinopril
C. Amlodipine
D. Hydrochlorothiazide
E. Minoxidil

The correct answer is D

Comment: Thiazides are known to produce mild hyperglycemia.[1] It is typically not of clinical consequence in nondiabetics and can be minimized by correcting any associated hypokalemia (the two side effects appear to be linked). The effect on plasma glucose is typically very small, with the low doses of thiazides typically prescribed for treating hypertension because low doses have minimal natriuretic effects.

Clinical Presentation 20

A definite contraindication for the use of ACEIs and ARBs includes which one of the following?

A. Asthma
B. Bilateral renal artery stenoses
C. Diabetes
D. Tachycardia
E. Hypokalemia

The correct answer is B

Comment: Angiotensin II (Ang II) is necessary for maintaining efferent arteriole resistance in this setting. Reducing Ang II levels, or Ang II effects, can reduce GFR and cause kidney failure in this setting. In general, contraindications to ACEI use include hyperkalemia (>5.5 mmol/L), renal artery stenosis, pregnancy, or prior adverse reaction to ACEIs including angioedema.[1]

Clinical Presentation 21

A 4-year-old boy was admitted to our hospital because of hyperpigmented macules in 2008. The pigmentations were present when he was born, but this was his first hospital admission. On physical examination, axillary freckling and multiple café-au-lait spots ≥5 mm in size were revealed, spread over the skin of the trunk. His height was 100 cm (10–50th percentile), and weight was 15 kg (10–25th percentile). He was normotensive. Slit-lamp examination showed the presence of more than 10 Lisch nodules for each eye. Patient was diagnosed as having NF1. The p.R304 pathogenic mutation (also known as c.910C > T), located in coding exon 9 of the *NF1* gene, was detected in the genetic examination of NF1.

When the patient was 5 years old, he was admitted to the hospital because of epistaxis in 2009. His blood pressure was 170/100 mm Hg and heart rate was 108/min. Bilateral radial/femoral pulses were bounding. There were no abdominal and carotid bruits. Electrocardiogram was normal. Clinical laboratory investigations revealed that kidney and liver function tests, blood cell counts, urinalysis, serum electrolytes, and 24-hour urine levels of catecholamines were all within normal ranges, but plasma renin activity was elevated, >500 (1–6.5 ng/mL/h). Kidney Doppler ultrasound showed bilateral renal arterial stenosis. Abdominal computed tomography (CT) angiography revealed a severe right ostial renal artery stenosis, total occlusion of the left renal artery and the celiac trunk, and moderate stenosis of the superior mesenteric artery and collateral circulation for these arteries. Amlodipine and propranolol were initiated. Percutaneous transluminal renal angioplasty (PTRA) was performed. During PTRA, contour irregularity and minimal stenosis in the ostium of the right renal artery and perivascular diaphragmatic collateral arteries at the level of the left renal artery orifice were observed. A coronary balloon catheter was used for the right renal artery. For the left renal artery, surgery was performed, and the occluded segment was removed and anastomosis was made. After these procedures, BP returned to normal levels. Previously initiated amlodipine and propranolol were discontinued.

After a few years, his BP became moderately high. An echocardiographic examination revealed hypertrophy of the interventricular septum, and an ophthalmological examination revealed grade 1 to 2 hypertensive retinopathy. Ophthalmic fundus examination showed tiny veins twisted into a spiral shape and corkscrew retinal vessels. Antihypertensive treatment was initiated again (amlodipine and metoprolol). When he was 17 years old, he was admitted to the hospital because of 150/100 mm Hg BP. Conventional angiography was performed. Abdominal aorta was low in caliber. The celiac truncus was markedly dilated and its branches were patent. It was occluded at the ostium of the superior mesenteric artery and was filled from celiac truncus via the dilated pancreaticoduodenal arch, and its branches were patent. The segment containing the previously placed intravascular stent at the level of the right renal artery ostium was patent. Aorto-left renal artery neoanastomosis was patent and showed smooth wall features. In the nephrogram phase, both kidneys showed smooth contours and homogeneous opacifications. In the right carotid system, the communicating segment of the internal carotid artery was obstructed/severely stenotic, and collateral flow was monitored. The posterior cerebral artery was also patent. The anterior cerebral artery segment was hypoplastic. In the left carotid system, there was an aneurysm 2 mm in size on the posterior wall of the ophthalmic segment of the left internal carotid artery.

What is the cause of hypertension in the patient?

A. Renal vascular disease
B. Mutation in the *NF1* gene
C. Overactivity of the renin-angiotensin system (RAS)
D. Carotid artery stenosis

The correct answer is B

Comment: HTN is a frequent finding in patients with NF1 and may develop during childhood.[1] If the vascular stenosis resulting from loss of neurofibromin expression occurs in the renal arteries, the patient develops renovascular HTN. The RAS plays an important role in the development of HTN.[2] In unilateral RAS, decreased kidney blood flow stimulates the production of renin, angiotensin II, and aldosterone. Aldosterone production causes sodium and water retention, but these excesses of sodium and water are rapidly excreted by the contralateral kidney by pressure natriuresis. But in bilateral RAS, as in our patient, although there is water and salt retention with a similar mechanism, natriuresis cannot be achieved because of decreased blood flow in both kidneys. The increased plasma volume suppresses plasma renin activity, and it causes volume-mediated HTN not renin-mediated.[3] HTN in NF1 is a complicated problem. Approximately 15% of NF1 patients have HTN, either primary HTN or secondary HTN because of RAS. Because of stenosis, kidney blood flow decreases and plasma renin level is measured as high.[4,5]

In our patient, because the plasma renin level was high and bilateral RAS was detected, treatment was started with antihypertensive medications, then PTRA was performed and a stent was placed in a renal artery. The patient was normotensive in the follow-up period, and antihypertensive drugs were discontinued. However, over the years, our patient developed mild HTN, and RAS overactivity developed again in follow-up. In our patient, the renin level was normal, and it was seen that renal artery blood flow was patent after PTRA. HTN was seen to regress.

Clinical Presentation 22

A 16-year-old female (162 cm tall, weight 77 kg, and 160 cm tall) is diagnosed with stage I hypertension. Her BP averages 135/85 mm Hg. She has no other comorbid conditions and is otherwise in excellent health.

What initial therapy would be most appropriate for her?

A. Clonidine
B. Diltiazem
C. Hydrochlorothiazide
D. Prazosin
E. Lifestyle modification

The correct answer is E

Comment: Patients with stage I hypotension (BP 130–139/80–89 mm Hg) who are at low risk for cardiovascular (CV) disease should be initially treated with nonpharmacologic, lifestyle improvements, with reassessment after 3 to 6 months to determine if they have met their BP goal of <130/<80 mm Hg.[1]

Clinical Presentation 23

A 14-year-old male was recently diagnosed with stage I hypertension. His history is unremarkable except that both parents and a grandparent died from systolic heart failure at a relatively early age.

Which antihypertensive drug would be best at preventing heart failure if prescribed to this patient?

A. An ACEI
B. A beta-blocker
C. An alpha-blocker
D. A CCB
E. A thiazide diuretic

The correct answer is E

Comment: The correct answer is a thiazide diuretic. Studies have shown that alpha-blockers actually double the risk of heart failure compared with a diuretic, and both CCBs and ACEIs are also inferior to a diuretic for preventing congestive heart failure (CHF).[1]

Among patients selected for antihypertensive drug treatment, therapy should be initiated with either one drug (i.e., monotherapy) or two drugs (i.e., combination therapy, preferably in a single pill to improve adherence).[1,2]

In general, patients with a SBP 10 to 20 mm Hg above goal and/or a diastolic BP 10 mm Hg above goal should have antihypertensive drug therapy initiated with low to moderate doses of two agents with complementary mechanisms of action.[2] Some experts begin with two agents in patients with stage II hypertension (i.e., SBP ≥140 mm Hg and/or diastolic BP ≥90 mm Hg), whereas other experts would initiate therapy with two drugs in patients whose SBP is ≥150 mm Hg and/or diastolic BP is ≥90 mm Hg.

Clinical Presentation 24

A 16-year-old female has recently been diagnosed with HTN by her primary care physician. Her BP during the past two visits has averaged 145/95 mm Hg. She is 85 kg, 162 cm tall, and exercises regularly. Her electrocardiogram indicates mild left ventricular hypertrophy. Her plasma lipids and fasting glucose are normal. She is a smoker (one pack per day). She is advised to enter a smoking cessation program to reduce cardiovascular risk, adopt a DASH diet, and maintain her daily routine of 30 minutes per day of aerobic exercise, with the target of losing at least 5 kg over the next 6 months. Her physician then discusses the options for drug therapy.

Which of the following is the *most* appropriate drug selection for this patient?

A. Furosemide plus losartan
B. Hydralazine
C. Hydrochlorothiazide plus ramipril
D. Hydrochlorothiazide
E. Amlodipine plus metoprolol

The correct answer is C

Comment: This patient will need at least two drugs to reduce her SBP from 145 to <130 mm Hg. If she is successful in losing weight, with concomitant reduction of BP, one of the two drugs can be reduced in dosage or discontinued. The 2017 American College of Cardiology/American Heart Association recommends therapy with two drugs consisting of either a thiazide, an ACEI (or ARB), and a CCB.[1] Note that the side effects of the thiazide (mild hypokalemia) can be countered by either an ACEI or an ARB (which can produce mild hyperkalemia).

Combination therapy lowers BP more than monotherapy and increases the likelihood that target BP will be achieved in a reasonable time. In addition, using two drugs may lead to attainment of goal BP with lower doses of each medication, and this reduces the risk of dose-related side effects.[2]

Regardless of whether treatment is begun with one or two drugs, the initial drug dose should generally be low. However, by far the most important strategy for ultimately achieving BP control is to avoid therapeutic inertia. Therapeutic inertia is defined as failing to initiate or adjust/intensify prescribed drug therapy despite the recognition of uncontrolled HTN.

When two drugs are used, they should be from different antihypertensive drug classes. In most patients, the drugs should be selected from among the three preferred classes (i.e., ACEIs [or ARBs], CCBs, and thiazide diuretics).

Clinical Presentation 25

An 18-year-old overweight adolescent male was recently diagnosed with hypertension (143/92 mm Hg) and type 2 diabetes.

Which of the following would be the best drug of first choice to manage his hypertension?

A. Atenolol
B. Hydrochlorothiazide
C. Lisinopril
D. Nifedipine
E. Metoprolol

The correct answer is C

Comment: Patients with a history of either diabetes or kidney disease should be given an ACEI or an ARB to prevent the development, or further progression, of kidney disease.[1]

Patients treated with antihypertensive drug therapy should be evaluated (either in person or by telehealth) every 2 to 4 weeks until their BP is at goal. Waiting 4 weeks to reevaluate after starting or intensifying therapy is typically appropriate to permit long-acting antihypertensive drugs enough time to manifest their full BP-lowering effect. If BP is uncontrolled, we typically escalate doses of individual antihypertensive drugs to at least half the maximum recommended dose (i.e., to a moderate or high dose) before adding additional therapy. After goal BP is attained, we usually follow patients every 3 to 6 months.

Clinical Presentation 26

A 17-year-old man presents with HTN, asthma, and atrial fibrillation. He is able to walk six blocks before stopping to rest, and his echocardiogram shows an ejection fraction of 57%. His rhythm is irregularly irregular, with a ventricular response between 110 and 160/min.

Which of the following agents would be the safest in treating his HTN and controlling his ventricular response?

A. Atenolol
B. Benazepril
C. Hydrochlorothiazide
D. Losartan
E. Verapamil

The correct answer is E

Comment: This is the best choice. It would increase the atrioventricular node's effective refractory period and slow his ventricular rate, while also reducing arterial BP. This is an example of treating a patient with a comorbid condition atrial fibrillation (AF).[1]

AF is an increasingly prevalent condition and the most common sustained arrhythmia encountered in ambulatory and hospital practice. Several clinical risk factors for AF include age, sex, valvular heart disease, obesity, sleep apnea, heart failure, and HTN.

Of all the risk factors, hypotension is the most commonly encountered condition in patients with incident AF.

The RAA system has been demonstrated to be a common mechanistic link in the pathogenesis of hypertension and AF.

Clinical Presentation 27

An 18-year-old woman with a history of mild HTN is planning to begin a family with her husband in the immediate future. She is currently being treated with a combination of hydrochlorothiazide and losartan.

Which agent could she be switched to that has a well-established track record for safety in the treatment of essential hypertension during pregnancy?

A. Aliskiren
B. Captopril

C. Candesartan
D. Methyldopa
E. Propranolol

The correct answer is D

Comment: Methyldopa has the best, most well-established track record for safety as an antihypertensive drug in pregnancy.[1]

ARBs are *contraindicated* in pregnancy. Women contemplating pregnancy should be counseled to discontinue these medications before conception. Exposure to such drugs may result in a decrease in placental blood flow, which can result in oligohydramnios, renal failure, low birth weight, cardiovascular anomalies, spontaneous abortions, and other abnormalities.

Clinical Presentation 28

A 16-year-old patient was admitted to the emergency department for severe chest pain and was found to have severe hypertension (197/119 mm Hg).

What intravenous medication would you choose to manage his condition?

A. Atenolol
B. Furosemide
C. Phenylephrine
D. Sodium nitroprusside

The correct answer is D

Comment: Intravenous sodium nitroprusside is one of the drugs of choice for rapid lowering of SBP to <120 mm Hg (within 20 minutes) in the setting of a dissecting aorta. Most other hypertensive emergencies do not call for such rapid changes in BP because of the overriding concern about reductions in cerebral blood flow associated with rapid drops in BP.[1]

The traditional drug of choice for therapy of hypertensive emergencies is sodium nitroprusside.

Intravenous labetalol produces a prompt, controlled reduction in BP and is a promising alternative.

Other agents used are diazoxide, trimethaphan camsylate, hydralazine, nitroglycerin, and phentolamine. However, all these agents have disadvantages, including unpredictable antihypertensive effects, difficult BP titration, and serious potential adverse effects such as profound hypotension, reduced renal blood flow, and increased myocardial workload. Most patients with hypertensive urgencies can be effectively treated with orally or sublingually administered agents. Older regimens of reserpine, methyldopa, or guanethidine, with their slow onsets and long durations of action, have been largely replaced by clonidine and nifedipine. Captopril and minoxidil have also been used with some success. Despite the lack of comparative trials with traditional agents, demonstrated efficacy and desirable pharmacologic characteristics have made several new agents acceptable for therapy of hypertensive crises.

Clinical Presentation 29

Smoking increases arterial BP and accelerates vascular injury by which *one* of the following mechanisms?

A. Promoting endothelial dysfunction
B. Retention of sodium
C. Increased aldosterone protein

D. Activation of adducing gene
E. increases the production of catecholamines

The correct answer is A

Comment: Tobacco smoking is a potent promoter of endothelial dysfunction and activates vasoconstriction by inhibition of endothelium-dependent vasodilatation.[1]

Clinical Presentation 30

A 15-year-old male indicates that his BP during the past year routinely stayed above 150/90 mm Hg despite limitation of sodium intake and regular exercise.

Antihypertensive therapy for the past 4 years consisted of thiazide diuretics with BP readings that averaged approximately 134/82 mm Hg. Current medications include amiloride/hydrochlorothiazide (5/50 mg daily); ramipril (10 mg daily), and diltiazem (240 mg daily).

On examination, the pertinent findings were BP 35 156/98 mm Hg, pulse 72 beats/min, weight 81 kg, and BMI 28 kg/m^2. No ankle edema noted. Serum creatinine was 1.4 mg/dL; Na 146 mEq/L, K 3.4 mEq/L, Cl 95 mA/L, and CO_2 28 mEq/L. An electrocardiogram showed left ventricular hypertrophy and urinalysis trace protein.

Which *one* of the following studies is most likely to clarify the reason for his resistance to therapy?

A. GFR
B. Plasma aldosterone to renin ratio
C. Plasma catecholamines
D. Urinary microalbumin

The correct answer is B

Comment: The elevated serum sodium, high serum bicarbonate, and low serum potassium levels reflect a high probability of mineralocorticoid effect, which would explain the recent development of resistant hypertension.[1] Therefore, measurements of aldosterone and renin are most likely to reveal this disturbance. Measurement of GFR, catecholamines, and microalbuminuria would not explain the electrolyte changes and are far less likely to add useful information regarding identifying the cause of treatment resistance, making options A, C, and D incorrect.

Clinical Presentation 31

Which *one* of the following statements is *true* regarding BP reduction in a hypertensive patient with normal renal function who is consuming a high-potassium, low-sodium (60 mEq/day) diet?

A. They will decrease their SBP by 12 to 14 mm Hg within a few months.
B. They will decrease their SBP by 12 to 14 mm Hg within a few months.
C. The diet has little effect on SBP but decreases diastolic BP by >10 mm Hg within a few months.
D. The diet is well tolerated, and thus no significant BP response is noted.
E. This diet increases the need for diuretics because of the high potassium load.

The correct answer is B

Comment: A review of the DASH diet studies indicates that the greatest benefit was seen among African-American women who were hypertensive, and the least significant effect on BP reduction in normotensive women.[1] The DASH diet lowers BP but not weight or glucose control.

Clinical Presentation 32

A 16-year-old female with a BMI of 35 kg/m^2 and BP of 154/90 mm Hg is referred to you for albuminuria. Urine albumin/creatinine ratio is 370 mg/g creatinine (normal <30 mg/g). For the past 2 years, she has been receiving metoprolol 50 mg/day, and before that she had never been told she was hypertensive. On this visit, you note all laboratory tests are normal except for her fasting glucose of 124 mg/dL. Her current BP is 155/92 mm Hg and her pulse is 68 beats/min and regular.

Which *one* of the following choices provides for the patient's *best* management?

A. Stay on a 1200 calorie/day (American Diabetic Association diet).
B. Stop the beta-blocker and begin an ACEI/diuretic combination and titrate to BP goal.
C. Increase metoprolol and titrate to BP goal.
D. Add an ACEI to her current regimen.
E. Recommend exercise for weight loss.

The correct answer is B

Comment: Clearly, this patient is obese and has impaired glucose tolerance. Moreover, she has HTN and is being treated with a drug at a very low dose, given her body size, that worsens glucose tolerance. Getting her to lose weight will take a long time, and even if successful, it will increase her total BP load over time. Increasing the dose of metoprolol will increase the likelihood of diabetes and worsen her morbidity. Adding an ACEI to an underdosed beta-blocker such as metoprolol does not alleviate the risk for diabetes development and, although it may improve HTN, will not have the same effect as a drug combination that is well documented in having additional BP-lowering effects in such patients.[1]

Clinical Presentation 33

A 6-year-old girl has been hospitalized twice in the past 6 months with symptoms of CHF. A magnetic resonance angiogram showed complete occlusions of the right renal artery and high-grade stenosis (>90% narrowing of the left renal artery). Current medications include ramipril 5 mg daily and furosemide 40 mg daily. Physical examination shows BP 155/80 mm Hg, pulse 64 beats/min, lungs with occasional rhonchi, third heart sound appreciated, and a 2+ peripheral edema noted. Laboratory studies show hemoglobin 12 g/dL, serum creatinine 1.0 mg/dL, Na 139 mEq/L, K 3.9 mEq/L, and normal urinalysis.

Which *one* of the following recommendations would be most appropriate for this patient's care?

A. Stenting of the left renal artery
B. Laparoscopic nephrectomy of right kidney
C. Withdrawal of ACEI
D. Improve BP to <129/80 mm Hg before any surgical intervention
E. Bilateral nephrectomy followed by renal replacement therapy

The correct answer is A

Comment: Stenting of the left renal artery reflects the benefit of renal revascularization when renal stenosis affects the entire functioning mass for patients with recurrent CHF.[1] ACEIs have established survival benefits and should be continued, not stopped. Unilateral nephrectomy of the occluded kidney might lower BP levels, but low BPs are counterproductive and may worsen fluid retention when the remaining kidney has high-grade vascular disease.

Clinical Presentation 34

Which of the following choices most accurately describe(s) the role that ambulatory BP monitoring (ABPM) would play in a patient with white coat HTN (select all that apply)?

A. Average BP readings <140/90 mm Hg would confirm the presence of office or white coat hypertension.
B. Failure to lower nocturnal BP would signify higher risk of left ventricular hypertrophy.
C. The difference between day and night BP measurements would guide the choice of antihypertensive therapy.
D. Home BP reading can accurately predict white coat HTN.
E. Persistent elevations in nighttime readings of BP require the exclusion of sleep apnea as a cause for hypertension.

The correct answers are B and E

Comment: Sleep apnea interferes with the nocturnal fall in BP. Lack of nocturnal fall in BP predicts risk of left ventricular hypertrophy. ABPM BP readings are lower than those obtained under office conditions, and normal levels are below 135/85 mm Hg, not 140/90 mm Hg. The use of ABPM defines white coat HTN rather than home BPs, and the specific range of day-night variability does not guide specific drug therapy.[1,2]

Clinical Presentation 35

A 9-year-old girl presents to the emergency department with acute onset of severe headache and a BP of 180/80 mm Hg. She is given 10 mg of sublingual nifedipine twice over 1 hour, with a reduction in pressure to 150/80 mm Hg. At this time, her only complaint is that she feels tired. Her physical examination is unremarkable other than a round face and short stature. An echocardiogram is normal.

Additional evaluation includes a renal ultrasound, urinalysis, blood urea nitrogen (BUN) and creatinine, plasma cortisol, and a 24-hour urine for metanephrines and catecholamines, all of which are within the normal range. Serum sodium is 142 mEq/L, potassium 3.1 mEq/L, chloride 92 mEq/L, and bicarbonate 29 mEq/L. A random urine chloride is 89 mEq/L. She is placed on 20 mg/day enalapril, 25 mg/day of hydrochlorothiazide, 10 mg/day of amlodipine, and 60 mEq of potassium daily. One month later, she presented with chest pain and a BP of 175/83 mm Hg.

Which *one* of the following laboratory tests would provide the greatest likelihood of making a correct diagnosis?

A. Renal angiogram
B. Peripheral plasma renin-to-aldosterone ratio
C. Dexamethasone suppression test
D. 24-hour urinary aldosterone
E. Thyroid function studies

The correct answer is D

Comment: This patient has systolic HTN associated with hypokalemic metabolic alkalosis with normal renal function. Given the patient's history and existing laboratory studies, the most likely diagnosis is either primary hyperaldosteronism or pseudo-hyperaldosteronism (Liddel syndrome).

The most sensitive and specific test to rule out primary aldosteronism is a 24-hour urinary aldosterone level.[1] Other tests, such as plasma renin or aldosterone, have many problems, and their value in this setting has not been validated.

Clinical Presentation 36

A 6-year-old girl presents with a BP of 194/116 mm Hg. Her baseline laboratory values include BMI of 23 kg/m^2, glycated hemoglobin of 5%, microalbuminuria of 320 mg/g creatinine, serum creatinine of 1.0 mg/dL, BUN of 33 mg/dL, bicarbonate of 24 mEq/L, and potassium of 3.8 mEq/L. Urinalysis is otherwise normal. Echocardiogram shows left ventricular hypertrophy with no evidence for the coarctation of the aorta. She is receiving an ACEI, a CCB, and thiazide diuretic for BP management.

Which *one* of the following would be appropriate as a next step in her evaluation?

A. Perform renal ultrasound.
B. Order echocardiogram.
C. Measure urine microalbumin excretion.
D. Restrict sodium intake and add a loop diuretic.
E. Order magnetic resonance angiography to assess renal arteries.
F. Add clonidine.

The correct answer is E
Comment: This patient has severe hypertension. The clinical and laboratory findings suggest renal vascular hypertension. The best choice for a study would be a magnetic resonance angiography.[1]

Clinical Presentation 37

A 17-year-old girl presents for a second opinion regarding her BP control and medicine regimen. She was told that she has renal insufficiency, but she feels fine. Her physical examination is unremarkable, and she currently receives an ACEI, thiazide diuretic, and nondihydropyridine calcium antagonist for her BP control. Her sitting BP is 146/84 mm Hg, with an abnormal pulse of 78. Laboratory tests demonstrate serum potassium of 3.5 mEq/L and serum creatinine of 1.4 mg/dL.

A 24-hour urine contains 108 mEq of sodium (adequate urine collection).

Which *one* of the following antihypertensive medications would help reduce mortality by inhibiting fibrosis of the heart and helping achieve her BP goal?

A. An ARB
B. A long-acting beta-blocker
C. An aldosterone receptor antagonist
D. Hydralazine
E. Clonidine

The correct answer is C
Comment: In this patient, low potassium is a clear contributor to persistent HTN. Potassium channels tend to close when hypokalemia is present, causing vasoconstriction that leads to a sustained elevation in BP. This patient needs potassium supplementation along with a potassium-sparing diuretic such as spironolactone.[1]

Clinical Presentation 38

A 16-year-old White female presented to the emergency department with severe HTN and evidence of neurologic deficits. Her BP was 210/120 mm Hg, pulse was 88 beats/min, and she had a regular and continuous bruise over her left lateral abdominal area. Her serum creatinine level was 1.6 mg/dL, potassium 3.9 mEq/L, sodium 139 mEq/L, chloride 104 mEq/L, and bicarbonate 24 mEq/L. A chest x-ray was normal. She was given 10 mg of sublingual nifedipine and started on intravenous nitroprusside. She died suddenly in the process of being transferred to the intensive care unit.

Which of the following choices describes what should have been the best approach for this patient's management?

A. Nothing different should have been done because she had a fatal cardiac arrhythmia.
B. Intravenous fenoldopam should have been substituted for nitroprusside because of her renal insufficiency.
C. Both intravenous labetalol and intravenous fenoldopam should have been given.
D. Intravenous nitroprusside and intravenous furosemide should have been administered.

The correct answer is C
Comment: It is clear from the physical examination that the patient has an abdominal aneurysm and renal insufficiency. Attempting to lower this patient's pressure with vasodilators that will cause reflex tachycardia could result in further stress to the aortic wall and rupture the aneurysm, which is exactly what happened to this patient. The use of intravenous beta-blockers is ideal therapy in patients with a selective dopamine-1 receptor agonist to vasodilate without increasing heart rate.[1]

Clinical Presentation 39

A 14-year-old boy with end-stage renal disease (ESRD) is dialyzed on the morning shift, at which his SBP is consistently between 150 to 170 mm Hg. After each treatment, his SBP remains above 140 mm Hg. A 24-hour BP monitor demonstrates that his average BP during the day is 148/72 mm Hg. At night, it averages 144/78 mm Hg.

He currently receives all his medications (ACEI, CCB, and beta-blocker) in the morning, but he does not take them on the morning of dialysis.

Which *one* of the following choices *most* accurately describes his cardiovascular risk?

A. He is at the same risk as the average ESRD patient.
B. He is at much higher risk than those ESRD patients whose BP manifests a nighttime dip.
C. His most likely time to have a cardiovascular event is in the late evening.
D. His prognosis will not improve if he converts to Dipper.
E. There is no known therapy that will convert him to dipping status.

The correct answer is B
Comment: Studies have shown that dialysis patients, like those non-dippers with normal renal function (i.e., those failing to decrease their normal SBP by at least 20 mm Hg), have a higher risk of CV events and death than do dippers.[1]

Clinical Presentation 40

A 15-year-old girl with a BMI of 35 kg/m^2 and BP of 146/90 mm Hg is referred to you for new-onset microalbuminuria (59 mg/g creatinine; normal <20 mg/g). She has been on antihypertensive medications (50 mg/day of metoprolol) for the past 3 years. On this visit, you note all laboratory tests are normal except her fasting blood glucose of 124 mg/dL. Her current BP is 149/92 mm Hg and pulse is 68 and regular.

Which of the following is (are) the *best* management approach(es) for this patient?

A. Tell her to lose weight and put her on a 1200-calorie/day diet.
B. Increase metoprolol dose to achieve BP goal.
C. Add an ACEI to current medication.
D. Stop the beta-blocker and start an ACEI/diuretic and titrate to BP goal.

The correct answers are A and D

Comment: In addition to losing weight and modifications in lifestyle, based on her cardiovascular risk factor profile, the elevated BP, the ideal therapy for her would be an ACEI with a diuretic.[1]

Clinical Presentation 41

A 13-year-old boy presents for a second opinion regarding difficulty in controlling his BP. He has taken an ACEI and an ARB at maximal doses but experienced only 8 to 10 mm Hg reduction in SBP. He is currently on maximal doses of a CCB and an ACEI with a sitting BP of 148/92 mm Hg.

Which *one* of the following genotypes might help predict an appropriate antihypertensive drug class to achieve the BP goal for this patient?

A. ACE gene
B. Angiotensinogen gene
C. Aldosterone synthase gene
D. Alpha-adducin gene
E. 11-beta hydroxy steroid dehydrogenase gene

The correct answer is D

Comment: Adducin 1 (*ADD1*) is a protein coding gene. Diseases associated with *ADD1* include HTN and essential and esophageal atresia. Among its related pathways are activation of cAMP-dependent protein kinase A (PKA) and unfolded protein response. Gene ontology annotations related to this gene include RNA binding and protein heterodimerization activity. An important paralog of this gene is ADD3.[1]

In an analysis of almost 1000 patients, it was noted that carriers of the adducin variant had a lower risk for CV events or stroke when they received diuretic therapy compared with other antihypertensive drugs. It was also noted that those with the adducin variant had greater reductions in BP in response to a diuretic compared with other therapies.[1,2] None of the other genotypes listed has been associated with this type of relationship to BP response and outcomes with a particular class of agents.

Clinical Presentation 42

A 15-year-old adolescent female presents to the emergency department with profound weakness and polyuria. Her past medical history is unremarkable. She is taking no medications. Family history is negative. Her temperature is 37°C, blood pressure 145/89 mm Hg, heart rate 84 beats/min, respiration rate 12 breaths/min, and BMI 25 kg/m^2.

Serum sodium is 142 mEq/L, potassium 2.9 mEq/L, chloride 106 mEq/L, bicarbonate 29 mEq/L, BUN 12 mg/dL, and creatinine 0.5 mg/dL. Serum aldosterone is 2.2 ng/dL and plasma renin activity is less than 0.1 ng/mL/h.

Urinalysis shows a specific gravity of 1.025, pH 8, otherwise negative with unremarkable sediment. Random urinary potassium to creatinine is 2.1.

Generalized weakness and electrolyte abnormalities persisted despite treatment with large doses of oral potassium supplements and spironolactone.

Which of the following options at this point would best fit the patient's conditions?

A. Obtain serum cortisol level.
B. Measurement of the ratio of cortisol to cortisone in a 24-hour urine
C. Measurement of urinary 17-hydroxysteroid
D. Measurement of serum Mg concentration
E. Switch spironolactone to amiloride.

The correct answer is E

Comment: Constellation of hypertension and hypokalemic metabolic alkalosis associated with decreased serum aldosterone and plasma renin activity, unresponsive to spironolactone, is strongly suggestive of Liddle syndrome.

An improvement in HTN and correction of hypokalemia and metabolic alkalosis is expected following amiloride administration (option E),[1,2] although genetic testing is the gold standard and can identify congenital defects.

Clinical Presentation 43

You are asked to see a 4-year-old with heart failure and reduced systolic ejection fraction from aortic. He has no edema. His blood pressure is 154/98 mm Hg.

Which of the following is the preferred choice for the management of hypertension in this patient?

A. ACEI or ARB in combination with a thiazide diuretic
B. ACEI or ARB in combination with CCB, spironolactone, and a low-sodium diet
C. ACE or ARB and spironolactone with a low-sodium diet
D. Labetalol and CCB in combination with a thiazide diuretic

The correct answer is C

Comment: Treatment of HTN in children with heart failure must be tailored, depending on the pathophysiology mechanism, status of systolic or diastolic function of the heart, severity of HTN, presence of end-organ damage, and coexisting renal abnormalities.

Our patient presents with congestive heart failure associated with low cardiac output or reduced systolic ejection fraction. About half of the patients with CHF have systolic dysfunction and develop the classical symptoms of CHF, including edema. Systolic dysfunction is best treated with beta-blockers, ACEIs, ARB, and spironolactone plus a low-sodium diet (option C).[1] A loop diuretic is recommended in the presence of edema.

For patients who have normal systolic fraction ejection with left ventricular hypertrophy or diastolic dysfunction, ACE or ARB and CCB tend to induce significantly more regression than beta-blockers.[1]

Clinical Presentation 44

A 20-month-old girl with a history of polydipsia (more than 3 L/day), polyuria (more than 3 L/day), and weight loss (12–10.6 kg) that started 4 months ago, with an initial impression of Bartter syndrome, was transferred from another hospital. Laboratory blood tests performed at the previous hospital revealed metabolic alkalosis, hyponatremia, and hypokalemia with a high transtubular potassium gradient (TTKG). Her BP was measured to be 90/60 mm Hg initially. However, the BP checked on arrival at our hospital was as high as 190/120 mm Hg. Her height and weight were 86 cm (50th–75th percentile) and 11.07 kg (25th–50th percentile), respectively. Dehydrated lips and a large palpable abdominal mass were found on physical examination. There was no family history of inherited kidney diseases or hypertension.

Laboratory study results were as follows: serum sodium 131 mmol/L, potassium 2.9 mmol/L, chloride 92 mmol/L, osmolality 265 mOsm/kg, bicarbonate 28.4 mmol/L, blood pH 7.57, BUN 4 mg/dL, creatinine 0.23 mg/dL, and estimated GFR 154.25 mL/min/1.73 m^2. She had proteinuria (urine protein/creatinine ratio 3.4 mg/mg) without hematuria or glucosuria. Urine electrolyte analysis showed diluted urine with osmolarity 157 mOsm/kg, sodium 27 mmol/L, chloride 32 mmol/L, and a TTKG of 5. Hormone studies for malignant hypertension revealed elevated plasma renin and aldosterone levels (renin 37 ng/mL/h, aldosterone 182 ng/dL), normal vanillylmandelic acid levels, and normal levels of plasma and urine catecholamines. Abdominal CT showed a large mass on the left kidney, encasing the left renal artery. Left ventricular hypertrophy was detected by echocardiography. A biopsy of the kidney mass revealed Wilms tumor and other imaging evaluations confirmed no evidence of metastasis.

Several antihypertensive medications failed to control hypertension. Hyponatremia and hypokalemia were transiently improved with intravenous fluid and oral electrolyte supplementation. After the left radical nephrectomy, BP and electrolyte imbalance were normalized, and no further medication was necessary.

What is the pathophysiology of this condition?

A. Apparent mineralocorticoid excess
B. Liddle syndrome
C. Hyperaldosteronism
D. Hyperactivation of the RAA system

The correct answer is D

Comment: The patient presented with polydipsia, polyuria, weight loss, and HTN. HTN was sufficiently severe in both cases to develop hypertensive cardiomyopathy and/or hypertensive retinopathy. Serum and urine laboratory tests revealed hyponatremia, hypokalemia with a high TTKG, hypochloremia, metabolic alkalosis, and proteinuria. Unilateral renal artery stenosis was found in imaging studies. Wilms tumor was the culprit of this case. This condition is known as hyponatremic-hypertensive syndrome.

Hyperactivation of the RAA axis is regarded to be the key pathophysiologic mechanism behind specific symptoms and electrolyte imbalances in hyponatremic-hypertensive syndrome.[1] If unilateral RAS is severe enough to induce renal ischemia in the affected kidney, the ischemic kidney secretes a large amount of renin, which leads to increased levels of Ang II, a potent vasoconstrictor. Arterial pressure rises, and hyperfiltration in the contralateral kidney results in hyponatremia and volume depletion, known as pressure natriuresis. Increased aldosterone levels, another effect of Ang II, lead to hypokalemia. Both Ang II and volume depletion stimulate antidiuretic hormone secretion, which is responsible for thirst and polydipsia, further worsening hyponatremia. Proteinuria is a result of glomerular hyperfiltration and the proteinuric effect of Ang II.[2]

Clinical Presentation 45

A 15-year-old girl with no significant past medical history presented for evaluation of a left neck mass. The mass had been growing for approximately 1 year. Contrast-enhanced CT of the neck showed a well-circumscribed cystic mass originating from the left carotid space extending into the left parotid space, with associated mass effect and near-complete effacement of the upper internal jugular vein. She was scheduled for surgical excision of the mass; however, while in the preoperative anesthesia care unit, she became hypertensive to 170/110 mm Hg. She remained hypertensive even after receiving midazolam for induction of anesthesia, so surgical excision of the mass was postponed.

Serum electrolytes, urea, creatinine, calcium, and uric acid concentrations were normal. Urinalysis showed specific gravity 10.17, pH 6.0 no blood or protein.

After recovery from anesthesia, she was alert, talkative, and in no acute distress. She had normal pupils that were reactive to light. Her left parotid area was notable for a firm 4-cm immobile mass, deep to the left earlobe and outwardly displacing the ear. There was neither significant tenderness nor lymphadenopathy, and there were no carotid bruits. Her laboratory results were unremarkable. The patient was admitted to the nephrology service for further evaluation and management. A transthoracic echocardiogram and Doppler ultrasound of the kidney and bladder were normal. MRI of the neck redemonstrated a well-defined, highly vascular mass, centered in the left parotid space with mass effect on the left internal jugular vein and parotid gland.

Further history revealed that at an outpatient visit 3 weeks prior, the patient's systolic BP was elevated to 160 mm Hg, and she had a previous emergency room visit for dizziness, nausea, and abdominal pain where her BP was 130/80 mm Hg. She also endorsed daily frontal headaches for the past few months, associated with phonophobia and resolving with acetaminophen. Her last headache was on the day before admission.

What is the likely cause of hypertension in this patient?

A. Mineralocorticoid excess renal artery stenosis and renal parenchymal disease
B. Coarctation of the aorta
C. Renal artery stenosis
D. Pheochromocytoma

The correct answer is D

Comment: In this patient with a parotid mass, headaches, and episodic hypertension, considerations include catecholamine-secreting tumors as well as a mass effect on the sympathetic ganglion or vascular supply resulting in compensatory hypertension to maintain cerebral perfusion. Plasma metanephrines were sent and a 24-hour urine collection for catecholamines was started. The results of her plasma and urinary metanephrines confirmed a catecholamine-secreting tumor. She underwent a subsequent positron emission tomography Ga68-DOTATE scan, which showed that her neck mass, along with multiple lesions in the chest and abdomen, were all somatostatin-receptor-rich, consistent with a metastatic catecholamine-secreting paraganglioma.

Pheochromocytomas and paragangliomas are rare tumors that are seen in approximately 2% of children who present with hypertension.[1] A patient with a pheochromocytoma and paraganglioma typically presents with intermittent, recurrent symptoms of catecholamine excess, such as hypertension, headaches, or diaphoresis. Other, less specific symptoms include anxiety and panic attacks, as well as nausea, vomiting, and tremors. Although most patients will present with hypertension and headaches, up to 25% of cases will be entirely asymptomatic.[2,3]

Pheochromocytomas and paragangliomas can be diagnosed with blood tests and imaging. The most sensitive biochemical tests are plasma-free metanephrines and normetanephrine, the breakdown products of catecholamines, which have a sensitivity of up to 100% in children.[4] Urinary metanephrines can be used in equivocal cases, with sensitivities that are similarly high in many studies.[5] If biochemical testing shows elevated levels of catecholamines, contrast-enhanced CT of the abdomen, specifically protocolized to the adrenal gland, is a reasonable first imaging study. This can be followed by MRI, which is more sensitive for the detection of extraadrenal masses.[4] If neither of these studies visualizes any masses despite biochemical evidence of disease, functional iodine-123 metaiodobenzylguanidine scintigraphy can be considered.[5] Alternatively, positron emission tomography with fluorine-18-labeled dihydroxyphenylalanine may offer better sensitivity than metaiodobenzylguanidine because of better visualization of anatomy and less radiographic artifact and is preferred in patients with metastatic disease.[5]

Clinical Presentation 46

A 19-year-old man was admitted for elective surgery for resection of a brain mass resulting from metastatic melanoma. He had a history of prostate cancer treated with resection 6 years ago and resection of a small-bowel carcinoid tumor that had recurred with peritoneal nodules. Nephrology was consulted for the evaluation of persistent hypokalemia and metabolic alkalosis. The patient denied abdominal pain, headache, fever, vomiting, or diarrhea. He did not use over-the-counter or herbal medications. Home medications included omeprazole 20 mg and daily and monthly octreotide injections. In the hospital, he was receiving omeprazole 20 mg daily; levetiracetam 1000 mg twice per day for seizure prophylaxis after his brain surgery; and subcutaneous heparin 5000 units twice per day for deep venous thrombosis prophylaxis. On physical examination, the patient's temperature was 37.3°C (99.1°F), heart rate was 90 beats/min, BP was 155/95 mm Hg, respiration rate was 14 breaths/min, and oxygen saturation was 97% on room air. Cardiac examination findings were unremarkable. Lungs were clear bilaterally. His abdomen was soft with no visceromegaly or tenderness. There was no edema. There were no focal neurologic findings.

Laboratory investigation showed sodium 144 mEq/L, potassium 2.8 mEq/L, chloride 99 mEq/L, bicarbonate 33 mEq/L, urea nitrogen 18 mg/dL, creatinine 0.8 mg/dL, calcium 7.9 mg/dL 7.9, albumin 3.8 g/dL, glucose 95 mg/dL Additional studies included arterial blood gas pH 7.52 PCO_2 38 mm Hg, PO_2 90 mm Hg, and HCO_3 32 mEq/L. Urine potassium (random) 104 mEq/L, urine chloride (random) 60 mEq/L. Plasma renin 0.6 ng/m (normal, 1.06 (range 0.25–5.82)), plasma aldosterone 1 ng/dL (normal, 3–16), plasma cortisol (morning) 41 mcg/dL (normal, 6–26), 24-hour urine cortisol 1062 (normal, 4–50 24-hours), urine creatinine 1.1 g/24 hours (0.63–2.50), Plasma corticotropin 92 pg/mL (normal, 92 (range 6–50)).

What is the most likely cause of this patient's hypokalemia, metabolic alkalosis, and hypertension?

A. Liddle syndrome
B. Syndrome of apparent mineralocorticoid excess
C. Congenital adrenal hyperplasia
D. Cushing syndrome

The correct answer is D

Comment: Hypokalemia is generally due to either urinary or gastrointestinal tract losses, a shift from the extracellular to intracellular fluid compartment, or in rare cases, decreased oral intake. In our patient, renal losses were thought to be most likely given the elevated urinary potassium concentration.[1]

Metabolic alkalosis is often classified as chloride responsive (urine chloride <20 mEq/L) or chloride resistant (urine chloride >20 mEq/L). When urine chloride excretion is <20 mEq/L, the metabolic alkalosis is usually saline responsive. In metabolic alkalosis, urine chloride concentration may be a more accurate indicator of intravascular volume depletion than urine sodium concentration because bicarbonaturia in early stages of development of a chloride-depletion metabolic alkalosis results in sodium and potassium excretion in urine (as accompanying cations with bicarbonate). Thus, urine sodium and potassium concentrations may be elevated in the first 24 to 72 hours of volume depletion, then decline subsequently. Urine chloride concentration will remain low because of ongoing sodium and chloride reabsorption in the proximal tubule from activation of the RAA axis and other factors in response to volume depletion.

Our patient developed chloride-resistant metabolic alkalosis (urine chloride >20 mEq/L). Given the presence of hypertension along with urine potassium excretion >20 mEq/L and low levels of both serum renin and aldosterone, the differential diagnosis includes Liddle syndrome, syndrome of apparent mineralocorticoid excess, Cushing syndrome, congenital adrenal hyperplasia, and excessive licorice use.[2]

Given the patient's elevated morning cortisol level, markedly increased 24-hour urine cortisol excretion, and high serum corticotropin (ACTH) level, ACTH-dependent Cushing syndrome was diagnosed.[1,2]

ACTH-dependent Cushing syndrome could result from either an ACTH-secreting pituitary tumor or an ectopic ACTH-secreting tumor. Findings from MRI of the pituitary gland and CT of the chest were unremarkable. CT of the abdomen revealed peritoneal nodules consistent with his history of recurrent carcinoid tumor. Ectopic ACTH-dependent Cushing syndrome, most likely from the active carcinoid tumor, was diagnosed. There are few case reports that describe Cushing syndrome attributed to the presence of carcinoid tumor.[3] What are treatment options for this patient? Cortisol has the capacity to bind mineralocorticoid receptors in principal cells of the cortical collecting duct. Normally, this is limited by conversion of cortisol to cortisone, which is unable to bind to the mineralocorticoid receptor, by the enzyme 11 hydroxysteroid dehydrogenase type 2. Excess production of cortisol, as in our patient, saturates the enzyme, allowing cortisol to persist and activate mineralocorticoid receptors. This causes translocation of epithelial sodium channel proteins into the luminal membrane, increasing basolateral adenosine triphosphatase sodium/potassium pump activity and increasing renal outer medullary potassium channel activity, leading to sodium reabsorption and hypertension, hypokalemia, and metabolic alkalosis.

Clinical Presentation 47

A 14-year-old female with no significant medical or familial history was evaluated for 1 week of intermittent bouts of mild flank pain, occasionally associated with nausea and vomiting. The patient denied fever, chills, or hematuria. On physical examination, BP was 150/100 mm Hg and bilateral flank fullness and tenderness were noted. Laboratory tests showed serum creatinine level of 0.85 mg/dL, corresponding to estimated GFR of 65 mL/min/1.73 m^2. Urinalysis showed hematuria (+), white blood cells (+), and proteinuria (++). Microscopic examination of urine sediment showed three to five white blood cells/high-power field, five to nine red blood cells/high-power field, scattered dysmorphic red blood cells, tubular epithelial cells, and fatty casts. A 24-hour urinary protein measurement was 0.9 g, up from 0.5 g 1 year earlier. Abdominal ultrasound showed enlarged kidneys (left measuring 12.2 cm; right, 13.51 cm) with abnormal appearance. A CT showed bilateral kidney parenchymal thinning with peripelvic and perirenal fluid attenuation collections. These lesions could not be enhanced with contrast. Scalloping of both kidneys also was noted. Magnetic resonance urography showed multiloculated cysts and fibrous septae within both kidneys, with the lesions giving high signal intensity on the T2-weighted image.

What is the clinical pathologic diagnosis?

A. Renal lymphangiectasia
B. Polycystic kidney disease
C. Multicystic renal tumor
D. Medullary sponge kidney

The correct answer is A

Comment: Based on clinical features and imaging findings, a diagnosis of renal lymphangiectasia was made. Needle aspiration of the perinephric fluid was performed, with laboratory analysis showing a predominance of lymphocytes. The differential diagnosis must include polycystic kidney disease as well as cystic renal tumors (especially multilocular cystic renal tumors). Polycystic kidney disease commonly has a familial history, with multiple cysts arising from the renal parenchyma and often within the liver. Most cystic kidney tumor lesions are solitary and arise from renal parenchyma with solid content in contrast CT. In uncertain cases, fine-needle biopsy is useful to establish the diagnosis.

Renal lymphangiectasia is a rare benign disorder of lymphatic malformation characterized by disruption of the perirenal lymphatic system. The renal capsule lymphatics and perinephric tissue empty into the renal sinus lymphatics, which drain into the para-aortic, paracaval, and interaortic nodes. The lymph then flows through the lumbar trunk and thoracic duct before emptying into the left brachiocephalic vein, superior vena cava, and right heart. Renal sinus drainage disturbances lead to an ectatic perirenal, peripelvic, and intrarenal lymphatic system, which explains the classic imaging findings.[1] Clinically, renal lymphangiectasia can be detected incidentally by ultrasonography or CT in patients who undergo abdominal imaging procedures. The most common concerns are flank pain and abdominal distension, but hematuria, proteinuria, cyst hemorrhage, hypertension, fever, and, rarely, decreased kidney function can develop.[2] On occasion, renal lymphangiectasia can present with infection and bleeding that result in acute pain. The clinical evolution and prognosis of renal lymphangiectasia are unclear. Owing to the rarity of the condition, no standard treatment is established. Asymptomatic and localized cases can be managed conservatively because the condition does not affect kidney function.[1] If kidney function decreases or collections become symptomatic, percutaneous drainage can relieve compression.[3] Recurrent collections may require marsupialization into the peritoneum.[4] In severe uncontrollable cases, nephrectomy may be performed.[5] Our patient's perinephric collections were large and resulted in discomfort, so percutaneous drainage was performed to relieve compression and protect kidney function. After 1 month, drainage decreased to 5 mL per day and the tubes were removed. No fluid reaccumulation appeared during 6 months of follow-up.

Clinical Presentation 48

A 19-year-old woman presented with HTN. Two years earlier, she had been evaluated for elevated BP of 150–170/110–120 mm Hg and found to have a serum potassium level of 2.6 mmol/L and plasma renin concentration of 362 mIU/L (reference range, 2.8–40 mIU/L) in the supine position. She underwent renal angiography, for which there were no findings of note. The patient was prescribed amlodipine 5 mg and irbesartan 150 mg/d, and her BP responded promptly by decreasing to 115/70 mm Hg. On presentation, the patient denied symptoms aside from nocturia. She had no headache, chest pain, or edema. Her family history was not notable for any diseases or syndromes. She was not taking antihypertensive medication, and BP was 156/110 mm Hg. The rest of her examination findings were unremarkable, and she had no apparent obesity. She had a serum potassium level of 3.0 mmol/L, serum bicarbonate level of 23 mmol/L, serum creatinine level of 0.64 mg/dL (57 mmol/L; corresponding to eGFR 90 mL/min/1.73 m^2), and spot urine albumin-creatinine ratio of 42 mg/mmol. Plasma renin concentration was 846 mIU/L (reference range, 2.8–40 mIU/L) in the supine position, and serum aldosterone level was 2370 pmol/L (reference range, 30–444 pmol/L) in the supine position.

What is (are) the cause(s) of hypertension in this patient?

A. Cushingoid syndrome
B. Juxtaglomerular cell tumor
C. Primary hyperaldosteronism
D. Apparent mineralocorticoid excess

The correct answer A

Comment: The most common causes of hypertension in young women are essential hypertension or hypertension as part of metabolic syndrome. Secondary causes include fibromuscular dysplasia, overproduction of aldosterone, and hormonal causes such as those related to oral contraceptive use or pregnancy-induced hypertension. In this age group, additional endocrine explanations for secondary hypertension include thyroid or parathyroid disorders and low vitamin D levels. A rare but important cause is coarctation of the aorta. Finally, exogenous factors such as licorice consumption, substantial alcohol intake, and use of nonsteroidal antiinflammatory drugs should be investigated and/or ruled out.

In the present case, the patient was pregnant, but hypertension in gestational week 7 should not be regarded as gestational hypertension or preeclampsia.

Renin is produced by juxtaglomerular cells in the kidney and plays a major role in BP regulation by inducing the RAA system. Hypertensive high renin states can be secondary or primary. Secondary causes of a high renin state include renovascular disease, most commonly fibromuscular dysplasia of the renal artery in young women. Additionally, hypertensive states per se are associated with a slight increase in renin levels, but this is much more pronounced in the malignant hypertensive condition. This might be explained by renovascular ischemia resulting from intimal hyperplasia. As for primary causes of hypertensive high renin states, renin-producing renal tumors can be seen with simultaneous high aldosterone levels. Duplex ultrasound examination of the kidneys and echocardiography were performed to exclude renal artery stenosis and coarctation of the aorta. Magnetic resonance tomography of the upper abdomen identified a mass in the caudal area of the left kidney. Plasma renin and aldosterone concentrations in the left renal vein were 1230 mIU/L and 3900 pmol/L, respectively. In a peripheral vein, values were 726 mIU/L and 1330 pmol/L, respectively.

This high secretion of renin from the left tumor-containing kidney supports the diagnosis of reninoma.

^{111}In-octreotide scintigraphy was performed, showing high uptake of the radionuclide in the left renal mass. This uptake is due to the high expression of somatostatin receptor type 2 (SSTR2) by tumor cell.[1] This was further supported by immunohistochemical analysis of the surgical specimen, which demonstrated strong membranous staining of tumor cells by a monoclonal anti-SSTR2 antibody.[2] Most reninomas are benign, but metastatic cases have been reported.[3] The patient underwent surgical resection of the tumor with normalization of BP (110/70 mm Hg without medication) and renin and aldosterone levels (18.0 mU/L and 232 pmol/L, respectively). Because the tumor was clearly visible on ^{111}In-octreotide scintigraphy and expressed SSTR on immunohistochemical staining, a neuroendocrine phenotype for the tumor was identified. This suggests the opportunity to control hormone secretion and tumor cell proliferation in these tumors by long-acting somatostatin analogues or targeted radiotherapy in the case of unresectable masses.[3,4] The final diagnosis was hypertension from a juxtaglomerular cell tumor (reninoma) secreting large amounts of renin.

References

Clinical Presentation 1

1. Kenny D, Polson J, Martin R, et al. Hypertension and coarctation of the aorta: an inevitable consequence of developmental pathophysiology. *Hypertens Res*. 2011;34:543–547.

Clinical Presentation 2

1. Arnett DK, Blumenthal RS, Albert MA, et al. 2019 ACC/AHA guideline on the primary prevention of cardiovascular disease: a report of the American College of Cardiology/American Heart Association task force on clinical practice guidelines. *Circulation*. 2019;140(11):e596–e646. https://doi.org/10.1161/CIR.0000000000000678.

2. Blumenthal JA, Babyak MA, Hinderliter A, et al. Effects of the DASH diet alone and in combination with exercise and weight loss on blood pressure and cardiovascular biomarkers in men and women with high blood pressure: the ENCORE study. *Arch Intern Med.* 2010;170(2):126–135.

Clinical Presentation 3

1. Assadi F, Brackbill EL. Bilateral pheochromocytomas and congenital anomalies associated with a de novo germline mutation in the von Hippel-Lindau gene. *Am J Kidney Dis.* 2003;41(1):E3. https://doi.org/10.1053/ajkd.2003.50021.

Clinical Presentation 4

1. Acelajado MC, Hughes ZH, Oparil S, Calhoun DA. Treatment of resistant and refractory hypertension. *Circ Res.* 2019;124(7):1061–1070.

Clinical Presentation 5

1. Overlack A. ACE inhibitor-induced cough and bronchospasm. Incidence, mechanisms and management. *Drug Saf.* 1996;15(1):72–78. https://doi.org/10.2165/00002018-199615010-00006.

Clinical Presentation 6

1. Funder JW, Carey RM, Fardella C, et al. Case detection, diagnosis, and treatment of patients with primary aldosteronism: an endocrine society clinical practice guideline. *J Clin Endocrinol Metab.* 2008;93:3266–3281.
2. Kempers MJ, Lenders JW, van Outheusden L, et al. Systematic review: diagnostic procedures to differentiate unilateral from bilateral adrenal abnormality in primary aldosteronism. *Ann Intern Med.* 2009;151:329–337.
3. Karagiannis A, Tziomalos K, Papageorgiou A, et al. Spironolactone versus eplerenone for the treatment of idiopathic hyperaldosteronism. *Expert Opin Pharmacother.* 2008;9:509–515.

Clinical Presentation 7

1. Funder JW, Carey RM, Fardella C, et al. Case detection, diagnosis, and treatment of patients with primary aldosteronism: an endocrine society clinical practice guideline. *J Clin Endocrinol Metab.* 2008;93:3266–3281.
2. Kempers MJ, Lenders JW, van Outheusden L, et al. Systematic review: diagnostic procedures to differentiate unilateral from bilateral adrenal abnormality in primary aldosteronism. *Ann Intern Med.* 2009;151:329–337.
3. Karagiannis A, Tziomalos K, Papageorgiou A, et al. Spironolactone versus eplerenone for the treatment of idiopathic hyperaldosteronism. *Expert Opin Pharmacother.* 2008;9:509–515.

Clinical Presentation 8

1. Funder JW, Carey RM, Fardella C, et al. Case detection, diagnosis, and treatment of patients with primary aldosteronism: an endocrine society clinical practice guideline. *J Clin Endocrinol Metab.* 2008;93:3266–3281.
2. Kempers MJ, Lenders JW, van Outheusden L, et al. Systematic review: diagnostic procedures to differentiate unilateral from bilateral adrenal abnormality in primary aldosteronism. *Ann Intern Med.* 2009;151:329–337.
3. Karagiannis A, Tziomalos K, Papageorgiou A, et al. Spironolactone versus eplerenone for the treatment of idiopathic hyperaldosteronism. *Expert Opin Pharmacother.* 2008;9:509–515.

Clinical Presentation 9

1. Funder JW, Carey RM, Fardella C, et al. Case detection, diagnosis, and treatment of patients with primary aldosteronism: an endocrine society clinical practice guideline. *J Clin Endocrinol Metab.* 2008;93:3266–3281.
2. Kempers MJ, Lenders JW, van Outheusden L, et al. Systematic review: diagnostic procedures to differentiate unilateral from bilateral adrenal abnormality in primary aldosteronism. *Ann Intern Med.* 2009;151:329–337.
3. Karagiannis A, Tziomalos K, Papageorgiou A, et al. Spironolactone versus eplerenone for the treatment of idiopathic hyperaldosteronism. *Expert Opin Pharmacother.* 2008;9:509–515.

Clinical Presentation 10

1. Funder JW, Carey RM, Fardella C, et al. Case detection, diagnosis, and treatment of patients with primary aldosteronism: an endocrine society clinical practice guideline. *J Clin Endocrinol Metab.* 2008;93:3266–3281.
2. Kempers MJ, Lenders JW, van Outheusden L, et al. Systematic review: diagnostic procedures to differentiate unilateral from bilateral adrenal abnormality in primary aldosteronism. *Ann Intern Med.* 2009;151:329–337.
3. Karagiannis A, Tziomalos K, Papageorgiou A, et al. Spironolactone versus eplerenone for the treatment of idiopathic hyperaldosteronism. *Expert Opin Pharmacother.* 2008;9:509–515.

Clinical Presentation 11

1. Yaxley JP, Thambar SV. Resistant hypertension: an approach to management in primary care. *J Family Med Prim Care.* 2015;4(2):193–199.

Clinical Presentation 12

1. Blanchette E, Flynn JT. Implications of the 2017 AAP clinical practice guidelines for management of hypertension in children and adolescents: a review. *Curr Hypertens Rep.* 2019;21(5):35.

Clinical Presentation 13

1. Flynn JT, Kaelber DC, Baker-Smith CM, et al. Clinical practice guideline for screening and management of high blood pressure in children and adolescents. *Pediatrics.* 2017;140(3):e20171904. https://doi.org/10.1542/peds.2017-1904.

Clinical Presentation 14

1. Mann JFE. Overview of hypertension in acute and chronic kidney disease. UpToDate. May 2024. Accessed 23 March 2023.
2. Unger T, Borghi C, Charchar F, et al. 2020 International Society of Hypertension global hypertension practice guidelines. *J Hypertens.* 2020;38(6):982–1004.

Clinical Presentation 15

1. Taddei S. Combination therapy in hypertension: what are the best options according to clinical pharmacology principles and controlled trial evidence? *Am J Cardiovasc Drugs.* 2015;15:185–194.

Clinical Presentation 16

1. Adams M, Bellone J, Wright BM, Rutecki GW. Evaluation & pharmacologic approach to patients with resistant hypertension. *Postgrad Med.* 2012;124:74–78.
2. Williams B, Macdonald TM, Morant S, et al. Spironolactone versus placebo, bisoprolol, and doxazosin to determine the optimal treatment for drug-resistant hypertension (PATHWAY-2): a randomized, double-blind, crossover trial. *Lancet.* 2015;386:2059–2068.

Clinical Presentation 17

1. Gradman AH, Parise H, Lefebvre P, et al. Initial combination therapy reduces the risk of cardiovascular events in hypertensive patients: a matched cohort study. *Hypertension.* 2013;61:309–318.

Clinical Presentation 18

1. Mann JF, Flack JM. Choice of drug therapy in primary (essential) hypertension. UpToDate. Literature review current through March 2023.

Clinical Presentation 19

1. Papaccio G, Esposito V. Hyperglycemic effects of hydrochlorothiazide and propranolol. A biochemical and ultrastructural study. *Acta Diabetol Lat.* 1987;24(4):325–330.

Clinical Presentation 20

1. Schoolwerth AC, Sica DA, Ballermann BJ, Wilcox CS. Council on the Kidney in Cardiovascular Disease and the Council for High Blood Pressure Research of the American Heart Association. Renal considerations in angiotensin converting enzyme inhibitor therapy: a statement for healthcare professionals from the Council on the Kidney in Cardiovascular Disease and the Council for High Blood Pressure Research of the American Heart Association. *Circulation.* 2001;104(16):1985–1991. https://doi.org/10.1161/hc4101.096153.

Clinical Presentation 21

1. Dubov T, Toledano-Alhadef H, Chernin G, et al. High prevalence of elevated blood pressure among children with neurofibromatosis type 1. *Pediatr Nephrol.* 2016;31:131–136.
2. Fossali E, Signorini E, Intermite RC, et al. Renovascular disease and hypertension in children with neurofibromatosis. *Pediatr Nephrol.* 2000;14:806–810.
3. Sattur S, Prasad H, Bedi U, et al. Renal artery stenosis—an update. *Postgrad Med.* 2013;125:43–50.
4. Duan L, Feng K, Tong A, Liang Z. Renal artery stenosis due to neurofibromatosis type 1: case report and literature review. *Eur J Med Res.* 2014;19:17.
5. Lu J, Liu H, Zhang L, Ma L, Zhou H. Corkscrew retinal vessels and retinal arterial macroaneurysm in a patient with neurofibromatosis type 1: a case report. *Medicine (Baltimore).* 2018;97:e11497.

Clinical Presentation 22

1. Mann JF, Flack JM. Choice of drug therapy in primary (essential) hypertension. UpToDate. Literature review current through March 2023.

Clinical Presentation 23

1. Levy H. Hypertension from Framingham to ALLHAT: translating clinical trials into practice. Cleveland Clinic. *J Med.* 2007;74(9):672–678.
2. Mann JF, Flack JN. Choice of drug therapy in primary (essential) hypertension. UpToDate. Literature review current through March 2023.

Clinical Presentation 24

1. Whelton PK, Carey RM, Aronow WS, et al. ACC/AHA/AAPA/ABC/ACPM/AGS/APhA/ASH/ASPC/NMA/PCNA Guideline for the Prevention, Detection, Evaluation, and Management of High Blood Pressure in Adults: a report of the American College of Cardiology/American Heart Association Task Force on Clinical Practice Guideline. *Hypertension.* 2018;71:e13–e115.
2. Mann JF, Flack JN. Choice of drug therapy in primary (essential) hypertension. UpToDate. Literature review current through March 2023.

Clinical Presentation 25

1. Mann JF, Flack JN. Choice of drug therapy in primary (essential) hypertension. UpToDate. Literature review current through March 2023.

Clinical Presentation 26

1. Dzeshka MS, Shantsila A, Shantsila E, Lip GYH. Atrial fibrillation and hypertension. *Hypertension.* 2017;70:854–861.

Clinical Presentation 27

1. Li D-K, Yang C, Andrade S, Tavares B, Ferber JR. Maternal exposure to angiotensin converting enzyme inhibitors in the first trimester and risk of malformations in offspring: a retrospective cohort study. *BMJ.* 2011;34:d5931. https://doi.org/10.1136/bmj.d5931.

Clinical Presentation 28

1. Stumpf JL. Drug therapy of hypertensive crises. *Clin Pharm.* 1988;7(8):582–591.

Clinical Presentation 29

1. Ritz E, Benck U, Franek E, et al. Effects of smoking on renal hemodynamics in healthy volunteers and in patients with glomerular disease. *J Am Soc Nephrol.* 1998;9:1798–1804.

Clinical Presentation 30

1. Mulatero P, Stowasser M, Loh KC. Increased diagnosis of primary aldosteronism, including surgically correctable form, in centers from five continents. *J Clin Endocrinol Metab.* 2004;89:1045–1050.

Clinical Presentation 31

1. Sacks FM, Svetkey LP, Vollmer WM, et al. Effects on blood pressure of reduced dietary sodium and the Dietary Approaches to Stop Hypertension (DASH) diet. DASH-Sodium Collaborative Research Group. *N Engl J Med.* 2001;344(1):3–10.

Clinical Presentation 32

1. Bakris GL, Gaxiola E, Messerli FH. Clinical outcomes in the diabetes cohort of the INVEST. *Hypertension*. 2003;44:637.

Clinical Presentation 33

1. Gray BH, Olin JW, Childs MB, Sullivan TM, Bacharach JM. Clinical benefit of renal artery angioplasty with stenting for the control of recurrent and refractory congestive heart failure. *Vas Med*. 2002;7:275–279.

Clinical Presentation 34

1. Bur A, Herkner H, Vlcek M, et al. Classification of BP levels by ambulatory BP in hypertension. *Hypertension*. 2002;40:817–822.
2. Logan AC, Perlikowski SM, Mente A. Prevalence of unrecognized sleep apnea in drug- resistant hypertension. *J Hypertension*. 2001;19:2271–2277.

Clinical Presentation 35

1. Young WF Jr. Primary aldosteronism: management issues. *Ann NY Acad Sci*. 2002;970:61–76.

Clinical Presentation 36

1. Schoenberg SO, Knopp MV, Londy F, et al. Morphologic and functional magnetic resonance imaging of renal artery stenosis: a multireader tricenter study. *J Am Soc Nephrol*. 2002;13:158–169.

Clinical Presentation 37

1. Tobian L. Dietary sodium chloride and potassium have effects on the pathophysiology of hypertension in humans and animals. *Am J Clin Nutr*. 1997;65:606S–611S.

Clinical Presentation 38

1. Mansoor GA, Frishman WH. Comprehensive management of hypertensive emergencies and urgencies. *Crit Care Clin*. 2001;17:435–451.

Clinical Presentation 39

1. Liu M, Takahashi H, Morita Y, et al. Non-dipping is a potent predictor of cardiovascular mortality and is associated with autonomic dysfunction in hemodialysis patients. *Nephrol Dial Trans*. 2003;18:563–569.

Clinical Presentation 40

1. Wright JT, Bakris GL, Greene T, et al. Effect of BP lowering and antihypertensive drug class on progression of hypertensive kidney disease: results from the AASK trial. *JAMA*. 2002;288:2421–2431.

Clinical Presentation 41

1. Gong Y, McDonough CW, Padmanabhan S, et al. Hypertension pharmacogenetics. In: *Handbook of Pharmacogenomics and Stratified Medicine*. Elsevier, London; 2014:747–748. https://doi.org/10.1016/B978-0-12386882-4.00042-3.
2. Province MA, Arnett DK, Hunt SC, et al. Association between the α-adducin gene and hypertension in the HyperGEN study. *AM J Hypertens*. 2000;13(6):710–718.

Clinical Presentation 42

1. Assadi F, Kimura R, Subramarian U, Patel S. Liddle syndrome in a newborn infant. *Pediatr Nephrol*. 2002;17:609–611. https://doi.org/10.1007/s0046-002-0897-z.
2. Assadi F, Hooman N, Mazaheri M, Ghane Sharbaf F. Endocrine hypertension: discovering the inherited causes. In: Pappachan JM, Fernandez CJ, eds. *Endocrine Hypertension: From Basic Science to Clinical Practice*. London: Elsevier Academic Press; 2022:127–148.

Clinical Presentation 43

1. Rad EM, Assadi F. Management of hypertension in children with cardiovascular disease and heart failure. *Int J Prev Med*. 2014;5(Suppl 1):S10–S16.

Clinical Presentation 44

1. Brown JJ, Davies DL, Lever AF, et al. Plasma renin concentration in human hypertension. 1. Relationship between renin, sodium, and potassium. *Br Med J*. 1965;2:144–148.
2. Ding JJ, Lin SH, Lai JY, et al. Unilateral renal artery stenosis presented with hyponatremic-hypertensive syndrome—case report and literature review. *BMC Nephrol*. 2019;20:64.

Clinical Presentation 45

1. Wyszyńska T, Cichocka E, Wieteska-Klimczak A, et al. A single pediatric center experience with 1025 children with hypertension. *Acta Paediatr*. 1992;81:244–246.
2. Manger WM, Gifford RW. Pheochromocytoma. *J Clin Hypertens (Greenwich)*. 2002;4:62–72.
3. Mazzaglia PJ. Hereditary pheochromocytoma and paraganglioma. *J Surg Oncol*. 2002;106:580–585.
4. Chen H, Sippel RS, O'Dorisio MS, et al. The North American Neuroendocrine Tumor Society consensus guideline for the diagnosis and management of neuroendocrine tumors: pheochromocytoma, paraganglioma, and medullary thyroid cancer. *Pancreas*. 2010;39:775–783.
5. Lenders JW, Duh QY, Eisenhofer G, et al. Pheochromocytoma and paraganglioma: an endocrine society clinical practice guideline. *J Clin Endocrinol Metab*. 2014;99:1915–1942.

Clinical Presentation 46

1. Gennari FJ. Hypokalemia. *N Engl J Med*. 1998;339:451–458.
2. Lococo F, Margaritora S, Cardillo G, et al. Bronchopulmonary carcinoids causing Cushing syndrome: results from a multicentric study suggesting a more aggressive behavior. *Thorac Cardiovasc Surg*. 2016;64:172–181.

Clinical Presentation 47

1. Ramseyer LT. Case 34: renal lymphangiectasia. *Radiology*. 2001;219(2):442–444.
2. Cadnapaphomchai MA, Ford DM, Tyson RW, Lum GM. Cystic renal lymphangiectasis presenting as renal insufficiency in childhood. *Pediatr Nephrol*. 2000;15(1–2):129–131.
3. Ozmen M, Deren O, Akata D, Akhan O, Ozen H, Durukan T. Renal lymphangiomatosis during pregnancy: management with percutaneous drainage. *Eur Radiol*. 2001;11(1):37–40.
4. Wani NA, Kosar T, Gojwari T, Qureshi UA. Perinephric fluid collections due to renal lymphangiectasia. *Am J Kidney Dis*. 2011;57(2):347–351.
5. Ashraf K, Raza SS, Ashraf O, Memon W, Memon A, Zubairi TA. Renal lymphangiectasia. *Br J Radiol*. 2007;80(954):e117–e118.

Clinical Presentation 48

1. Weckbecker G, Lewis I, Albert R, Schmid HA, Hoyer D, Bruns C. Opportunities in somatostatin research: biological, chemical and therapeutic aspects. *Nat Rev Drug Discov*. 2003;2(12):999–1017.
2. Körner M, Waser B, Schonbrunn A, Perren A, Reubi JC. Somatostatin receptor subtype 2A immunohistochemistry using a new monoclonal antibody selects tumors suitable for in vivo somatostatin receptor targeting. *Am J Surg Pathol*. 2012;36(2):242–252.
3. Corvol P, Pinet F, Plouin P-F, Bruneval P, Menard J. Renin secreting tumors. *Endocrinol Metab Clin North Am*. 1994;23:255–270.
4. Theodoropoulou M, Stalla GK. Somatostatin receptors: from signaling to clinical practice. *Front Neuroendocrinol*. 2013;34(3):228–252.

CHAPTER 8

Tubulointerstitial Disease

Clinical Presentation 1

A 3-month-old male infant presented to pediatric emergency with poor oral feeding, frequent vomiting, and poor activity for 1 day. He was born at full term with a birth weight of 4410 g from a mother with preeclampsia and gestational diabetes. Because of birth asphyxia, he developed hypoxic-ischemic encephalopathy with epilepsy, which was treated with phenobarbital. He was fed standard formula milk without a supplement. There was no family history of renal disease.

His pulse rate was 131 beats/min, blood pressure (BP) 83/41 mm Hg, respiratory rate 34/min, and body temperature 37.0°C. Physical examination revealed drowsiness, delayed capillary refill time, and multiple firm subcutaneous nodules with no discoloration of overlying skin on his back and neck. There was no dysmorphic feature, heart murmur, or other abnormality. The most striking laboratory anomaly was profound hypercalcemia (total calcium 15.1 mg/dL) with hypercalciuria (urine calcium-to-creatinine ratio of 3.1 mg/mg, normal range [NR], <0.8 mg/mg). The remainder of blood tests revealed Na^+ 139 mmol/L, K^+ 5.6 mmol/L, Cl^- 105 mmol/L, inorganic phosphate 5.2 mg/dL, blood urea nitrogen (BUN) 19 mg/dL, and creatinine 0.61 mg/dL. Hormone profiles showed low intact parathyroid hormone (iPTH; <2.5 pg/mL; NR, 7–53) but normal $1,25(OH)_2$ vitamin D_3 (44 ng/mL; NR, 15–55), thyroid function, and cortisol levels. Ultrasonography of the neck clearly demonstrated marked skin thickness and increased echogenicity of the subcutaneous fat layer. Renal ultrasound revealed bilateral diffuse hyperechogenicity of the pyramids, typical for medullary nephrocalcinosis.

What is the underlying cause of hypercalcemia?

A. Accelerated bone calcium reabsorption (resorbtive hypercalcemia)
B. Increased intestinal calcium absorption (absorbtive hypercalcemia)
C. Subcutaneous fat necrosis with hypercalcemia
D. Increased renal calcium reabsorption (renal hypercalciuria)

The correct answer is C

Comment: The clinical features of hypercalcemia in infants may range from polyuria, hypovolemia, weakness, hypotonia, and impaired consciousness to seizure attacks. Early recognition of hypercalcemia is critical to prevent catastrophic events. In general, the heterogeneous causes of hypercalcemia can be divided into three categories[1,2]:

Increased renal tubular calcium reabsorption (reabsorptive hypercalcemia)
Accelerated bone calcium resorption (resorptive hypercalcemia)
Enhanced gastrointestinal calcium absorption (absorptive hypercalcemia)

Detailed patient history and complete physical examination, measurement of the urinary calcium excretion rate, serum iPTH, and $1,25(OH)_2$ vitamin D_3 levels provide a rapid differentiation of these three categories. The patient's marked hypercalciuria, low serum iPTH, but inappropriately high serum $1,25(OH)_2$ vitamin D_3 concentration pointed to absorptive hypercalcemia. He did not receive exogenous vitamin D supplements, such as fortified milk formulas, the most common cause of hypercalcemia in children.

The pathological findings from the biopsy of subcutaneous neck nodules showed he had subcutaneous fat necrosis causing absorptive hypercalcemia. He was treated with intravenous hydration and furosemide with oral potassium citrate. His serum calcium level was normalized within 5 days, followed by the resolution of subcutaneous nodules 3 weeks later and improvement of medullary nephrocalcinosis during a 6-month follow-up.

Clinical Presentation 2

A 3-year-old boy presented at the age of 2 with a urinary tract infection (UTI) associated with a febrile illness. Urine culture grew *Escherichia coli* at >10^5 organisms/mL. He received a treatment course of antibiotics and was then commenced on antibiotic prophylaxis. An initial renal ultrasound performed 1 week after treatment of the UTI was normal, demonstrating kidneys measuring 5.1 cm on the right and 6 cm on the left. A Technetium-99 m (^{99m}Tc)-dimercaptosuccinic acid (DMSA) scan carried out 6 weeks after treatment of the UTI demonstrated only a small amount of uptake by both kidneys. Renal function was normal based on serum creatinine measurement of 0.4 mg/dL. The DMSA scan was repeated 6 months later because of the unusual appearance of the kidneys on the first scan. Once again, the scan demonstrated no fixation of ^{99m}Tc-DMSA in the kidneys, and again the child's renal function was normal, with a creatinine measurement of 0.3 mg/dL. Following these unusual findings, a MAG3 renogram was conducted, which confirmed that both kidneys were functioning normally, based on normal perfusion, uptake, and excretion of the radioisotope. Relative uptake at 3 minutes was 49% on the left and 51% on the right. A micturating cystourethrogram showed no vesicoureteric reflux.

Urinary albumin/creatinine ratios on repeated occasions were elevated, ranging from 65 to 112 mg/mg. A 24-hour urine collection at 12 months of age indicated hypercalciuria at 5.9 mg/kg/day. An early morning urine osmolality was normal. The patient's urine demonstrated a mild generalized aminoaciduria. Urinary retinol binding protein was also found to be elevated in this child at 220 mg/L (normal range, 0–15 mg/L). White cell cystine was 0.05 nmol half-cystine/mg protein (normal range <0.3 half-cystine/mg protein), thereby excluding a diagnosis of nephropathic cystinosis. The tubular phosphate reabsorption was normal.

Clinically, the child did not have any features of renal disease, and his growth was normal. Ophthalmic review excluded any corneal or retinal changes. A renal biopsy was performed, and 73 glomeruli were obtained; 3 of these were small and sclerosed and associated with some interstitial fibrosis and tubular atrophy. The glomeruli were otherwise unremarkable and normal in appearance, and the appearance suggested a mild focal atrophy that was nonspecific and may have represented scarring. There was no evidence of tubular disease. The biopsy did not provide any further information that would explain the absence of ^{99m}Tc-DMSA uptake by the kidneys of this boy. In view of the proteinuria, the patient was started on enalapril. A repeat ultrasound 8 months later demonstrated that the kidneys were growing appropriately. Because there was no evidence of vesicoureteric reflux noted on the micturating cystourethrogram and no further UTIs had occurred, prophylactic antibiotics were stopped at age 2 years, 5 months. Growth was maintained and the child continues to be asymptomatic and normotensive. A further renal ultrasound scan at the age of 6 years showed nephrocalcinosis.

What is the cause for the poor uptake of ^{99m}Tc-DMSA in this patient?

A. Fanconi syndrome
B. Tubulointerstitial disease secondary to Dent disease
C. Idiopathic tubular proteinuria
D. Lowe syndrome

The correct answer is B

Comment: ^{99m}Tc-DMSA is a renal cortical imaging agent. Static renal scintigraphy using ^{99m}Tc-DMSA obtains information about the overall morphology of the functional renal unit and split renal function and detects parenchymal abnormalities. It is a highly useful imaging technique for identifying renal cortical scarring or defects. ^{99m}Tc-DMSA is a dithiol and localizes to the renal cortex by binding to sulfhydryl groups in the proximal tubules.[1] Renal uptake of ^{99m}Tc-DMSA approximates the functional renal cortical mass, which depends on renal blood flow and proximal tubular membrane transport function. Renal scintigraphy using ^{99m}Tc-MAG3 is a dynamic scan. It allows simultaneous investigation of renal perfusion and the presence of any obstruction. To have a complete absence of uptake of ^{99m}Tc-DMSA despite a normal ^{99m}Tc-MAG3, there must be a defect in the transport mechanism into the proximal tubular cells of ^{99m}Tc-DMSA in this child. This DMSA abnormality led to the early diagnosis of Dent disease in this child before any symptoms appearing.

The differential diagnosis in this case includes idiopathic autosomal-dominant idiopathic Fanconi syndrome, mitochondrial disorder, and iatrogenic secondary to aminoglycoside use. Patients with idiopathic tubular proteinuria present with asymptomatic low-molecular-weight proteinuria with normal renal function and show similar poor renal accumulation of ^{99m}Tc-DMSA.[2]

Lowe syndrome was unlikely because the patient did not have the other features of bilateral congenital cataracts, renal Fanconi syndrome, and intellectual disability.[3] Tubular proteinuria secondary to aminoglycoside treatment is usually transient. Cytotoxic agents including ifosfamide and cisplatin can cause renal tubular injury that can present with reduced uptake of ^{99m}Tc-DMSA before clinical deterioration.[4]

Dent disease is part of a spectrum of hereditary renal tubular disorders known as X-linked hypercalciuric nephrolithiasis. These include Dent disease, X-linked recessive nephrolithiasis, X-linked recessive hypophosphatemic rickets, and low-molecular-weight proteinuria, and are caused by mutations in the *CLCN5* gene.[5] It was first described by Dent and Friedman in 1964.[4] Dent disease causes a renal Fanconi syndrome with proximal renal tubular defects, including low-molecular-weight proteinuria, hypercalciuria, nephrolithiasis/nephrocalcinosis, metabolic bone disease, and progressive renal failure. Female carriers are asymptomatic but have low-molecular-weight proteinuria, and approximately half have hypercalciuria. Low-molecular-weight proteinuria is uniformly present in disorders of proximal tubular function such as Dent, and its absence excludes the diagnosis.

Subsequent genetic analysis in our patient has revealed a mutation p.Gly57Arg in the *CLCN5* gene, confirming the diagnosis. This mutation has not been described before but is believed to be pathogenic because pGly57Val has previously been identified as a pathogenic mutation.[1]

The *CLCN5* gene encodes for the voltage-gated chloride channel and chloride/proton exchanger (CIC-5). CIC-5 is predominantly expressed in the proximal tubule of the kidney, where it is thought to be involved in endosomal acidification. Nonsense and missense mutations in the *CLCN5* gene reduce or abolish CIC-5 chloride currents. CIC-5 knockout mice have been shown to have reduced levels of two apical cell surface receptors, megalin and cubilin. These receptors are involved in the uptake of proteins into the cells of the proximal tubule by endocytosis and reduced recycling of megalin and cubilin leads to low-molecular-weight proteinuria. Dent patients have been shown to be deficient in urinary megalin.[6]

It has been proposed that ^{99m}Tc-DMSA is filtered in the glomeruli and then reabsorbed by megalin and cubilin endocytosis in the proximal renal tubule. This explains the reduced ^{99m}Tc-DMSA uptake seen in Dent patients.[7] ^{99m}Tc-DMSA has a molecular size of 24 to 28 kDa, which is within the range of low-molecular-weight proteins.[8]

Calcium crystals are removed from the collecting duct apical cell surface by endocytosis. This is impaired in Dent patients because of an increase in plasma membrane annexin A2, a crystal-binding molecule. This may be why Dent patients may develop nephrocalcinosis even in the absence of hypercalciuria.[9]

Treatment with thiazide diuretics has been proven to improve the hypercalciuria, but it is uncertain whether this improves renal survival, although they are associated with adverse events including hypovolemia and electrolyte abnormalities particularly at higher doses.[10] Future therapeutic options may include reduction of inflammation and immunomodulation, but this has not been established.[6] The use of an angiotensin-converting enzyme inhibitor may also delay the reduction in renal function as in other tubulopathies, although the value in normotensive patients is uncertain.[11]

Clinical Presentation 3

A 7-year-old male patient was admitted with intermittent gross hematuria and dysuria of 1 month's duration. He had been treated with several antibiotics despite negative urine cultures. He had no history of any allergies, genitourinary problems, or external trauma. According to his medical history, he had been diagnosed with autism 2 years previously and had been treated with valproic acid since then. His family history was insignificant.

There were no pathological findings on physical examination. Macroscopically, the urine was red. Urinalysis revealed hematuria, minimal proteinuria, and no pyuria or casts. Urine culture was negative. Spot urine calcium/creatinine ratio was normal (0.04 mg/mg).

Laboratory studies revealed a white blood cell (WBC) count of 7,900/mm^3 with peripheral eosinophilia (10%). The serum creatinine level was 0.42 mg/dL, BUN was 26 mg/dL, and electrolytes were normal. Immunological studies showed markedly elevated serum immunoglobulin E (IgE; 1050 IU/mL). Bladder wall thickness was 8 mm under ultrasound with no upper urinary tract and renal pathology. The etiology of gross hematuria remained uncertain; thus, further investigation was performed.

Cystoscopy revealed edematous and hyperemic bladder wall and urethra but no petechia or bleeding. Histopathological examination showed an infiltration of the mucosa and submucosa by numerous eosinophils.

What is the most likely diagnosis?

A. Eosinophilic cystitis (EC)
B. UTI
C. Idiopathic benign hematuria
D. IgA nephritis

The correct answer is A

Comment: Eosinophilic cystitis is an inflammatory disorder caused by eosinophilic infiltration of the bladder wall. Immunological factor associated with EC is thought to be the IgE-mediated formation of antigen-antibody complex that attacks eosinophils at the bladder wall. Many etiologies have been proposed including allergy; asthma; drugs such as cyclophosphamide, sulfonamides, warfarin, nonsteroidal antiinflammatory drugs (NSAIDs), antihistamines, and penicillin; and UTI and vesicoureteral reflux.[1,2]

The presenting symptoms of EC is similar to those of UTI, such as frequency, urgency, dysuria, gross hematuria, and suprapubic pain. Some patients have microscopic hematuria, urinary retention, and nocturia. Urinalysis in EC commonly shows proteinuria and microscopic hematuria. Urine cultures are usually sterile.

Diagnosis of EC requires tissue biopsy for histological examination, which will reveal eosinophilic infiltration of the lamina propria and muscularis in the acute phases and variable degrees of fibrosis in more long-standing disease.[1,2]

Clinical Presentation 4

A 14-year-old girl with a history of primary hypoparathyroidism and unstable calcium and phosphorus levels and on ongoing treatment was admitted to the department of pediatric nephrology because of the onset of nephrocalcinosis and difficulties achieving normocalcemia. The obstetric, neonatal, and developmental history was unremarkable. The child was born at full term after a normal seventh pregnancy and fifth delivery, with a birth weight of 3150 g and an Apgar score of 10. An adenoidectomy was performed at the age of 6 years. The first symptoms of the disease appeared at the age of 9 years and consisted of several episodes of syncope and seizures. At presentation, apart from a white-coated tongue, dental caries, and enamel hypoplasia, the clinical, neurological, cardiovascular, and ophthalmic examinations were normal. Laboratory tests revealed hypocalcemia, hyperphosphatemia, and low serum parathyroid hormone. Computed tomography (CT) and magnetic resonance imaging (MRI) revealed bilateral calcifications in the basal ganglia and the frontal lobes. The thyroid gland was slightly heterogeneous on ultrasound, and antithyroid peroxidase antibodies were present, without any other clinical or biochemical features of hypothyreosis. A treatment of primary hypoparathyroidism based on calcium supplementation and 1-α-hydroxycholecalciferol administration was prescribed. During a period of 3 years (2011–2014), the dosage had to be progressively increased because of persisting hypocalcemia, to a maximum of 4.0 g of calcium carbonate and 1.75 μg of 1-α-hydroxycholecalciferol daily. In January 2015, the patient was hospitalized because of dyspnea, generalized weakness, polydipsia, nausea, and tachycardia. She was severely hypercalcemic at that moment but recovered rapidly after intensive fluid therapy, loop diuretics, and temporary withdrawal of the vitamin D and calcium. The doses were ultimately reduced to 1.25 μg and 3.0 g, respectively. Renal sonography remained normal. In September 2015, however, features of mild nephrocalcinosis appeared, with increased echogenicity of the borders of the renal pyramids, which led to her referral to the nephrology department. On admission, the girl was in good general condition. Physical examination showed the same oral findings as described previously, with the confirmation of candidiasis in swab culture. Laboratory tests showed biochemical findings similar to the aforementioned: low level of serum parathyroid hormones (PTH), 25-OH-vitamin D, and alkaline phosphatase; hyperphosphatemia; and clearly decreased levels of total and ionized calcium. Persistent hypercalciuria was observed, with an elevated calcium-to-creatinine ratio in a morning urine sample of 0.24 mg/mg, and a decreased magnesium-to-calcium ratio of 0.25 mg/mg. The other results were within the normal range, including an estimated glomerular filtration rate (eGFR) by the Schwartz formula of 92 mL/min/1.73 m^2. A bone densitometry (total body and lumbar region) was appropriate for age. During hospitalization, the girl reported transient acute pain in her right knee. X-ray imaging showed no pathological changes. Ultrasound examination revealed, besides mild nonprogressive bilateral nephrocalcinosis, a duplex left kidney with a mild dilatation of the upper-pole collecting system of 10 mm in sagittal dimension.

What is the likely diagnosis?

A. Hyperparathyroidism
B. Autoimmune polyglandular syndrome type 1
C. Vitamin D intoxication
D. Hypoparathyroidism

The correct answer is B

Comment: The coexistence of hypoparathyroidism, oral candidiasis, dental enamel hypoplasia, and subclinical Hashimoto disease in our patient is strongly suggestive of autoimmune polyglandular syndrome type 1.[1,2] One of the clinical implications of this diagnosis is the high probability of future occurrence of adrenal insufficiency, emphasizing the importance of maintaining a high level of suspicion with the onset of symptoms such as weakness, fainting, hypotonia, or hyperkalemia. Addison disease would in fact represent quite a challenge in terms of the future management of this patient.

Clinical Presentation 5

A 7-year-old boy presented to a community clinic looking generally unwell. He was referred to our hospital and found to have end-stage kidney disease.

He was born at 40 + 3 weeks' gestation to nonconsanguineous parents by normal vaginal delivery following spontaneous onset of labor after a maternal antepartum hemorrhage. His antenatal ultrasounds were normal at 12, 20, 22, 30, 32, and 34 weeks. He was born in good condition, with a birth weight of 4 kg, and discharged on day 2 of life.

From the time he was discharged home, his mother was concerned about nystagmus, and at 8 weeks he was referred to the ophthalmologist, as he was not fixing and following. He was reviewed by both a developmental pediatrician and an ophthalmologist on a monthly basis and was diagnosed with hypermetropia requiring glasses at 9 months of age. He had a cranial MRI scan at 11 months of age that was reported to be normal.

He was noted to have global developmental delay. Blood tests were taken at the age of 2 years as part of a genetics workup, and these showed normal renal function (plasma creatinine 36 μmol/L, urea 3.5 mmol/L, sodium 141 mmol/ L, potassium 4.5 mmol/L, and hemoglobin 121 g/L). He did not walk independently until the age of 4.5 years and was diagnosed with an autistic spectrum disorder at 7 years of age (he only had four words at 9 years of age).

He was diagnosed with pharyngitis and given oral antibiotics by his general practitioner at the age of 7.5 years. A few weeks later, he presented to a community clinic looking generally unwell and was noted to be pale with a flow murmur. He was referred to the hospital, and on admission his weight and height were 22.3 kg (>ninth percentile) and 117.1 cm (<ninth percentile), respectively, and he was hypertensive with systolic BP of 155 mm Hg. His urine protein/creatinine ratio was 124 mg/mmol, and his blood tests revealed a plasma creatinine level of 8.6 mg/dL, urea 98 mg/dL, sodium 142 mmol/L, potassium 4.2 mmol/L, corrected calcium 10.4 mg/dL, phosphorus 7.1 mg/dL, bicarbonate mmol/L, and hemoglobin 5.5 g/dL.

Following admission and stabilization, he was referred to a tertiary nephrology unit because of his deranged renal function, persistent hypocalcemia, and metabolic acidosis. A renal ultrasound scan showed loss of corticomedullary differentiation and increased echogenicity, with his right kidney measuring 8.2 cm and left kidney measuring 9.2 cm (fifth and 50th percentiles for age are 7.4 cm and 8.8 cm, respectively).

He then underwent a percutaneous renal biopsy under general anesthetic, which contained 41 glomerular profiles, of which 5 (12%) were globally sclerosed. Two showed periglomerular fibrosis, and a number of the others showed mild ischemic shrinkage. There was no mesangial thickening, hypercellularity, or segmental lesions. Glomerular basement membranes showed mild ischemic shrinking on silver stain only, with negative Congo red staining for amyloid. There was focal tubular atrophy and diffuse interstitial edema with a dense diffuse interstitial inflammatory infiltrate of lymphocytes. In several foci, lymphocytes were seen to infiltrate tubules, and tubular rupture was noted. There were no specific glomerular deposits as revealed by immunocytochemistry (IgG, IgA, IgM, or C3). Three sclerosed and one viable glomerulus were visible on electron microscopy examination, all of which showed some ischemic shrinkage and foot process fusion but no deposits. The conclusion drawn from the biopsy results was acute tubulointerstitial nephritis (TIN), with the presence of sclerosis and atrophy consistent with a degree of chronicity.

The patient was commenced on corticosteroid therapy, which he remained on for 4 months. Hemodialysis was started at presentation, and he has required this since. On referral to our quaternary pediatric nephrology service for transplant workup at the age of 9 years, his history was reviewed and it was felt that he exhibited a number of features of Joubert syndrome (JS). His previous MRI scan was reviewed again and confirmed the pathognomic sign of JS. The results of his genetics workup were sent, and further review also confirmed the diagnosis of JS.

What are the renal manifestations typically seen in JS including the radiological and histological findings?

A. Juvenile nephronophthisis (NPHP)
B. Tubulointerstitial disease
C. Glomerulopathy
D. Cystic kidney disease

The correct answers are A, B, and D

Comment: The renal manifestation in JS is similar to patients with NPHP. NPHP patients typically present with polyuria and polydipsia, and NPHP ultimately leads to progressive renal failure, usually within the first three decades of life.[1] The predominant form of NPHP is juvenile, although a much rarer infantile form also exists. The typical features revealed by ultrasonography are normal or reduced kidney size (note that normalized kidneys in end-stage renal disease is unusual), loss of corticomedullary differentiation, and small cysts at the corticomedullary junction.[2] On renal biopsy, structural tubulointerstitial abnormalities are seen including tubular atrophy, interstitial fibrosis, and tubular basement membrane defects.[3] In infantile NPHP, there can be enlarged kidneys on the ultrasound scan, and renal biopsy findings include cortical microcysts and normal tubular basement membrane.

Patients with JS present with developmental delay, hypotonia, abnormal ocular movement, colobomas, and cerebellar vermis agenesis evolving into ataxia.[4,5] Subsequently, a neuroradiological mid-hindbrain malformation, known as the "molar tooth sign," was identified. This malformation is caused by hypoplasia of the cerebellar vermis with fourth ventricle deformity and a sagittal vermian cleft from incomplete vermis fusion. Elongated and thickened superior cerebellar peduncles with a widened interpeduncular fossa are also present.[4] The absence of a normal vermis results in a midline cleft between the cerebellar hemispheres, resulting in the "bat wing" sign on an MRI scan.[5]

In general, juvenile NPHP presents with biopsy findings of severe chronic tubulointerstitial changes with secondary tubular dilatation but with minimal inflammation. Conversely, TIN usually shows marked interstitial inflammation with minimal chronic change. In this boy's biopsy, there was extensive lymphocytic infiltration of tubules and a dense interstitial inflammatory infiltrate of lymphocytes, presenting a histological picture of acute TIN rather than the expected picture of chronic change one would expect in NPHP.

Clinical Presentation 6

A previously healthy 15-year-old girl was admitted because of reddish discoloration of the urine, which presented after walking for approximately 30 minutes on a smooth road; she reported three similar episodes over the previous 2 months. Discoloration lasted for four to five urinations (~12 hours) in each episode, followed by complete disappearance of hemoglobulin/myoglobulin on urine dipstick. No other exercise-produced discoloration and no other symptoms were reported. The parents were unrelated, and the family history was negative for kidney and hematological diseases. On admission, physical examination was normal, including arterial BP (120/ 80 mm Hg).

Laboratory evaluation following the fourth and fifth episodes, respectively, revealed a reddish urine sample, with four to six and two to four red blood cells per high-power field (RBCs/HPF); no to two WBCs/HPF; and 3+ hemoglobin/myoglobin. Mildly elevated blood lactate dehydrogenase (453 U/L and 454 U/L; normal range, 115–230 U/L) and total bilirubin (1.6 and

1.8 mg/dL; normal range, 0.1–1.0 mg/dL) were identified. Hemoglobin was within normal limits (12.5 and 12.4 g/dL), as was total reticulocyte count (58 and 65 × $10^3/\mu L$). Blood smear analysis showed mild anisopoikilocytosis with stomatocytes (4%) and ovalocytes (4%). WBCs, platelet counts, serum creatinine, liver function tests, and serum electrolyte levels were all within normal range. Serum muscle enzymes, creatine kinase, alanine aminotransferase, and aldolase were measured twice, both at the time of urine discoloration and 24 hours later within normal limits. Her 24-hour urine analysis revealed protein excretion 3 mg/m^2 per hour, calcium excretion 2 mg/kg per 24 hours, and creatinine clearance 115 mL/min/1.73 m^2. Urinary tract ultrasound (US) and color Doppler US were normal.

What differential diagnosis would you consider?

A. Paroxysmal cold agglutinins hemoglobinuria
B. Paroxysmal nocturnal hemoglobinuria
C. Paroxysmal nocturnal hemoglobinuria
D. Glucose-6-phosphate dehydrogenase deficiency

The correct answers are A, B, C, and D

Comment: The presence of reddish urine discoloration with a positive dipstick test for hemoglobinuria after walking and after exclusion of other causes of hemoglobinuria, and otherwise normal erythrocytes, is most likely secondary to march hemoglobinuria.[1,2]

The repetitive reddish discoloration of the urine in his patient was associated with hemoglobinuria or myoglobinuria, based on the positive dipstick test and the absence of RBCs on microscopic urine examination. The normal levels of serum blood muscle enzymes, creatine kinase, and alanine aminotransferase ruled out the diagnosis of myoglobinuria.

A detailed laboratory evaluation ruled out other causes of hemoglobinuria, such as paroxysmal nocturnal hemoglobinuria (presence of CD55 and CD59 on peripheral erythrocytes by flow cytometry), cold agglutinin disease and paroxysmal cold hemoglobinuria (negative direct antiglobulin test, absence of cold agglutinins and Donath-Landsteiner antibody), glucose-6-phosphate dehydrogenase deficiency (normal levels of the enzyme), and congenital unstable hemoglobinopathies (normal hemoglobin electrophoresis).[1]

Erythrocyte membrane disorders, such as hereditary spherocytosis, stomatocytosis, and ovalocytosis, were excluded by osmotic fragility testing, and the results of the flow cytometric eosin-5′-maleimide-binding test and the spectrin/band3 and ankyrin/band3 ratios were within the normal range. Pyrimidine 5′ nucleotidase deficiency was also ruled out with the use of a specific screening test (OD260/OD280 absorbance ratio). The levels of other enzymes involved in erythrocyte metabolism were within the normal range (i.e., hexokinase, glucose phosphate isomerase, phosphofructokinase, glyceraldehyde-P-dehydrogenase, phosphoglycerate kinase, pyruvate kinase, 6-phosphogluconate dehydrogenase, and adenylate kinase).

Because of the presence of reddish urine discoloration with a positive dipstick test for hemoglobinuria after walking, exclusion of other causes of hemoglobinuria, and otherwise normal RBCs, the most likely diagnosis is march hemoglobinuria.

The patient was advised to avoid long walks, to take frequent rest breaks even during short walks, and to use appropriate footwear for walking. No other episodes of urine discoloration occurred during the next 8 months.

Clinical Presentation 7

A 12-month-old male infant was admitted with concerns of fever, excessive irritability, and inconsolable cry while micturating for 2 days. The baby was hemodynamically stable and normotensive. Examination revealed microcephaly (head circumference 39 cm) with bipyramidal signs (spastic quadriparesis and exaggerated muscle stretch reflexes) and visual inattention. The weight was 8.3 kg (10th percentile) and length was 74 cm (between 25th and 50th percentiles). The developmental examination showed global developmental delay, with no head control and maternal recognition. The anterior fontanelle had closed. Facial dysmorphism (broad nasal bridge, prominent cheeks, long philtrum) was noted. No other gross congenital anomalies were evident. Lens dislocation was absent; the retina was normal. The urinalysis showed numerous pus cells with no red blood cells or proteinuria. Urine nitrite dipstick was positive. Urine culture grew *E. coli* and intravenous cefoperazone-sulbactam was administered for 10 days. The blood urea (25 mg/dL) and serum creatinine (0.19 mg/dL) were normal for age. Serum calcium (9.5 mg/dL), phosphorus (4.5 mg/dL), and magnesium (2.1 mg/dL) were normal. Serum uric acid levels were consistently low (0.4 mg/dL) and fractional excretion of uric acid was low (1.1%). The 24-hour urine calcium and oxalate levels were within normal limits. Sodium nitroprusside test performed on the urine sample was negative. Ultrasonogram showed normal-sized kidneys (right kidney, 52 mm; left kidney, 56 mm) with multiple calculi in bilateral renal pelvis, with no hydronephrosis or ureteral dilatation.

The passage of a stone in the urine was noted by the caregivers during a hospital stay. The past history was significant. He was born to second-degree consanguineous parents at 38 weeks of gestation by vaginal delivery and weighed 3.5 kg at birth. The perinatal period had been eventful with delayed crying at birth and seizures from day 3 onward. The child cried after tactile stimulation, and unequivocal evidence of neonatal encephalopathy was not forthcoming. Documented evidence of sepsis, hypoglycemia, or dyselectrolytemia were absent, and the neonatal seizures responded to phenobarbitone. There were no neurocutaneous markers on examination. Brain MRI on day 7 after birth revealed multicystic changes in bilateral frontal regions and was reported to be secondary to probable hypoxic-ischemic encephalopathy. The serum T3, T4, and thyroid-stimulating hormone levels were normal. He was later admitted at 8 months of age at another hospital with concerns of developmental delay and multifocal seizures, for which therapy with levetiracetam had been initiated. Detailed family history revealed similar history and clinical features in an elder male sibling with global developmental delay with multifocal refractory seizures who expired at 7 months of age (2 years ago). There was no history of renal stones in that baby.

Given the consanguinity, sibling death, and unexplained neurological features with cystic changes on MRI, inborn errors of metabolism were strongly considered. Plasma homocysteine was low (1.2 μmol/L; reference value, 4–12 μmol/L). Samples were sent for targeted genetic analysis by next-generation sequencing. Reproductive counseling was offered to the parents, and the child was initiated on neurorehabilitation with antiepileptic and antispastic measures. The passed stone was sent for a Fourier transform infrared spectroscopy stone analysis, which revealed it was 100% xanthine.

What is (are) the cause(s) of urolithiasis wherein hypouricemia is encountered?

A. Cystinuria
B. Primary hyperoxaluria
C. Distal renal tubular acidosis
D. Hereditary renal xanthiuria

The correct answer is D

Comment: Our patient had xanthine stones with hypouricemia and hypouricosuria. The genetic analysis by next-generation sequencing of our patient revealed a homozygous missense variation in exon 2 of the *MOCS2* gene (c.45T>A) that resulted in the amino acid substitution of arginine for serine at codon 15 (p.Ser15Arg; ENST00000450852).[1–4] Xanthine renal stones are uncommon in infants and children, out of which hereditary renal xanthiuria (HX) type I and HX type II contribute to a majority of their etiology.

Clinical Presentation 8

A 12-year-old girl presented with a 10-day history of left lumbar and flank pain. The pain had started in association with mild dysuria and was increasing in intensity so she needed continued analgesia with several drugs. She had been studying at her local hospital. UTI and renal lithiasis had been ruled out. The patient was submitted to our unit for further explorations and difficulty in pain relief. She denied hematuria, fever, chills, weight loss, or gynecological complaints. She had nausea and vomiting, loss of appetite, and orthostatic hypotension. Past medical history was remarkable for asthma, repeated episodes of dysuria without confirmation of urinary tract infection, and dysmenorrhea. Four years before, she had undergone a laparotomy for recurrent abdominal pain, with intestinal bridles being the only significant finding. During early childhood, the patient grew up in an unfavorable social environment resulting from affective family problems. Family history included a father with renal urolithiasis and a mother with clinical depression.

Vital signs were normal. Physical examination was unremarkable with no abdominal tenderness, bruits, or signs of organomegaly, but the patient was affected by the pain and noticeably tried to keep a fetal position. She refused to eat and did not tolerate standing.

Laboratory workup revealed repeatedly normal complete blood count, and biochemistry, including hepatic, pancreatic, and renal functions, and a negative pregnancy test. Procalcitonin, C-reactive protein, and erythrocyte sedimentation rate were normal as well. Urinalysis was normal, without hematuria or proteinuria, in six separate determinations. Fecal calprotectin was also normal. Kidney US revealed retroaortic double left renal vein (LRV). Bone and renal scans were normal. Other imaging tests were performed subsequently.

What further diagnostic test is necessary to establish a diagnosis?

A. CT scan of kidney and urinary bladder
B. Intravenous pyelogram
C. Doppler ultrasound
D. Renal biopsy

The correct answer is A

Comment: Differential diagnosis must consider potential causes of left lumbar and flank pain of severe intensity including (1) nephrourologic diseases, such as acute pyelonephritis, urolithiasis, cystic kidney diseases, and renal vascular alterations; (2) infectious, traumatic, or tumoral disorders involving spinal column; (3) gynecological diseases such as endometriosis, and pelvic inflammatory disease; (4) abdominal inflammation or ischemia, including inflammatory bowel disease and acute intermittent porphyria; and (5) psychosomatic problems.[1–3]

The finding of a retroaortic LRV is a condition known as nutcracker anatomy. This anatomical position of the LRV not leading to symptoms is called the nutcracker phenomenon, but the presence of symptoms and signs related to LRV outflow obstruction defines the nutcracker syndrome. LRV entrapment may be of two types: anterior or posterior. The anterior one is more common and corresponds to the entrapment of the LRV between the abdominal aorta and superior mesenteric artery.

Clinical manifestations include hematuria (microhematuria or macroscopic); orthostatic proteinuria; left flank pain; abdominal pain; varicocele; dyspareunia; dysmenorrhea; fatigue; orthostatic intolerance; and symptoms of autonomic dysfunction such as hypotension, syncope, and tachycardia.[4] The pain can be strong and prolonged and become relentless, and the use of chronic narcotics may be required for adequate analgesia.

Clinical Presentation 9

A 10-year-old boy was evaluated for recurrent cystitis resulting from *Enterococcus faecalis*. The boy had a history of autoimmune gastritis, constipation with encopresis, and primary enuresis. An US scan ruled out the presence of a urinary tract malformation, showing a mild wall thickening of both the bladder and the rectum. The MRI study evoked the suspicion of a possible rectourethral fistula. To confirm this hypothesis, combined cystoscopy and colonoscopy were scheduled, under general anesthesia with sevoflurane, fentanyl, and propofol. Cystoscopy was performed while irrigating the rectum with methylene blue, to assist the detection of any fistulous tract. Despite the instillation of a large amount of dye, the test proved negative. A colonoscopy was eventually performed after washing the rectum, showing no evidence of inflammation. The night following the procedure, the boy referred to voiding bluish urine. During the following day, a greenish hue of the urine was noted, which gradually faded within a few days. Urinalysis was otherwise unremarkable.

What is the differential diagnosis for a child with green urine?

A. Rectal enema containing methylene blue
B. Recto-urethral fistula
C. Hartnup disease
D. Blue diaper syndrome

The correct answer is A

Comment: The observation of green urine in this child raised further concerns about a recto-urethral fistula; however, this hypothesis was made unlikely by the lack of findings during cystoscopy, despite the irrigation of the rectum with a large amount of methylene blue. The differential diagnosis of green urine was therefore advocated.

Congenital conditions potentially responsible for greenish discoloration of urine (namely Hartnup disease, blue diaper syndrome) were easily ruled out based on the sudden occurrence of the phenomenon in adolescent age. Biliverdinuria and urinary tract infections were excluded by the normal urinalysis results. Among the different drugs potentially involved, propofol was taken into account: however, very low induction doses were used in this child, who had been sedated with propofol before without displaying any similar findings. Finally, a dye-related urine discoloration was considered: based on previous reports, the occurrence of green urine in this child was attributed to the administration of methylene blue through a rectal enema. As expected, the urine discoloration eventually faded over few days. The history of recurrent cystitis was attributed to severe constipation.

The diagnosis of dye-related urine discoloration is clinical and does not require any additional test. Urinalysis can assist in the exclusion of urinary tract infections, potentially responsible for the urine of greenish hue. The awareness of the benign nature of this condition prevented this child from undergoing further unnecessary invasive investigations.[1–3]

Clinical Presentation 10

A 6-year-old boy was referred because of abnormal kidney function tests performed following vomiting and diarrhea lasting for 5 days before admission. The family denied a decrease in urine. There was no consanguinity between the parents, nor did he have a known disease in his medical history. In his medical records, his serum creatinine was 0.6 mg/dL 6 months before admission. He had a body weight of 21.4 kg (25th–50th percentile), height of 118.5 cm (25th–50th percentile), body temperature of 36.7°C, BP of 158/100 mm Hg (>95th percentile +12), heart rate of 104/min, and respiratory rate of 26/min. The patient was oriented and cooperative. In his physical examination, he had +1 pretibial pitting edema. Respiratory sounds were normal. There was no splenomegaly or hepatomegaly.

A urinary catheter was inserted, but no urine was observed. The urine output was 0.3 mL/kg/h after forced diuresis. There was no finding in favor of active infection in serology including COVID-19. Kidney biopsy revealed global sclerosis in three, cellular/fibrocellular crescents in four, fibrous crescents in four, ischemic collapse in 10 or 11, and segmental sclerosis in one glomerulus of the 43 glomeruli. Basement membranes and mesangial cellularity were normal. A mixed type of inflammatory cell infiltration with dense lymphoplasmacyte cells, containing mild-to-moderate eosinophils, was observed in the tubulointerstitial area. In addition to active tubulitis findings including loss of brush border epithelium, localized shedding of epithelial cells, tubular dilatation with proteinous hyaline casts, moderate tubular atrophy, and severe interstitial fibrosis attributable to chronic tubulointerstitial nephritis (CTIN) were noted. In the immunofluorescence study, there was +2 fine granular IgG staining in the basement membranes and a segmental +1 nonspecific IgM staining in the basement membranes in some glomeruli. Ophthalmologic examination was normal.

What could be the cause of CTIN in this patient (list all that apply)?

A. Malignancy
B. Nephrocalcinosis
C. Autoimmune diseases
D. IgG4-related kidney disease

The correct answers are A, B, C, and D

Comment: In cases of CTIN, the causes of systemic and chronic inflammation must be reviewed.[1] Drug use is the leading chronic cause. Antibiotics, NSAIDs, analgesics, proton pump inhibitors, calcineurin inhibitors, and chemotherapeutic agents are the most common underlying factors.[2] Heavy metals such as lead, bismuth, cadmium, and aristolochic acid can cause CTIN.[2] Infection-related causes including chronic pyelonephritis, malakoplakia, and xanthogranulomatous pyelonephritis are among the other common causes of CTIN.[3] In addition, systemic diseases such as dysproteinemias, lymphoproliferative diseases, sickle cell disease, inflammatory bowel disease, cystinosis, and atheroembolic diseases; metabolic diseases such as oxalate nephropathy, uric acid nephropathy, nephrocalcinosis, and hypokalemic nephropathy; autoimmune diseases including Sjögren syndrome, sarcoidosis, systemic lupus erythematosus, tubulointerstitial nephritis and uveitis (TINU), and scleroderma; and IgG4-related disease are among the other differential diagnoses of CTIN.[3]

To evaluate these diseases, medical history, anti-nuclear-antibody (ANA), anti-dsDNA, C3 and C4, p-antineutrophil cytoplasmic antibody (ANCA), c-ANCA, immunoglobulin levels, urine electrolytes, urine cultures, ophthalmologic examination, and abdominal US should be performed in such a patient as the first step. These were performed and resulted in normal ranges in our patient. There was no drug use or known toxic substance exposure.

The IgE levels in our patient were remarkably high, with 26,400 IU/mL at admission and 31,000 IU/mL in the control. In such a case with severely high levels of IgE without eosinophilia, primary and secondary causes of immune deficiencies, and systemic diseases including allergic, skin, infectious, inflammatory, and although rare in children, neoplastic problems including gammopathies should be ruled out.[4] There was no evidence suggesting primary or secondary immunodeficiency in his medical history or flow cytometric lymphocyte panel. Serum immunofixation electrophoresis demonstrated no paraprotein associated with IgD or IgE. Contrast-enhanced thoracal and abdominal tomography revealed no tumoral mass in any cavity of the body.

High IgE levels, CTIN, and glomerular pathologies with crescents pointed at IgG4-related disease as the underlying cause.[5] The patient serum IgG4-related disease was 2.42 g/L (normal, 0.012–1.699). Accordingly, immunohistochemical IgG4 staining of the biopsy specimens resulted in more than 10 IgG4 (+) plasma cells per HPF.

High IgG4 levels and lymphoplasmacytic infiltration with IgG4 (+) plasma cells >10/HPF in the kidney biopsy were suggestive of IgG4-related kidney disease.[5]

Clinical Presentation 11

A 3-year-old boy was admitted to our pediatric urology department for further investigation of dysuria. He was previously healthy and had thrived. Macroscopic and microscopic urinary assessment did not reveal any pathologic features. A sonography of the boy's urinary tract revealed urinary bladder wall thickening (up to 2 cm) with heterogeneous echogenicity. Further imaging with MRI scans unraveled these heterogeneous wall thickenings as polypus endoluminal concavities. The only other abnormal finding on routine examination was peripheral eosinophilia (28% of peripheral leukocytes and 2470/mm^3 absolute eosinophil count) in the boy's blood count. Eosinophilia is defined as the presence of higher absolute and relative counts of eosinophils in the peripheral blood (>5% of peripheral leukocytes and >500/mm^3 absolute eosinophil count).[1] Causes for eosinophilia are highly diverse and include primary (clonal) forms caused by hematologic neoplasms and the more common secondary (reactive) forms resulting from allergic disorders (e.g., asthma, atopic dermatitis), parasitic and fungal infections, rheumatological diseases (e.g., systemic lupus, and vasculitis), respiratory diseases (e.g., eosinophilic pneumonia), other neoplasms (e.g., solid tumors, lymphomas), dermatologic disorders (e.g., Wells syndrome), disorders of immune regulation (e.g., hyper-IgE syndrome), gastrointestinal disorders (e.g., eosinophilic esophagitis), and drugs.[2] Through clinical, serological, urinary, and fecal examinations, we could not identify any secondary causes for eosinophilia.

For the first and most important step to rule out bladder malignancy (i.e., rhabdomyosarcoma), and to either diagnose or rule out collagen vascular diseases, the boy underwent cystoscopy and subsequent biopsy of the polypus endoluminal concavities. Histologic analysis described an inflammatory eosinophilic-dominated infiltrate with no signs of malignant disease. Symptomatic treatment with oxybutynin (0.1 mg/kg three times per day) for the boy's dysuria and pollakisuria was initiated. Initially, the boy's symptoms were relieved, and the urinary bladder wall thickening declined after 1 month of treatment from 2 to 0.27 cm. However, about 3 months after diagnosis, urinary bladder wall thickening increased to 0.5 cm. The boy also experienced constipation, a common side effect of treatment with oxybutynin, and initial symptoms returned, with peripheral eosinophilia still at high levels (18% of peripheral leukocytes and 1900/mm^3 absolute eosinophil count). At the end of the fourth month of oxybutynin treatment, bladder wall thickening increased to 1.2 cm and the boy presented with weight loss of 2.3 kg over 4 months, abdominal distention, and markedly decreased subcutaneous fat. Laboratory tests revealed hypoalbuminemia and deficiencies of iron, vitamin D, and vitamin A.

To rule out other reasons for the weight loss, we performed further analysis that revealed IgA antibodies against transglutaminase 2 of more than 10 times the upper reference value (>200 U/mL) and positivity for endomysial antibodies (1:640). Together with positivity for endomysial antibodies (1:640) and the at-risk human leukocyte antigen (HLA)-DQ2: A1*0505, B1*0202 genotype, the diagnosis of celiac disease was established.

What is the diagnosis and what is its most likely etiology (select all that apply)?

A. Allergies
B. Eosinophilic cystitis
C. Medications
D. Fibroblast growth factor receptor 1

The correct answers are A, B, C, and D

Comment: The patient has eosinophilic cystitis, which developed because of eosinophilia triggered by celiac disease. Under normal conditions, eosinophils are mainly found in the bone marrow, lymphoid organs, the mucosa of the gastrointestinal tract, and the uterus, but very rarely in other organ tissues. Secondary (reactive) eosinophilia is mainly driven by cytokines, whereas primary (clonal) forms of eosinophilia are mostly caused by tyrosine kinase gene fusions, involving the coding genes for platelet-derived growth factor receptor alpha (*PDGFRA*), beta (*PDGFRB*), or fibroblast growth factor receptor 1 (*FGFR1*). Secondary (reactive) eosinophilia has multiple causes, such as allergy, drugs, parasitic disease, and respiratory, gastrointestinal, and rheumatologic disorders.[1]

Regardless of its cause, prolonged or marked activation of eosinophils may lead to migration of eosinophils into other organ tissues, such as the heart, lung, skin, or urinary tract, resulting in tissue and subsequent end-organ damage. Therefore, evaluation for the presence of other end-organ damage is essential. Based on individual signs and symptoms, chest x-ray, electrocardiogram, echocardiography, abdominal US, tissue biopsies, and other evaluations should be performed.[1,2]

Clinical Presentation 12

A 9-month-old male infant, first child of a third-degree consanguineous marriage, was admitted to our center with history of recurrent high-grade fever since 5 months of age for which he had been admitted and treated with intravenous antibiotics three times.

On examination, the child had severe failure to thrive with weight and height both <3 *Z* score for age and oculo-cutaneous albinism with hypopigmented hair. Ocular examination revealed nystagmus and retinal hypopigmentation. The infant also had pallor with mild pedal edema along with hepatosplenomegaly and a large perianal abscess.

He was diagnosed as a case of Chediak Higashi syndrome because of the presence of classic clinical features and observation of giant granules in neutrophils, lymphocytes, monocytes, and platelets.[1] The diagnosis was further confirmed by the identification of homozygous frameshift mutation of the *LYST* gene (c.5731_5734delinsTAT) on molecular testing by next-generation sequencing.

Initial investigations revealed severe anemia and thrombocytopenia, elevated serum ferritin, triglycerides, and lactate dehydrogenase with normal kidney functions. Bone marrow aspirate was suggestive of hemophagocytosis.

The child was managed with intravenous vancomycin and meropenem along with incision and drainage of the abscess. However, the infant continued to have high-grade fever, and on further evaluation, both blood and urine culture revealed *Candida tropicalis* sensitive to caspofungin and amphotericin. The child was given 4 weeks of intravenous caspofungin on which he improved symptomatically with no growth on repeat blood and urine cultures. The patient was discharged on oral fluconazole and cotrimoxazole-trimethoprim prophylaxis. The parents were counseled about the nature of the disease and the need for a bone marrow transplant.

The child remained asymptomatic on follow-up except for low-to-moderate–grade fever recorded once or twice a week. Two weeks after discharge, however, investigations done on an outpatient basis revealed deranged kidney function tests. The blood and urine culture was sterile, and urine output was normal, so repeat investigation after another 2 weeks and follow-up was planned.

The infant was returned, however, after a week with progressively increasing edema and found to have pallor, tachypnea, and anasarca on examination.

Ultrasonography of the abdomen and kidneys revealed bilateral enlarged kidneys with normal to mildly raised echogenicity and poor corticomedullary differentiation with no focal lesions.

In view of the unexplained gross derangement of kidney functions and nonresolution of acute kidney injury (AKI) after 4 weeks of admission with no obvious cause, US-guided kidney biopsy was performed, and the core sent for light microscopy, immunofluorescence, and electron microscopy.

The kidney biopsy showed 18 glomeruli with all glomeruli displaying normal morphology. The tubulointerstitial compartment showed dense inflammation with numerous epithelioid cells and granulomas with foci of central necrosis with no caseation. There was also evidence of acute tubular necrosis with the presence of hyaline casts. No acid-fast bacilli were identified on Ziehl-Neelsen stain, and no fungal hyphae/spores were seen on periodic acid–Schiff stain.

What are the causes of glomerulointerstitial nephritis (GIN) in this patient (select all that apply)?

A. Tuberculosis-induced GIN
B. Fungal-induced GIN
C. Drug-induced GIN
D. Sarcoidosis-induced GIN

The correct answers are A, B, and C

Comment: The cause of AKI in this child could be a granulomatous infection of the kidneys causing progressive derangement of the kidney function tests and enlarged kidneys. In this clinical setting of an immunocompromised child who has been on multiple antibiotics for a prolonged period, deep-seated fungal infection or infection with *Mycobacterium* appears to be a strong possibility.

Our child had pancytopenia and hemophagocytosis with no evidence of lymphocytic infiltration of organs when he presented with a bacterial infection and developed a secondary fungal infection. Hemophagocytosis and pancytopenia in this case could be secondary to severe infection because no evidence of lymphocytic infiltration of any organ was evident. The kidney biopsy also showed granulomatous interstitial nephritis without lymphocytic infiltration and, as mentioned earlier, was secondary to an infectious cause.

Our patient developed GIN most likely due to fungal infection or tuberculosis. Renal tuberculosis is rarely reported in infants, but given the background of the child's immunocompromised status, it merits consideration. Drug-induced GIN is also reported rarely in pediatric cases and has been usually shown to respond to steroid therapy, but in this case, it will be a diagnosis of exclusion as discussed earlier.[1,2]

Clinical Presentation 13

A 14-year-old boy presented to the pediatric nephrology clinic with complaints of dull, mildly aching pain in the left flank for 2 days. The pain was nonspasmodic and without radiation to any specific site. There was no history of fever, weight loss, cough, anorexia, red-colored urine, oliguria, dysuria, vomiting, or trauma. He also did not have headaches, seizures, or altered sensorium. There was no history of drug intake or recurrent UTIs. His bladder and bowel habits were regular. There was no past history of fractures, polydipsia, vomiting, tetany, seizures, night blindness, photophobia, dry skin, neck flop, or muscle weakness. The patient was born to second-degree consanguineous parents with uneventful antenatal and neonatal history. His scholastic performance had been good. There was no family history of kidney stones. Before presentation to our hospital, he had been evaluated at another hospital where a 4-mm calculus was detected in the left renal pelvis, without any hydronephrosis or ureteral dilatation. The parents were apprehensive about the stone detected on ultrasound, and the child had been referred to our hospital for further evaluation.

At presentation, the patient's anthropometric measurements were within the normal range with a weight of 54 kg (+0.29 Z), height 153 cm (−1.33 Z), and body mass index 23.1 (+1.14 Z). The Tanner sexual maturity rating was appropriate for age (Tanner stage 4). The pulse rate was 97/min, respiratory rate 22/min, capillary refill time was less than 2 seconds, BP was 110/70 mm Hg, and oxygen saturation was 95% while on room air. There was no pallor, icterus, edema, cyanosis, digital clubbing, bony deformities, rickets, or lymphadenopathy. Abdominal examination revealed no tenderness. There was no tenderness in the lumbar region. There was no hepatosplenomegaly. The rest of the systemic examination was unremarkable. The ophthalmological and ear-nose-throat examinations were normal.

The initial blood investigations revealed hypercalcemia, hypercalciuria, and hypophosphatemia. Ultrasound of the kidneys revealed a 4-mm calculus in the left renal pelvis. Both the kidneys were normal in size and had normal echoes. There was no dilatation of the pelvicalyceal system or ureteral dilatation.

What are the differential diagnoses for hypercalcemia in a child with urolithiasis (select all that apply)?

A. Distal renal tubular acidosis
B. Medullary sponge kidney
C. Dent disease
D. Hyperparathyroidism

The correct answers are A, B, and C

Comment: Conditions that cause hypercalciuria in the presence of normocalcemia include distal renal tubular acidosis, loop diuretic use, medullary sponge kidney and hyperalimentation. Dent disease is an example of hypercalciuria with low-molecular-weight proteinuria.

The hypercalcemic states associated with hypercalciuria that causing nephrolithiasis include primary hyperparathyroidism, hypervitaminosis D, sarcoidosis and other granulomatous diseases, prolonged immobilization, milk-alkali syndrome, and malignancy. Of all the aforementioned causes, primary hyperparathyroidism and hypervitaminosis D constitute the most important etiologies for hypercalcemia causing urolithiasis in children.[1]

In our patient, hypercalcemia and hypophosphatemia prompted us to investigate for primary hyperparathyroidism. Serum PTH level in our index case was elevated (249 ng/mL [normal, <64 ng/mL]), which was responsible for hypercalcemia and hypophosphatemia. The 25-hydroxycholecalciferol level was 33.1 ng/mL (normal for age), thereby ruling out hypervitaminosis D as the underlying etiology of urolithiasis in our patient. The patient did not have any features suggestive of sarcoidosis or other chronic granulomatous conditions that could produce a hypercalcemic state by increased production of calcitriol. Other etiologies such as prolonged immobilization, milk-alkali syndrome, and malignancy were not forthcoming in this case. Hence, primary hyperparathyroidism was the most likely etiology of hypercalcemia and urolithiasis. In view of the elevated PTH levels, further workup was done to unveil the underlying cause. Ultrasonography of the neck revealed a 10 × 6-mm well-defined hypoechoic lesion with polar vessels from the inferior thyroid artery noted in the corresponding site, which indicated a possibility of adenoma or hyperplasia. Contrast-enhancing CT of the neck revealed a well-defined hypodense enhancing soft tissue lesion in the right tracheaesophageal groove anterior to C7 vertebra measuring 7 × 4 mm, consistent with an adenoma. A ^{99m}Tc scan was done for the parathyroid gland, which showed ectopic right superior parathyroid adenoma. As a part of the workup for primary hyperparathyroidism, evaluation for the involvement of other endocrine organs was carried out.

Blood glucose and serum T3, T4, and thyroid-stimulating hormone were normal. Contrast-enhancing CT of the abdomen was done to rule out pancreatic involvement as in multiple endocrine neoplasia type 1. Clinical exome sequencing was also done, which was normal. The patient was finally diagnosed with primary hyperparathyroidism secondary to a parathyroid adenoma. A biopsy report of the parathyroid gland (after excision) confirmed parathyroid adenoma.[1–3]

Clinical Presentation 14

A 17-year-old woman presents with complaints of fevers, sore throat, rhinorrhea, mild conjunctivitis, and nonproductive cough. She has no past medical history and is otherwise healthy. On examination, the temperature is 38.3°C and her oropharynx is erythematous without plaques or ulcers. There is no lymphadenopathy, and her conjunctiva has mild bilateral erythema. A rapid strep test is negative. She was treated with Augmentin and sent home. One week later, she presented to the emergency department with low-grade fever and maculopapular skin rash on her chest. Her sore throat, cough, and conjunctivitis have improved. She denies the use of NSAIDs or herbal medications. Laboratory values were sodium 138 mmol/L, potassium 4.2 mmol/L, chloride 108, HCO_3 21, BUN 18 mg/dL, creatinine 1.9 mg/dL, calcium 9.1, glucose 82, albumin 4.0 g/dL, WBC 8.7 (13% eosinophil), hemoglobin 12.7 g/dL, hematocrit 37%, and platelets 307 k. Urinalysis pH 6.0, specific gravity 1.015, negative glucose, trace protein, negative blood, 10 WBC, zero to five RBCs, no casts, and urine culture negative. Further workup reveals urine protein 150 mg/dL, urine albumin 11 mg/dL, and urine creatinine 144 mg/dL. Fractional excretion of beta-2 microglobulin is high. Her renal US and chest radiograph unremarkable. Her Augmentin was discontinued and 2 days later her serum creatinine was 1.4 mg/dL.

At this point, which one of the following would you recommend?

A. Recommend supportive care.
B. Perform a renal biopsy.
C. Consult ophthalmology for slit marks lamp examination.
D. Order an IgG-4 level.
E. Order an angiotensin-converting enzyme level.

The correct answer is C

Comment: TINU is a rare form of bilateral anterior uveitis found in patients with acute kidney inflammation. The uveitis is usually mild and the nephritis is self-limited. However, cases of chronic uveitis and renal failure have been reported.

Although the cause of TINU is unknown, research has revealed various associations. Certain HLA genotypes increase the relative risk of developing TINU in certain populations.[1] Medications such as NSAIDs and antibiotics have also been implicated, the drug causing hypersensitivity reaction or hapten-induced cytokine production and immune reaction. Another possibility links dysfunction or targeted disruption of similar enzymes in the renal tubule and ciliary epithelium.

TINU occurs predominately in young females. The median age of onset is 15 years old with patient's ages ranging from 9 to 74. It affects both sexes, with an overall predominance of females but a trend toward a male predominance in younger age groups.

Patients will usually present with typical anterior uveitis symptoms including eye pain, redness, decreased vision, photophobia, fever, malaise, fatigue, and flank pain.

In addition to ophthalmology findings, increased levels of serum and blood urinary beta-2 microglobulin, pyuria, hematuria, glycosuria, and presence of eosinophils may be noted. However, a definitive diagnosis of TIN can only be made with renal biopsy. Pathology will demonstrate eosinophilic and mononuclear cellular infiltrates with glomerular sparing. Blood urea nitrogen and creatinine are elevated in renally compromised patients.

A number of other conditions can present with both renal manifestations and uveitis. These include systemic lupus erythematosus, Sjögren syndrome, syphilis, sarcoidosis, granulomatosis with polyangiitis (formerly Wegener), Behcet disease, Epstein-Barr virus-associated infectious mononucleosis, tuberculosis, toxoplasmosis, brucellosis, histoplasmosis, and hyper-IgG4 disease.

Standard treatment for anterior uveitis with topical steroids can be effective. However, with the high frequency of recurrent disease, long-term follow-up is recommended for these patients. If kidney functions do not quickly normalize, a short course of high-dose intravenous or oral steroids is often used. Steroid-sparing immunomodulatory therapy may be needed for severe inflammation.

Long-term ocular complications are rare.

Uveitis will often persist longer than the nephritis and may require long-term local therapy, rarely lasting more than a year. Recurrence of uveitis can occur in patients with TINU, as high as

40%. Most recurrences occur within the first few months of stopping therapy but have occurred as late as 2 years later. Renal outcomes are also generally good, with nephritis often spontaneously resolving, but there have been cases of chronic renal failure following TINU. In contrast to uveitis, nephritis rarely recurs.

Clinical Presentation 15

A 16-year-old woman presents for evaluation of acute kidney injury. Four days ago, she presented with bilateral burning of her eyes and blurry vision. A slit-lamp examination revealed bilateral anterior uveitis. Laboratory studies drawn the next day were normal except for a serum creatinine of 1.8 mg/dL. She was taking no medications or supplements. Her urinalysis revealed 1+ protein, glycosuria, and pyuria. The urine culture was negative and her serum angiotensin-converting enzyme, ANCA, ANA, SSA/SSB, IgG-4, and chest radiograph were negative or normal. A renal biopsy demonstrated acute lymphocytic interstitial nephritis with monocytes. The glomeruli were uninvolved. The ophthalmologist began topical steroids for her uveitis.[1]

Which one of the following would you recommend at this time?

A. Begin mycophenolate mofetil.
B. Begin oral prednisone.
C. Begin rituximab.
D. Agree with topical steroids alone because they will be effective for uveitis.
E. Begin intravenous immunoglobulin.

The correct answer is D

Comment: TIN and TINU syndrome is a rare disease. The renal prognosis is generally thought to be better in children with TINU syndrome than in adults.

The median age at diagnosis of TINU syndrome is from 15 to 17 years, but the exact incidence and prevalence remain undetermined and are probably underestimated, as the condition could be underdiagnosed.

Patients with TINU syndrome have been treated successfully with corticosteroids, but the use of systemic steroids may be restricted in patients with significant tubulointerstitial injury. However, uveitis must be treated because of its poor prognosis. Some patients require additional immunosuppressive drugs such as azathioprine, methotrexate, cyclosporine, or rituximab if steroid resistance, recurrence of uveitis, or significant steroidal side effects occur.

Clinical Presentation 16

The pathogenesis of TINU is most likely related to which one of the following mechanisms?

A. Autosomal recessive condition affecting the epithelial sodium channel leading to cyst development and tubulointerstitial disease
B. Autosomal dominant condition affecting the epithelial sodium channel leading to cyst development and tubulointerstitial disease
C. T-cell response to an inciting trigger generating a cascade of inflammation in the uvea and renal tubulointerstitium including cytokines and recruited B cells in genetically susceptible individuals based on HLA clustering
D. X-linked condition that affects the genes that encode for type IV collagen present in the tubular epithelium and uvea

The correct answer is C

Comment: The pathogenesis of TINU is likely multifactorial, with contributions from genetic, infectious, autoimmune, and iatrogenic factors. The nephrology literature has made the most headway in exploring the links between these factors and acute interstitial nephritis. Work in this field has identified a role for allergy-mediated immune mechanisms in drug-induced interstitial nephritis and mutations in genes encoding the "tubulointerstitial nephritis antigen" leading to chronic disease. However, the mechanistic links underlying the ocular disease or tying together the nephritis and uveitis remain largely unknown. Two promising areas of investigation are focused on understanding the dysregulation of cell-mediated immunity and humoral immunity in patients with TINU.[1–3]

Loss of T-cell tolerance in the pathogenesis of TINU is suggested by multiple studies identifying a strong link between TINU and certain class II HLA subtypes, such as HLA-DQA1*01, HLA-DQB1*05, and HLA-DRB1*01, with a relative risk as high as 167.1 for HLA-DRB1*0102. The latter HLA gene is an independent risk factor for TINU, particularly of younger onset. These HLA subtypes confer variable risks based on the population studied. Because HLA class II molecules are involved with exogenous antigen presentation to CD4+ T-helper cells, molecular mimicry between exogenous infectious antigens and ocular antigens could explain the HLA association with this disease. Other potential mechanisms could include an insufficient or poorly functioning antigen-specific regulatory T-cell population. However, there is controversy about the role of regulatory T cells in autoimmune uveitis and no TINU-specific studies have been reported.[1–4]

The role of humoral immunity in TINU pathogenesis has been suggested by the identification of autoreactive antibodies directed against renal and ocular antigens in TINU patients. One study identified elevated titers of anti-monomeric C-reactive protein (anti-mCRP) antibodies in the serum of patients with active TINU. Serum from healthy subjects, and from active patients with isolated acute interstitial nephritis (AIN, idiopathic or drug-related), ANCA-vasculitis, IgA-nephropathy, minimal change disease, Sjögren syndrome, or amyloidosis was also tested. This study found that elevated titers of anti-mCRP antibodies were not unique to patients with TINU, but the percentage of patients with elevated titers was significantly higher in the TINU group (9/9, 100%) when compared with all other groups. The only disease category with more than two patients that also demonstrated an elevated titer was AIN (4/11, 36%). It is not known if these patients with AIN were screened for eye disease, their follow-up course, or if any did ultimately proceed to TINU, but it is interesting that other forms of kidney disease other than interstitial nephritis did not lead to the development of anti-mCRP antibodies. This suggests that these antibodies may have disease-specific relevance. In addition to elevated serum anti-mCRP antibodies, the authors also showed an increase in the extent of mCRP found in kidney biopsies by immunohistochemistry when compared with normal kidneys.[1–4]

In the eye, mCRP was identified in normal human iris and ciliary body collected at the time of trabeculectomy by immunohistochemistry. Serum obtained from patients with active TINU colocalized with mCRP staining in these normal tissues further suggests a mechanistic link between this protein and disease pathogenesis. mCRP is the dissociated monomer of the parent acute phase reactant pentamer (C-reactive protein) and is involved in the activation and regulation of the complement pathway, but no tissue-specific role for the protein has been identified.[1] Therefore, it is not clear if mCRP is truly a specific antigen involved in ocular and renal disease, or if these findings represent an autoantibody that develops to this acute phase reactant as a result of chronic inflammation as has been reported previously in lupus nephritis. Understanding the role of humoral immunity in uveitis has become more important as we try to explain the success of rituximab, a B-cell–depleting biologic therapy, on certain forms of recalcitrant uveitis. A more thorough understanding of TINU pathogenesis may also uncover an important role for humoral immunity in other forms of uveitis.[1–4]

Another interesting question in TINU pathogenesis is whether the disease is a sequential process where an initial renal (or potentially uveal) insult incites an inflammatory cascade with secondary effects on the other organ, or if both tissues share a common target for a single underlying mechanism. However, there is evidence to suggest that the kidney is the primary target. One study found that in patients with AIN, elevated anti-mCRP antibodies were predictive of subsequent uveitis development. Thus, a reasonable hypothesis for disease pathogenesis begins with exposure of the kidney to an inciting agent that stimulates a HLA class II response that targets the immune system to a common antigen in both organs. Most likely this antigen is a native protein in the uvea and renal interstitium that shares a common epitope. However, the mCRP data also suggest the antigen could be an acute phase reactant that deposits in the eye and kidney. Experimental animal models will be required to address these possible hypotheses.[1–4]

Clinical Presentation 17

Which of the following is the most common cause of acute tubulointerstitial nephritis?

A. Allergic reaction to a drug
B. Certain types of blood cancer
C. Damage from a drug (not an allergic reaction)
D. Heavy metal toxins

The correct answer is A

Comment: Allergic reaction to a drug is the most common cause of acute tubulointerstitial nephritis is an allergic reaction to a drug. Antibiotics such as penicillin and sulfonamides, diuretics, and NSAIDs, including aspirin, may trigger an allergic reaction.[1] Options B, C, and D are other causes of both acute and chronic forms of tubulointerstitial nephritis.

Clinical Presentation 18

A 15-year-old Hispanic woman was referred to the outpatient nephrology clinic for a recent increase in serum creatinine level.

The patient's medical history included gastric ulcers, cutaneous psoriasis diagnosed at the age of 11 years, treated with adalimumab 40 mg every 2 weeks for the past 12 months, and acute pyelonephritis 2 months before the current referral. At that time, URI was complicated by *E. coli* septicemia, severe sepsis, and AKI with a creatinine level at admission of 5.73 mg/dL (corresponding to eGFR of 8 mL/min/1.73 m^2 as calculated by the Chronic Kidney Disease Epidemiology Collaboration equation, versus 0.6 mg/dL (eGFR, 111 mL/min/1.73 m^2) on a laboratory test performed 15 months earlier. Systematic workup ruled out urinary tract obstruction, and the patient was treated with crystalloid intravenous hydration, ceftriaxone, and withdrawal of adalimumab treatment. Her condition improved rapidly, and she was discharged on day 21, when serum creatinine level was 1.98 mg/dL (eGFR, 30 mL/min/1.73 m^2).

At the outpatient clinic 45 days later, the patient's BP was 120/80 mm Hg and physical examination findings were unremarkable. Medications included pantoprazole 40 mg once daily and oral iron supplementation. Laboratory tests showed serum creatinine level of 1.94 mg/dL (eGFR, 31 mL/min/1.73 m^2) and mild proteinuria of tubular origin; urinary sediment was bland and culture results were negative. Extensive viral and autoimmune screening gave negative results. An US of the abdomen showed normal-sized kidneys, and there was no lymphadenopathy on chest x-ray. A kidney biopsy was performed.

What does the biopsy show and what is your pathologic diagnosis?

A. Membranous glomerulonephritis (GN)
B. Membranoproliferative GN
C. Granulomatose interstitial nephritis (GIN)
D. Mesangial proliferative GN

The correct answer is C

Comment: Light microscopy showed diffuse interstitial inflammation with lymphocytes, edema, tubulitis, and atrophic tubules with the presence of an epithelioid, nonnecrotic, noncaseating granuloma leading to the diagnosis of GIN. Two of the 12 glomeruli available for analysis were sclerotic, whereas the others appeared normal. No immune deposit was detectable by immunofluorescence.[1,2]

Clinical Presentation 19

What is your differential diagnosis and how would you proceed?

A. Infectious disease
B. Autoimmune disorders
C. Allergic reaction to drugs
D. Sjögren disease

The correct answer is A

Comment: Tubulointerstitial nephritis often results in kidney failure. It may be caused by various diseases, drugs, toxins, or radiation that damages the kidneys. Damage to the tubules results in changes in the electrolytes with the kidney's ability inability to concentrate urine, resulting in urine that is too diluted.[1,2]

Problems concentrating urine causes an increase in daily urine volume (polyuria) and difficulty maintaining the proper balance of water and electrolytes in the blood.

The most common cause of acute tubulointerstitial nephritis is an allergic reaction to a drug. Antibiotics such as penicillin and the sulfonamides, diuretics, and NSAIDs, including aspirin, may trigger an allergic reaction. The interval between the exposure to the allergen that caused the reaction and the development of acute tubulointerstitial nephritis varies usually from 3 days to 5 weeks.

Drugs can also cause tubulointerstitial nephritis through nonallergic mechanisms. For example, NSAIDs can directly damage the kidney, taking up to 18 months to cause chronic tubulointerstitial nephritis.

UTIs can also cause acute or chronic tubulointerstitial nephritis.

Tubulointerstitial nephritis may be caused by immunologic disorders that primarily affect the kidney, such as antitubular basement membrane antibody-associated interstitial nephritis.

When tubulointerstitial nephritis develops suddenly, the urine may be almost normal, with only a trace blood or protein, but often the abnormalities are striking. The urine may show large numbers of WBCs, including eosinophils. Eosinophils do not normally appear in the urine, but when they do, a person may have acute tubulointerstitial nephritis caused by an allergic reaction. In such cases, blood tests may show that the number of eosinophils in the blood is increased.

When tubulointerstitial nephritis develops gradually, the first symptoms to appear are those of kidney failure, such as itchiness, fatigue, decreased appetite, nausea, vomiting, and difficulty breathing. BP is normal or only slightly above normal in the early stages of the disease. Most patients manifest polyuria, nocturia, hypokalemia, and hyponatremia with elevated BUN and serum creatinine concentrations.

The main causes of GIN include drugs, infections, and immune disorders. In our patient, recent antibiotic therapy and pantoprazole treatment were considered as potential causative agents, and proton pump inhibitor treatment was withdrawn. Extensive serologic testing for bacteria, parasites, fungi, viruses, and immune disorders returned negative results. Ziehl-Nielsen staining, Lowenstein culture, and DNA polymerase chain reaction (PCR) on kidney biopsy and three independent urinary samples found no evidence of *Mycobacterium tuberculosis* infection.

However, tumor necrosis factor α–blocking agents such as adalimumab facilitate the progression from latent to active tuberculosis (TB) and are associated with a 5- to 25-fold increase in risk for TB infection stressing the need for additional investigations in our patient. Interferon γ release assay was suggestive of either latent or active TB infection, and positron emission tomography showed hypermetabolic lymph nodes in the abdomen and retroperitoneum. A biopsy of a retrogastric lymph node was performed, and a diagnosis of infection caused by Mycobacterium tuberculosis was made based on both culture and PCR results.

Although classic renal TB is characterized by unilateral gross tissue scarring and calcification of the kidneys and urinary and genital tracts. TB-related GIN was recently identified as an emerging alternative presentation of mycobacterial kidney disease.

This insidious and progressive form of renal TB is characterized by bilateral involvement, absence of calcification, and lesions of GIN.

The correct diagnosis is challenging and frequently delayed; in the vast majority of cases, mycobacteria are undetectable by Ziehl-Nielsen staining of the kidney biopsy, culture, and PCR testing. However, the high frequency (~50%) of extrarenal lesions may provide an opportunity for diagnosis and timely initiation of treatment, especially in high-risk patients.

Clinical Presentation 20

How would you manage this patient?

A. Rifampin, isoniazid, pyrazinamide, and ethambutol
B. Rifampin, isoniazid, and ethambutol
C. Isoniazid, ethambutol, and pyrazinamide
D. Isoniazid, pyrazinamide, and ethambutol
E. Rifampin, pyrazinamide, and ethambutol

The correct answer is A

Comment: Modern anti-TB treatment, based on an initial induction period of three to four drugs including rifampicin, followed by a continuation phase, is effective for the treatment of renal TB, including GIN. However, the optimal duration of treatment and potential role of a short course of corticosteroids is not established. In our patient, a 10-month standard regimen led to significant improvement in kidney function (serum creatinine, 1.07 mg/dL; eGFR, 63 mL/min/1.73 m^2) and normalization of positron emission tomography imaging. Secukinumab, a human monoclonal antibody selectively targeting interleukin 17A, which has not been associated with TB reactivation, was introduced because of persistence of severe psoriasis.[1,2]

Clinical Presentation 21

A 17-year-old male presented to the hospital with a 2-week history of progressive malaise, myalgia, fever, nausea, vomiting, diarrhea, polyuria, and polydipsia. He had a history of gastroesophageal reflux that did not respond to ranitidine. He had started taking oral pantoprazole (40 mg daily) 6 weeks earlier. He reported having taken ibuprofen (400 mg) for myalgia no more than three times over the 2-week period before presentation. He had no history of renal disease or drug allergies.

On presentation, the patient was afebrile (temperature, 36.5°C), with a BP of 127/82 mm Hg, a pulse of 72 beats/min, a respiratory rate of 18 breaths/min, and an oxygen saturation of 97% in room air. The jugular venous pressure was measured at the sternal angle. His chest sounds were normal, and there was no pericardial friction rub or peripheral edema. The results of a dermatological examination were unremarkable.

The results of laboratory tests revealed a serum creatinine level of 2.5 mg/dL. He had mild hyperkalemia, but his electrolyte levels were otherwise normal. His leukocyte and eosinophil counts were normal. The ratio of protein to creatinine in his urine was 28 (normal, 0–23), and the protein level in a 24-hour urine collection was 410 (normal, <150) mg. Protein electrophoresis showed that the protein in the urine was predominantly albumin. When analyzed by use of Wright stain, the first urine sample was negative for eosinophils, but 1% of the leukocytes in the second sample were eosinophils. US showed that both of the patient's kidneys were of normal size, and that there was normal echogenicity with no hydronephrosis.

A kidney biopsy showed moderate-to-severe patchy interstitial infiltrates, predominantly plasma cells with some lymphocytes and occasional eosinophils. Immunofluorescence was negative for IgG, IgA, IgM, C3, C1q, and fibrin antibodies. These results supported the diagnosis of acute interstitial nephritis.

How would you manage this patient (select all that apply)?

A. Begin high-dose prednisone with gradual tapering.
B. Stop pantoprazole.
C. Initiate treatment with rituximab.
D. Give intravenous immunoglobulin.

The correct answers are A and B

Comment: Our patient was diagnosed with acute interstitial nephritis likely caused by the use of pantoprazole. The key features leading to this diagnosis were acute renal failure from a renal cause with associated proteinuria and eosinophiluria, as well as a renal biopsy that showed interstitial inflammation and a lack of evidence for other causes of renal failure.

Treatment included volume repletion and discontinuation of pantoprazole. The patient was prescribed high-dose oral prednisone (1 mg/kg daily) with stepwise tapering.[1,2] After 6 weeks on steroid treatment, the patient's creatinine level had decreased and plateaued at 0.8 mg/dL and his BP was normal. Prednisone was discontinued at this point.

Esophagogastroduodenoscopy was performed to evaluate the patient's reflux disease. The results suggested severe esophagitis with a benign lower esophageal ulcer. The patient was given both ranitidine and domperidone, and he was instructed not to take any proton pump inhibitors or NSAIDs, except for acetylsalicylic acid (81 mg daily). As of the patient's last visit, his reflux was controlled with ranitidine (300 mg twice daily) and calcium carbonate tablets (750 mg twice daily).

Clinical Presentation 22

A 16-year-old-female was brought to the emergency department with a history of nausea, vomiting, poor oral intake, and decreased urination for 3 to 4 days. Past medical history was significant for type 2 diabetes mellitus and hypertension, well controlled on metformin and lisinopril, respectively.

She denied use of any over-the-counter pain pills or antibiotics.

Patient was afebrile and hemodynamically stable and denied any fever, rash, joint pains, cough, abdominal pain, difficulty urination, or discoloration of urine. Physical examination was normal with clear lungs, normal heart sounds, soft nontender abdomen without organomegaly, clear skin, and normal joints. Initial workup was significant for elevated WBC count of 10.1/mm, BUN of 56 mg/dL, and creatinine of 7.4 with electrolytes within normal range. Urinalysis showed 2+ proteinuria, sterile pyuria with seven to eight white blood cells, and eosinophils positive for Hensel stain. The patient was admitted, and supportive treatment for AKI was started. By the second day, her condition deteriorated with further increase in serum creatinine along with severe drop in urine output. The patient developed severe respiratory distress from fluid overload and pulmonary edema leading to acute respiratory failure, requiring institution of mechanical ventilation and continuous renal replacement therapy.

Laboratory tests performed to discover the etiology of the AKI showed low C3, normal C4, and positive ANA (1:80 titer). Other tests including C-ANCA, P-ANCA, liver function tests, hepatitis panel, anti-streptolysin O titers, peripheral smear, and blood cultures were normal. Renal US and transesophageal echocardiogram showed normal findings. Meanwhile, renal function and fluid status began improving on renal replacement therapy, and her respiratory distress resolved.

The patient was found to have a raised WBC to 16.7 with predominant neutrophils, and empiric treatment for infection with vancomycin and piperacillin plus tazobactam was started.

The patient described a mild jaw pain that had persisted for more than a week; on examination, she was found to have a tender dental abscess.

Imaging revealed a periodontal abscess with infected tooth, which was drained along with extraction of the tooth. Cultures from the abscess grew anaerobic streptococci, and the patient was started on clindamycin.

A renal biopsy revealed patchy interstitial inflammatory infiltrates with prominent eosinophilic component most consistent with AIN.

What is the most likely etiology of AKI in this patient?

A. Infection-associated acute interstitial nephritis
B. Vancomycin-induced acute renal injury
C. Clindamycin-induced acute renal injury
D. Piperacillin-induced acute renal injury

The correct answer is A

Comment: Infection-associated AIN is likely to develop during the course of many systemic infections from bacterial, viral, and parasitic organisms. It has a variable clinical presentation depending on the causative organism along with renal impairment ranging from mild self-limiting renal dysfunction to progressive renal impairment resulting in CKD. Laboratory results are usually nonspecific. Renal biopsy showing interstitial edema and predominant lymphocytic interstitial infiltrates remains the definitive test for diagnosis for any type of AIN. Infection-associated AIN shows prominent neutrophilic infiltration and tends to be negative on immunofluorescence microscopy. Extensive interstitial damage can result in irreversible tubulointerstitial fibrosis leading to the progression of AKI into CKD.[1,2]

Basic principles of management in infection-associated AIN are similar to other cases of AKI, which is mainly renal supportive therapy with a special focus on limiting the inflammatory damage by controlling the causative infection and by achieving immunosuppression.

Steroid therapy started early in the course likely limits the inflammatory cellular infiltration and edema, thereby preventing the fibrosis and scarring and promoting faster recovery of renal function without long term complications.[1,2]

In summary, it is essential to consider AIN in the differential for unexplained AKI. Initial management should include conservative therapy by withdrawing any suspected causative agent. Renal biopsy is needed for confirmation in cases where kidney function fails to improve within 5 to 7 days on conservative therapy. A trial of corticosteroids can be started in biopsy-proven patients with AKI for <3 weeks. Steroid therapy is usually maintained for 4 to 6 weeks and dosage is tapered over the next 4 weeks.

Clinical Presentation 23

A 17-year-old male was brought into the emergency department because of weakness, fever, and confusion. Assessment in the emergency department revealed the patient was lethargic with dry mucous membranes, 1+ peripheral pulses, delayed capillary refill, 2+ pitting edema in both lower extremities, bilateral crackles, and Foley output of 15 mL/h of dark amber urine.

Vital signs were as follows: BP 91/60 mm Hg (MAP 70), heart rate 120/min, respiration 25/min, O_2 saturation 88%, and temperature 39°C.

He has a history of chronic kidney disease stage 2 and hypertension. He had been taking ibuprofen for many years for headaches.

Laboratory tests revealed diminished renal function (BUN 55 mg/dL, creatinine 2.7mg/dL, GFR of 52 mL/min/1.73 m^2, hyperkalemia 5.8 mEq/L, eosinophilia (3.5%), and metabolic acidosis (pH 7.25, $PaCO_2$ 30, HCO_3 10 mEq/L). A urine analysis demonstrated a urine sodium of 15, osmolality of 800, and specific gravity of 1.9. A renal biopsy confirmed diagnosis of drug induced-acute interstitial nephritis with 50% interstitial fibrosis and RIFLE criteria of stage 2 failure.

What are this patient's risk factors for AKI (select all that apply)?

A. Preexisting renal insufficiency
B. History of hypertension
C. Extracellular fluid volume (ECFV)
D. Hypotension
E. Chronic use of ibuprofen

The correct answers are A, B, C, D, and E

Comment: AIN represents a frequent cause of AKI, accounting for 15% to 27% of renal biopsies performed because of this condition. By and large, drug-induced AIN is currently the most common etiology of AIN, with antimicrobials and NSAIDs being the most frequent offending agents. Pathogenesis is based on an immunologic reaction against endogenous nephritogenic antigens or exogenous antigens processed by tubular cells, with cell-mediated immunity having a major pathogenic role. The characteristic interstitial infiltrates, mostly composed of lymphocytes, macrophages, eosinophils, and plasma cells, experience a rapid transformation into areas of interstitial fibrosis. A significant proportion of AIN has an oligosymptomatic presentation, although specific extrarenal symptoms such as fever, skin rash, arthralgias, and peripheral eosinophilia have important roles in orientating clinical diagnosis. Identification and removal of the offending drug are the mainstay of the treatment, but recent studies strongly suggest that early steroid administration (within 7 days after diagnosis) improves the recovery of renal function, decreasing the risk of chronic renal impairment.[1]

Clinical Presentation 24

How is tubulointerstitial nephritis treated (select all that apply)?

A. Corticosteroids
B. Mycophenolate mofetil
C. NSAIDs
D. All of the above

The correct answers are A and B

Comment: Corticosteroids have been a mainstay of therapy for tubulointerstitial nephritis, but mycophenolate mofetil may also have a role. Ultimately, however, treatment depends on the underlying etiology.[1]

Most patients presenting with renal insufficiency, proteinuria, and/or acid-base electrolyte disorders require consultation with a nephrologist. These patients may require inpatient care until stabilization or resolution.

Hypertensive patients should be on a low-sodium diet. For all patients with early renal disease, recommend general guidelines for a healthy diet (i.e., a low-fat [low-cholesterol] diet rich in fresh fruits and vegetables such as the Dietary Approaches to Stop Hypertension [DASH] diet).

Provide patients with acute interstitial nephritis with follow-up care until resolution. Patients who do not recover renal function and those with chronic tubulointerstitial nephritis should receive long-term follow-up care to ensure that optimal control of BP is achieved and to protect kidneys from further potentially nephrotoxic therapies and/or interventions.

Clinical Presentation 25

Which of the following histological findings is *not* characteristic of tubulointerstitial nephritis?

A. Interstitial fibrosis
B. Diffuse proliferative glomerulonephritis
C. Active inflammatory mononuclear and eosinophils infiltrate
D. Tubular atrophy

The correct answer is B

Comment: Kidney biopsy is the definitive test for diagnosing acute allergic interstitial nephritis, particularly in cases in which the clinical diagnosis is difficult.[1] Because the differential diagnosis of acute tubulointerstitial nephritis encompasses multiple etiologies, consider kidney biopsy when the diagnosis is not obvious.

Kidney biopsy shows mononuclear and often eosinophilic cellular infiltration of the renal parenchyma with sparing of the glomeruli. Sometimes, interstitial changes such as fibrosis and atrophy are also present.

The renal cortex shows a diffuse interstitial, predominantly mononuclear, inflammatory infiltrate with no changes to the glomerulus. Tubules in the center of the field are separated by inflammation and edema, compared with the more normal architecture in the right lower area.

Findings on kidney biopsy in chronic tubulointerstitial nephritis usually show varying degrees of interstitial fibrosis, tubular atrophy, fibrosis, arteriolar sclerosis, and, occasionally, patchy mononuclear cell infiltration. Often, the findings are nonspecific and the etiology is not discernible from the biopsy; some diseases, such as sarcoidosis, show noncaseating granulomas, and, in viral diseases, immunostaining can yield clues to the cause.

Clinical Presentation 26

Which one of the following conditions is *not* part of the etiology of tubulointerstitial disease?

A. Heavy metal intoxication
B. Sjögren disease
C. Infectious diseases
D. Ureteropelvic junction obstruction
E. Hypercalcemia
F. Hypouricemia

The correct answer is F

Comment: Tubulointerstitial diseases of the kidney encompass diverse etiologies and pathophysiologic processes, and the patient can present with acute or chronic conditions. Many forms of tubulointerstitial injury involve exposure to drugs or other nephrotoxic agents such as heavy metals and, rarely, infection. By far the most common form of tubulointerstitial inflammation is a hypersensitivity reaction to medications, termed allergic interstitial nephritis.

The following are the causes of tubulointerstitial disease:

1. Any drugs can cause acute allergic and hypersensitivity reactions involving the kidney.
2. Immunologic diseases (e.g., lupus, Sjögren syndrome, primary glomerulopathies, sarcoidosis, vasculitis, ANCA-associated vasculitis)
3. Metabolic diseases such as hyperglycemia, hypercalcemia, and hypokalemia
4. Infectious diseases
5. Neoplasia
6. Genetics (medullary cystic disease, Alport syndrome)
7. Heavy metals exposure
8. Obstructive uropathy
9. Nephrolithiasis
10. Vesicoureteral reflux

In a study by Maripuri et al., kidney biopsies in 24 patients with primary Sjögren syndrome who also had kidney dysfunction revealed that 17 individuals had tubulointerstitial nephritis as the primary lesion[1] and 11 of those 17 patients had the chronic form of this nephritis. The investigators suggested these results support the notion that in patients with primary Sjögren syndrome, chronic tubulointerstitial nephritis is the most frequent cause of renal impairment found through kidney biopsy.

Similarly, a prospective study by Jain et al. of renal involvement in 70 patients with primary Sjögren syndrome reported that tubulointerstitial nephritis was the most common disorder found on kidney biopsy. Tubulointerstitial nephritis was identified in 9 of 17 biopsies in this study.[2]

Clinical Presentation 27

Which one of the following biomarkers is the most diagnostic-sensitive screening tool for detecting tubulointerstitial syndrome in children with uveitis?

A. Urinalysis
B. Serum creatinine
C. eGFR
D. Serum and urinary β2-microglobulin
E. Kidney US

Correct answer is D

Comment: Urinary β2-microglobulin and serum creatinine levels are sensitive and relatively simple diagnostic screening tools for detecting renal dysfunction to diagnose tubulointerstitial nephritis in young patients with uveitis.[1]

Clinical Presentation 28

Which type of cancer occurs at 40 times the normal rate in people with Sjögren syndrome?

A. Lymphoma
B. Breast cancer
C. Skin cancer
D. Colon cancer

The correct answer is A

Comment: Lymphoma, a cancer of the lymphatic system, is more common in people with Sjögren syndrome than in the general population. People with Sjögren syndrome develop non-Hodgkin lymphoma at 40 times the normal rate. Options B, C, and D: These cancers are not more common in people with Sjögren syndrome.[1]

Clinical Presentation 29

A 15-year-old male presents with cough and shortness of breath. SARS-CoV-2 infection is confirmed. In 24 hours, he undergoes intubation for worsening pulmonary function. Within 8 hours of intubation, AKI ensues. He is on steroids and tocilizumab. He is started on remdesivir, vitamin C, and pantoprazole. Within the next 24 hours, he requires kidney replacement therapy.

What is the *most* common kidney pathology findings in patients with COVID-19–associated AKI?

A. Acute tubulointerstitial injury
B. AKI
C. Collapsing focal segmental hyalinosis
D. Membranous nephropathy
E. Acute tubular necrosis

Correct answer is A

Comment: AKI is common among hospitalized patients with COVID-19, with the occurrence of AKI ranging from 0.5% to 80%. Both live kidney biopsies and autopsy series suggest acute tubular necrosis as the most commonly encountered pathology.[1] Collapsing glomerulopathy and thrombotic microangiopathy are other encountered pathologies noted in both live and autopsy tissues. Other rare findings such as anti-neutrophil cytoplasmic antibody vasculitis, anti-glomerular basement membrane disease, and podocytopathies have been reported.[1]

Clinical Presentation 30

A 19-year-old White woman presents with chronic kidney disease (serum creatinine 3.1 mg/dL). She is asymptomatic. Her history is unremarkable except that she takes an over-the-counter NSAID (Ibuprofen) for a few days each month for menstrual cramps and over-the-counter Chinese herbs for weight loss. Six months ago during a routine examination, her serum creatinine was 1.1 mg/dL. Her physical examination reveals a BP of 144/82 mm Hg and obesity (weight 129 kg; height 160 cm). No other abnormal findings are present. Urinalysis shows 8 to 10 erythrocytes (all isomorphic), 4 to 6 leukocytes per HPF, and trace proteinuria. Serum electrolytes, albumin, globulin, calcium, and phosphorous are normal. Serum cholesterol is 200 mg/dL. A renal ultrasound shows that both kidneys are at the lower limits of normal size and have increased echogenicity. One small cyst is seen in the cortex of the kidney. No dilatation of the ureters or renal pelvis is present.

A renal biopsy is likely to reveal which *one* of the following lesions?

A. Interstitial noncaseating granuloma
B. Hypocellular interstitial fibrosis and tubular atrophy
C. Lymphocytic interstitial inflammation and tubular atrophy
D. Small-vessel vasculitis
E. Focal and segmental glomerulosclerosis

The correct answer is B

Comment: TIN is a frequent cause of AKI that can lead to CKD. TIN is associated with an immune-mediated infiltration of the kidney interstitium by inflammatory cells, which may progress to fibrosis. Patients often present with nonspecific symptoms, which can lead to delayed diagnosis and treatment of the disease.[1]

The etiology of TIN can be drug-induced, infectious, idiopathic, genetic, or related to a systemic inflammatory condition such as TINU syndrome, inflammatory bowel disease, or IgG4-associated immune complex multiorgan autoimmune disease. It is imperative to have a high clinical suspicion for TIN to remove potential offending agents and treat any associated systemic diseases. Treatment is ultimately dependent on underlying etiology. Although there are no randomized controlled clinical trials to assess treatment choice and efficacy in TIN, corticosteroids have been a mainstay of therapy, and recent studies have suggested a possible role for mycophenolate mofetil. Urinary biomarkers such as alpha1-microglobulin and beta2-microglobulin may help diagnose and monitor disease activity in TIN.[1,2] Screening for TIN should be implemented in children with inflammatory bowel disease, uveitis, or IgG4-associated multiorgan autoimmune disease.

Clinical Presentation 31

A 17-year-old presents to the emergency department with pain radiating to the right testicle. The pain began as a dull ache in the right flank approximately 6 hours prior while he was sitting at his desk at school. The pain rapidly progressed increasing in intensity steadily over a period of 1 hour. It was subsequently associated with radiation along the inguinal canal into the groin and the right testicle. This is the first time the patient has experienced these symptoms. He does admit to some nausea and vomiting in the past several hours but denies chills, fever, dysuria, or urgency. Current medication includes atenolol 25 mg once daily for mild hypertension. On examination the vital signs are normal. He weighs 70 kg. Examination of head, ears, eyes, and throat (HEENT) is normal. The chest is clear to auscultation and percussion. The heart size is normal and there are no murmurs. The abdomen is soft, nontender, and slightly distended with hypoactive bowel sounds. There is no organomegaly, no masses, rebound, or guarding. No bruits are heard and there are no hernias. There is moderate costovertebral angle tenderness to palpation on the right side. There is no edema. Laboratories studies show hemoglobin 14 g/dL; head circumference (HC) 44%; WBC 5600 cells/umL; sodium 140 mEq/L; potassium 4 mEq/L; chloride 105 mEq/L; CO_2 25 mEq/L; BUN 15 mg/dL; and creatinine 1.0 mg/dL. Urinalysis revealed pH 5.0; specific gravity (SG) 1.016; 4+ blood; 1+ protein; no glucose; too many to count RBCs; no casts; and multiple calcium oxalate crystals.

Which of the following studies is most likely to provide the correct diagnosis and should be done first in this situation?

A. Non–contrast-enhanced helical CT scan
B. Abdominal plain film
C. Intravenous pyelogram (IVP)
D. Ultrasonography

The correct answer is A.[1,2]

Clinical Presentation 32

A helical CT scan demonstrates a 3-mm stone in the right ureter.

Which of the following is the likely diagnosis?

A. Calcium phosphate nephrolithiasis
B. Calcium oxalate nephrolithiasis
C. Uric acid nephrolithiasis
D. Cystine nephrolithiasis

The correct answer is B.[1,2]

Clinical Presentation 33

What would be the best management approach at this time for this patient (select all that apply)?

A. Urology consultation
B. Hospitalization
C. Intravenous fluids
D. Intravenous antibiotics
E. Intravenous analgesics

The correct answers are C and E.[1,2]

Clinical Presentation 34

The patient experienced significant pain relief after intravenous analgesics and tolerated oral medications and fluids.

What orders would you write now (select all that apply)?

A. Hospitalization.
B. Discharge to home.
C. Low-calcium diet.
D. Maintain increased oral fluid intake.
E. Strain the urine.
F. Schedule a follow-up intravenous pyelogram (IVP) for the following week.
G. Schedule a 24-hour urine collection for calcium and creatinine.

The correct answers are B, D, and E.[1,2]

Clinical Presentation 35

Which of the following studies should be included in this evaluation (select all may apply)?

A. 24-hour urine for calcium
B. 24-hour urine for uric acid
C. 24-hour urine for oxalate
D. 24-hour urine for citrate
E. 24-hour urine for cystine
F. 24-hour urine for creatinine
G. 24-hour urine for phosphorous
H. Serum calcium
I. Serum uric acid
J. Serum albumin
K. Serum creatinine
L. Serum electrolytes

The correct answers are A, B, C, D, F, H, J, K, and L

Comment: Nephrolithiasis is a common health problem across the globe with a prevalence of 15% to 20%. Idiopathic hypercalciuria is the most common cause of nephrolithiasis, and calcium oxalate stones are the most common type of stones in idiopathic hypercalciuric patients. Calcium phosphate stones are frequently associated with other diseases such as renal tubular acidosis type 1, UTIs, and hyperparathyroidism. Compared with flat abdominal film and renal sonography, a noncontrast helical CT scan of the abdomen is the diagnostic procedure of choice for the detection of small and radiolucent kidney stones with sensitivity and specificity of nearly 100%. Stones smaller than 5 mm in diameter often pass the urinary tract system and rarely require surgical interventions.

The main risk factors for stone formation are low urine output, high urinary concentrations of calcium, oxalate, phosphate, and uric acid compounded by a lower excretion of magnesium and citrate. A complete metabolic workup to identify the risk factors is highly recommended in patients who have passed multiple kidney stones or those with recurrent disease. Calcium oxalate and calcium phosphate stones are treated by the use of thiazide diuretics, allopurinol, and potassium citrate. Strategies to prevent kidney stone recurrence should include the elimination of the identified risk factors and a dietary regimen low in salt and protein, rich in calcium and magnesium, with adequate fluid intake.[1,2]

Clinical Presentation 36

An 18-year-old woman was admitted with right flank pain, fever, and chills that had begun the day before. She had a history of recurrent hypokalemia: it first had been detected incidentally at her annual examination 3 years earlier, but she did not receive either regular clinic follow-up or formal evaluation thereafter. She reported no use of diuretics or laxatives. She was slim, weighing 47 kg with a body mass index of 19 kg/m^2. Temperature was 39.3°C, and BP was 110/70 mm Hg. Laboratory examinations showed leukocytosis and a potassium level of 2.3 mEq/L. An abdominal sonogram showed hyperechoic lesions with acoustic shadowing and mild hydronephrosis in the right kidney. A kidneys, ureters, and bladder (KUB) radiograph showed no radiopaque lesion, but an intravenous urogram detected a filling defect over the right ureteropelvic junction with hydronephrosis. Urine culture grew *E. coli*. After antibiotic treatment and potassium chloride repletion, the patient underwent extracorporeal shock wave lithotripsy and double-J stent placement. On discharge, she was maintained on potassium chloride supplements (48 mEq/d) and advised to avoid unnecessary over-the-counter drugs. Two months later, the patient was readmitted with recurrent right flank pain and fever.

Serum pH was 7.47, sodium 134 mEq/L, potassium 2.4 mEq/L, chloride 93 mEq/L, bicarbonate 32.9 mEq/L, magnesium 1.6 mEq/L, calcium 9.2 mg/dL, phosphorus 2.8 mg/dL, uric acid 5 mg/dL urea nitrogen 23 mg/dL, creatinine 1.1 mg/dL, and eGFR 56 mL/min/1.73 m^2. Urine pH was 6.5 sodium 156 mEq/L, potassium 22 mEq/L, chloride 38 mEq/L, magnesium 2.4 mEq/L, calcium 3.2 mg/dL, phosphorus 177 mg/dL, uric acid 57.2 mg/dL, urea nitrogen 1025 mg/dL, and creatinine 190 mg/dL.

Radiologic studies again showed bilateral nonopaque lesions with right hydronephrosis. She underwent retrograde ureteroscopy, and the encrusted double-J stent was removed. She subsequently voided a 1.5-cm white-brown and smooth oval calculus.

What is the differential diagnosis of the kidney stones?

A. Uric acid stone
B. Cysteine stone
C. Ammonium urate stones
D. Calcium oxalate stone

The correct answer is C

Comment: Kidney stones can be classified broadly into two categories: radiopaque and radiolucent. Calcium- and uric acid–containing calculi are the most common types of radiopaque and radiolucent stones, respectively. Imaging studies such as KUB radiography, abdominal sonography, intravenous urography, and non-contrast CT help separate the density, size, location, and obstruction of stones. The formation of various kidney stones also is influenced strongly by urinary pH. Alkaline urine (pH 7) suggests calcium phosphate or struvite stones, whereas acidic urine (pH 5.3) can produce pure uric acid or cystine stones.

In this patient, radiologic studies showed radiolucent lesions on KUB radiograph, but hyperechoic lesions with acoustic shadow on abdominal sonography and relatively alkaline urine (pH 6.5). This profile made pure uric acid or cysteine stones less likely.[1]

With relatively alkaline urine, high urate excretion, and negative urine anion gap suggestive of ammonium, but low urine sodium excretion and the morphologic finding of brown-tinged radially striated spherical crystals, a clinical diagnosis of ammonium urate stones was made and then confirmed by infrared spectrophotometry.

The cause of ammonium urate stones can be endemic or sporadic. Endemic cases often occur in developing countries where a diet is enriched in grain (rice) and low in animal protein. Sporadic cases are prevalent in patients with inflammatory bowel disease, ileostomy diversion, laxative abuse, or urinary infection.[2] In this patient, low urine potassium (potassium-creatinine ratio 0.08 0.15 mEq/mg) and sodium (6 mEq/L) excretion, combined with relatively high chloride (58 mEq/L) and ammonium levels suggested electrolyte losses through the colon.[3] The patient admitted to using a stimulant laxative (bisacodyl) habitually for weight control for 7 years, with an increase to 10 to 15 tablets daily during the preceding 4 months. Laxative abuse, especially with bowel stimulant (diphenylmethane derivatives [bisacodyl] and anthraquinones [senna and cascara]), increasingly has been reported to cause ammonium urate stones.[4] The resulting hypokalemia with proximal tubular intracellular acidosis increases ammonium excretion, increases urinary pH, and decreases citrate excretion in urine. The low urinary sodium excretion resulting from volume depletion in the relatively alkalized urinary milieu contributes to stone formation.

The management of laxative-associated ammonium urate stones with obstructive pyelonephritis is aimed at controlling infection, relieving obstruction, and preventing recurrence. The supersaturation and crystallization of ammonium urate can occur rapidly, in as short a period as 1 day. Given its rapidly forming characteristics, recurrent ammonium urate stones may promptly encrust and obstruct stents, leading to obstruction and recurrent infection. Volume repletion with sufficient potassium supplementation and complete cessation of stimulant laxatives are needed to avoid recurrence and complication.

Clinical Presentation 37

A 19-year-old man presented with worsening kidney function. Serum creatinine level was 1.1 mg/dL (eGFR, 53.2 mL/min/1.73 m^2 when he underwent a physical checkup at the age of 14 years) but increased to 2.5 mg/dL (eGFR, 21.4 mL/min/1.73 m^2) and 5.0 mg/dL (eGFR, 10.0 mL/min/1.73) at the time of presentation. He had two prior occurrences of urolithiasis, and one of his uncles had recurrent urolithiasis. On physical examination, no costovertebral angle tenderness was noted. Urinalysis was negative for both protein and occult blood, and repeated urinary sediment examination showed only hyaline casts with numerous small brown crystals. Additional laboratory tests showed uric acid level of 5.5 mg/dL (327 mol/L), calcium level of 9.4 mg/dL, phosphate level of 4.2 mg/dL (1.36 mmol/L), and a slight increase in beta-2 microglobulin level. Abdominal x-ray showed no calcification within the kidneys or urinary tract, whereas ultrasound examination showed normal-sized kidneys with a slightly irregular surface, absence of hydronephrosis, and no increase of resistive indices (0.68 ± 0.04; normal range, 0.70). Fine-needle kidney biopsy was performed. Light microscopy identified large crystals within the lumen of a distended atrophied urinary tubule, with reactive interstitial nephritis. The crystals were shaped like cogwheels or sea urchins, negative for von Kossa stain, and doubly refractile. Electron microscopy showed a lancet-shaped crystal penetrating into the tubular cell.

What is the differential diagnosis and what is needed to confirm the diagnosis?

A. Crystal nephropathy caused by medications
B. Crystal nephropathy caused by distal renal tubular acidosis
C. Crystal nephropathy caused by type I adenin phosphoribosyltransferase (APRT) deficiency
D. Crystal nephropathy caused by cystinuria

The correct answer is C

Comment: Virtually any disease that causes urolithiasis can cause crystal nephropathy. The histochemical reaction known as von Kossa stain is specific for phosphates. Absence of reaction with the von Kossa stain indicates that the crystals do not contain calcium phosphate salts, but there are several different potential causes of von Kossa–negative stones. Adult-onset congenital metabolic defects cannot be ruled out as a primary cause. Primary hyperoxaluria and cystinuria are frequently associated with kidney stones. Although stones from primary hyperoxaluria are sometimes von Kossa positive, stones formed of most pure oxalates are negative by means of von Kossa stain. Stones associated with disorders of purine metabolism are phosphate free and have a characteristic shape. Stones associated with acute hyperoxaluria caused by ethylene glycol or ascorbic acid intoxication also are possibly negative by means of von Kossa stain.[1] An increased incidence of kidney stones and renal failure in infants has been reported in China, believed to be associated with the ingestion of infant formula contaminated with melamine.[2] To the best of our knowledge, no biopsy specimens have been obtained from human cases, but melamine and cyanuric acid intoxication was found to cause rather circular von Kossa–negative crystal formation in animals.[3] Drugs, such as acyclovir or protease inhibitors, as well as infection, also can cause crystals.[4]

In addition to patient history, stone analysis is necessary for the diagnosis; however, not enough urinary stones were obtained from our patient. Instead, a urinary analysis was performed by using gas chromatography and mass spectrometry for a broad screening of congenital metabolic defects.[5] Urine samples from our patient showed marked increases in adenine and its metabolite, 2,8-dihydroxyadenine (2,8-DHA). Subsequent genetic examination showed that the patient was homozygous for the APRTQ0 allele, that is, the null allele of the adenine phosphoribosyltransferase gene. The patient therefore was identified as having a type I APRT deficiency.[6] APRT deficiency is an autosomal recessive inherited disorder of purine metabolism.[6] Age at diagnosis has ranged from 5 months to 74 years, and this disease affects only the kidney and urinary tract.[6] Two types of APRT deficiency have been described. Patients with type I, predominantly White, feature undetectable enzyme activity in erythrocyte lysate and are either homozygotes or compound heterozygotes for a variety of null alleles, collectively referred to as APRTQ0.[6] The inability to salvage adenine in APRT deficiency results in the accumulation of its alternative metabolite, 2,8-DHA, by means of xanthine dehydrogenase. This extremely insoluble and nephrotoxic product generates crystals in affected individuals. In addition to adenine restriction and hydration, allopurinol is used as a treatment for this condition.[6] Tubular crystal deposition in patients with APRT deficiency is not a well-known cause of acute kidney injury or chronic kidney disease.[7] APRT deficiency usually is identified by the detection of urinary stones, whereas urinary stones have not been detected in some patients with chronic kidney disease, possibly because of diminished clearance of 2,8-DHA.[7]

Clinical Presentation 38

A 2-year-old male preterm infant (36 weeks), small for gestational age, was born to a 24-year-old mother. Labor was induced because of maternal urinary infection, which led to a cesarean birth. The patient presented no symptoms at a routine visit. As a habitual medical conduct, a urine test was ordered, which revealed a urinary infection caused by *Proteus mirabilis*. Because of that result,

US was ordered of the kidneys and urinary tract, which revealed normally positioned kidneys with usual contours and preserved corticomedullary ratio. The left kidney was enlarged in its general size (70.4 × 38.5 × 28.7 mm) in comparison with the right kidney (67.8 × 29.3 × 23.8 mm). In the distal mid-third of the left kidney, we identified the presence of confluent hyperechogenic structures, which caused posterior acoustic shadowing, generating segmental dilatations of calyceal structures. Based on the alteration in the test, the patient was referred to a pediatric nephrologist. Tests were performed for assessment of metabolic disorders, such as hypercalciuria and hypocitraturia, with urine measurements: citrate/creatinine ratio = 1.11; and calcium/creatinine ratio = 0.39, both normal for the patient age group. Renal US and urodynamic tests were also conducted, with no evidence of alterations in the kidney and urinary tract in the right side of the patient's body. On the other hand, the left kidney presented a hyperechogenic structure with posterior acoustic shadowing following part of the pelvis and calyces of the lower third, compatible with staghorn calculus, measuring 30 × 13 × 8.5 mm in the longest axes.

A mild dilatation of the renal pelvis and the other calyces was noted both majors and minors. The ipsilateral ureter presented normal caliber in the proximal portion and it was slightly increased in the distal, with absent calculi. The examination showed the right kidney with normal echography size and aspect, whereas the left kidney size revealed normal parenchyma and staghorn calculus, with mild dilatation of the pyelocalyceal system and distal ureter. The bladder contained debris, which could correspond to crystalluria, hematuria, or pyuria. A CT scan was suggested of the abdomen and pelvis. That examination revealed kidneys of the usual shape, contours, and size, as well as the presence of a staghorn calculus to the left with a density of 1147 UH, measuring 26 × 19 mm in the pelvis and in the lower calyceal group. It also identified the presence of hydronephrosis on the left and the bilateral dilatation of the ureters, greater on the left, measuring about 7 mm in the anteroposterior diameter, without signs of ureterolithiasis. The other abdominal and pelvic hollow organs evaluated presented with the usual characteristics. The dynamic renal scintigraphy revealed high obstruction to the left, with diagnosis of ureteropelvic junction stenosis. The definitive conduct was pyelolithotomy, followed by pyeloplasty and surgical placement of a double-J catheter unilaterally. The patient evolved well postoperatively, remaining asymptomatic during chemoprophylaxis, with an isolated episode of hematuria.

Which of the following surgical interventions would you recommend?

A. Extracorporeal lithotripsy (ECL)
B. Endoscopic lithotripsy using US
C. Open pyelolithotomy
D. Percutaneous nephrolithotomy (PCNL)

The correct answer is D

Comment: Staghorn calculi are a specific type of lithiasis in which the calculus occupies the pelvis and renal calyces, taking the form of a coral.[1,2] Staghorn nephrolithiasis is characterized as a disease of rapid growth that, if not treated, will possibly evolve into destruction of the affected kidney and sepsis.[2,3]

In the pediatric patient, the clinical picture of the disease can be nonspecific, which requires much attention, because just a minority will clinically exteriorize the urinary calculus as classical renal colic.[4] Considering its significant morbidity and mortality, this disease demands early evaluation and treatment.[5] The gold-standard treatment for staghorn calculi is surgery and aims at obtaining a stone-free collecting system, besides preserving renal function.[6] PCNL is the treatment of choice for staghorn calculi with the best treatment rates.[6]

Staghorn calculi chemical condition is variable: it can be formed of calcium oxalate, uric acid, cystine, and struvite.[7] Struvite staghorn calculi are composed of magnesium, ammonium, and phosphate and are closely related to UTIs.[8] The infections that mostly associate to the pathogenesis of staghorn calculi are those caused by organisms producing the urease enzyme, promoting the generation of ammonia and hydroxide from urea such as *Proteus*, *Klebsiella*, *Pseudomonas*, and *Staphylococcus*.[8] This relationship occurs because of the dependent coexistence of pH 7.2 and ammonia for the crystallization of struvite in urine. There is another mechanism for which UTI can induce the formation of those calculi: association with increased adherence of crystals; yet, this thesis is still not fully clarified. Such a hypothesis justifies the fact that *E. coli* is related to 13% of the struvite calculi,[10] although that bacterium causes 85% to 90% of UTIs.[11] Staghorn calculi are uncommon in the pediatric population and pose challenges and singular difficulties for surgical treatment.[12] This illness can occur in patients of any age, with the mean age at diagnosis among children being 7 to 10 years.[4] Those calculi represent a substantial concern because the combination of infection and the increased potential obstruction can induce damage to renal parenchyma.[12] Around 75% to 85% of children with urolithiasis present risk factors, such as metabolic disorders, recurrent infections, and/or congenital abnormalities of the urinary tract.[8] Staghorn calculus, in turn, is associated with delay in diagnosis and treatment of UTI. This happens because the recognition of these infections in the child can be difficult, as symptoms are nonspecific or absent, especially in infants. In this group, fever is the main manifestation and many times the only sign.[3] When diagnosis of urinary lithiasis is made due to a casual finding, the metabolic study of the patient must be conducted, because it is a risk factor for the development of urolithiasis. In the presence of this occasional finding in the reported patient, we continued with metabolic investigation, which did not show significant results. Besides, one must readily evaluate and treat nephrolithiasis,[2] especially because of the importance and the severity of staghorn calculus. Removal, eradication of infection, and correction of eventual metabolic disorders and anatomical abnormalities causing urinary stasis are the bases for treatment. This can be clinical, interventional, or demand association with other therapies. The clinical approach must be considered in combination with surgery for those patients with prohibitive surgical risk, because conservative treatment presents a mortality rate of 28% in 10 years and 36% risk of developing severe kidney failure.[5]

The interventional treatment includes ECL, endoscopic lithotripsy using the ultrasound, open pyelolithotomy, and PCNL. The intervention is chosen according to the calculus location and its effects on the kidneys.[4] Moreover, decisions must be individualized, considering aspects related to the age and health status of each patient.[6] With the development of minimally invasive surgeries, the number of open surgeries decreased, especially in pediatric patients. At a large series, PCNL for the treatment of staghorn calculus revealed rates of partial and complete removals of 98.5% and 71%, respectively.[8] In spite of the high popularity of this surgical technique, there are just two randomized clinical essays that assess its therapeutic value and prove the superiority of PCNL over ECL, so the first is recommended as the preferential treatment for struvite staghorn calculi.[6] Pyeloplasty is the indicated treatment for correction of ureteropelvic junction stenosis. Such stenosis is characterized as the ureter narrowing in its cranial portion, close to the renal pelvis, which, by causing urinary stasis, can develop into progressive hydronephrosis. Pictures of hydronephrosis are not rare in children and, in their majority, occur because of congenital uropathies.[9–13] Pyelolithotomy is the removal of calculus by means of an incision in the posterior face of the renal pelvis. This practice became obsolete after the appearance of CL and PCNL. However, in the case of our patient, the adoption of these procedures was not possible. Although nowadays open surgery is not frequently used, it is recommended for complex cases. Among its indications for the treatment of urinary lithiasis, the main recommendations are cases of large staghorn calculi in patients with complex collecting systems,[14] as in the described clinical case. Its morbidity is related to the incision, surgical infection, and vascular and parenchymal lesions, which can cause renal atrophy.[14] Ureteral obstruction is a frequent complication in renal surgeries because of local inflammation that can occur with adherence of ureteral walls. For such, the insertion of a double-J catheter[15–16] is indicated. The adequate and early treatment is directly associated with the maintenance of renal function; therefore, the information presented here is very useful to avoid complications, such as kidney failure in children.

Clinical Presentation 39

A 14-year-old girl was admitted for evaluation of fever, malaise, and polyuria of 3 weeks duration. One month before admission, she had been treated with antibiotics (azithromycin) and acetaminophen (paracetamol) for upper respiratory infection. In the meantime, being a vegetarian, she had been taking different "homemade" herbal mixtures of some local plants. Her past medical history was unremarkable with normal growth and development. At the age of 7 years, she had been evaluated for urinary infection. Intravenous urography and micturating cystography were normal. There were no renal or metabolic diseases and no smokers in her family.

On admission, she was febrile with pale skin without rash or edema, and normotensive (BP 110/70 mm Hg). Laboratory investigations showed an elevated erythrocyte sedimentation rate (ESR) of 120 mm/h, hemoglobin of 11.7 g/dL, WBC count of 11.4 × 10^9 cells/L with 5% to 10% eosinophilia, and positive C-reactive protein (3+). Her serum creatinine was 245 μmol/l (normal, 80%), and mild uricosuria expressed by uric acid/creatinine ratio of 0.5 (normal, >0.57).[2] An outstanding feature of tubular dysfunction was elevated excretion of ß2-MG of 3.410 μg/L (normal range, 5–154 μg/L) and NAG/creatinine ratio of 26.5 U/g (normal, <4.2 U/g).

Throat swabs and blood and urine cultures were sterile. Anti-streptolysin O titer, C3, C4, and serum IgE were normal. Serology tests for hepatitis B, cytomegalovirus, Epstein-Barr, and Hantaan virus were negative. Systemic diseases were excluded by negative titer of antinuclear antibodies, negative antiglomerular basement membrane, antitubular basement membrane, and antinuclear cytoplasmic antibodies. However, serum IgG of 26.9 g/L (normal, 8–17 g/L), IgM of 3.19 g/L (normal, 0.6–2.8 g/L), and lymphocyte subpopulations expressed as CD4/CD8 ratio of 3.04 (normal, 1–2.5) were slightly elevated. Renal US showed enlarged edematous kidneys without corticomedullar differentiation and no evidence of obstructive uropathy or nephrocalcinosis. Ophthalmological examination was normal with no signs of uveitis. Renal biopsy revealed interstitial edema and abundant mononuclear infiltrates of inflammatory cells, partly dilated tubules, and unchanged glomeruli. Abundant mononuclear cell infiltrate comprised lymphocytes, plasma cells, macrophages, and a few eosinophils, with severely damaged tubular cells, consistent with hypersensitive ATIN. Immunofluorescence studies were unremarkable.

What is the likely cause of acute tubulointerstitial disease in this case?

A. Drug-induced acute tubulointerstitial disease (ATID)
B. Heavy metal intoxication
C. Autoimmune disease
D. Idiopathic ATID

The correct answer is D

Comment: Children presenting with acute renal failure usually exhibit a number of clinical symptoms. Laboratory findings relative to recent medical history enable the clinician to differentiate between acute glomerulonephritis and systemic disease, mainly lupus nephritis and ATIN.[1,2] Very often, renal biopsy is mandatory for diagnosis. Renal biopsy findings of interstitial mononuclear cellular infiltration with eosinophils, interstitial edema, and changed tubular cells but intact vessels and glomeruli are characteristic of ATIN.[2] Drugs represent the most frequent cause of ATIN, most commonly in association with beta-lactams and NSAIDs, even in children.[2,3] Typical clinical signs of drug-induced ATIN, such as fever and skin rash, are not always present. Renal manifestations range from completely asymptomatic urinary abnormalities to acute renal failure with tubular dysfunction.[1] The magnitude of renal damage depends on the localization and extent of interstitial inflammation affecting different segments of nephrons. In children, isolated glycosuria, mild tubular proteinuria, and hyposthenuria seem to be the only constant manifestations of tubular dysfunction.[2] Peripheral eosinophilia and eosinophiluria, although nonspecific findings, usually support the clinical diagnosis of drug-induced ATIN. However, the definite diagnosis of ATIN has to be based on renal biopsy findings, with a clear distinction between acute and chronic changes characterized by tubular atrophy and interstitial fibrosis.[4]

Despite the abundance of clinical elements correlating with ATIN caused by drugs in our patient, the drug directly responsible for actual renal damage could not be identified, and heavy metal intoxication was suspected.

Heavy metal analyses of serum and urine were normal, except for the high urinary excretion of cadmium. Cadmium excretion was 13.52 μg/24 hours (normal, <2 μg/24 h), which was sixfold higher than the normal range. A serum cadmium concentration of 1.7 μg/L (normal, <1.5 μg/L) was slightly elevated but insignificant according to our laboratory. In an attempt to explain the presence of such high levels of urinary cadmium, the assessment of cadmium in four herbal preparations that she had consumed was undertaken. The analyzed plants were *Hypericum perforatum*, *Melissa officinalis*, *Achillea millefolium*, and *Plantago media*. The estimated cadmium concentration of analyzed herbs ranged from 0.034 to 0.36 mg/kg (limits of detection up to 0.02 mg/kg) and was assigned to the category of high metal concentration but considered insignificant according to low-average consumption.[5] Two weeks following admission and after she stopped taking the herbal mixtures, her impaired renal function remained unchanged. According to renal biopsy findings consistent with drug-induced ATIN, therapy with pulse methylprednisolone (three pulses) was introduced, followed by prednisolone 1 mg/kg per day.[12] Her serum creatinine normalized promptly within 3 weeks, followed by normalization of ESR, negative C-reactive protein, and disappearance of glycosuria, phosphaturia, and uricosuria after 4 weeks. Mild proteinuria, elevated ß2-MG, and elevated urinary cadmium persisted for 6 months. After normalization of serum creatinine, her steroid regimen was changed to alternate-day therapy, with tapering of the dose for the next 2 months. Closely followed for the next 3 years, her renal function remained stable. Control urinary cadmium was 10.7, 1.8, and 0.7 μg/24 h after 3 months, 6 months, and 3 years, respectively. Currently, the girl is asymptomatic, in good health, and not receiving any therapy.

The published data about the safety of azithromycin[5] led us to consider a possible adverse reaction to acetaminophen (paracetamol), despite a relatively short period of treatment and no evidence of nephrotic syndrome, as has been reported sporadically in children receiving NSAIDs.[3]

Besides drugs, our vegetarian patient had been consuming different "homemade" herbal mixtures composed of some local plants. Reports dealing with herbal mixtures point to the dangers of misidentification, adulteration, and contamination.[6] Based on the plants listed in this particular case, poisoning from natural chemistry was not likely, although individual susceptibility depending on age, state of health, and the concomitant use of other drugs[7] could not be excluded. The unexpected finding of elevated urinary cadmium led us to consider possible contamination of consumed herbs. Any herbal product can be contaminated during production and processing, especially by insecticides, fungicides, or heavy metals, including cadmium.[6,7] Cadmium as an environmental or occupational toxin can cause severe toxicity in a variety of organs, with the kidney as the principal target. The renal toxicity of cadmium documented in highly exposed populations in occupational settings is characterized by irreversible tubular and glomerular dysfunction and the tendency to disease progression even after a reduction in environmental cadmium exposure.[8] In a recently published Cadmibel study, increased cadmium body burden resulting from environmental pollution was not associated with progressive renal dysfunction.[9] As reported, the renal effects of cadmium ranged from weak, stable, and reversible changes after reduced exposure. The intake of cadmium through food varies geographically and is generally low in most European countries (1–2 μg/day). However, slight cadmium-induced renal effects on the kidney have been reported in Germany and Sweden.[10] Predisposing factors such as dietary habits, including contaminated vegetables and low body iron stores, enhance the absorption of cadmium from the gastrointestinal tract.[11] The signs of cadmium toxicity rarely give rise to symptoms and clinical disease, even if different segments of the nephron are affected by cadmium.[12] Because urinary concentrations associated with renal effects vary, besides an increased excretion of low-molecular-weight proteins, urinary β2-MG and NAG excretion have been proposed as indirect but sensitive biological indicators of cadmium accumulation in the kidney.[12] However, the mechanism underlying the increased excretion of these markers and the mechanisms by which cadmium leads to multiple tubular abnormalities remain uncertain.[11] Irrespective of the causative agent of ATIN,[13] the recommended therapy is still controversial.[2] Reported benefits from steroid therapy in drug-induced ATIN are not generally approved. In certain situations, when the simple exclusion of the offending drug has no influence on the compromised renal function, a trial of steroids has to be undertaken.[2]

The kidney is especially susceptible to toxic injury, either from drugs or other toxins. In cases of ATIN occurring in patients treated by more than one potentially nephrotoxic agent, it is sometimes difficult to discern which one is responsible for renal damage, as in the presented case of drug-induced ATIN and the simultaneous occurrence of elevated urinary cadmium. A search of the relevant literature did not reveal a single report of environmental exposure to toxic metals or cadmium-induced reversible renal failure in children. The cadmium-induced renal damage in our patient was documented by elevated urinary cadmium, ß2-MG, and NAG excretion. These findings cannot be considered accidental, but rather a complementary cause of drug-induced ATIN. The presence of cadmium in the urine and all analyzed herb preparations, despite the low concentrations, had to be regarded as responsible for the actual renal damage. If renal effects of cadmium in cases of low environmental exposure are reversible,[9] why should this not be the case with temporary consumption of herbal preparations containing cadmium in concentrations defined as high but harmless because of low average consumption?[13] In any case, the multiple tubular dysfunction may not be solely attributed to drugs but also to cadmium in patients with vegetarian habits.

Clinical Presentation 40

A 19-year-old male was admitted because of a decreased GFR. The decreased GFR had been detected during a routine health check 2 years earlier, but no further examinations were performed. One year previously, his kidney function had deteriorated. Fetal ultrasonography of his sister revealed agenesis of the right kidney and multiple cysts in the left kidney, and her estimated GFR was 50 mL/min/1.73 m^2. His father has diabetes mellitus and chronic kidney disease. His history included tonsillitis and appendicitis as a child and depression for the previous 2 years. His depression was treated at an outpatient clinic with paroxetine, olanzapine, and flunitrazepam.

On admission, the patient was 162 cm tall and weighed 59.8 kg. BP was 123/84 mm Hg; heart rate, 75 beats/min; and body temperature, 35.8°C. Edema was not present in the lower extremities. Results of laboratory tests were as follows: serum creatinine, 1.64 mg/dL; urea nitrogen, 18 mg/dL; eGFR, 38.8 mL/min/1.73 m^2; hemoglobin A1c, 6.2%, and total urinary protein excretion, 0.04 g/d. Urine sediment contained fewer than 1 erythrocyte per HPG. MRI showed multiple small cysts in the corticomedullary and medullary areas of bilateral kidneys. Total kidney volume was 291 mL (right kidney, 143 mL; left kidney, 148 mL). CT showed pancreatic hypoplasia with deficiency of the pancreatic body and tail.

Because of the patient's decreased GFR, an echo-guided percutaneous kidney biopsy of the right kidney was performed. In light microscopy of the biopsy specimen, 70% of the total kidney cortical region was replaced by tubulointerstitial fibrosis, and there was thinning of the cortex. Almost all tubules were narrowed, and duplication and swelling of the tubular basement membrane were definite. Cystic lesions were not present in the specimen. Global sclerosis was observed in 15 of 21 glomeruli, mainly in the outer cortical region. The remaining glomeruli were intact. Fibroelastosis of the intralobular arteries was moderate, but arteriolar hyalinosis was not noted. Immunofluorescence was negative for IgG, IgA, IgM, C3, C4, and C1q. Electron microscopy did not reveal any abnormality in glomeruli or tubular basement membranes but showed that mitochondria in tubular epithelial cells were small, rounded, and swollen, with shortened cristae. Although the individual had borderline diabetes mellitus, the glomerular basement membrane was not thickened (width, 330–380 nm; normal width, <430 nm) and was not consistent with diabetic nephropathy.

What is the underlying cause of tubulointerstitial disease in this patient?

A. Autosomal dominant tubulointerstitial disease
B. Drug-induced tubulointerstitial disease
C. Medullary cystic kidney disease
D. All of the above

The correct answer is A

Comment: This patient had a reduced GFR, borderline diabetes mellitus, multiple small kidney cysts bilaterally, and pancreatic hypoplasia. He also had a family history of diabetes and kidney cystic lesions, which are HNF1B-associated phenotypes, and genetic analysis revealed a novel variant of HNF1B. The kidney biopsy demonstrated not only tubulointerstitial fibrosis but also abnormal mitochondrial morphology in tubular cells. These findings represent autosomal dominant tubulointerstitial kidney disease (ADTKD)-HNF1B and genetic analysis revealed a missense variant of HNF1B.[1,2]

ADTKD is a chronic tubulointerstitial kidney disease caused by a gene variant. The subtype hepatocyte nuclear factor 1β (HNF1B) is caused by a variant in the *HNF1B* gene and is referred to as ADTKD-HNF1B. This subtype has a variety of extrarenal manifestations, such as pancreatic hypoplasia, hyperparathyroidism, hypomagnesemia-like Gitelman syndrome, and genital tract malformation, as well as kidney cysts, unilateral kidney agenesis, and hypoplasia.[1,2] It is closely related to early-onset diabetes mellitus with a familial history, in particular maturity-onset diabetes of the young type 5 (MODY5).[3] Cystic formation is present in 73% of patients with ADTKD-HNF1B; cysts are usually small and often arise within the kidney cortex.[1] However, previous reports have not described the pathology of the kidney in ADTKD-HNF1B.

Medullary cystic kidney disease, which is characterized by cyst formation in the corticomedullary and medullary areas, is a morphologic classification based on radiologic features. Genetic analyses of medullary cystic kidney and related disease have revealed variants of five different genes, including *MUC1*, uromodulin (*UMOD*), *REN*, *HNF1B*, and more rarely, *SEC61A1*.[4–6] Kidney Disease: Improving Global Outcomes redefined the disease concept of medullary cystic kidney disease as ADTKD, which involved a change from morphologic classification to genetic classification of the disease.

In individuals with ADTKD-HNF1B, hypoplasia of the pancreatic body and tail and a slightly atrophic pancreatic head are involved in the development of diabetes.[3] Diabetes with onset before the age of 25 years in families with this autosomal dominant inheritance is called MODY, and the type caused by the variant of HNF1B is called HNF1BMODY (MODY5). In 2014, Faguer et al.[6,7] described an HNF1B score that can be calculated from clinical, imaging, and biological variables. The cutoff threshold for a negative predictive value to rule out HNF1B variants is 8 points. Our patient scored at least 20 points, indicating that our diagnosis of ADTKD-HNF1B was correct.[6]

Although ADTKD is defined as tubulointerstitial nephropathy, few reports have described the kidney biopsy and pathologic features of ADTKD. Ayasreh Fierro et al.[8] reported that kidney specimens of patients with ADTKDUMOD showed interstitial fibrosis, tubular atrophy, normal glomeruli, and tubular dilatation with tubular microcystis. However, kidney biopsy of ADTKD-HNF1B has not been reported.

The findings in the kidney biopsy of this patient may support previous findings. For example, Connor et al.[9] showed that variants in mitochondrial DNA also caused tubulointerstitial kidney disease. Furthermore, Casemayou et al.[10] reported that HNF1B regulated transcription factor peroxisome proliferator-activated receptor-γ expression and regulated mitochondrial morphology and respiration in proximal tubule cells in mice.

Through genetic analysis, a novel heterozygous missense variant of HNF1B (NM_000458.3: c.865A>C, p.(Asn289- His)) was detected in both the individual and his daughter. Faguer et al.[11] reported a variant (NM_000458.2: c.865A>G, p.(Asn289Asp)) and submitted the variant to the Human Gene Mutation Database (CM117494). This patient showed the same site variant. According to American College of Medical Genetics and Genomics guidelines, this variant meets PM1, PM2, PP1, and PP3 so that this variant is "likely pathogenic" of ADTKD-HNF1B. In conclusion, this patient presented with both kidney cystic lesions and diabetes and had a family history of kidney cystic lesion and diabetes, which are HNF1B-associated phenotypes, and genetic analysis revealed a novel variant of HNF1B.

This patient presented with both kidney cystic lesions and diabetes and had a family history of kidney cystic lesion and diabetes, which are HNF1B-associated phenotypes, and genetic analysis revealed a novel variant of HNF1B. We performed a kidney biopsy of his cystic kidney, and this is the first report of the kidney biopsy on ADTKD-HNF1B. This case also showed tubulointerstitial fibrosis and abnormal mitochondrial morphology in tubular cells.

Clinical Presentation 41

A 15-year-old White male, previously in excellent health except for obesity, developed malaise, anorexia, nausea, and vomiting. Other family members had similar symptoms that resolved spontaneously. The patient remained ill and subsequently developed thirst, frequency, nocturia, and weight loss. There was no fever, skin rash, exposure to medications or toxins, or other symptoms of systemic disease. The serum creatinine level was found to be 9.8 mg/dL and the patient was admitted to the hospital. On admission, the patient was afebrile and his BP was 150/90 mm Hg. Other than obesity, the physical examination was unremarkable. There was no skin rash. Admitting laboratory data were BUN 86 mg/dL, creatinine 10.9 mg/dL, uric acid 4.8 mg/dL, phosphorus 5.4 mg/dL, albumin 4.1 g/dL, glucose 134 mg/dL, sodium 137 mEq/L, potassium 3.3 mEq/L, CO_2 14 mmol/L, chloride 104 mEq/L, hematocrit 31%, WBC count 6500 with 2% eosinophils, and the ESR was 59 mm/h. Urinalysis revealed a specific gravity of 1.007, pH 5.5, 1+ glucose, 1+ protein, renal tubular epithelial cells, WBCs, and many granular casts. A renal ultrasound and diethylenetriaminepentaacetic acid scan showed normal-sized unobstructed kidneys. A trial of volume expansion failed to improve renal function. Because the obscure origin of the renal failure, a percutaneous renal biopsy was performed and processed by routine methods for light, immunofluorescent, and electron microscopy. There were 10 glomeruli that were essentially normal, except for a slight increase in mesangial matrix. The striking finding was diffuse marked cellular infiltration of the interstitium, with lymphocytes, plasma cells, and occasional eosinophils. There was also prominent interstitial edema and tubular necrosis. In some tubules, lymphocytes were seen between the tubular basement membrane and the tubular epithelial called tubulitis. Immunofluorescence revealed only minor nonspecific staining for IgG and C3. Immunoperoxidase failed to stain lymphocytes invading tubular epithelium for IgG, IgM, and muramidase, suggesting that these were T lymphocytes. Electron microscopy confirmed marked tubulointerstitial inflammation and tubular necrosis, and there were no deposits. No cause could be found for the tubulointerstitial nephritis. The following tests were negative or normal: chest x-ray, blood and urine cultures, cold agglutinins, heterophile, cytomegalovirus, toxoplasmosis and leptospiral antibodies, hepatitis B profile, antistreptolysin-O titer, serum protein electrophoresis, IgE level, heavy metal screen, ANA, and complement levels. A 24-hour urine contained 2122 mg protein, 937 mg uric acid, 639 mg phosphorus, 17 g glucose, and generalized aminoaciduria. The fractional excretions of phosphorus, uric acid, and glucose were 76%, 113%, and 60%, respectively. Urine protein electrophoresis showed only a trace of albumin, with no monoclonal protein. Prednisone 60 mg daily was begun and renal function improved dramatically. Within 1 week, the creatinine had decreased to 6.0 mg/dL, and by 1 month decreased to 1.8 mg/dL. Steroids were gradually tapered over the next 2 months at which time the creatinine was 1.4 mg/dL. Approximately 2.5 months following hospitalization, the patient complained of redness and discomfort in the right eye. Eye examination revealed right episcleritis and mild bilateral uveitis. He was treated with topical steroids and experienced complete resolution. Now, more than 2 years after presentation, the patient's serum creatinine is 1.11 mg/ dL. The urine sediment shows five to 10 WBCs per HPF. A 24-hour urine contains 98 mg protein, 343 mg glucose, 1127 mg phosphorus, and 1004 mg uric acid. The fractional excretions of uric acid, phosphorus, and glucose are 10.4%, 13.5%, and 0.18%, respectively. Aminoaciduria is no longer present, and first-morning urine osmolality is 758 mOsm/kg.

What is the underlying cause of tubulointerstitial nephritis?

A. Autoimmune disease
B. Idiopathic
C. Drug-induced
D. Hereditary

The correct answer is B

Comment: Acute tubulointerstitial nephritis (ATIN) is characterized histologically by inflammation of the renal interstitium, with relative sparing of glomeruli.[1,2] This lesion may account for 10% to 15% of cases of unexplained acute renal failure investigated with renal biopsy.[3,4] Acute tubulointerstitial nephritis be caused by drugs, infections, or systemic disease, but sometimes no cause is found.[5] Because cases of ATID are rarely diagnosed, clinical experience with them is limited and optimal therapy is unknown. In particular, whereas steroid therapy has been used with apparent success,[6–8] its true value remains unproven. This report will review the clinical and pathologic features of acute idiopathic tubulointerstitial nephritis and report two additional cases. Our patients presented with severe azotemia and evidence of generalized proximal tubular dysfunction. Both patients responded dramatically to steroid therapy.

Acute idiopathic tubulointerstitial nephritis must be considered in the differential diagnosis of acute renal failure. Although there is a predominance of females, both sexes and all ages are affected. In the majority of cases, there is a prodrome consisting of nonspecific constitutional symptoms, and a few patients experience flank or abdominal pain. Unlike drug-induced acute interstitial nephritis, fever and skin rash are usually absent. There is no history of preceding drug or toxin exposure, nor are there signs or symptoms of a specific systemic disease. However, some cases have been associated with uveitis and bone marrow and lymph node granulomas.[6–8]

Patients often present with moderate to severe renal failure, which is usually nonoliguric. BP is almost always normal. There is usually mild anemia, and the ESR is almost always elevated, but routine cultures and serologic markers of rheumatologic and infectious disease are negative. Complement levels are usually normal. Eosinophilia is seen only in a minority of patients, and IgE levels, when measured, have been either normal or increased. Proteinuria is generally <2g/24 h, and only occasional RBCs, WBCs, and granular casts are seen on urinalysis. Only four patients with heavy proteinuria have been reported, and all had glomerular involvement on biopsy.[9] The kidneys are of normal size and are not obstructed. Our patients presented with severe renal failure and evidence of generalized proximal tubular dysfunction, with impaired reabsorption of glucose, amino acids, uric acid, and phosphorus.[9] The recognition of proximal tubular dysfunction is more difficult when the glomerular filtration rate is reduced[10]; however, renal failure alone cannot explain all the findings in our patients. Both patients had marked elevations of the fractional excretion of uric acid, much greater than that associated with renal failure alone.[11] Moreover, both patients had marked renal glycosuria and generalized aminoaciduria, useful markers of proximal tubular dysfunction, which are not features of renal failure alone.[10,12] During an exacerbation, case 2 demonstrated full Fanconi syndrome, including a hypokalemia hyperchloremic acidosis, hypophosphatemia, hypouricemia, renal glycosuria, and generalized aminoaciduria. Although there are only two previous reports of generalized proximal tubular dysfunction[6] and Fanconi syndrome[10] in acute idiopathic tubulointerstitial nephritis, many other cases have had glycosuria on routine urinalysis.[8] Many of these patients would have manifested other features of the Fanconi syndrome had these been sought. As previously suggested,[6] the finding of glycosuria in the presence of a normal blood glucose is an important clue to the diagnosis of acute tubulointerstitial nephritis, but its absence does not exclude the diagnosis.[13] Histologically, an intense inflammatory interstitial infiltrate is seen, with relative sparing of the glomeruli. The majority of infiltrating cells are lymphocytes and plasma cells-eosinophils are prominent only occasionally. Lymphocytes may be seen between the basement membrane and tubular cells, so-called tubulitis.[14] There may be tubular necrosis, loss of tubular basement membrane, and varying degrees of interstitial edema and fibrosis. In most cases, immunofluorescence has been negative or has shown only nonspecific staining, and electron microscopy confirms tubular injury and has usually not revealed deposits.[1] The prognosis of acute idiopathic tubulointerstitial nephritis has generally been favorable with or without steroid therapy. Only one patient has been described who required permanent dialysis,[15] although several patients have required dialysis during the acute illness. Many patients reported were left with some degree of renal impairment. However, their ultimate outcome is unclear because follow-up was short. The etiology of this condition is unknown. Its frequent prodrome raises the possibility of an infectious origin. In fact, in our first case, other family members had similar symptoms. However, attempts to demonstrate viral, bacterial, and fungal infections have been unsuccessful in all reported cases. Similarly, no systemic disease has emerged during follow-up of these patients. The lack of specific immunofluorescence and the demonstration that the majority of infiltrating cells are T-lymphocytes[5] suggest a role for cell-mediated immunity in this disorder. If cell-mediated immunity is responsible for the injury pattern, then steroids would be rational therapy.[16] In several cases, steroids were used and led to dramatic improvements of renal function,[17–22] usually within 1 to 2 months. However, because there have been reports of spontaneous recovery,[6–8] the value of steroids remains open to question. Our two cases shed further light on this issue. Both patients' renal function improved dramatically after steroid therapy was begun. Moreover, our second case is the first reported in which renal function initially improved on steroids, deteriorated when steroids were withdrawn, and then improved a second time with reinstitution of steroid therapy. This leaves little doubt that steroids were both effective and instrumental in reversing the tubulointerstitial nephritis in this patient. Similarly, Frommer et al.[23] described a patient who was on dialysis for 31 months before a renal biopsy demonstrated interstitial nephritis; the creatinine decreased to 2 mg/100 mL after the institution of steroid therapy. Thus, although the prognosis of acute idiopathic tubulointerstitial nephritis is generally good with or without therapy, steroids are effective and may be necessary to improve renal function[1] in some patients. Therefore, in the absence of contraindications, we believe a short course of high-dose steroid therapy is indicated in patients with severe renal failure. During follow-up, markers of proximal tubular dysfunction should be monitored in addition to the serum creatinine. In our second case, despite near normalization of serum creatinine, glycosuria persisted after the first course of steroid therapy; such findings signal the need for close observation and perhaps continued therapy.[24] Finally, we emphasize that such cases demonstrate the value of renal biopsy in acute renal failure of obscure origin. Although gallium scanning may be suggestive,[25] only through biopsy can acute tubulointerstitial nephritis be diagnosed definitively. Left undetected, this potentially treatable lesion can lead to end-stage renal disease.

References

Clinical Presentation 1

1. Mahe E, Girszyn N, Rabia SH, et al. Subcutaneous fat necrosis of the newborn: a systemic evaluation of risk factors, clinical manifestations, complications and outcome of 16 children. *Br J Dermatol.* 2007;156:709–715.
2. Dudink J, Wakther FJ, Beekman RP. Subcutaneous fat necrosis of the newborn: hypercalcemia with hepatic and atrial myocardial calcification. *Arch Dis Child Fetal Neonatal Ed.* 2003;88:F343–F345.

Clinical Presentation 2

1. Lloyd SE, Gunther W, Pearce SH, et al. Characterisation of renal chloride channel, CLCN5, mutations in hypercalciuric nephrolithiasis (kidney stone) disorders. *Hum Mol Genet.* 1997;8:1233–1239.
2. Suzuki S, Suzuki J, Kume K, et al. Poor renal accumulation of ^{99m}Tc-DMSA in idiopathic tubular proteinuria. *Nephron.* 1999;81:49–54.
3. Lee BH, Lee SH, Chol HJ, et al. Decreased renal uptake of ^{99m}Tc-DMSA in patients with tubular proteinuria. *Pediatr Nephrol.* 2006;24:2211–2216.
4. Caglar M, Yaris N, Akyuz C. The utility of (99m)Tc-DMSA and Tc(99m)-EC scintigraphy for early diagnosis of ifosfamide induced nephrotoxicity. *Nuc Med Comm.* 2001;22:1325–1332.
5. Muller-Suur R, Gutsche HU. Tubular reabsorption of technetium-99m-DMSA. *J Nucl Med.* 1995;36(9):1654–1658.
6. Ludwig M, Utsch B, Monnens LA. Recent advances in understanding the clinical and genetic heterogeneity of Dent's disease. *Nephrol Dial Transplant.* 2006;21:2708–2717.
7. Lee BH, Lee SH, Chol HJ, et al. Decreased renal uptake of (99m)Tc-DMSA in patients with tubular proteinuria. *Pediatr Nephrol.* 2006;24:2211–2216.
8. Suzuki S, Suzuki J, Kume K, et al. Poor renal accumulation of ^{99m}Tc-DMSA in idiopathic tubular proteinuria. *Nephron.* 1999;81:49–54.
9. Ludwig M, Utsch B, Balluch B, et al. Hypercalciuria in patients with CLCN5 mutations. *Pediatr Nephrol.* 2006;21:1241–1250.
10. Raja KA, Schurman S, D'mello RG, et al. Responsiveness of hypercalciuria to thiazide in Dent's disease. *J Am Soc Nephrol.* 2002;13:2938–2944.
11. Levtchenko E, Blom H, Wilmer M, et al. ACE inhibitor enalapril diminishes albuminuria in patients with cystinosis. *Clin Nephrol.* 2003;60:386–389.

Clinical Presentation 3

1. Ficarra V, Beltrami P, Giusti G, et al. Spontaneous bladder perforation due to eosinophilic cystitis: a case report. *Prog Urol.* 1997;7:1012–1014.
2. Van den Ouden D. Diagnosis and management of eosinophilic cystitis: a pooled analysis of 135 cases. *Eur Urol.* 2000;7:386–394.

Clinical Presentation 4

1. Peterson P, Peltonen L. Autoimmune polyendocrinopathy syndrome type 1 (APS 1) and AIRE gene: new views on molecular basis of autoimmunity. *J Autoimmun.* 2005;25:49–55.
2. Halonen M, Eskelin P, Myhre AG, et al. AIRE mutation and human leukocyte antigen genotypes as determinants of the autoimmune polyendocrinopathy—candidiasis—ecodermal dystrophy phenotype. *J Clin Endocrinol Metab.* 2002;87:2568–2574.

Clinical Presentation 5

1. Maria BL, Quisling RG, Rosainz LC, et al. Molar tooth sign in Joubert syndrome: clinical, radiologic, and pathologic significance. *J Child Neurol.* 1999;14:368–376.
2. Simms RJ, Eley L, Sayer JA. Nephronophthisis. *Eur J Hum Genet.* 2009;17:406–416.
3. Patel S, Barkovich AJ. Analysis and classification of cerebellar malformations. *Am J Neuroradiol.* 2002;23:1074–1087.

4. Hildebrandt F, Zhou W. Nephronophthisis-associated ciliopathies. *J Am SocNephrol.* 2007;18:1855–1871.
5. Zollinger HU, Mihatsch MJ, Edefonti A, Gaboardi F, Imbasciati E, Lennert T. Nephronophthisis (medullary cystic disease of the kidney). A study using electron microscopy, immunofluorescence, and a review of the morphological findings. *Helv Paediatr Acta.* 1980;35:509–530.

Clinical Presentation 6

1. Khalighi MA, Henriksen KJ, Chang A, et al. March hemoglobinuria-associated acute tubular injury. *Clin Kidney J.* 2014;7:488–489.
2. Tobal D, Olascoaga A, Moreira G, et al. Rust urine after intense hand drumming is caused by extracorpuscular hemolysis. *Clin J Am Soc Nephrol.* 2008;3:1022–1027.

Clinical Presentation 7

1. Hoppe B, Kemper MJ. Diagnostic examination of the child with urolithiasis or nephrocalcinosis. *Pediatr Nephrol.* 2010;25:403–413.
2. Mantan M, Bagga A, Virdi VS, Menon S, Hari P. Etiology of nephrocalcinosis in northern Indian children. *Pediatr Nephrol.* 2007;22:829–833.
3. Tanaka ST, Pope JC. Pediatric stone disease. *Curr Urol Rep.* 2009;10:138–143.
4. Rönnefarth G, Misselwitz J. Nephrocalcinosis in children: a retrospective survey. Members of the Arbeitsgemeinschaft für pädiatrische Nephrologie. *Pediatr Nephrol.* 2000;14:1016–1021.

Clinical Presentation 8

1. Velasquez CA, Saeyeldin A, Zafar MA, et al. A systematic review on management of nutcracker syndrome. *J Vasc Surg Venous Lymphat Disord.* 2018;6:271–278.
2. Kurklinsky AK, Rooke TW. Nutcracker phenomenon and nutcracker syndrome. *Mayo Clin Proc.* 2010;85:552–559.
3. Skeik N, Gloviczki P, Macedo TA. Posterior nutcracker syndrome. *Vasc Endovascular Surg.* 2011;45:749–755.
4. Takemura T, Iwasa H, Yamamoto S, et al. Clinical and radiological features in four adolescents with nutcracker syndrome. *Pediatr Nephrol.* 2000;14:1002–1005.

Clinical Presentation 9

1. Leclercq P, Loly C, Delanaye P, et al. Green urine. *Lancet.* 2009;373:1462.
2. Ku BD, Park KC, Yoon SS. Dark green discoloration of the urine after prolonged propofol infusion: a case report. *J Clin Pharm Ther.* 2010;36:734Y736.
3. Assadi FK. Clinical quiz. Evaluation and management of a dark and purple-colored urine. *Pediatr Nephrol.* 1996;10(3):393–394. http://doi.org/10.1007/BF00866792.

Clinical Presentation 10

1. Oliva-Damaso N, Oliva-Damaso E, Payan J, et al. Acute and chronic tubulointerstitial nephritis of rheumatic causes. *Rheum Dis Clin N Am.* 2018;44:619–633.
2. Perazella MA, Markowitz GS. Drug-induced acute interstitial nephritis. *Nat Rev Nephrol.* 2010;6:461–470.
3. Perazella MA. Clinical approach to diagnosing acute and chronic tubulointerstitial disease. *Adv Chronic Kidney Dis.* 2017;24:59.
4. Oettgen HC. Fifty years later: emerging functions of IgE antibodies in host defense, immune regulation, and allergic diseases. *J Allergy Clin Immunol.* 2016;137:1631.
5. Quattrocchio G, Roccatello R. IgG4-related nephropathy. *J Nephrol.* 2016;29:487–493.

Clinical Presentation 11

1. Butt NM, Lambert J, Ali S, et al. Guideline for the investigation and management of eosinophilia. *Br J Haematol.* 2017;176:553–572.
2. Popescu OE, Landas SK, Haas GP. The spectrum of eosinophilic cystitis in males: case series and literature review. *Arch Pathol Lab Med.* 2009;133:289–294.

Clinical Presentation 12

1. Nerli RB, Kamat GV, Alur SB, Koura A, Vikram P, Amarkhed SS. Genitourinary tuberculosis in pediatric urological practice. *J Pediatr Urol.* 2008;4:299–303.
2. Tong JE, Howell DN, Foreman JW. Drug-induced granulomatous interstitial nephritis in a pediatric patient. *Pediatr Nephrol.* 2007;22:306–309.

Clinical Presentation 13

1. Craven BL, Passman C, Assimos DG. Hypercalcemic states associated with nephrolithiasis. *Rev Urol.* 2008;10:218–226.
2. Hulton SA. Evaluation of urinary tract calculi in children. *Arch Dis Child.* 2001;84:320–323.
3. Ramya K, Krishnamurthy S, Sivamurukan P. Etiological profile of nephrocalcinosis in children from Southern India. *Indian Pediatr.* 2020;57:415–419.

Clinical Presentation 14

1. Amaro D, Carreño E, Steeples LR, et al. Tubulointerstitial nephritis and uveitis (TINU) syndrome: a review. *Br J Ophthalmol.* 2020;104(6):742–747.

Clinical Presentation 15

1. Chevalier A, Duflos C, Clave S, et al. Renal prognosis in children with tubulointerstitial nephritis and uveitis syndrome. *Kidney Int Rep.* 2021;6(12):3045–3053.

Clinical Presentation 16

1. Mackensen F, Billing H. Tubulointerstitial nephritis and uveitis syndrome. *Curr Opin Ophthalmol.* 2009;20:525–531.
2. Abed L, Merouani A, Haddad E, et al. Presence of autoantibodies against tubular and uveal cells in a patient with tubulointerstitial nephritis and uveitis (TINU) syndrome. *Nephrol Dial Transplant.* 2008;23:1452–1455.
3. Gorroño-Echebarría MB, Calvo-Arrabal MA, Albarrán F, et al. The tuberculointerstitial nephritis and uveitis (TINU) syndrome is associated with HLA-DR14 in Spanish patients. *Br J Ophthalmol.* 2001;85:1010–2011.
4. Yeh S, Li Z, Forooghian F, et al. CD4+Foxp3+ T-regulatory cells in noninfectious uveitis. *Arch Ophthalmol.* 2009;127:407–413.

Clinical Presentation 17

1. Mackensen F, Billing H. Tubulointerstitial nephritis and uveitis syndrome. *Curr Opin Ophthalmol.* 2009;20:525–531.

Clinical Presentation 18

1. Nasr SH, Koscica J, Markowitz GS, et al. Granulomatous interstitial nephritis. *Am J Kidney Dis.* 2003;41:714–719.
2. Mackensen F, Billing H. Tubulointerstitial nephritis and uveitis syndrome. *Curr Opin Ophthalmol.* 2009;20:525–531.

Clinical Presentation 19

1. Nasr SH, Koscica J, Markowitz GS, et al. Granulomatous interstitial nephritis. *Am J Kidney Dis.* 2003;41:714–719.
2. Mackensen F, Billing H. Tubulointerstitial nephritis and uveitis syndrome. *Curr Opin Ophthalmol.* 2009;20:525–531.

Clinical Presentation 20

1. Nasr SH, Koscica J, Markowitz GS, et al. Granulomatous interstitial nephritis. *Am J Kidney Dis.* 2003;41:714–719.
2. Mackensen F, Billing H. Tubulointerstitial nephritis and uveitis syndrome. *Curr Opin Ophthalmol.* 2009;20:525–531.

Clinical Presentation 21

1. Gonzalez E, Gutierrez E, Galeano C, et al. Early steroid treatment improves the recovery of renal function in patients with drug-induced acute interstitial nephritis. *Kidney Int.* 2008;73:940–946.
2. Rossert J. Drug-induced acute interstitial nephritis. *Kidney Int.* 2001;60:804–817.

Clinical Presentation 22

1. Praga M, González E. Acute interstitial nephritis. *Kidney Int.* 2010;77(11):956–961. http://doi.org/10.1038/ki.2010.89.

2. Ramachandran R, Kumar K, Nada R, et al. Drug-induced acute interstitial nephritis: a clinicopathological study and comparative trial of steroid regimens. *Indian J Nephrol.* 2015;25(5):281–286. http://doi.org/10.4103/0971-4065.147766.

Clinical Presentation 23

1. Praga M, González E. Acute international nephritis. *Kidney Int.* 2010;77(11):956–961.

Clinical Presentation 24

1. Praga M, González E. Acute international nephritis. *Kidney Int.* 2010;77(11):956–961.

Clinical Presentation 25

1. Praga M, González E. Acute interstitial nephritis. *Kidney Int.* 2010;77(11):956–961. http://doi.org/10.1038/ki.2010.89.

Clinical Presentation 26

1. Maripuri S, Grande JP, Osborn TG, et al. Renal involvement in primary Sjögren's syndrome: a clinicopathologic study. *Clin J Am Soc Nephrol.* 2009;4(9):1423–1431.
2. Jain A, Srinivas BH, Emmanuel D, et al. Renal involvement in primary Sjogren's syndrome: a prospective cohort study. *Rheumatol Int.* 2018;38(12):2251–2262.

Clinical Presentation 27

1. Kalinina Ayuso V, de Boer JH, Byers HL, et al. Intraocular biomarker identification in uveitis associated with juvenile idiopathic arthritis. *Invest Ophthalmol Vis Sci.* 2013;54(5):3709–3720.

Clinical Presentation 28

1. Vitali C, Minniti A, Pignataro F, et al. Management of Sjögren's syndrome: present issues and future perspectives. *Front Med (Lausanne).* 2021;8:676885. http://doi.org/10.3389/fmed.2021.676885.

Clinical Presentation 29

1. Sharma P, Ng JH, Bijol V, et al. Pathology of COVID-19-associated acute kidney injury. *Clin Kidney J.* 2021;14(Suppl 1):i30–i39. http://doi.org/10.1093/ckj/sfab003.

Clinical Presentation 30

1. Agnes B, Fogo AB, Lusco MA, Najafian B, Alpers CE. Acute international nephritis. *Am J Kidney Dis.* 2016;67(6):e35–e36.
2. Iványi B, Hamilton-Dutoit SJ, Olsen S, et al. Acute tubulointerstitial nephritis: phenotype of infiltrating cells and prognostic impact of tubulitis. *Vichows Archiv A Pathol Anat.* 1996;428:5–12.

Clinical Presentation 31

1. Assadi F, Moghtaderi M. Preventive kidney stones: continue medical education. *Int J Prev Med.* 2017;8:67. http://doi.org/10.4103/ijpvm.IJPVM_17_17.
2. Assadi FK, Scott CI Jr, McKay CP, et al. Hypercalciuria and urolithiasis in a case of Costello syndrome. *Pediatr Nephrol.* 1999;13(1):57–59. http://doi.org/10.1007/s004670050563.

Clinical Presentation 32

1. Assadi F, Moghtaderi M. Preventive kidney stones: continue medical education. *Int J Prev Med.* 2017;8:67. http://doi.org/10.4103/ijpvm.IJPVM_17_17.
2. Assadi FK, Scott CI Jr, McKay CP, et al. Hypercalciuria and urolithiasis in a case of Costello syndrome. *Pediatr Nephrol.* 1999;13(1):57–59. http://doi.org/10.1007/s004670050563.

Clinical Presentation 33

1. Assadi F, Moghtaderi M. Preventive kidney stones: continue medical education. *Int J Prev Med.* 2017;8:67. http://doi.org/10.4103/ijpvm.IJPVM_17_17.
2. Assadi FK, Scott CI Jr, McKay CP, et al. Hypercalciuria and urolithiasis in a case of Costello syndrome. *Pediatr Nephrol.* 1999;13(1):57–59. http://doi.org/10.1007/s004670050563.

Clinical Presentation 34

1. Assadi F, Moghtaderi M. Preventive kidney stones: continue medical education. *Int J Prev Med.* 2017;8:67. http://doi.org/10.4103/ijpvm.IJPVM_17_17.

2. Assadi FK, Scott CI Jr, McKay CP, et al. Hypercalciuria and urolithiasis in a case of Costello syndrome. *Pediatr Nephrol.* 1999;13(1):57–59. http://doi.org/10.1007/s004670050563.

Clinical Presentation 35

1. Assadi F, Moghtaderi M. Preventive kidney stones: continue medical education. *Int J Prev Med.* 2017;8:67. http://doi.org/10.4103/ijpvm.IJPVM_17_17.
2. Assadi FK, Scott CI Jr, McKay CP, et al. Hypercalciuria and urolithiasis in a case of Costello syndrome. *Pediatr Nephrol.* 1999;13(1):57–59. http://doi.org/10.1007/s004670050563.

Clinical Presentation 36

1. Teotia M, Sutor DJ. Crystallisation of ammonium acid urate and other uric acid derivatives from urine. *Br J Urol.* 1971;43(4):381–386.
2. Soble JJ, Hamilton BD, Streem SB. Ammonium acid urate calculi: a reevaluation of risk factors. *J Urol.* 1999;161(3):869–873.
3. Lin SH, Davids MR, Halperin ML. Hypokalemia and paralysis. *QJM.* 2003;96(2):161–216.
4. Roerig JL, Steffen KJ, Mitchell JE, Zunker C. Laxative abuse: epidemiology, diagnosis and management. *Drug.* 2010;70(12):1487–1503.

Clinical Presentation 37

1. Seshan SV, D'Agati VD, Appel GA, Churg J. Tubulo-interstitial and vascular lesions associated with metabolic diseases. In: *Renal Disease Classification and Atlas of Tubulointerstitial and Vascular Diseases.* New York, NY: Lippincott Williams & Wilkins; 1999:231–259.
2. World Health Organization. *Melamine and Cyanuric Acid: Toxicity, Preliminary Risk Assessment and Guidance on Levels in Food.* Geneva, Switzerland: World Health Organization; 2008.
3. Brown CA, Jeong KS, Poppenga RH, et al. Outbreaks of renal failure associated with melamine and cyanuric acid in dogs and cats in 2004 and 2007. *J Vet Diagn Invest.* 2007;19:525–531.
4. Perazella MA. Crystal-induced acute renal failure. *Am J Med.* 1999;106:459–465.
5. Kuhara T. Gas chromatographic-mass spectrometric urinary metabolome analysis to study mutations of inborn errors of metabolism. *Mass Spectrom Rev.* 2005;24:814–827.
6. Sahota A, Tischfield JA, Kamatani N, Simmonds HA. Adenine phosphoribosyltrasferase deficiency and 2,8- dihydroxyadenine lithiasis. In: Scriver CR, Beaudet AL, Sly WS, Valle D, Vogelstein B, Childs B, eds. *The Metabolic and Molecular Basis of Inherited Disease.* 8th ed. NewYork, NY: McGraw Hill; 2001:2571–2584.
7. Edvardsson V, Palsson R, Olafsson I, Hjaltadottir G, Laxdal T. Clinical features and genotype of adenine phosphoribosyltransferase deficiency in Iceland. *Am J Kidney Dis.* 2011;38:473–480.

Clinical Presentation 38

1. Horuz R, Sarica K. The management of staghorn calculi in children. *Arab J Urol.* 2012;10(3):30–35.
2. Preminger GM, Assimos DG, Lingeman JE, et al. AUA guideline on management of staghorn calculi: diagnosis and treatment recommendations. *J Urol.* 2005;173(6):1991–2000.
3. Marques JJ, Muresan C, Lúcio R, et al. Litíase coraliforme: caso clínico raro e complicado. *Acta Urológica.* 2011;4:58–61. http://hdl.handle.net/10400.17/675.
4. Penido MGMG. Litíase urinária na infância. In: Júnior DC, Burns DAR, Lopez FA, eds. *Tratado de pediatria: Sociedade Brasileira de Pediatria.* 3rd ed. Barueri, SP: Manuele; 2014:1685–1696.
5. Koga S, Arakaki Y, Matsuoka M, et al. Staghorn calculi-long-term results of management. *Br J Urol.* 1991;68:122–124.
6. Diri A, Diri B. Management of staghorn renal stones. *Ren Fail.* 2018;40(1):357–362.
7. Herring LC. Observations of 10,000 urinary calculi. *J Urol.* 1962;88:545–547.
8. Krzemień G, Szmigielska A, Jankowska-Dziadak K, PańczykTomaszewska M. Renal staghorn calculi in small children—presentation of two cases. *Dev Period Med.* 2016;20(1):23–29.
9. Gleeson MJ, Griffith DP. Struvite calculi. *Br J Urol.* 1993;71:503–511.
10. Holmgren K, Danielson BG, Fellström B, Ljunghall S, Niklasson F, Wikström B. The relation between urinary tract infections and stone composition in renal stone formers. *Scand J Urol Nephrol.* 1989;23(2):131–136.
11. Malheiros DMAC, Cavalcanti FBC, Testagrossa LA, David DSR. Sistema urinário. In: Brasileiro Filho G, ed. *Bogliolo Patologia.* 8th ed. Rio de Janeiro: Guanabara Koogan; 2011:519–585.

12. Schults AJ, Jia W, Ost MC, Oottamasathien S. Combination of extracorporeal shockwave lithotripsy and ureteroscopy for large staghorn calculi in a pediatric patient: case report. *J Endourol Case Rep.* 2017;3(1):64–66.
13. Chibber PJ. Percutaneous nephrolithotomy for large and staghorn calculi. *J Endourol.* 1993;7(4):293–295.
14. Yiee J, Wilcox D. Management of fetal hydronephrosis. *Pediatr Nephrol.* 2008;23(3):347.
15. Assimos DG. Anatrophic nephrolithotomy. *Urology.* 2001;57(1):161–165.
16. Cavalli AC, Tambara Filho R, Slongo LE, Cavalli RC, Rocha LC. The use of double-J catheter decreases complications of retroperitoneoscopic ureterolithotomy. *Rev Col Bras Cir.* 2012;39(2):112–118.

Clinical Presentation 39

1. Toto RD. Review: acute tubulointerstitial nephritis. *Am J Med Sci.* 1990;299:392–410.
2. Smoyer WE, Kelly CJ, Kaplan BS. Tubulointerstitial nephritis. In: Holliday MA, Barratt TM, Avner ED, eds. *Pediatric Nephrology.* 3rd ed. Baltimore: Williams and Wilkins; 1994:890–907.
3. Dharnidharka VR, Rosen S, Somers MJG. Acute interstitial nephritis presenting as presumed minimal change nephrotic syndrome. *Pediatr Nephrol.* 1998;12:576–578.
4. Dillon MJ. Tubulointerstitial nephropathy. In: Edelmann CM, ed. *Pediatric Kidney Disease.* Boston: Little Brown; 1992:1627–1639.
5. Treadway G, Pontani D. Pediatric safety of azithromycin: worldwide experience. *J Antimicrob Chemother.* 1996;37(Suppl C):143–149.
6. Huxtable RJ. The myth of beneficent nature: the risks of herbal preparations. *Ann Intern Med.* 1992;117:165–166.
7. Atherton JD, Rustin HM, Brostoff J. Need to correct identification of herbs in herbal poisoning. *Lancet.* 1993;341:637–638.
8. Fels LM. Risk assessment of nephrotoxicity of cadmium. *Renal Fail.* 1999;21:275–281.
9. Hotz P, Buchet JP, Bernard A, et al. Renal effects of low-level environmental cadmium exposure: 5-year follow-up of a subcohort from Cadmibel study. *Lancet.* 1999;354:1508–1513.
10. Skerfving S, Bencko V, Vahter M, Schütz A, Gerhardsson L. Environmental health in the Baltic region—toxic metals. *Scand J Work Environm Health.* 1999;25(Suppl 3):40–64.
11. Fels LM. Risk assessment of nephrotoxicity of cadmium. *Renal Fail.* 1999;21:275–281.
12. Linshaw M, Aigbe M, Kaskel F. The mineral disorders in pediatrics. *Semin Nephrol.* 1998;18:280–294.
13. Council of Europe. *Lead, cadmium and mercury in food: assessment of dietary intakes and summary of heavy metal limits of foodstuffs. Health protection of the consumer.* Strasbourg: Council of Europe Press; 1994:9–21.

Clinical Presentation 40

1. Clissold RL, Hamilton AJ, Hattersley AT, et al. HNF1B-associated renal and extra-renal disease—an expanding clinical spectrum. *Nat Rev Nephrol.* 2015;11:102–112.
2. Verhave JC, Bech AP, Wetzels JFM, et al. Hepatocyte nuclear factor 1β-associated kidney disease: more than renal cysts and diabetes. *J Am Soc Nephrol.* 2016;27:345–353.
3. Horikawa Y. Maturity-onset diabetes of the young as a model for elucidating the multifactorial origin of type 2 diabetes mellitus. *J Diabetes Investig.* 2018;9:704–712.
4. Ishiwa S, Sato M, Morisada N, et al. Association between the clinical presentation of congenital anomalies of the kidney and urinary tract (CAKUT) and gene mutations: an analysis of 66 patients at a single institution. *Pediatr Nephrol.* 2019;34:1457–1464.
5. Nagano C, Morisada N, Nozu K, et al. Clinical characteristics of HNF1B-related disorders in a Japanese population. *Clin Exp Nephrol.* 2019;23:1119–1129.
6. Devuyst O, Olinger E, Weber S, et al. Autosomal dominant tubulointerstitial kidney disease. *Nat Rev Dis Prim.* 2019;5:1–20.
7. Faguer S, Chassaing N, Bandin F, et al. The HNF1B score is a simple tool to select patients for HNF1B gene analysis. *Kidney Int.* 2014;86:1007–1015.
8. Ayasreh Fierro N, Miquel Rodríguez R, Matamala Gaston A, Ars Criach E, Torra Balcells R. A review on autosomal dominant tubulointerstitial kidney disease. *Nefrologia.* 2017;37:235–243.
9. Connor TM, Hoer S, Mallett A, et al. Mutations in mitochondrial DNA causing tubulointerstitial kidney disease. *PLoS Genet.* 2017;13:1–17.
10. Casemayou A, Fournel A, Bagattin A, et al. Hepatocyte nuclear factor-1b controls mitochondrial respiration in renal tubular cells. *J Am Soc Nephrol.* 2017;28:3205–3217.

11. Faguer S, Decramer S, Chassaing N, et al. Diagnosis, management, and prognosis of HNF1B nephropathy in adulthood. *Kidney Int.* 2011;80:768–776.

Clinical Presentation 41

1. Appel GB, Kunis CL. Acute tubulo-interstitial nephritis. Idiopathic acute interstitial nephritis. In: Cotran RS, Brenner BM, Stein JH, eds. *Tubulo-interstitial Nephropathies.* New York, NY: Churchill Livingstone; 1983:176–178.
2. Heptinstall RH. Interstitial nephritis. In: Heptinstall RH, ed. *Pathology of the Kidney.* Boston: Little Brown; 1983:1149–1193.
3. Linton AL, Clark WF, Driedger AA, et al. Acute interstitial nephritis due to drugs. Review of the literature with a report of nine cases. *Ann Intern Med.* 1980;93:735–741.
4. Wilson DM, Turner DR, Cameron JS, et al. Value of renal biopsy in acute intrinsic renal failure. *Br Med J.* 1976;2:459–461.
5. Bender WL, Whelton A, Beschorner WE, et al. Interstitial nephritis, proteinuria, and renal failure caused by nonsteroidal anti-inflammatory drugs. *Am J Med.* 1984;76:1006–1012.
6. Burghard R, Brandis M, Hoyer PF, et al. Acute interstitial nephritis in childhood. *Eur J Pediatr.* 1984;142:103–110.
7. Chazan JA, Garella S, Esparza A. Acute interstitial nephritis. A distinct clinico-pathological entity? *Nephron.* 1972;9:10–26.
8. Dobrin RS, Vernier RL, Fish AJ. Acute eosinophilic interstitial nephritis and renal failure with bone marrow-lymph node granulomas and anterior uveitis. *Am J Med.* 1975;59:325–333.
9. Ellis D, Fried WA, Yunis EJ, et al. Acute interstitial nephritis in children: a report of 13 cases and review of the literature. *Pediatrics.* 1981;67:862–870.
10. Roth KS, Foreman JW, Segal S. The Fanconi syndrome and mechanisms of tubular transport dysfunction. *Kidney Int.* 1981;20:705–716.
11. Lee DBN, Drinkard JP, Rosen VN, et al. The adult Fanconi syndrome. Observations on etiology, morphology, renal function and mineral metabolism in three patients. *Medicine.* 1971;51:107–138.
12. Steele TH, Rieselbach RE. The contribution of residual nephrons within the chronically diseased kidney to urate homeostasis in man. *Am J Med.* 1967;43:876–886.
13. Laberke HG, Bohle A. Acute interstitial nephritis: correlations between clinical and morphological findings. *Clin Nephrol.* 1980;14:263–273.
14. Ooi BS, Jao W, First MR, et al. Acute interstitial nephritis. A clinical and pathologic study based on renal biopsies. *Am J Med.* 1975;59:614–629.
15. Hyun J, Galen MA. Acute interstitial nephritis. A case characterized by increase in serum IgG, IgM, and IgE concentrations. Eosinophilia, and IgE deposition in renal tubules. *Arch Intern Med.* 1981;141:679–681.
16. Kida H, Abe T, Tomosugi N, et al. Prediction of long term outcome in acute interstitial nephritis. *Clin Nephrol.* 1984;22:55–60.
17. Klassen J, Andres GA, Brennan JC, et al. An immunologic renal tubular lesion in man. *Clin Immunol Immunopathol.* 1972;10:69–83.
18. Laberke HG, Bohle A. Acute interstitial nephritis: correlations between clinical and morphological findings. *Clin Nephrol.* 1980;14:263–273.
19. Levy P, Guesry P, Loirat C. Immunologically mediated tubulo-interstitial nephritis in children. *Contrib Nephrol.* 1979;16:132–140.
20. Nakamoto Y, Kida H, Mizumura Y. Acute eosinophilic interstitial nephritis with bone marrow granulomas. *Clin Immunol Immunopathol.* 1979;14:379–383.
21. Pamukcu R, Moorthy AV, Singer JR, et al. Idiopathic acute interstitial nephritis: characterization of the infiltrating cells in the renal interstitium as T helper lymphocytes. *Am J Kidney Dis.* 1984;4:24–29.
22. Steinman TI, Silva P. Acute interstitial nephritis and iritis. Renal-ocular syndrome. *Am J Med.* 1984;77:189–191.
23. Frommer P, Vldall R, Fay Wp, Deveber GA. A case of acute interstitial nephritis successfully treated after delayed diagnosis. *Can Med Assoc J.* 1979;121:585–586, 591.
24. Wood BC, Sharma IN, Germann DR, et al. Gallium citrate Ga 67 imaging in noninfectious interstitial nephritis. *Arch Intern Med.* 1978;138:1665–1666.
25. Bergstein J, Litman N. Interstitial nephritis with antitubular-basement-membrane antibody. *N Engl J Med.* 1975;292:875–878.

CHAPTER 9

Urinary Tract Infection

Clinical Presentation 1

The backward flow of urine in patients with vesicoureteral reflux (VUR) makes which of the following conditions more likely to develop (select all that apply)?

A. Chronic kidney disease
B. Incontinence
C. Hydronephrosis
D. Urinary tract infections

The correct answers are A, C, and D
Comment: Vesicoureteral reflux makes UTIs more likely to occur. Kidney damage may also occur, leading to reflux nephropathy. High-grade reflux can cause hydronephrosis as well.[1]

Clinical Presentation 2

What percentage of children with a UTI will also have vesicoureteral reflux?

A. 5%
B. 10%
C. 20%
D. 40%

The correct answer is D

Clinical Presentation 3

What is the expected bladder capacity of a 3-year-old child?

A. 30 mL
B. 60 mL
C. 150 mL
D. 240 mL

The correct answer is C

Clinical Presentation 4

What grade of reflux is demonstrated with contrast refluxing into the proximal renal collecting system without dilatation?

A. Grade 1
B. Grade 2
C. Grade 3
D. Grade 4

The correct answer is B

Clinical Presentation 5

Reflux is typically seen during early filling of the bladder.

A. True
B. False

The correct answer is B

Clinical Presentation 6

A preliminary kidneys, ureters, and bladder film is not necessary in the voiding cystoureterogram (VCUG) examination because it results in unnecessary radiation.

A. False
B. True

The correct answer is A

Comment: Bladder capacity (ounces) = age (years) + 2 predicts normal bladder capacity.[1]

VUR, a congenital anomaly characterized by either a unilateral or bilateral reflux of urine from the bladder to the kidneys, is common in young children. Approximately 30% of children younger than 5 years of age with VUR are identified by routine voiding cystourethrogram after UTI, and 9% to 20% of prenatal hydronephrosis with VUR are detected postnatally. For most, VUR resolves spontaneously. About 20% to 30% will have further infections, and only a few will experience long-term renal sequelae.

It is well known that the severity of renal scarring is associated with the severity of VUR. Previous studies have identified that the older age of VUR diagnosis (≥5 years), higher grade of VUR, and higher number of UTIs were risk factors for renal scarring. Similarly, other studies showed a direct relationship between male sex, high-grade VUR, and renal dysplasia. Thus, efforts to prevent renal scarring should be directed toward a rapid diagnosis and treatment of VUR.

Few reports have focused on the prevalence and risk factors for deteriorating renal function associated with VUR. According to data from North American Pediatric Renal Trials, there is an estimate of 3.5% to 5.2% of children in renal replacement therapy because of VUR nephropathy.

In addition to the prevalence of chronic kidney disease (CKD) among VUR patients, findings regarding the predictive risk factors for the development and progression of CKD in children with VUR have been conflicting; furthermore, it is debated whether VUR is a benign or nonbenign condition. Grade V VUR, bilateral renal damage, and a delay in the diagnosis of VUR 12 months after UTI were independent predictors of CKD. The older the age, the higher the CKD stage and the history of UTI are significant risk factors for CKD progression in children with VUR.

Renal function deterioration tends to be inversely correlated with the increasing degree of VUR and bladder dysfunction.

Clinical Presentation 7

Which of the following statements is incorrect?

A. VUR is found in 35% of children who have a febrile UTI.
B. VUR by itself does not cause UTI and UTI does not cause reflux.

C. Patients with high-grade VUR might need to take antibiotics to prevent infection.
D. VUR is more common in girls than boys.
E. VUR will often disappear by 6 years of age.
F. VUR is often associated with costovertebral angle (CVA) tenderness and flank pain.

The correct answer is F

Comment: VUR is a condition in which urine flows backward from the bladder into the ureters during urination. VUR is found in 35% of children who have a UTI with fever. When children have recurrent UTIs, VUR is thought to increase the risk of kidney damage.

In most children, reflux is a birth defect caused by an abnormal attachment between the ureter and bladder with a short, ineffective valve. In some children, an infrequent urination pattern may cause reflux to occur. A child with VUR is more likely to develop a kidney infection, which can lead to kidney damage.

Because VUR does not cause pain, discomfort, or problems with urination, it is a silent abnormality that usually goes undetected unless there is a UTI. The average age of diagnosis is 2 to 3 years, and approximately 75% of children treated for reflux are girls.

Although surgery is sometimes required, reflux will often gradually disappear by age 5 or 6 years. Imaging studies can determine the grade of the VUR condition. High grades of VUR may require a daily low dose of an antibiotic, given, sometimes for several years, in hope of preventing recurrent UTIs and kidney damage.[1]

Clinical Presentation 8

A 2-year-old girl presents with bilateral VUR, discovered after a UTI 2 months ago.

What would you recommend?

A. Careful follow-up without antibiotics
B. Repair of the vesicoureteral reflux
C. Long-term antibiotic prophylaxis
D. Nonantibiotic probiotic prophylaxis

The correct answer is D

Comment: Febrile infants with UTIs should undergo renal and bladder ultrasonography to detect anatomic abnormalities that require further evaluation.

VCUG should not be performed routinely after the first febrile UTI; VCUG is indicated if renal bladder ultrasound (US) reveals hydronephrosis, scarring, or other findings that would suggest either high-grade VUR or obstructive uropathy, as well as in other atypical or complex clinical circumstances. Further evaluation should be conducted if there is a recurrence of febrile UTI.[1]

Probiotics are effective and safer than antibiotics at reducing the risk of recurrent UTI in children with a normal urinary tract after their first episode of febrile UTI.[2]

Clinical Presentation 9

A fetus has VUR if routine prenatal ultrasonography shows which of the following in the fetus?

A. Dilated ureter
B. Hydroureteronephrosis
C. Distended bladder
D. Urine leaking into amniotic fluid

The correct answers are A and B

Comment: The presence of hydronephrosis is highly suspicious of either ureteropelvic junction, obstruction, hydrometer, or VUR.[1]

Clinical Presentation 10

An 18-year-old female presents to her primary care physician with a report of urinating more frequently and pain with urination. She denies blood in her urine, fevers, chills, flank pain, and vaginal discharge. She reports having experienced similar symptoms a few years ago and that they went away after a course of antibiotics. The patient has no other past medical problems.

Pertinent history reveals she has been sexually active with her boyfriend for the past 4 months and uses condoms for contraception. She reports two lifetime partners and no past pregnancies or sexually transmitted diseases. Her last menstrual period was 1 week ago.

On physical examination, the patient is afebrile, normotensive, and nontachycardic. She appears well on observation. She has a soft, nondistended abdomen with normoactive bowel sounds. On palpation, she has moderate discomfort in her suprapubic region but no CVA tenderness. A pelvic examination is normal with no evidence of abnormal vaginal or cervical discharge or inflammation.

Which diagnosis is most likely and why?

A. Acute cystitis
B. Vaginitis
C. Cervicitis
D. UTI
E. Acute pyelonephritis

The correct answers are A and D

Comment: The most likely diagnosis in this patient is a UTI, specifically, acute cystitis. Classic UTI symptoms include urinary frequency urgency and dysuria. Other complaints could include suprapubic pain or discomfort, hesitancy, nocturia, and even gross hematuria. Urinary tract infections are classified by the anatomical location in which the infection and inflammation occur. Risk factors that this patient possesses, which will be discussed later, are female sex, age, recent sexual activity, and a history of prior UTI, which we can infer from her report of previous similar symptoms.[1]

Vaginitis and cervicitis should also be considered in this patient given her history of sexual activity. However, the patient has no reported vaginal discharge or signs of these infections on the pelvic examination. Another important diagnosis to consider is pyelonephritis, which involves infection of the upper urinary tract. This is also not likely given her lack of fever, flank pain, and other key symptoms which will be discussed in a later section.

Clinical Presentation 11

Which populations age are at higher risk of contracting a UTI and why?

A. Postmenopausal age
B. Female gender
C. Sexual activity
D. All of the above

The correct answer is D

Comment: Urinary tract infections are due to the colonization of the urinary tract by microbes. Certain populations are at higher risk of infections of the urinary tract. Women are among those most affected by UTIs, with a lifetime incidence rate of almost 50%. The difference between the sexes is attributed to women's shorter urethral length. Women who are sexually active are also at risk of UTI because of the proximity of the urethral meatus to the flora-rich anus. If the patient is a premenopausal, otherwise healthy, and nongravid female, as in this case, she has developed an "uncomplicated" infection.

Patients who are predisposed to conditions that make colonization more likely or are exposed to microbes that are more facile in evading the body's natural protective mechanisms are more apt to contract UTIs, and their infections can be more difficult to treat. These patients have "complicated" infections. Numerous conditions make a patient more susceptible to UTI. These include underlying medical problems or structural abnormalities of the urinary tract such as urinary obstruction, vesicoureteral reflux, underlying urinary tract disease, diabetes, renal papillary necrosis, immunosuppression (medically induced or as a result of HIV infection), treatment with antibiotics, pregnancy, menopause, and spinal cord injuries.

The elderly are also at increased risk of UTI, particularly men, many of whom develop obstructive uropathy from benign prostatic hypertrophy.[1]

Clinical Presentation 12

Which of the following statement(s) is (are) most appropriate for catheter-associated UTI (CAUTI)?

A. Patients should have signs and symptoms of UTI.
B. Culture of the patient's urine sample should yield greater than 10,000 colony-forming units (CFU)/mL.
C. Culture of the patient's urine sample should yield greater than 100,000 CFU/mL.
D. Patients who are catheterized are at increased risk of infection with fungal organisms as well as bacterial infections.

The correct answers are A, B, and D

Comment: According to the Infectious Diseases Society of America, both clinical and laboratory criteria should be met to make the diagnosis of a CAUTI. The patient should have signs or symptoms of a UTI and no other known source of infection. Culture of the patient's urine sample should yield greater than 103 CFU/mL of at least one species of bacteria. The cultured urine should be from a single specimen in those patients who are still catheterized. CAUTI can also be diagnosed in those who have had a catheter removed within the preceding 48 hours, in which case a midstream voided urine is the appropriate specimen.

CAUTIs are a type of complicated UTI and are among the most common nosocomial (hospital-acquired) infections in the United States. Urinary catheters facilitate the ascent of microbes into the urinary tract. There are different methods of catheterization: for example, clean intermittent catheterization, indwelling urethral catheters, and suprapubic catheters. Microorganisms can be introduced during the procedure of catheterization despite implementing sterilization methods. Also, without appropriate catheter care, these indwelling devices can become a nidus for infection, permitting various other flora to travel along the tube and into the urinary tract.

Escherichia coli is the most common causative organism of acute cystitis in uncomplicated UTIs. It is also the most commonly isolated organism in CAUTI. However, patients with catheters are at higher risk of infection by organisms less commonly seen in noncatheterized patients. Patients who are catheterized for both short and long periods are at increased risk of infection with fungal organisms as well as Enterobacteriaceae such as *Klebsiella*, *Serratia*, *Enterobacter*, *Pseudomonas*, *Enterococcus*, and *Proteus* species. These organisms are exceptionally well adapted for invasion given the ability many of them possess to form biofilms. The longer a patient is catheterized, the more likely they are to develop bacteriuria, a symptomatic infection, and potentially colonization of the urinary tract. Thus, timely removal of catheters when no longer necessary is wise.[1]

Clinical Presentation 13

Which laboratory studies should be performed initially to evaluate a potential UTI (select all that apply)?

A. Urine dipstick
B. Urinalysis with microscopy
C. Urine culture and gram stain with sensitivity testing
D. Voiding cystourethrogram
E. Kidney and bladder US

The correct answers are A, B, and C

Comment: Laboratory tools are commonly used in the investigation of UTIs for patients with a complicated UTI, recurrent infections, or an unclear diagnosis based purely on history and physical examination. Again, test results should always be correlated with clinical findings because false-positive or false-negative results can occur through multiple avenues. Available tests include a urine dipstick, urinalysis with microscopy, and culture and gram stain with sensitivity testing. The first two of these have the potential to be performed in physicians' offices. A clean-catch midstream specimen should be submitted to avoid contamination from vaginal or penile microorganisms. Patients should be given a 2% castile soap towelette and instructed in appropriate specimen collection. Men should cleanse the glans, retracting the foreskin first if uncircumcised. Women should cleanse the periurethral area after spreading the labia. Identification of lactobacilli and epithelial cells from the vagina suggest contamination.

General features of the urine can first be examined to include the color, clarity, and odor; but these features are nonspecific. For example, cloudy urine can be caused by the presence of white blood cells (WBCs) and/or bacteria in a UTI, but it can also be caused by numerous other pathologic and nonpathologic substances.

Urine dipstick studies, primarily searching for leukocyte esterase and nitrites, are useful when the pretest probability of UTI is high. Leukocyte esterase is an enzyme possessed by WBCs; thus, a positive urine dipstick for leukocyte esterase indicates the presence of inflammatory cells in the patient's urinary tract. Inflammatory cells in the urine are not specific for a UTI because leukocytes can also be present in other situations such as glomerulonephritis and vaginal contamination. Nitrite is a breakdown product of nitrates, which are normally found in a healthy patient's urine. The dipstick test for nitrite is specific for gram-negative organisms that possess an enzyme enabling them to reduce nitrates. It follows, then, that this test is less useful in the setting of potential gram-positive microbe infection. Also notable is that the nitrite test can be falsely negative in a patient with abundant fluid intake and frequent urination.[1] Multiple other factors including medications, diet, and specimen handling can affect urine dipstick results, such as inappropriate handling or expiration of test strips.

Urinalysis with microscopy provides a window into the kidney and urinary tract. The presence of red blood cells, WBCs, casts, crystals, and bacteria aid in many diagnoses. Specific to UTI, the presence of WBCs and red blood cells indicates inflammation and, potentially, infection in the urinary tract. Pyuria, the presence of leukocytes in the urine, is not specific to UTIs as noted previously, but the absence of leukocytes should cause one to question a diagnosis of UTI unless the culture is positive. The identification of crystals might suggest the presence of renal calculi, which can serve as a nidus for infection. In fact, some stones (e.g., struvite) are the direct result of infection with urea-splitting organisms. Overall, urinalysis is useful; however, the clinical history still plays a key role to avoid under- and overdiagnosis.

Urine culture is the gold-standard diagnostic tool for diagnosing UTIs. As stated previously, in patients with a convincing clinical history and physical examination consistent with uncomplicated cystitis, no culture is necessary. However, in patients with complicated, severe upper urinary tract, or recurrent, UTIs, urine culture should not be foregone, because it is necessary for determining the causative organism and, consequently, for guiding appropriate therapeutic intervention. Furthermore, growth of the organism in culture facilitates sensitivity studies, in which pharmacologic agents are tested on the microbe isolated from the patient. This testing provides medical personnel with information regarding the efficacy of potential therapeutic options in the form of minimal inhibitory concentrations. This information guides the narrowing of antibiotic choice from whichever broad-spectrum treatment was initiated when a UTI was first suspected. Some organisms such as *Ureaplasma* may not be grown on routine cultures, so a false-negative result is possible. False-positive results are rare, other than from contamination, which should be suspected in most cases with the growth of multiple types of bacteria or vaginal flora.[1]

Clinical Presentation 14

When should a diagnosis of pyelonephritis be suspected (select all that apply)?

A. Fever, chills
B. Flank pain
C. Voiding dysfunction
D. Hypotension, tachycardia, and tachypnea

The correct answers are A, B, C, and D
Comment: Infection of the kidney is termed *pyelonephritis*. These patients tend to present acutely with "upper tract signs," including fever, chills, flank pain, and CVA tenderness. Symptoms of lower UTI can also be present; however, this is not usually the case. The clinical presentation may vary and can be life-threatening. In the most severely ill, patients may present in septic shock, with hypotension, tachycardia, and tachypnea, especially when infected with a gram-negative organism.[1]

Clinical Presentation 15

Which of the following are the potential complications of UTIs (select all that apply)?

A. Acute kidney injury
B. CKD
C. Septic shock
D. Perinephric abscess
E. Kidney stones

The correct answers are A, B, C, D, and E
Comment: Urinary tract infections can be complicated by several conditions depending on the severity and chronicity of the infection and the implicated organism. Severe upper UTIs can lead to acute kidney injury and, if not treated, can lead to permanent kidney damage and fibrosis. Similarly, upper UTIs can be complicated by renal or perinephric abscesses. Renal abscesses are mostly found in patients with preexisting kidney disease. Patients infected by a urea-splitting organism are at risk of struvite stones, which are commonly found in the upper urinary tract.[1]

Clinical Presentation 16

Which of the following antibiotics are appropriate to give patients with UTI (select all that apply)?

A. Nitrofurantoin monohydrate
B. Trimethoprim-sulfamethoxazole
C. Trimethoprim
D. Fesfomycin
E. Pivmecillinam

The correct answers are A, B, C, D, and E

Comment: The choice of therapy for a UTI depends on the clinical treatment setting and whether it is a complicated or uncomplicated UTI. An optimal outpatient antibiotic can be taken orally, has a tolerable side effect profile, and is concentrated to a therapeutic level in the patient's urine. Antibiotics that fit this profile are appropriate to give patients who have a low risk for infection with a multidrug-resistant strain. Options for therapy include nitrofurantoin monohydrate, trimethoprim-sulfamethoxazole, fosfomycin, and pivmecillinam.

Recent infectious disease guidelines reflect growing concern for infection with multidrug-resistant organisms. When therapy needs to be escalated because of infection with a multidrug-resistant organism or tissue-invasive disease with bacteremia, options remain for oral therapy. In these situations, it is advantageous to obtain urine culture and microbe antibiotic sensitivities to better eliminate the infection. If hospitalization is indicated and the patient requires parenteral antibiotics, empiric therapy should be initiated. After microorganism sensitivities return, antibiotic therapy can be narrowed to one of the following: a carbapenem, third-generation cephalosporin, fluoroquinolone, ampicillin, or gentamicin.

Pharmacotherapy for complicated UTIs should begin with broad-spectrum therapy and then be narrowed by sensitivities when possible.[1] The grouping that places the patient in the "complicated" category plays a role in treatment selection. For example, UTIs in men typically involve the prostate as well as the bladder, so treatment should target the infection in both organs. Patients who are pregnant require antibiotics that are safe for the fetus. Some complicated UTIs, especially in the case of upper UTIs, are managed in an inpatient setting with intravenous antibiotics because of the presence of tissue-invasive disease or bacteremia. In this case, the concentrations of antibiotic in the blood and the urine are important. This differs from the treatment of uncomplicated UTIs, which are dependent on the concentration of the pharmacotherapeutic agent in the urine.

Potential correction of modifiable risk factors for UTIs, if present, can also be addressed to prevent recurrent infection. This may include correction of an anatomic or structural abnormality of the urinary tract, consideration of alternative birth control types in a woman who uses a diaphragm with spermicide, removing a urinary catheter, or simply counseling a woman to attempt urination after sexual intercourse.[1]

Clinical Presentation 17

Which microorganisms most commonly cause acute cystitis (select all that apply)?

A. *E. coli*
B. *Staphylococcus saprophyticus*
C. Group B *Streptococcus*
D. *Klebsiella*

The correct answers are A, B, C, and D

Comment: In general, gram-negative aerobic rods are the most commonly isolated pathogens implicated in UTIs. *Escherichia coli* is the most common causative organism of UTIs, especially in sexually active young women. Microorganisms such as uropathogenic *E. coli* with an enhanced ability to bind and to adhere to urinary tract epithelia are more capable of causing infection. Adhesins and pili resistant to the innate immune mechanisms of defense are among the advantageous traits that particularly virulent strains of uropathogenic *E. coli* possess.

A variety of other Enterobacteriaceae are also found in the setting of CAUTIs. However, gram-positive organisms are clinically significant in some settings. *Staphylococcus saprophyticus* is not infrequently implicated in uncomplicated UTIs in young, sexually active women. Group B *Streptococcus* (*Streptococcus agalactiae*) is of particular concern in pregnant patients. In one prospective study, Group B *Streptococcus* was the second most isolated pathogen behind *E. coli* in the urine of asymptomatic bacteriuric pregnant women. Screening pregnant women for asymptomatic bacteriuria plays an important role in decreasing the risk of pyelonephritis during pregnancy.[1]

Clinical Presentation 18

What is asymptomatic bacteriuria?

A. Positive urine culture $<10^5$ CFU/mL
B. Positive urine culture $\geq 10^5$ CFU/mL
C. Dysuria and frequency
D. Bedtime wetting

The correct answer is B

Comment: The diagnosis of asymptomatic bacteriuria requires two criteria: (1) the urine is culture-positive; and (2) the patient does not have symptoms or signs of a UTI. The level of bacteria in culture should reach ≥105 CFU/mL, although it can be lower in catheterized patients (≥102 CFU/mL). Asymptomatic bacteriuria is only treated in some groups of patients, including those who are pregnant or undergoing urologic procedures because it otherwise does not correlate with symptomatic disease or complications.[1]

Clinical Presentation 19

A 19-year-old woman undergoes consultation for recurrent symptomatic lower UTI. She has increased frequency over the past 3 years to a rate of about two times per night. She has been unable to relate onset to any specific activity. Symptoms resolve quickly with initiation of prescribed antibiotics. She is otherwise well.

Which of the following is the most appropriate management?

A. Daily cranberry tablets
B. Daily D-mannose supplementation
C. Nightly prophylaxis with low-dose ciprofloxacin
D. Self-treatment with nitrofurantoin
E. Urination immediately after sexual intercourse

The correct answer is D

Comment: Self-treatment of each infection with nitrofurantoin is appropriate for this patient (option D). One-quarter to one-third of women who recover from an episode of cystitis will develop another symptomatic infection within 6 months. Recurrent infections that return within 2 weeks of finishing appropriate antibiotic therapy for uncomplicated cystitis and involve the same cultured bacteria are categorized as relapsed.

Recurrent UTIs occurring weeks after successful antibiotic treatment and often involving bacterial strains different from the original are termed *reinfections*. This type of recurrent UTI is defined by three culture-positive infections in the previous 12 months or two infections within 6 months. Contributing factors for reinfection in premenopausal women include sexual activity, diaphragm and spermicide use, delayed urinary habits, and douching. Diminished estrogen levels and, to a lesser extent, increases in residual bladder urine volume and incontinence play much larger roles in UTIs in postmenopausal women. Episodic self-diagnosis and treatment with a first-line, short-course regimen such as nitrofurantoin is an appropriate initial strategy. Single-dose postcoital antibiotics are effective in reducing bladder infections if infection is temporally related to coitus; avoidance of spermicides has also proven beneficial.

Anecdotal claims of the benefits of ingestion of daily cranberry juice or tablets (option A), presumably by inhibiting the adherence of *E. coli* to uroepithelial cells, lack randomized clinical trial confirmation.

Adhesion blockers such as D-mannose (option B), theorized to block *E. coli* adhesion to mannosylated uroepithelial receptors, have not been tested in clinical trials.

Antimicrobial prophylaxis should be reserved for women with frequent recurrent cystitis, defined as three or more infections within 12 months that have not lessened after attempts using nonantimicrobial strategies.

Placebo-controlled trials using nightly doses of antibiotics demonstrated an approximate 95% reduction in infection recurrence. A 6-month trial is recommended; however, the previous pattern of recurrent infection occurs in nearly 50% of women when antibiotic prophylaxis is discontinued. Preferred prophylactic regimens include nitrofurantoin (50–100 mg), trimethoprim-sulfamethoxazole (single strength), and cephalexin (125–250 mg). Ciprofloxacin (option C) or other fluoroquinolone antibiotics are no longer recommended because of long-term safety concerns.

Urination soon after sexual intercourse (option E) is often recommended but is an unproven strategy to prevent recurrent UTI.[1]

Clinical Presentation 20

In teenagers, urethritis occurs when organisms that gain access to the urethra acutely or chronically colonize the structures of the urethra. This infection can be associated with sexually transmitted pathogens.

Which of the following pathogens is most common in this scenario?

A. E. coli
B. *Chlamydia trachomatis*
C. *Lactobacillus* species
D. *Helicobacter pylori*

The correct answer is B
Comment: Options A, C, and D are commonly associated with other types of infections.[1]

Clinical Presentation 21

CAUTIs account for more than 80% of all intensive care patients treated with an indwelling urinary tract catheter during their hospital stay.

Because of the high incidence rate of morbidity and mortality, urinary catheterization should be avoided unless there is a medical necessity, and when no longer necessary, the catheter should be removed immediately. Medical indications for urinary catheter placement include bladder outlet obstruction, acute urinary retention, neurogenic bladder, following pelvic surgery, patients with diabetes mellitus, malnutrition, CKD, and immune deficiency who are at higher risk for CAUTIs.

Which of the following preventive measures should be avoided in patients with an indwelling urinary catheter in place?

A. Antibiotic prophylaxis
B. Urethral cleaning with povidone-iodine solution or soap and water
C. Use of antibiotic-coated catheter
D. Maintaining unobstructed urine flow and closed sterile drainage system
E. Daily catheter irrigation with normal saline or antibiotic-containing-containing solution

The correct answer is D

Comment: Maintaining a sterile, closed unobstructed urinary drainage should be used with indwelling catheters. The indwelling catheter and collecting system should not be disconnected. Breaking the collecting system to obtain urine specimens for analysis and bacterial culture should be avoided. To obtain urine specimens, the sampling port for the urine collection must be used (option D is correct).

Most studies suggest that antimicrobial prophylaxis is not useful in the prevention of CAUTIs in asymptomatic patients (option A is incorrect).

Urethral cleaning with povidone-iodine solution or soap and water has not been shown to prevent CAUTIs. There is evidence that frequent urethral cleaning can lead to mucosal irritation and breakdown that may increase the risk of infection (option B is incorrect).[1]

Antibiotic-coated catheter has not been shown to decrease CAUTIs and should be used as a routine prevention measure (option C is incorrect). Routine irrigation with normal saline or antibiotic-containing solution should be avoided unless obstruction is suspected (option E is incorrect).[1]

Clinical Presentation 22

A previously healthy 4-month-old male infant presents to the emergency department with decreased oral intake, increased fussiness, and fever. His parents state that he has not been taking feeds well for the past 2 days and has a decreased number of wet diapers daily. He has had no vomiting. Temperature at home was 101.4°F rectally this morning. He has become increasingly more irritable and seems to cry each time he urinates. The parents have not noticed any blood in the urine or on the diaper. Physical examination reveals heart rate of 155 beats/min, blood pressure 90/50 mm Hg, sunken anterior fontanel, and sticky oral mucous membranes. Blood cultures and a catheterized urine specimen are obtained for culture. Urinalysis reveals the presence of leukocyte esterase and nitrites. Microscopic urine evaluation shows greater than 50 WBC/high-power field (HPF). You diagnose a UTI complicated with dehydration and admit the patient for intravenous fluid and antibiotic therapy.

After initiation of therapy, the patient's clinical condition rapidly improves. Urine culture shows greater than 100,000 CFU of *E. coli*. Renal US is normal. A repeat urine culture after 10 days of appropriate antibiotic therapy was sterile, after initiating appropriate antibiotic therapy.

What is the *most* appropriate next step in the management of this patient?

A. VCUG to evaluate for VUR along with initiation of oral prophylactic antibiotic therapy.
B. Reassure the patient's parents that this is unlikely to occur again; observe without further surveillance testing.
C. Reassure the patient's parents and order repeat urine cultures monthly as surveillance for a recurrent UTI.
D. Start prophylactic oral antibiotics until a dimercaptosuccinic acid (DMSA) renal scan is obtained.

E. Start nonantibiotic prophylactic therapy with probiotics and instruct the patient's parent that if fever, irritability, poor feeding, vomiting, or diarrhea occurs again, there would be need for further surveillance testing.
F. Urology referral for cystoscopy to evaluate for urinary tract obstruction along with initiation of oral prophylactic antibiotic therapy.

The correct answer is E

Comment: In 2016, the American Academy of Pediatrics (AAP) reaffirmed its 2011 UTI clinical practice guideline and recommended that VCUG should not be performed routinely after the first febrile UTI and indicated that VCUG is warranted if renal US reveals hydronephrosis, scarring, or other findings that would suggest either high-grade VUR or obstructive uropathy.

Furthermore, AAP recommended that antimicrobial prophylaxis should not be given to children aged 2 to 24 months after their first febrile UTI if the results of renal and bladder ultrasonography are normal. According to the AAP guidelines, the use of routine antibiotic prophylaxis seems to be ineffective in preventing the recurrence of febrile UTI and also it promotes the growth of bacterial-resistant microorganisms.

The high recurrent UTI rates in infants and young children increase the potential risk for the development of bacterial resistance, as has been reported in a recent randomized controlled clinical trial.[1]

The study results concluded that probiotic compared to no treatment (placebo) was more effective in preventing UTI recurrence after the first febrile UTI in young children with normal urinary tract system (option E).[2]

Clinical Presentation 23

How would your answer change if hydronephrosis were found on US?

A. Start prophylactic antibiotic therapy.
B. Follow-up serum creatinine level
C. Order cystoscopy.
D. Annual renal US

The correct answer is A

Comment: UTI associated with urinary upper tract dilatation should be given prophylactic antibiotics and undergo further imaging studies including a diuretic renogram or VCUG if clinically indicated.[1]

Clinical Presentation 24

Which of the following statements is true regarding acute uncomplicated UTI (select all that apply)?

A. Acute uncomplicated cystitis rarely progresses to severe disease, even if untreated; thus, the primary goal of treatment is to ameliorate symptoms.
B. Ecologic adverse effects of an antimicrobial agent (selection for antimicrobial-resistant organisms) should be considered along with efficacy in selecting antimicrobial therapy.
C. With respect to both ecologic adverse effects and efficacy, nitrofurantoin, trimethoprim-sulfamethoxazole, fosfomycin, and pivmecillinam are considered first-line agents for cystitis, even though there are concerns about increasing resistance (trimethoprim-sulfamethoxazole) and suboptimal efficacy (of fosfomycin and pivmecillinam).
D. Recurrent cystitis should be managed with prophylactic antimicrobial therapy only when nonantimicrobial preventive strategies are not effective.
E. Fluoroquinolones have other important indications and thus should be considered second-line agents for cystitis, but they are the drugs of choice for empirical treatment of pyelonephritis.

The correct answers are A, B, C, D, and E

Comment: Acute UTIs are relatively common in children. The most common pathogen is *E. coli*, accounting for approximately 85% of UTIs in children. Renal parenchymal defects are present in 3% to 15% of children within 1 to 2 years of their first diagnosed UTI. Clinical signs and symptoms of a UTI depend on the age of the child, but all febrile children aged 2 to 24 months with no obvious cause of infection should be evaluated for UTI (with the exception of circumcised boys older than 12 months). Evaluation of older children may depend on the clinical presentation and symptoms that point toward a urinary source (e.g., leukocyte esterase or nitrite present on dipstick testing; pyuria of at least 10 WBCs per HPF and bacteriuria on microscopy). Increased rates of *E. coli* resistance have made amoxicillin a less acceptable choice for treatment, and studies have found higher cure rates with trimethoprim-sulfamethoxazole. Other treatment options include amoxicillin-clavulanate and cephalosporins. Prophylactic antibiotics do not reduce the risk of subsequent UTIs, even in children with mild to moderate vesicoureteral reflux. Constipation should be avoided to help prevent UTIs. Ultrasonography, cystography, and a renal cortical scan should be considered in children with UTIs. Options A, B, C, D, and E are in agreement with the AAP's Clinical Practice Guideline.[1,2]

Clinical Presentation 25

A 15-year-old male presented with a 3-day history of dysuria, urinary frequency, hesitancy, dribbling of urine, and transient hematuria. He denied fever, chills, nausea, vomiting, scrotal pain, or back pain. He is not sexually active. Urine dipstick test results were positive for leukocyte esterase and nitrates. The patient was prescribed a 7-day course of nitrofurantoin empirically for suspected cystitis. In 24 hours, urine culture results were positive for *E. coli*, susceptible to all tested antimicrobial agents. The patient's symptoms resolved in a few days.

In addition to antibiotic therapy, what would be the best next course of action?

A. Kidney and bladder sonography
B. VCUG
C. Diuretic renogram
D. Cystoscopy

The correct answer is A

Comment: UTI in men without an indwelling urethral catheter is uncommon. Once a male patient is confirmed to have a first UTI, evaluation of the upper and lower urinary tract is recommended given the high prevalence of urologic abnormalities among men who present with a UTI. Residual urine volume should be assessed by means of noninvasive ultrasonography. Although there is no clear cutoff, a residual volume exceeding 100 mL raises suspicion for a urinary tract obstruction distal to the bladder.

Either computed tomography with intravenous contrast or ultrasonography is the diagnostic modality of choice in evaluating the anatomy of the urogenital tract. These investigations are especially high yield in febrile UTI cases.[1,2]

Clinical Presentation 26

A 17-month-old female presents with 5 days of crying with voids, lower abdominal tenderness, increased urinary frequency, pink urine, and fever to 38.3°C.

Pre- and postnatal medical and prenatal kidney abnormalities are unremarkable. Family history of urogenital anomalies and urologic conditions is negative.

A clean catch showed leukocyte esterase, nitrites, blood, specific gravity 1.025, pH 8; microscopy confirms 50 to 100 WBC/HPF and bacteria. A catheterized urine sample is sent for culture. You initiate amoxicillin while awaiting for the culture. There was no clinical improvement after 24 hours on amoxicillin. The culture returns, and you need to change amoxicillin due to resistant *E. coli*. You choose first-generation cephalosporin while waiting for culture antibiogram and sensitivity for local pathogens.

What should you do next?

A. Renal-bladder US
B. Voiding cystoureterogram
C. DMSA renal scan
D. Intravenous pyelogram

The correct answer is A

Comment: According to the AAP, renal-bladder US is mandated for screening after the first febrile UTI. Voiding cystourethrogram should be obtained if screening US demonstrates collecting system dilatation or renal parenchymal abnormality, or if second febrile UTI occurs. A renal DMSA nuclear scan should be obtained either acutely or within 3 months if screening US shows cortical thickening and irregularities or if a second febrile UTI occurs. A DMSA nuclear scan will indicate upper tract involvement by photopenic areas, which may become areas of permanent scar or may return to normal by the 3 months.

A clean-catch urine test positive for leukocyte esterase, nitrites, blood, and containing 50 to 100 WBC/HPF and bacteria under microscopic examination should be considered highly suspicious of bacterial infection and warrant imperative intravenous antibiotic therapy.

Ideally, there is a need to obtain a catheterized sample for culture, so that there would be no question about the diagnosis because of significant implications for the child/workup.

If unable to catheterize, send the sample for culture. In any case, >50,000 CFU/mL of a single pathogen confirms the diagnosis of pyelonephritis.

Most community UTIs are *E. coli*, but about half may be resistant to ampicillin/amoxicillin. Therefore, you could choose first-generation cephalosporin or trimethoprim-sulfamethoxazole; adjust after culture/sensitivity.

Consider the patient's age and ability to clear the antibiotic (e.g., renal, hepatic function) when selecting a medication. Consult institutional antibiogram for local pathogens and antibiotic coverage.

Await culture (48–72 hours to result). Support symptom amelioration with analgesics, increased fluids, and antipyretics.

Repeat culture or urinalysis for test of cure is not indicated in the absence of persistent symptoms.

If a structural abnormality is suspected or found on US, you may want to proceed to VCUG. If VUR is detected and US demonstrates upper tract dilation, initiate prophylactic antibiotics. However, avoid using prophylactic antibiotics in a child with the first febrile UTI with normal kidney-bladder US. In this situation, consider a nonantibiotic, probiotic therapy.

In older children, check for functional bladder or bowel dysfunction and aggressively work on correcting constipation, elimination avoidance behaviors, and hydration. Failure to correct will lead to continued risk of UTI, no matter what else may be wrong.[1,2]

Clinical Presentation 27

A 14-year-old male who underwent orthotopic heart transplant 2 years ago is admitted for an elective percutaneous endoscopic gastrostomy (PEG) tube placement. Medical history is significant for respiratory failure resulting from H1N1 influenza pneumonia from tracheostomy and ventilator dependency, end-stage renal disease on hemodialysis three times/week, and hypertension.

A left internal jugular tunneled catheter has been in place for dialysis and a condom catheter was present, draining clear amber urine.

The patient was taken to the operating room for elective placement of the PEG tube and tolerated the procedure well. He was transferred to the surgical intensive care unit because of his ventilator requirement.

His temperature was an icy 37.2°C. Lungs were clear bilaterally And the PEG site was oozing serosanguinous drainage.

A stool specimen collected for abdominal pain and diarrhea and was positive for *Clostridium difficile*, and metronidazole was started.

Eighteen hours postoperatively, the patient had a temperature of 38.3°C. The PEG site is clean and dry. There is no evidence of inflammation or drainage at the left IJ tunneled catheter site, and lungs are clear bilaterally. Blood, urine, and sputum cultures are sent.

The urinalysis is reported as 3+ leukocyte esterase, WBC too numerous to count, and moderate bacteria. The patient continues with fever to 38°C. Co-trimoxazole is started, and the patient receives hemodialysis.

On day 2 after surgery, urine culture reported as positive for 60,000 CFU/mL gram-negative bacilli, which are subsequently identified as *Providencia stuartii*. Blood and sputum cultures are negative. Peripheral WBC is 25,000. Computed tomography of the abdomen is suggestive of colitis and the patient continues to have a temperature of 38°C.

Blood cultures are repeated and reported as positive for gram-negative bacilli, which are subsequently identified as *P. stuartii*.

Does the patient have a CAUTI?

A. No, there were no symptoms present, so the patient does not have a CAUTI.
B. Yes, this is a CAUTI.
C. No, the patient was not catheterized.

The correct answer is C

Comment: Although the patient meets the criteria for a UTI, it is not a CAUTI because no indwelling catheter was present in the 48 hours before the infection. An indwelling catheter is defined as a "drainage tube that is inserted into the urinary bladder through the urethra." A condom catheter does not meet this definition.[1,2]

Clinical Presentation 28

An 18-year-old woman just back from her honeymoon has urinary frequency, urgency, painful voiding of small volumes of urine, and lower abdominal pain. Urine culture was positive (100,000 colonies for *E. coli*). Her blood pressure, kidney US, and renal functions are normal.

What is the most likely diagnosis?

A. Uncomplicated UTI
B. UTI from urinary tract obstruction
C. Asymptomatic bacteriuria
D. Early pregnancy

The correct answer is A

Complicated UTI is defined as when the infection is associated with obstructive hydronephrosis, hypertension, impaired renal function, or vesicoureteral reflux.[1]

Clinical Presentation 29

A 4-year-old White female presents in the pediatric clinic with complaints of urinary urgency and foul-smelling urine. Her mother describes symptoms of rushing to the bathroom and minor urine leakage during the day over the past 48 hours. She also wet the bed the past two nights. She does not complain of pain with urination, and there has been no fever.

Her mother reports her concern regarding multiple UTIs over the past year. One infection was associated with fever, flank pain, and vomiting. The mother is very frustrated that this continues to be a problem.

She also reports that her daughter voids infrequently; she sometimes goes up to 2 hours after awakening in the morning before she urinates. During the day, she holds it until the last minute, and sometimes they see her squatting or crossing her legs to avoid going to the bathroom. She has occasional damp spots in her underwear during the day but is typically dry at night; during infections, she has accidents both day and night. Her first infection was approximately 9 to 10 months ago. A clean-catch midstream specimen grew 100,000 *E. coli*. She did not have a fever, flank pain, nausea, or vomiting. The mother had taken the child to a clinic because of the incontinence. She was treated with amoxicillin, and her symptoms resolved. Six weeks later, the mother noticed she had an episode of nocturnal enuresis. At that time, a repeat culture was done, which grew less than 50,000 *E. coli*. She was treated again, but still had occasional day accidents.

Mom reports the daughter's bowel movements are infrequent and hard to pass. She has stool streaks in her underwear.

Approximately 2 months before this clinic visit, the patient was seen in the local emergency department with a fever of 102°F. She complained of generalized abdominal pain, nausea, and a headache. She vomited several times. She was started on antibiotics and treated as an outpatient. Her urine culture grew greater than 100,000 *Klebsiella pneumoniae*.

The mother had a history of urinary tract infections as a child but does not recall being evaluated.

On physical examination you find the patient has no specific abnormalities. Her abdomen is soft and nontender; there is no evidence of a mass. Stool is palpable in the right lower quadrant. She denies CVA tenderness. You palpate her lower spine and it is normal. There is no visual evidence of any abnormality, no sacral dimple, discolorations, asymmetry, or hair patch. Her feet are not high-arched and her toes are straight. She has no complaints of back pain, lower extremity pain, or weakness. She has full range of motion and ambulates with a normal gait. The external genitalia yield separate urethral and vaginal openings; the perineum is normal aside from some minor irritation. Her vital signs are within normal limits. She is afebrile.

Patient urinalysis is both leukocyte and nitrite positive and was sent to the laboratory for culture and sensitivity.

What is your differential diagnosis (select all that apply)?

A. Urinary tract infection
B. Cystitis
C. External perineal irritation
D. External elimination syndrome
E. Pinworms
F. Renal calculi
G. Hypercalciuria
H. Constipation
I. Vesicoureteral reflux or bladder outlet obstruction.

The correct answers are A, D, and I

Comment: History and physical findings are consistent with the diagnoses of a UTI and dysfunctional elimination syndrome. The urinalysis is both leukocyte and nitrite positive.

How a specimen is collected directly correlates to its validity: the most valid is suprapubic bladder aspirate, the second is sterile urethral catheterization, and the third is clean-catch midstream. The least reliable is the bagged specimen.[1]

The patient has no known allergies. She has delayed voiding, posturing to prevent enuresis, and constipation, which are symptoms consistent with dysfunctional elimination syndrome. There is one documented upper UTI with fever, nausea, and vomiting. Pyelonephritis may be indicative of structural abnormality and warrants additional evaluation. Structural abnormalities such as VUR, obstruction, or other anatomical defects may present as UTIs.

In children, it is important to discover anatomical sources for bacterial persistence that may necessitate surgical intervention. A renal and bladder US should be obtained in any child with a febrile UTI and a VCUG should be obtained in children with hydronephrosis and in children with the second febrile UTI.[1]

Clinical Presentation 30

Which of the following antibiotics do you now recommend for this patient?

A. Trimethoprim-sulfamethoxazole
B. Gentamicin
C. Vancomycin
D. Ceftriaxone
E. Amoxicillin
F. Furadantin

The correct answer is A

Comment: The patient should be started on antibiotics empirically. Two months ago, she was seen in the emergency department at which time her urine specimen grew greater than 100,000 colonies of *K. pneumoniae*. She was treated with a single dose of ceftriaxone and discharged on oral cephalexin. The culture was sensitive to the prescribed treatment and sulfamethoxazole. On this admission, her clinical symptoms are consistent with a lower tract bladder infection; she does not have fever, flank pain, nausea, or vomiting, which are symptoms of pyelonephritis. She is started on trimethoprim-sulfa; when she finishes the treatment dose, she will be started on prophylaxis. Trimethoprim-sulfa is a good choice; it is inexpensive, does not need to be refrigerated, has a relatively long shelf life, and is unlikely to cause gastrointestinal upset. The side effect profile overall is low.

Trimethoprim-sulfamethoxazole can be used in children older than 2 months of age. The treatment dose is based on trimethoprim 6 to 12 mg/kg/day given twice per day for 10 days. The prophylaxis dose is also based on trimethoprim, but at 1 to 2 mg/kg/day. Trimethoprim-sulfamethoxazole diffuses into vaginal fluid and decreases bacterial colonization.

Macrodantin or Furadantin elixir is another effective treatment and/or prophylactic agent. It does not achieve high blood levels and should not be used for systemic or febrile infections. The most common side effect is gastrointestinal upset. To help prevent this problem, the medication should be given with food. The liquid form is not tolerated well by children. The capsules can be opened and sprinkled on applesauce, yogurt, or pudding. It can be given to children older than 2 months of age, and the treatment dose is 5 to 7 mg/kg/day given four times per day. Prophylaxis is 1 to 2 mg/kg/day in a single dose.

Amoxicillin is also used to treat urinary tract infections and is often used for prophylaxis in children younger than 3 months of age. It is tolerated well and has a low side effect profile but can cause candidiasis in high doses. The suspension has to be refilled every 14 days, which makes it less convenient for families to use. Prophylaxis is 20 mg/kg/day in a single dose. Treatment dosing of amoxicillin is variable based on age and severity of infection. Cephalosporins can also be used for treatment and/or prophylaxis.

Antibiotic management of pediatric UTIs is always done with caution. Age-related dosing restrictions, comorbid conditions, and severity of infection must be considered before treatment is recommended. These issues also affect the decision of whether to use inpatient intravenous therapy versus outpatient oral management. Children who appear toxic and those younger than 2 months of age who have suspected pyelonephritis should receive intravenous treatment. Ampicillin and aminoglycoside (if there is no known drug allergy) are started until culture and sensitivity results are final. Fluoroquinolones have been approved by the Food and Drug Administration for the treatment of complicated UTIs in children. In children who present with a febrile UTI but do not appear toxic, 1 to 2 days of intramuscular ceftriaxone can provide coverage until culture results are final and appropriate oral therapy is determined.

The family should be educated on the signs and symptoms of a UTI at this appointment. They should be able to differentiate between a significant upper tract or kidney infection and lower tract symptoms or bladder infection. With a history of vesicoureteral reflux, at the first sign of infection, the child should be evaluated. The signs and symptoms of UTI should be revisited when discussing the x-ray evaluation with the family. If a urinalysis is positive, treatment should be started before culture results have been received to prevent the development of pyelonephritis. Vesicoureteral reflux should be evaluated by ultrasound and VCUG every 12 to 18 months. As long as the child has good overall renal growth, no evidence of scarring, no infections while on prophylaxis, and no worsening reflux, the child can be managed conservatively. If they have breakthrough infections or upper tract changes, alternate management would need to be considered. This would warrant a referral to a pediatric urologist. Other variables that might lead to surgical management are allergies to multiple antibiotics and poor compliance with medical management.

Antibiotic prophylaxis is appropriate for a child with a history of recurrent febrile infection until she has been evaluated fully. She is at risk for anatomical abnormalities and should be maintained on prophylaxis until her x-ray evaluation is complete.

Dysfunctional elimination must be addressed regardless of the results of her x-ray evaluation. She needs to be placed on a timed voiding regimen during the day. She is in the habit of holding her urine to the point of having urge incontinence. Often, these children have difficulty relaxing the external sphincter and do not take time to void to completion. This is complicated by constipation, which increases colonization of the intestinal flora and may create difficulty with voiding to completion.

You explain to the mother that her daughter's dysfunctional elimination will be managed by placing her on a strict timed voiding schedule during the day, every 2 hours by the clock, whether she has the urge to urinate or not. You suggest using a simple behavioral modification chart with days of the week and times of the day for scheduled voiding, which can be created with stickers to recognize her cooperation with the plan.

There are rare cases in which children with dysfunctional elimination, UTI, and reflux have symptoms that persist or worsen, even with appropriate management. This outcome could indicate a neurologic abnormality, so evaluation of the lower spine by magnetic resonance imaging may need to be done. Other symptoms that can be associated with neurologic issues are chronic back and lower extremity pain, gait abnormalities, and stool incontinence. Physical evidence of bony abnormalities can sometimes be seen on plain radiographs, or as sacral dimples, gluteal asymmetry, lower spine discolorations, or a sacral hair patch.[1]

Clinical Presentation 31

Which one of the following is *not* a risk factor for recurrent UTI in a woman?

A. Previous UTI
2. Sexual activity
3. Changes in the bacteria that live inside the vagina, or vaginal flora
C. Age (older adults and young children are more likely to get UTIs)
D. Structural problems in the urinary tract, such as hydronephrosis
E. Poor hygiene
F. Vitamin D deficiency

The correct answer is F

Comment: Some people are at higher risk of getting a UTI. UTIs are more common in females because their urethras are shorter and closer to the rectum. This makes it easier for bacteria to enter the urinary tract. Changes in the vaginal bacterial flora, such as during menopause or the use of spermicides, can cause these bacterial changes. So can poor hygiene, for example in children who are toilet training and primary or secondary vesicoureteral reflux.[1]

Clinical Presentation 32

A 19-year-old woman was married a year ago. Since then, she has experienced five attacks of acute cystitis, all characterized by dysuria, increased frequency, and urgency. Each case was diagnosed on the basis of the clinical picture and a laboratory urinalysis finding of bacteriuria. The urine bacterial counts in these cases ranged from 104 to 106 organisms/mL. Laboratory tests indicated that the first, second, and fifth infections were caused by *E. coli*, whereas the third infection was caused by an enterococcus, and the fourth infection was caused by *Proteus mirabilis*.

Each infection responded to short-term treatment with trimethoprim-sulfamethoxazole. The recurrences occurred at intervals of 3 weeks to 3 months following completion of antibiotic therapy.

For the past 2 days, she has once again been experiencing dysuria, with increased frequency and urgency, so she is going to see her physician. Her vital signs are temperature 37.2°C, pulse 100/min, respiratory rate 18/min, and blood pressure 110/70 mm Hg. Physical examination reveals a mild tenderness to palpation in the suprapubic area but no other abnormalities. A bimanual pelvic examination reveals a normal-sized uterus with no apparent adnexal tenderness. No vaginal discharge is noted. The cervix appears normal.[1]

What is the differential diagnosis?

A. Acute cystitis
B. Urethritis
C. UTI
D. Vaginitis
E. All of the above

The correct answer is E

Comment: The differential includes acute cystitis, a more extensive UTI, vaginitis, and urethritis. Urethritis would most likely be caused by a sexually transmitted pathogen. There are no other symptoms that would point to a sexually transmitted disease, and the patient's history does not suggest this alternative. Vaginitis is also a reasonable possibility, but the physical examination did not reveal any obvious symptoms of this type of infection. There are no indications of an upper UTI (e.g., fever, flank pain), so it would appear that the patient simply has yet another case of acute cystitis.[1]

Clinical Presentation 33

What is your preliminary diagnosis?

A. Acute cystitis
B. Urethritis
C. UTI
D. Vaginitis
E. All of the above

The correct answer is C

Comment: In women who present with one or more symptoms of UTI, the probability of infection is approximately 50%. Specific combinations of symptoms (e.g., dysuria and frequency without vaginal discharge or irritation) raise the probability of UTI to more than 90%, effectively ruling in the diagnosis based on history alone.[1]

Clinical Presentation 34

What tests should you order to confirm your preliminary diagnosis (select all that apply)?

A. Urinalysis
B. Urine culture
C. Complete blood count with differential
D. Serum electrolytes

The correct answers are A, B, and C

Comment: The most appropriate tests would include urinalysis with microscopic evaluation of clean-catch urine for bacteria and pyuria, a urine culture, and a complete blood count with differential.[1]

Clinical Presentation 35

Laboratory tests indicate a hemoglobin of 13.6 g/dL, hematocrit 40.7%, mean corpuscular volume 84, and WBC count 10,910/μL. White blood cells and bacteria are evident in the urine sediment. A urine culture indicates approximately 106 bacterial cells/mL. A gram stain of the urine reveals gram-positive cocci. The gram-positive bacterium is isolated and is found to be catalase-positive and coagulase-negative.

Do the test results support your preliminary diagnosis?

A. Urolithiasis
B. Acute cystitis
C. UTI
D. Vaginitis

The correct answer is C

Comment: The results support a diagnosis of acute cystitis. Enterococci, group B streptococci, and some staphylococci are known to cause UTIs. The positive catalase test eliminates enterococci and Group B streptococci. The negative coagulase test eliminates *Staphylococcus aureus*. At present, the coagulase-negative *Staphylococcus* species that are most likely to cause cystitis in a young woman is *Staphylococcus saprophyticus*.[1]

Clinical Presentation 36

Which of the following must be considered when taking a sample for analysis in a case like this?

A. Early morning collection of the sample before ingestion of any fluid
B. Random urine at any time of the day

The correct answer is B

Comment: The method for obtaining urine for culture is a random collection taken at any time of day with no precautions regarding contamination. The sample may be dilute, isotonic, or hypertonic and may contain white cells, bacteria, and squamous epithelium as contaminants. In women, the specimen may contain vaginal contaminants such as trichomonads, yeast, and, during menses, red cells.

Early morning collection of the sample before ingestion of any fluid is usually hypertonic and reflects the ability of the kidney to concentrate urine during dehydration, which occurs overnight. If all fluid ingestion has been avoided since 6 p.m. the previous day, the specific gravity usually exceeds 1.022 in healthy individuals.

Clean-catch, midstream urine specimen is collected after cleansing the external urethral meatus.

A cotton sponge soaked with benzalkonium hydrochloride is useful and nonirritating for this purpose. A midstream urine is one in which the first half of the bladder urine is discarded and the collection vessel is introduced into the urinary stream to catch the last half. The first half of the stream serves to flush contaminating cells and microbes from the outer urethra before collection. This sounds easy, but it is not (try it yourself before criticizing the patient). It can be messy, which reduces compliance.

Catheterization of the bladder through the urethra is carried out only in special circumstances (i.e., in a comatose or confused patient). This procedure risks introducing infection and traumatizing the urethra and bladder, thus producing iatrogenic infection or hematuria.

When done under ideal conditions, suprapubic transabdominal needle aspiration of the bladder provides the purest sampling of bladder urine. This is a good method for infants and small children.[1]

Clinical Presentation 37

What are the possible causes of recurrent lower UTIs and which of the following is most likely in this case?

A. Urinary tract anatomical abnormalities
B. Vesico-ureteral reflux
C. Poor immune responses
D. Improper toilet hygiene
E. High urinary bladder residual volume

The correct answers are A, B, C, D, and E

Comment: Recurrence of UTI may be either a relapse (i.e., the reappearance of the original infection) or, far more commonly, reinfection, which is the occurrence of a new infection. Relapse is caused by the same organism that caused the original infection and usually occurs within 2 weeks following the completion of antibiotic therapy. The short time frame suggests that the causative organism has persisted in the urinary tract or nearby, possibly because of an anatomic problem such as a stone or obstruction. A subclinical kidney infection (pyelonephritis or renal abscess) is another possibility. This patient's history does not support a diagnosis of relapse because the identity of the infectious agent changes from one incident to the next and the recurrences did not occur soon enough after completing antibiotic therapy. Reinfections can be caused by a different organism or by the same organism that caused the original infection. They can occur at any time after the original infection and do not imply an anatomical abnormality. It is not at all unusual for young women to experience a series of recurrent UTIs that are unrelated to anatomical abnormalities or other conditions. In fact, 10% of all women experience this problem at some point in their lives.[1]

Clinical Presentation 38

How should this case be treated (select all that apply)?

A. Short-term antibiotics after intercourse
B. Continuous antibiotic therapy
C. Vaginal douche after each intercourse
D. Stop drinking alcohol
E. Quit smoking

The correct answers are A and B
Comment: The major goal here is to interrupt the cycle of colonization of the introitus and infection of the bladder. Success is achieved with drugs such as trimethoprim-sulfamethoxazole or some quinolones, which reach high concentrations not only in urine but also in vaginal secretions. Treatment generally requires long-term prophylaxis (low dose), which may be administered either continuously or after intercourse (preferred).[1,2]

Clinical Presentation 39

A 4-week-old male neonate with a known antenatal US diagnosis of fused horseshoe kidneys and bilateral renal hydronephrosis presented in the outpatient clinic with a history of jaundice since he was 1 week old. His mother reported a history of passing dark urine and pale stools. The mother also noticed that he was passing a smaller amount of urine and his abdomen was distended. Antenatally, the mother was free from any medical complications during pregnancy; the neonate was delivered by spontaneous vaginal delivery, with a birth weight of 3 kg.

Kidney US after delivery revealed fused horseshoe kidneys and mild left hydronephrosis. MCUG was performed, which showed no evidence of posterior urethral valve and vesicoureteral reflux. There was positive consanguinity but no family history of a similar condition or liver disease. He was transferred to the pediatric medical ward for further investigations and management.

Examination on admission revealed that he had deep jaundice but was not pale. The anterior fontanelle was normally opened, with no dysmorphic features. His vitals were as follows: heart rage, 104 beats/min; resting respiration, 44 cycle/min; blood pressure, 95/50 mm Hg; temperature, 36.5°C; and capillary blood glucose 58 mg/dL with oxygen saturation 100% in room air. His weight was 3 kg, height 52 cm, and head circumference 35 cm. He looks dehydrated with dry mucous membranes. His abdomen was slightly distended and the liver was palpable 2 cm below the costal margin. Other systemic reviews were unremarkable.

Investigation showed elevated white blood cell count 21,000 cell/mm^3 with 55% polymorphs and 35% lymphocytes, hemoglobin 9.5 g/dL reticulocyte was 3.32%, lactate dehydrogenase 180 units/L, platelets 356/mm^3, C-reactive protein 50 mg/L, serum total bilirubin 17.78 mg/dL, direct serum bilirubin 15.16 mg/dL, indirect serum bilirubin mg/dL 2.62, serum aspartate transferase 172 IU/L, serum alanine transaminase 162 IU/L, serum gamma-glutamyl transferase

252 IU/L, total serum proteins 5.2 g/dL, serum albumin 2.6 g/dL, serum sodium 123 mmol/L, and serum creatinine was within normal 0.2 mg/dL. Urine analysis showed presence of nitrate and leukocyte esterase 500 with WBC 65/hpf. Urine culture showed *Enterobacter cloacae*. Blood culture revealed no growth. Thyroid-stimulating hormone was 1.99 mIU/mL. TORCH titers revealed high immunoglobulin G levels of rubella and cytomegalovirus.

Abdominal US revealed a contracted gallbladder and right ectopic fused kidneys. There was mild hydronephrosis in the left kidney and no hydronephrosis in the right kidney. Both kidneys showed normal corticomedullary differentiation. The urinary bladder showed a thick wall with a turbid content, consistent with cystitis.

Abdominal plain radiography revealed a paucity of the bowel gas in the right side. There was no abnormal bowel loop dilatation. Air within the rectum was noted, without pneumoperitoneum or abnormal calcification.

The patient was started on intravenous fluid on admission. Then normal saline 3% was started with maintenance D5 normal saline solution to correct his depletional hyponatremia and intravenous antibiotic for 14 days based on the sensitivity pattern. He also received a packed red blood cell transfusion for 3 hours because of a drop in his hemoglobin to 5.8 g/dL sepsis and frequent blood sampling. Intravenous vitamin K 5 g was administered. Repeated urine culture showed no growth, and UTI treatment resolved jaundice completely. He started passing stool freely and was discharged, with regular follow-up.

What is the cause of jaundice?

A. Urosepsis
B. Congenital biliary atresia
C. Neonatal hepatitis
D. Physiologic hyperbilirubinemia

The correct answer is A

Comment: Neonatal jaundice is a common problem in infancy. It is seen in 60% of full-term and 80% of preterm newborns.[1] Most cases are due to an increase in the direct fraction of bilirubin, whereas only 0.04% to 0.2% are cholestatic jaundice.[2] Physiological hyperbilirubinemia is considered the most common cause of jaundice after the first day of life, accounting for 53.9% of cases.[3] Among breast-fed infants, 15% experience some sort of jaundice for more than 3 weeks.[4] However, only a few infants with neonatal jaundice are found to have pathological causes, including metabolic and endocrine diseases, underlying hemolytic causes, congenital deficiency of liver enzymes, and bacteremia or sepsis.[1] The latter may cause increased direct fraction of bilirubin in infancy after first week of life, with UTI being the most common cause.[5] Gram-negative organisms were isolated from most cases of sepsis-related jaundice, of which *E. coli* was the most common causative agent.[6] Infants with structural abnormalities in the urinary tract are more susceptible to hyperbilirubinemia associated with UTI. These findings were especially related to hydronephrosis and vesicoureteral reflux, which are consistent with our case report.[7,8]

Some studies have found that hyperbilirubinemia could be the first and only manifestation of neonatal sepsis and UTI.[9] As in our patient, this was the case for a 2-month-old neonate reported in Turkey in 2017. He presented with jaundice 1 week after birth, and urine culture was positive for *K. pneumonia,* but no other signs of sepsis or UTI, which is uncommon. However, his jaundice resolved completely after treating his UTI.[10] Another case was reported in an 8-year-old girl who presented with jaundice and UTI from *E. coli.* Jaundice also resolved completely after treating the UTI.[11]

Infants with UTI usually have an increased indirect fraction of bilirubin.[11,12] This might be due to hemolysin toxins secreted by certain strains of gram-negative bacteria and increased red blood cell fragility, which eventually causes hemolysis and unconjugated hyperbilirubinemia.[13]

However, in our case and the other case reports mentioned previously, there was an increase in the direct fraction of bilirubin, which is defined as a conjugated bilirubin concentration of more than 2 mg/dL or more than 20% of total bilirubin.[14] Several mechanisms have been suggested to explain cholestatic jaundice in a setting of UTI. Endotoxins secreted by gram-negative organisms are thought to be the main cause of UTI-related hyperbilirubinemia.[15] A marked decrease in multidrug resistance–associated protein 2, an ATP-dependent transporter involved in the bile- and salt-independent bile export system, under oxidative stress caused by lipopolysaccharide (LPS) endotoxins from the bacterial outer membrane, has been reported.[15–17] This causes bile stasis because of impaired excretion and indirectly damages hepatocytes.[13]

Another suggested mechanism is direct hepatocellular damage caused by the invasion of gram-negative bacteria during an episode of bacteremia. However, the latter mechanism is not reliable because cholestatic syndrome was documented even in the absence of bacteremia.[18] Moreover, LPS released in the bloodstream from gram-negative organisms causes suppression of the inner circular muscles of the intestinal wall. This is thought to be the cause of sepsis-associated ileus and could explain constipation in our case.[5,19]

Clinical Presentation 40

A previously healthy 7-month-old infant presented with a fever for 2 days. He had a runny nose for a week. Nasal wash for respiratory syncytial virus, influenza A, and influenza B antigens was negative. He was noted to be circumcised. Otherwise, the physical examination was normal.

Urinalysis showed 2 to 3 WBC per HPF. The urine dipstick for nitrites was negative. A diagnosis of viral infection was made and he was sent home. Urine culture (catheter specimen) subsequently grew 10^3 to 10^5 CFU/mL of *Staphylococcus epidermidis*. No treatment was given because the organism was considered a contaminant.

His fever persisted and he developed intermittent vomiting for 4 days. On admission, his temperature was 40.6°C; he was alert and in no distress. Laboratory data showed a WBC of 15,600/mm^3 (70% neutrophils, 2% bands, and 17% lymphocytes). C-reactive protein was 238 mg/L (normal, 105 CFU/mL). Urinalysis showed 3 to 4 WBC/HPF, and a catheterized urine sample was sent for culture. His electrolytes and renal function tests were normal.

He was started on intravenous ceftriaxone treatment. He continued to spike fevers over the next 48 hours. Cerebrospinal fluid showed no evidence of meningitis. Direct fluorescent antibody testing of respiratory secretions was negative for adenovirus and parainfluenza. Urine culture showed pure growth of *S. epidermidis*, >105 CFU/mL. The organism was sensitive to vancomycin, trimethoprim-sulfamethoxazole, and gentamicin but was resistant to ceftriaxone. His treatment was changed to intravenous trimethoprim-sulfamethoxazole. Blood and cerebrospinal fluid cultures were negative.

A US scan of the kidneys showed mild distention of the right urinary collecting system and mild prominence of the left pelvicalyceal system. The bladder was distended and contained multiple scattered areas of internal echoes. A VCUG revealed bilateral vesicoureteral reflux, grade 5 on the right and grade 4 on the left. His fever resolved 36 hours after changing the antibiotic treatment. He was discharged to complete 10 more days of oral trimethoprim-sulfamethoxazole treatment. Subsequently, he was maintained on prophylactic daily oral trimethoprim-sulfamethoxazole. (He has done well and was followed by the urology service.)

Should the initial isolation of *S. epidermidis* from urine (<10^5/CFU) in this infant be considered as a pathogen even in the absence of pyuria or negative urine nitrite test?

A. Yes
B. No

The correct answer is A

Comment: S. epidermidis commonly causes infections associated with indwelling central venous catheters, cerebrospinal fluid shunts, prosthetic heart valves, and peritoneal dialysis catheters. When *S. epidermidis* is isolated from blood or body fluids in patients without predisposing factors, it is often considered a contaminant. Urinary tract infections caused by *S. epidermidis* are often associated with instrumentation of the urinary tract in a hospital setting, including neonates in the neonatal intensive care unit.

Our patient was a previously healthy infant who presented with persistent fever and had elevated WBC and C-reactive protein. Urinalysis showed 105 CFU/mL of *S. epidermidis* on two separate occasions. Imaging studies revealed a smaller right kidney with evidence of cortical thinning and right-sided vesicoureteral reflux.[1–6]

Hall and Snitzer[7] described two children (a 6-year-old and a 7-year-old) who presented with fever and shaking chills. Urine culture from each of these patients grew *S. epidermidis* on two occasions. Imaging studies identified vesicoureteral reflux in both cases. It is noteworthy that in both of the aforementioned reports of *S. epidermidis* UTI, there was a lack of significant pyuria.[6,7] This was also noted in our patient where urine microscopy showed only 5 to 10 WBC/hpf. This finding and the absence of urine nitrites, which are predominantly produced by gram-negative bacteria, indicate that urine dip and microscopy are less helpful in diagnosing urinary tract infections from *S. epidermidis*. Previous studies have suggested that in view of the tendency of *Staphylococcus* to form clusters, a count of 103 CFU/mL may be a significant marker for UTI.[5] Urinary radiographic imaging in the previous two reports revealed underlying abnormalities in all three cases (vesicoureteral reflux). Our patient also has severe bilateral reflux.

Clinical Presentation 41

A 7-year-old male presented with acute dysuria, suprapubic pain, frequent urination, urgent urination, urgent incontinence, and macrohematuria. The patient had no history of allergies and had normal body development.

On admission, he had a normal blood pressure. Normal red blood cells and normal hemoglobin were observed in the peripheral blood smears. Routine blood tests revealed eosinophil ratios of 24.0, 33.0, and 29.0% (normal range, 0.5–5%) on day 1, at the end of week 1, and at the end of week 2, respectively. The patient was diagnosed as having a urinary infection and given antimicrobial treatment (cefmetazole, 100 mg/kg/d).

A urine culture test yielded negative results, whereas a routine urine test and microscopy revealed 3 to 5 WBCs and many red blood cells, too numerous to count. Urine sediment was negative. There was no proteinuria on dipstick. The specific gravity of the urine was 1.030, and a nitrite test in the urine yielded negative results. The patient's renal functions were normal, and the concentration of complement C3 was 109 mg/dL. Purified protein derivative (PPD) experiments yielded negative results, and urine polymerase chain reaction revealed no adenovirus or *Mycobacterium tuberculosis*. No clear allergens were observed in the allergen screening.

Computed tomography and retrograde angiography of the bladder revealed local mucosal lesions with thickening of each side and the posterior wall of the bladder (data not shown). Cystoscopy revealed that the bladder volume was reduced and the mucosa at the bladder floor and neck was red.

What is your diagnosis?

A. Hemorrhagic cystitis
B. Acute pyelonephritis
C. Eosinophilic cystitis (EC)
D. All of the above

The correct answer is C

Comment: Our patient symptoms included acute dysuria, suprapubic pain, frequent urination, urgent urination, urge incontinence, and macrohematuria in the absence of pyuria or urinary tract infection. His urinary symptoms disappeared 3 days after the start of antibiotic, and blood eosinophils were normal. The clinical manifestations in the case were consistent with EC.[1] Biopsy of the lesions through the urethra revealed infiltration of blood vessels and eosinophils into the muscular layer, accompanied by focal muscle necrosis.

EC is an uncommon primary inflammatory disorder of the bladder with uncertain etiology. The incidence of EC in male adults is increased compared with female adults. Similarly, the incidence of EC in male children is increased compared with females; the average age of onset in children is 6 years.[2] The exact cause of EC remains unclear; however, certain studies have suggested that anaphylaxis may be a trigger.[3] Allergens may include food, dust mites, pollen, condom antigens, iodine, and anesthetic creams. Asthma and celiac disease are also associated with EC.[4] In the present study, the patient in case 1 was sensitive to *Dermatophagoides pteronyssinus* and *Dermatophagoides culinae*, whereas the patient in case 2 had no specific allergies. The pathogenesis of EC involves immunoglobulin E–mediated eosinophil activation, with subsequent mast cell degranulation and muscle damage. Patients with EC often exhibit a series of urinary symptoms, including frequent urination, hematuria, suprapubic pain, dysuria, and daytime and nocturnal enuresis; children with EC may have a clear suprapubic mass. The clinical manifestations in the cases presented in the present study were consistent with EC; however, the clinical manifestations of EC are often varied and may be easily confused with nonspecific cystitis.[2] Children with suprapubic masses should also be differentiated from those with malignant bladder tumors. EC is a rare condition that can mimic invasive bladder cancer symptoms. EC diagnosis may be considered if a bladder tumor is associated with eosinophilia. The eosinophil count in the blood was significantly increased in each of the two cases, and a bone marrow biopsy revealed increased eosinophils. In a number of patients with EC, peripheral blood eosinophilia occurs without reaching the level of eosinophilia syndrome. Patient 2 only received treatment by antiinflammatory and cetirizine hydrochloride without steroid therapy. During hospitalization, the eosinophils were found to be decreased in a routine blood test, and the patient's symptoms gradually improved. It has previously been suggested that EC may also present a self-healing trend.[3] In the present study, patient 1 presented with similar symptoms 3 years earlier; an US revealed thickening of the bladder wall, and following 3 days of antiinflammatory treatment, the symptoms disappeared. In addition, patient 1 was allergen-positive. The authors hypothesize that the onset of the disease in case 1 was associated with allergens, and that with the elimination of inflammatory mediators, symptoms may disappear.[3] It has previously been reported that urine cultures are positive in EC patients.[4] However, the urine cultures in each of the cases presented herein were negative. Eosinophils are rarely observed in urine sediments and are rapidly degraded or rarely detached from the mucosa. Certain EC patients have hematuria symptoms.[5] If an imaging examination reveals bladder wall thickening, which is similar to mass infiltration, a tumor is suggested. Cystoscopy results usually suggest bladder rhabdomyosarcoma.[6] Intense inflammatory changes, including congestion and edema of the bladder wall, may result in intense inflammatory changes in the bladder wall, and associated with this, lesion may produce excrescences, which resemble vesical rhabdomyosarcoma.[7] Because EC is very rare in children, there are no ideal guidelines for its treatment and follow-up, and treatment is typically based on experience.[8] First-line treatments typically involve the removal of any suspected allergens, followed by the use of antihistamines and corticosteroids. It has been reported that corticosteroids may accelerate the remission of symptoms and stabilize lysosomal membranes because of their antiinflammatory effects.[9] For refractory cases, cyclosporine A is administered orally for 8 months.[10] For children with peripheral blood eosinophilia, montelukast sodium is used.[11] Researchers have also tried intravesical instillation of dimethyl sulfoxide twice per week.[11] EC in children is normally benign and self-limiting; however, it may still develop into bladder fibrosis and secondary urinary tract obstruction. The diagnosis and treatment of EC depend on clinical suspicions and histopathological examination.

In conclusion, EC in children is similar to a tumor; however, it has its own characteristics. Although it is a rare disease, it should be considered when urinary tract symptoms and bladder wall thickening are observed in children. Bladder biopsy and histopathological evaluation are important for the diagnosis of EC and allow for the selection of an appropriate treatment.

References

Clinical Presentation 1

1. Mattoo TK. Medical management of vesicoureteral reflux–quiz within the article. Don't overlook placebos. *Pediatr Nephrol.* 2007;22(8):1113–1120. https://doi.org/10.1007/s00467-007-0485-3.

Clinical Presentation 2

1. Mattoo TK. Medical management of vesicoureteral reflux–quiz within the article. Don't overlook placebos. *Pediatr Nephrol.* 2007;22(8):1113–1120. https://doi.org/10.1007/s00467-007-0485-3.

Clinical Presentation 3

1. Mattoo TK. Medical management of vesicoureteral reflux–quiz within the article. Don't overlook placebos. *Pediatr Nephrol.* 2007;22(8):1113–1120. https://doi.org/10.1007/s00467-007-0485-3.

Clinical Presentation 4

1. Mattoo TK. Medical management of vesicoureteral reflux–quiz within the article. Don't overlook placebos. *Pediatr Nephrol.* 2007;22(8):1113–1120. https://doi.org/10.1007/s00467-007-0485-3.

Clinical Presentation 5

1. Mattoo TK. Medical management of vesicoureteral reflux–quiz within the article. Don't overlook placebos. *Pediatr Nephrol.* 2007;22(8):1113–1120. https://doi.org/10.1007/s00467-007-0485-3.

Clinical Presentation 6

1. Mattoo TK. Medical management of vesicoureteral reflux–quiz within the article. Don't overlook placebos. *Pediatr Nephrol.* 2007;22(8):1113–1120. https://doi.org/10.1007/s00467-007-0485-3.

Clinical Presentation 7

1. Subcommittee on Urinary Tract Infection, Steering Committee on Quality Improvement and Management, Roberts KB. Urinary tract infection: clinical practice guideline for the diagnosis and management of the initial UTI in febrile infants and children 2 to 24 months. *Pediatrics.* 2011;128(3):595–610. https://doi.org/10.1542/peds.2011-1330.

Clinical Presentation 8

1. Subcommittee on Urinary Tract Infection, Steering Committee on Quality Improvement and Management, Roberts KB. Urinary tract infection: clinical practice guideline for the diagnosis and management of the initial UTI in febrile infants and children 2 to 24 months. *Pediatrics.* 2011;128(3):595–610. https://doi.org/10.1542/peds.2011-1330.
2. Sadeghi-Bojd S, Naghshizadian R, Mazaheri M, Ghane Sharbaf F, Assadi F. Efficacy of probiotic prophylaxis after the first febrile urinary tract infection in children with normal urinary tracts. *J Pediatric Infect Dis Soc.* 2020;9(3):305–310. https://doi.org/10.1093/jpids/piz025.

Clinical Presentation 9

1. Mattoo TK. Medical management of vesicoureteral reflux–quiz within the article. Don't overlook placebos. *Pediatr Nephrol.* 2007;22(8):1113–1120. https://doi.org/10.1007/s00467-007-0485-3.

Clinical Presentation 10

1. Okarska-Napierała M, Wasilewska A, Kuchar E. Urinary tract infection in children: diagnosis, treatment, imaging—comparison of current guidelines. *J Pediatr Urol.* 2017;13(6):567–573. https://doi.org/10.1016/j.jpurol.2017.07.018.

Clinical Presentation 11

1. Okarska-Napierała M, Wasilewska A, Kuchar E. Urinary tract infection in children: diagnosis, treatment, imaging—comparison of current guidelines. *J Pediatr Urol.* 2017;13(6):567–573. https://doi.org/10.1016/j.jpurol.2017.07.018.

Clinical Presentation 12

1. Okarska-Napierała M, Wasilewska A, Kuchar E. Urinary tract infection in children: diagnosis, treatment, imaging—comparison of current guidelines. *J Pediatr Urol.* 2017;13(6):567–573. https://doi.org/10.1016/j.jpurol.2017.07.018.

Clinical Presentation 13

1. Okarska-Napierała M, Wasilewska A, Kuchar E. Urinary tract infection in children: diagnosis, treatment, imaging—comparison of current guidelines. *J Pediatr Urol.* 2017;13(6):567–573. https://doi.org/10.1016/j.jpurol.2017.07.018.

Clinical Presentation 14

1. Okarska-Napierała M, Wasilewska A, Kuchar E. Urinary tract infection in children: diagnosis, treatment, imaging—comparison of current guidelines. *J Pediatr Urol.* 2017;13(6):567–573. https://doi.org/10.1016/j.jpurol.2017.07.018.

Clinical Presentation 15

1. Okarska-Napierała M, Wasilewska A, Kuchar E. Urinary tract infection in children: diagnosis, treatment, imaging—comparison of current guidelines. *J Pediatr Urol.* 2017;13(6):567–573. https://doi.org/10.1016/j.jpurol.2017.07.018.

Clinical Presentation 16

1. Okarska-Napierała M, Wasilewska A, Kuchar E. Urinary tract infection in children: diagnosis, treatment, imaging—comparison of current guidelines. *J Pediatr Urol.* 2017;13(6):567–573. https://doi.org/10.1016/j.jpurol.2017.07.018.

Clinical Presentation 17

1. Okarska-Napierała M, Wasilewska A, Kuchar E. Urinary tract infection in children: diagnosis, treatment, imaging—comparison of current guidelines. *J Pediatr Urol.* 2017;13(6):567–573. https://doi.org/10.1016/j.jpurol.2017.07.018.

Clinical Presentation 18

1. Okarska-Napierała M, Wasilewska A, Kuchar E. Urinary tract infection in children: diagnosis, treatment, imaging—comparison of current guidelines. *J Pediatr Urol.* 2017;13(6):567–573. https://doi.org/10.1016/j.jpurol.2017.07.018.

Clinical Presentation 19

1. Okarska-Napierała M, Wasilewska A, Kuchar E. Urinary tract infection in children: diagnosis, treatment, imaging—comparison of current guidelines. *J Pediatr Urol.* 2017;13(6):567–573. https://doi.org/10.1016/j.jpurol.2017.07.018.

Clinical Presentation 20

1. Okarska-Napierała M, Wasilewska A, Kuchar E. Urinary tract infection in children: diagnosis, treatment, imaging—comparison of current guidelines. *J Pediatr Urol.* 2017;13(6):567–573. https://doi.org/10.1016/j.jpurol.2017.07.018.

Clinical Presentation 21

1. Assadi F. Strategies for preventing catheter-associated urinary tract infections. *Int J Prev Med.* 2018;9:50. https://doi.org/10.4103/ijpvm.IJPVM_299_17.

Clinical Presentation 22

1. Sadeghi-Bodh S, Naghdhishadian R, Mazaheri M, et al. Efficacy of probiotic prophylaxis after the first febrile urinary tract in children with normal urinary tracts. *Pediatr Infect Dis Soc.* 2019;9(3):305–310. https://doi.org/10.1093/joids/piz025.

2. Subcommittee on Urinary Tract Infection, Roberts KB, Downs SM, et al. Reaffirmation of AAP Clinical Practice Guideline: the diagnosis and management of the initial urinary tract infection in febrile infants and young children 2–24 months of age. *Pediatrics.* 2016;138(6):e20163026. https://doi.org/10.1542/peds.2016-3026.

Clinical Presentation 23

1. Subcommittee on Urinary Tract Infection, Roberts KB, Downs SM, et al. Reaffirmation of AAP Clinical Practice Guideline: the diagnosis and management of the initial urinary tract infection in febrile infants and young children 2–24 months of age. *Pediatrics.* 2016;138(6):e20163026. https://doi.org/10.1542/peds.2016-3026.

Clinical Presentation 24

1. Subcommittee on Urinary Tract Infection, Roberts KB, Downs SM, et al. Reaffirmation of AAP Clinical Practice Guideline: the diagnosis and management of the initial urinary tract infection in febrile infants and young children 2–24 months of age. *Pediatrics.* 2016;138(6):e20163026. https://doi.org/10.1542/peds.2016-3026.
2. Hooton TM. Uncomplicated urinary tract infections. *New Engl J Med.* 2012;366:1028–1037.

Clinical Presentation 25

1. Nicolle LE, Bradley S, Colgan R, Rice JC, Schaeffer A, Hooton TM. Infectious Diseases Society of America guidelines for the diagnosis and treatment of asymptomatic bacteriuria in adults. *Clin Infect Dis.* 2005;40(5):643–654.
2. Hooton TM. Uncomplicated urinary tract infection. *N Engl J Med.* 2012;366(11):1028–1037.

Clinical Presentation 26

1. Sadeghi-Bojd S, Naghshizadian R, Mazaheri M, et al. Efficacy of probiotic prophylaxis after the first febrile urinary tract infection in children with normal urinary tracts. *J Pediatric Infect Dis Soc.* 2020;9(3):305–310. https://doi.org/10.1093/jpids/piz025.
2. Okarska-Napierała M, Wasilewska A, Kuchar E. Urinary tract infection in children: diagnosis, treatment, imaging—comparison of current guidelines. *J Pediatr Urol.* 2017;13(6):567–573. https://doi.org/10.1016/j.jpurol.2017.07.018.

Clinical Presentation 27

1. Assadi F. Strategies for preventing catheter-associated urinary tract infections. *Int J Prev Med.* 2018;9:50. https://doi.org/10.4103/ijpvm.IJPVM_299_17.
2. Nicolle LE. Catheter associated urinary tract infections. *Antimicrob Resist Infect Control.* 2014;3:23. https://doi.org/10.1186/2047-2994-3-23.

Clinical Presentation 28

1. Okarska-Napierała M, Wasilewska A, Kuchar E. Urinary tract infection in children: diagnosis, treatment, imaging—comparison of current guidelines. *J Pediatr Urol.* 2017;13(6):567–573. https://doi.org/10.1016/j.jpurol.2017.07.018.

Clinical Presentation 29

1. Okarska-Napierała M, Wasilewska A, Kuchar E. Urinary tract infection in children: diagnosis, treatment, imaging—comparison of current guidelines. *J Pediatr Urol.* 2017;13(6):567–573. https://doi.org/10.1016/j.jpurol.2017.07.018.

Clinical Presentation 30

1. Okarska-Napierała M, Wasilewska A, Kuchar E. Urinary tract infection in children: diagnosis, treatment, imaging—comparison of current guidelines. *J Pediatr Urol.* 2017;13(6):567–573. https://doi.org/10.1016/j.jpurol.2017.07.018.

Clinical Presentation 31

1. Okarska-Napierała M, Wasilewska A, Kuchar E. Urinary tract infection in children: diagnosis, treatment, imaging—comparison of current guidelines. *J Pediatr Urol.* 2017;13(6):567–573. https://doi.org/10.1016/j.jpurol.2017.07.018.

Clinical Presentation 32

1. Okarska-Napierała M, Wasilewska A, Kuchar E. Urinary tract infection in children: diagnosis, treatment, imaging—comparison of current guidelines. *J Pediatr Urol.* 2017;13(6):567–573. https://doi.org/10.1016/j.jpurol.2017.07.018.

Clinical Presentation 33

1. Okarska-Napierała M, Wasilewska A, Kuchar E. Urinary tract infection in children: diagnosis, treatment, imaging—comparison of current guidelines. *J Pediatr Urol.* 2017;13(6):567–573. https://doi.org/10.1016/j.jpurol.2017.07.018.

Clinical Presentation 34

1. Okarska-Napierała M, Wasilewska A, Kuchar E. Urinary tract infection in children: diagnosis, treatment, imaging—comparison of current guidelines. *J Pediatr Urol.* 2017;13(6):567–573. https://doi.org/10.1016/j.jpurol.2017.07.018.

Clinical Presentation 35

1. Okarska-Napierała M, Wasilewska A, Kuchar E. Urinary tract infection in children: diagnosis, treatment, imaging—comparison of current guidelines. *J Pediatr Urol.* 2017;13(6):567–573. https://doi.org/10.1016/j.jpurol.2017.07.018.

Clinical Presentation 36

1. Okarska-Napierała M, Wasilewska A, Kuchar E. Urinary tract infection in children: diagnosis, treatment, imaging—comparison of current guidelines. *J Pediatr Urol.* 2017;13(6):567–573. https://doi.org/10.1016/j.jpurol.2017.07.018.

Clinical Presentation 37

1. Okarska-Napierała M, Wasilewska A, Kuchar E. Urinary tract infection in children: diagnosis, treatment, imaging—comparison of current guidelines. *J Pediatr Urol.* 2017;13(6):567–573. https://doi.org/10.1016/j.jpurol.2017.07.018.

Clinical Presentation 38

1. Reid G. Potential preventive strategies and therapies in urinary tract infection. *World J Urol.* 1999;17:359–363.
2. Paudel S, John PP, Poorbaghi SL, Randis TM, Kulkarni R. Systematic review of literature examining bacterial urinary tract infections in diabetes. *J Diabetes Res.* 2022;2022:3588297.

Clinical Presentation 39

1. National Collaborating Centre for Women's and Children's Health (UK). *Neonatal Jaundice.* London: RCOG Press; 2010:98–99. www.rcog.org.uk17.
2. Benchimol EI, Walsh CM, Ling SC. Early diagnosis of neonatal cholestatic jaundice: test at 2 weeks. *Can Fam Physician.* 2009;55:1184–1192.
3. Alkhotani A, Eldin EE, Zaghloul A, et al. Evaluation of neonatal jaundice in the Makkah region. *Scientific Rep.* 2015;4:1–4.
4. Winfield CR, MacFaul R. Clinical study of prolonged jaundice in breast- and bottle-fed babies. *Arch Dis Childhood.* 1978;53(6):506–507.
5. Garcia FJ, Nager AL. Jaundice as an early diagnostic sign of urinary tract infection in infancy. *Pediatrics.* 2002;109(5):846–851.
6. Zia E, Sheikhha M. Investigation of urinary tract infection in neonates with hyperbilirubinemia. *J Med Sci.* 2007;7(5):909–912.
7. Xinias I, Demertzidou V, Mavroudi A, et al. Bilirubin levels predict renal cortical changes in jaundiced neonates with urinary tract infection. *World J Pediatr.* 2009;5(1):42–45.
8. Omar C, Hamza S, Bassem AM, et al. Urinary tract infection and indirect hyperbilirubinemia in newborns. *N Am J Med Sci.* 2011;3(12):544–547.
9. Pereira NM, Shah I. Neonatal cholestasis mimicking biliary atresia: could it be urinary tract infection? *SAGE Open Med Case Rep.* 2017;5:2050313X17695998.
10. Naveh Y, Friedman A. Urinary tract infection presenting as jaundice. *BMJ.* 1978;62:524–525.
11. Hernández-Bou S, De la Maza TS, Alarcón Gamarra M, et al. Etiology and clinical course of urinary tract infections in infants less than 3 months-old. *Enferm Infecc Microbiol Clín.* 2016;3:516–520.

12. Lee HC, Fang SB, Yeung CY, et al. Urinary tract infections in infants: comparison between those with conjugated vs unconjugated hyperbilirubinaemia. *Ann Trop Paediatr.* 2005;25:277–282.
13. Chiou FK, Ong C, Phua KB, et al. Conjugated hyperbilirubinemia presenting in first fourteen days in term neonates. *World J Hepatol.* 2017;9(26):1108–1114.
14. Utili R, Abernathy CO, Zimmerman HJ. Inhibition of Na+, K+-adenosinetriphosphatase by endotoxin: a possible mechanism for endotoxin-induced cholestasis. *J Infect Dis.* 1977;136(4):583–587.
15. Saek J, Sekine IS, Horie T. LPS-induced dissociation of multidrug resistance-associated protein 2 (Mrp2) and radixin is associated with Mrp2 selective internalization in rats. *Biochemical.* 2011;81(1):178–184.
16. Sekine S, Yano K, Saeki J, et al. Oxidative stress is a triggering factor for LPS-induced Mrp2 internalization in the cryopreserved rat and human liver slices. *Biochem Biophys Res Comm.* 2010;399(2):279–285.
17. Hayman J. Jaundice due to bacterial infection. *Gastroenterology.* 1979;77(2):362–374.
18. Eskandari MK, Kalff JC, Billiar TR, et al. Lipopolysaccharide activates the muscularis macrophage network and suppresses circular smooth muscle activity. *Am J Physiol.* 1977;273(3):G727–G734.
19. Eskandari MK, Kalff JC, Billiar TR, et al. LPS-induced muscularis macrophage nitric oxide suppresses rat jejunal circular muscle activity. *Am J Physiolo.* 1999;277(2):G478–G486.

Clinical Presentation 40

1. Lohr JA, Downs SM, Schlager YA. Urinary tract infections. In: Lon SS, Pickering LK, Prober CG, eds. *Principles and Practice of Pediatric Infectious Diseases.* 3rd ed. Philadelphia, PA: Churchill Livingstone; 2008:343–350.
2. Baciulis V, Eitutiene G, Cerkauskiene R, et al. Long-term cefadroxil prophylaxis in children with recurrent urinary tract infections. *Medicina.* 2003;39(suppl 1):59–63.
3. Marosvari J, Kery V. Urinary tract infections caused by Staphylococcus saprophyticus in children. *Orv Hetil.* 1990;131(47):2601–2602.
4. Schille R, Sierig G, Spencker FB, et al. Urinary tract infections due to Staphylococcus saprophyticus in a child. *Klin Padiatrie.* 2000;212(3):126–128.
5. Abrahamsson K, Hansson S, Jodal U, et al. Staphylococcus saprophyticus urinary tract infections in children. *Eur J Pediatr.* 1993;152(1):69–71.
6. McDonald JA, Loh JA. Staphylococcus epidermidis pyelonephritis in a previously healthy child. *Pediatr Infect Dis J.* 1994;13(12):1155–1156.
7. Hall DE, Snitzer JA 3rd. Staphylococcus epidermidis as a cause of urinary tract infections in children. *J Pediatr.* 1994;124(3):437–438.

Clinical Presentation 41

1. Saadi A, Bouzouita A, Ayed H, et al. Pseudotumoral eosinophilic cystitis. *Urol Case Rep.* 2015;3:65–67.
2. Thomas JC, Ross JH. Eosinophilic cystitis in a child presenting with a bladder mass. *J Urol.* 2004;171:1654–1655.
3. Li G, Cai B, Song H, Yang Z. Clinical and radiological character of eosinophilic cystitis. *Int J Clin Exp Med.* 2015;8:533–539.
4. Ladocsi LT, Sullivan B, Hanna MK. Eosinophilic granulomatous cystitis in children. *Urology.* 1995;46:732–735.
5. Chia D. Eosinophilic cystitis and haematuria: case report of a rare disease and common presentation. *Int J Surg Case Rep.* 2016;24:43–45.
6. Li G, Cai B, Song H, et al. Clinical and radiological character of eosinophilic cystitis. *Int J Clin Exp Med.* 2015;8:533–539.
7. Redman JF, Parham DM. Extensive inflammatory eosinophilic bladder tumors in children: experience with three cases. *South Med J.* 2002;95(9):1050–1052.
8. Castillo J Jr, Cartagena R, Montes M. Eosinophilic cystitis: a therapeutic challenge. *Urology.* 1988;32:535–537.
9. Gerharz EW, Grueber M, Melekos MD, et al. Tumor-forming eosinophilic cystitis in children: case report and review of literature. *Eur Urol.* 1994;25:138–141.
10. Aleem S, Kumar B, Fasano MB, et al. Successful use of cyclosporine as treatment for eosinophilic cystitis: a case report. *World Allergy Organ J.* 2016;9:222.
11. Zaman SR, Vermeulen TL, Parry J. Eosinophilic cystitis: treatment with intravesical steroids and oral antihistamines. *BMJ Case Rep.* 2013;2013:bcr2013009327.

INDEX

A

Abdominal compartment syndrome, 8
Abdominal decompression, 8
Acetazolamide, 128
Acid-base disturbance, 125
Acquired apparent mineralocorticoid excess, 148
Acute contrast nephropathy, 9
Acute cystitis, 382, 393
Acute kidney injury (AKI), 338, 348
  appropriate management of, 5–6
  best management plan for, 11–12
  biomarkers, 1
  cause of, 19, 339
  chemotherapy as risk factor of, 13
  classical clinical and biological symptoms, 19
  COVID-19-associated, 352
  CPT II deficiency in, 19
  crystal-induced, treatment of, 5
  diagnosis of, 15
  Doppler renal ultrasound, 26
  food poisoning and, 32
  laboratory tests, 25–26
  loop diuretics, 3–4
  in paroxysmal cold hemoglobinuria, 23
  proteinuria associated with, 68
  risk factors for, 17, 349
  treatment of, 14–17
Acute post-streptococcal glomerulonephritis (APSGN), 35–36
Acute renal failure (ARF), 8
  causes of, 18
  medications associated with, 2–3
  modality selection for RRT in, 9
  in rhabdomyolysis, 17
Acute tubulointerstitial disease, 360
Acute tubulointerstitial nephritis (ATIN), 365
Acute uncomplicated cystitis, 386
ADAMTS13 mutations, 197
Addison disease, 329–330
Adenine phosphoribosyltransferase (APRT) deficiency, 214, 357
Adrenocorticotropic hormone (ACTH)
  dependent Cushing syndrome, 317
  secreting pancreatic NET, 172–173
Adult-type polycystic kidney disease, 204
AE1 mutations, 194
Aldosterone, 145
ALG1 gene mutation, 253
Allergens, 400–401
Allergic interstitial nephritis (AIN), 6
  corticosteroids for, 36
  histological hallmarks of, 36
  normotensive nature of, 36
  secondary to streptococcal infection, 36
  treatment of, 6
Alport syndrome, 184, 351
Alport syndrome-diffuse leiomyomatosis contiguous gene syndrome, 189
Alström syndrome, 188
Ambulatory BP monitoring (ABPM), 309
American Academy of Pediatrics (AAP), 386
Amlodipine, 301–302
Ammoniagenesis, 106
Amoxicillin, 392
Angiotensin-converting enzyme (ACE), 328
  inhibitors, 104, 106–111, 115, 184, 294–295, 298, 300, 308, 312–313
    contraindications to, 301
Angiotensin-receptor blockers (ARB), 100, 104, 107–108, 110, 306, 313
  in pregnancy, 306
Anion gap, 144
Antibiotic-coated catheter, 385
Antibiotic prophylaxis, 392
Antibiotics, 345
Antibodies to complement-regulating proteins, 274
Anti-DNase antibody testing, 276
Antiglobulin test, 23
Antihypertensive drug classes, 304–305
Antineutrophil cytoplasmic antibody (ANCA), 236
  associated vasculitis, 269–270
Anti-phospholipid antibody syndrome, 239
Anti-PLA2R antibodies, 278
APRTQ0 allele, 357
Arthralgia, 230
Ascites in children, 22
Asthma, 400–401
Asymptomatic bacteriuria, 383
Atherosclerotic renovascular disease, 291
Atorvastatin, 7
ATP-dependent transporter, 398
Atrial fibrillation (AF), 305
Augmentin, 341
Autosomal dominant polycystic kidney disease, 56–57, 62, 184–185, 195–196, 211
  development of renal insufficiency in, 196
  genetic testing for, 190–191
  imaging criteria for diagnosis, 190
  PKD gene mutations in, 185, 189
  therapeutic interventions, 212
Autosomal recessive polycystic kidney disease, 57, 80, 211
  PKD1 gene, 57
  PKD2 gene, 57
Azathioprine, 98
Azithromycin, 99
Azotemia, 291

B

Baller-Gerold syndrome, 54
Bardet-Biedl syndrome, 55, 196–197, 206, 213–214
  genes associated with, 213–214
Barnes syndrome, 203
Bartter syndrome, 128–129, 144, 146–147, 161, 192, 194, 214
"Bear paw" sign, 76
Behcet disease, 341
Bicarbonate-based replacement fluids, 90
Bilateral anterior uveitis, 341
Bilateral upper tract obstruction
  fungus ball, 66–67
  medical treatment for, 67
  urinary microscopic examinations for, 67
Bilateral ureteritis, 40
Biliverdinuria, 335
Bisphosphonates, 114
Bladder
  computed tomography, 399
  dysfunction, 376
  retrograde angiography of, 399
Blood pressure
  ACEI/diuretic combination for, 308
  in bronchiolitis, 298
  control strategy, 93–94
  DASH diet and, 307
  effect of smoking, 307
Blood smear analysis, 332
Bone alkaline phosphatase, 118, 231
Bone biopsy, 118
Bone marrow aspirate, 338
Branchio-oto-renal syndrome, 187
Bronchiolitis, BP elevation in, 298
Budd-Chiari syndrome, 239

C

Cadmium-induced renal damage, 362
Calcific arteriolopathy, 118
Calcific uremic arteriopathy, 116
Calcific vasculopathy, 230
Calcimimetics, 235
  therapy, 233
Calciphylaxis, 230, 234
Calcitonin therapy, 114
Calcitriol therapy, 103–104
Candida tropicalis, 338
Captopril, 306
Cardiac rhabdomyomas, 204
Caroli disease, 189
Cataract-dental syndrome, 78
Catheter-associated UTI (CAUTI), 379
  diagnosis of, 379
  type of, 379
Caudal dysplasia syndrome, 55–56
Celiac disease, 400–401
Cephalosporins, 392
Cerebrospinal fluid, 398
Cervicitis, 378
CHARGE syndrome, 54, 58
  characteristics of, 58
  hypogonadotropic hypogonadism in, 58
  immune system problems, 58
  kidney abnormalities, 58
  limb abnormalities, 58
  nasal passages, 58
Chediak Higashi syndrome, 338
Chloride-resistant metabolic alkalosis, 317
"Christmas tree" appearance, 248–249
Chronic constipation, 219
Chronic kidney disease (CKD), 107
  alterations in bone and mineral metabolism in, 102
  BP control in, 104
  cardiovascular disease in, 109
  first-line therapy for, 298
  management of pain, 97
  metabolic acidosis in, 103
  prevalence of, 376
  with proteinuria, 298
  risk of progression to ESRD, 104
Chronic Kidney Disease Epidemiology Collaboration equation, 344
Chronic respiratory alkalosis, 125
Clarithromycin, 99
CLCN5 gene, 327
Clear-cell sarcoma, 76
Clonidine, 294
COL4A5 mutation, 198
Computed tomography, 329
Congenital AIDS
  treatment of, 7
Congenital chloride diarrhea (CLD), 160–161
  diagnosis of, 161
  features of, 161
  SLC26A3 gene mutations in, 161
Congenital cytomegalovirus infection, 202
Congenital kidney dysplasia, 230
Congenital mesoblastic nephroma (CMN), 81
Congenital syphilis, 202
Congenital ureter anomalies, 50
Congestive heart failure (CHF), 135
Conorenal syndrome, 251
Continuous renal replacement therapy (CRRT), 89
  benefits of, 90
  in children, 91
  clearance of solute, 91
  daily trauma induced by, 92–93
  extracorporeal circuits, 92
Continuous venovenous hemodialysis filtration (CVVHDF), 89–91
Continuous venovenous hemofiltration (CVVH), 3, 13, 89–90
  replacement solutions in, 90
  therapeutic goal of, 90
Corticosteroids, 349
  therapy, 330–331
Cortinarius poisoning, 32
  prognosis, 32

Costovertebral angle (CVA) tenderness, 377
COVID-19, 335–336
CPT II deficiency in AKI, 19
CPT II deficiency-related rhabdomyolysis, 19, 33–34
diagnosis of, 34
management of, 34
prevention of, 34
primary cause of, 34
C-reactive protein, 334, 343, 361, 396–397
Crescentic fibrillary glomerulonephritis (CFGN), 265
Crescentic glomerulonephritis, 266
Currarino syndrome, 54
Cushing syndrome, 139, 171–172
ACTH-dependent, 172
adrenal causes of, 172
endogenous, 171–173
hypertension in, 171
levels of aldosterone and renin, 148
Cutaneous and uterine leiomyomas, 191
Cyclophosphamide, 221
Cyclosporine, 98–99, 119, 222
CYP24A1 deficiency, 30–31
diagnosis of, 31
genetic testing, 31
management of, 31
vitamin D levels in, 31
Cysteamine, 141
therapy with, 220
Cystic renal cell carcinoma, 159
Cystinosis, 140, 195, 199, 219
pregnant women with, 220
types of, 220
Cystinuria, 214
Cystoscopy, 335
Cytomegalovirus retinitis, 129

D

DASH diet and, 307
Deafness in branchiootorenal syndrome, 188
Deletion 22q11.2 syndrome, 54
Dental enamel hypoplasia, 329–330
Dent disease, 78, 192, 194–195, 199, 214, 221, 327
Denys-Drash syndrome (DDS), 68
Dermatophagoides pteronyssinus, 400–401
Dexamethasone, 143
Diabetes insipidus, 219
Dialysis catheter-related bacteremia, 93
Dietary flavonoids, 148
Dietary phosphorus adequacy, evaluation of, 119
Dietary protein restriction in kidney disease, 105
Diffuse mesangial glomerulosclerosis, 202
Diffuse mesangial sclerosis (DMS), 205
DiGeorge syndrome, 59
medical problems, 59
number and severity of symptoms, 59
Dimercaptosuccinic acid (DMSA)
abnormality, 327
nuclear scan, 388
Dipstick test, 380
Diuretic abuse, 148
Diuretic therapy, 4
side effects of, 4
Dobutamine, 14
Donor kidney transplantation, 98
Dopamine
for prevention/treatment of ATN, 4–5
Drainage tube, 389
Drash syndrome, 204–205
Drug-induced GIN, 339
Drug-induced tubulointerstitial disease, 30
Dry cough, 293
Dysfunctional elimination, 392
Dysplastic kidneys, 207

E

Eagle-Barrett syndrome. *See* Prune belly syndrome
Ectopic ACTH syndrome
dependent Cushing syndrome, 139
diagnosis of, 150
treatment of, 150
Ectopic ureterocele, 50
Ectopic ureters, 50
Edema, 362
Ellis-van Creveld syndrome, 203
E-mediated eosinophil activation, 400–401
Enalapril, 240
Endocarditis-associated glomerulonephritis, 6
End-stage renal disease (ESRD), 223, 311
Enterobacteriaceae, 380, 383
Eosinophils, 345
Eplerenone, 297
Epstein-Barr virus-associated infectious mononucleosis, 341
Erythrocyte membrane disorders, 332
Escherichia coli, 379–380
Esophagogastroduodenoscopy, 347
Essential HTN, 291
Etidronate, 114

F

Facial angiofibromas, 191
Facial dysmorphism, 333
Familial adolescent *NPH-3*, 201
Familial hypomagnesemia hypercalciuria and nephrocalcinosis (FHHNC), 60–63, 72, 192, 214, 241–242
CLDN16 gene expression in, 61, 72
clinical course of, 73
genetic defects in, 63–64
laboratory findings, 71–72
ocular manifestations, 64
oral glucose tolerance test, 73
PTH levels in, 61, 72–73
recurrent urinary tract infections in, 63
treatment of, 64
urinary tract infections and, 61
Familial INPH-1, 201
Familial juvenile hyperuricemic nephropathy, 70–71, 194
causes of, 71

Familial juvenile medullary cystic kidney, 185–186
genetic mutations in, 185–186
Familial juvenile nephronophthisis, 201
Fanconi anemia, 54
Fanconi-Bickel syndrome, 242
Fanconi syndrome, 51–52, 131, 140, 155, 183, 199, 209
diagnosis of cystine crystals, 140–141
inherited renal, 220
photophobia with, 140
Fechtner syndrome, 188
Feingold syndrome, 54
Fenoldopam, 311
Fibroblast growth factor 23 (FGF-23), 120, 233
First-generation cephalosporin, 388
Focal segmental glomerulosclerosis (FSGS), 101–102, 117, 193, 221, 223
causes of, 223
nephrotic syndrome and, 223
steroid-resistant nephrotic syndrome with, 224
types of, 223
Foscarnet, 129
adverse effects of, 129–130
Fractional excretion of urate (FEurate), 126
Frasier syndrome, 68
Fryns syndrome, 54
Full-blown nephrotic syndrome, 221
Furosemide, 8–9, 11–13, 153–154
induced hypovolemia, 14

G

Gadodiamide, 236
omniscan-induced spurious hypocalcemia, 116
Gadolinium, average removal rates of, 94
Galactosemia, 219
Gastroparesis, 336
Genetic focal and segmental glomerulosclerosis, 223
Gentamicin-citrate catheter lock, 93
Gitelman syndrome, 128, 147, 193–194
Glomerular basement membrane (GBM), 221, 330
Glomerular-tubular balance, 2
Glomerulointerstitial nephritis (GIN), 339
Glomerulonephritis, 219
Glucocorticoid-remediable aldosteronism, 194, 201, 296
Glucocorticoids, 119
Glycosylation, congenital disorders of
renal manifestations of, 254
Glycyrrhetinic acid, 143
Gordon syndrome, 193, 200–201
GRADE (Grading of Recommendations, Assessment, Development, and Evaluations) approach, 114–115

H

Hantaviruses, 21–22
Heimler syndrome, 49
Hematuria, gross, 226
Hemodialysis, 229
average removal rates of gadolinium in, 94
cefazolin therapy, 96
mupirocin ointment therapy, 96
ultrafiltration strategy in reducing intradialytic hypotension, 96–97
weekly dialysis treatment, 96
Hemolytic uremic syndrome (HUS), 99
Hemorrhagic fever with renal syndrome, 21–22
Hemorrhagic interstitial nephritis, 36–37
Henderson-Hasselbach equation, 138
Henoch-Schönlein purpura, 40, 229
Hepatorenal syndrome, 8, 10, 15
AKI resulting from, 11
Hepatosplenomegaly, 166
Hereditary nephrotic syndrome (NPHS) 1, 255
Hereditary osteo-onycho-dysplasia, 252
Hereditary spherocytosis, 332
Hereditary vitamin D-resistant rickets (HVDRR), 186
Hexadactyly, 197
High-grade reflux, 375
Hinman syndrome, 75
HIV-associated nephritis (HIVAN)
features of, 227
kidney biopsy for, 227
HIV infection
active antiretroviral therapy, 5
HIV seropositive, 227
HLA-B27 ankylosing spondylitis, 69
Horseshoe kidney, 208
Hydralazine, 310
Hydrochlorothiazide, 73, 193, 299, 301
Hydronephrosis, 51, 82, 208, 375, 378, 386
cause of, 245
severity of, 51
Hyperactivation of RAA system, 314
Hypercalcemia, 31, 118
cause of, 325
vitamin D intoxication and, 166–167
Hyperchloremic metabolic acidosis, 195
Hypericum perforatum, 361
Hyperkalemia, 162
Hyperoxaluria, 28
accumulation of oxalate, 28
autoimmune antibody testing, 28
calcium and magnesium salts in, 28
dietary, 28
enteric, 28
treatment of, 28
urinalysis, 28
Hyperphosphatemia, 117–118, 231
prevention of, 232
Hyperphosphaturia, pathogenesis of, 120
Hypertension (HTN)
causes of, 302–303, 315, 319
essential, 291
factors contributing to development of, 297
gestational (preeclampsia), 319
imaging of, 310
impact on systolic BP, 292

Hypertension (HTN) *(Continued)*
lifestyle modification for managing, 303
management of, 294, 313
mild, 305
nonpharmacological interventions, 292
paroxysmal, 291
renovascular, 291
resistant, 297, 299
stage II, 300
treatment-resistant, 293
Hypocalcemia, 132
Hypoglycemia, 2
Hypokalemia, 139, 143, 149, 155, 313, 316
anion gap in, 144
diagnosis of, 142–143
evaluation of, 146
plasma aldosterone concentration in, 147
plasma aldosterone levels and PRA in, 143
plasma renin activity in, 147
Hypokalemic periodic paralysis (HypoPP), 145, 152, 164
treatment of, 165
Hypomagnesemia, 148
Hyponatremia, 125–126, 135
causes, 136–137
in SIADH, 137
Hypoparathyroidism, 329–330
Hypovolemia, 169
Hypoxanthine-guanine-phosphoribosyl-transferase, 205–206
deficiency, 70, 249–250
test, 25

I

Ibuprofen, 33, 155–156
Idiopathic membranous glomerulopathy, clinicopathologic diagnosis of, 224
Idiopathic nephrotic syndrome, 222, 228
kidney biopsy and, 223
treatment plan in patients, 223
IgA nephropathy, 39, 60, 101, 112–113
IgG4-related disease, 270, 336
IgG4-related sclerosing disease, 278
Immune complex-mediated membranoproliferative glomerulonephritis (IC-MPGN), 243
Immunologic diseases, 351
Indinavir, 5, 7
Infantile polycystic kidney disease, 204
Infantile Refsum disease, 49
Infectious Diseases Society of America, 379
Inflammatory bowel disease, 353
Inflammatory cells, 380
Inherited distal renal tubular acidosis (RTA), 194
International Study of Kidney Disease in Children, guidelines from, 222
Intradialytic hypotension, 96–97
Intrathoracic mass, investigation of, 65–66
Intravenous urography, 360
Ischemic acute tubular necrosis, treatment of, 4–5, 10
Isolated proximal RTA from *SLC4A4* mutations, 200
Ivemark syndrome, 203

J

Jaffe reaction, 2
Jeune syndrome, 203
nature and degree of renal involvement, 203
Joubert syndrome (JS), 53, 55, 206, 331
basal body genes mutations in, 53
ciliary disorders and, 53
treatment of, 53, 207
types of renal disease, 53
Juvenile hyperuricemic nephropathy, 250

K

Kallmann syndrome, 157
Kawasaki disease (KD), 26, 38
BUN levels, 26
coronary abnormalities, 27
features, 27
renal complications, 27
renal function, 26
respiratory symptoms, 39
serum creatinine level, 26
treatment of, 39
Ketoacidosis, 144
Ketoconazole, 150
Kidney biopsy, 350
Kidney Disease: Improving Global Outcomes (KDIGO), guidelines from, 222
Kidney dysplasia, 103
therapy for, 103–104
Kidney stones, 208, 355
Kidney transplantation, 184
Klebsiella pneumoniae, 390
Kossa stain, 357

L

Lactate-based replacement fluids, 90
L-carnitine, 95
Left ventricular hypertrophy, 104–105
Lesch-Nyhan syndrome, 25, 205–206
Leukocyte esterase, 380
Leukocytosis, 21
Licorice, 143
Liddle syndrome, 133, 147, 193–194, 313
diagnosis of, 200
levels of aldosterone and renin, 148
response to amiloride, 149
treatment of, 134
Light chain cast nephropathy (LCCN), 30
Lipopolysaccharide (LPS) endotoxins, 398
Long-chain fatty acids (LCFAs), 20
Loop diuretics, 3–4
Lowe syndrome, 77–78, 194–195, 199, 208–209, 327
cataracts in, 77
developmental and intellectual disabilities, 77–78

Lowe syndrome *(Continued)*
kidney and brain abnormalities, 77, 209
signs of, 78, 209
X-linked recessive trait, 77
Low-molecular-weight proteinuria, 327
Lupus nephritis, 225, 258
class V, 226
immunosuppressive therapy in patients with, 225
treatment of, 226
Lymphadenopathy, 166–167
Lymphangioleiomyomatosis, 188
LYST gene, 338

M

Magnetic resonance angiography, 310
Magnetic resonance imaging, 329
Mainzer-Saldino syndrome, 251
Malignant teratoma, 64–65
Mannitol, 13
McArdle disease, 20
Meacham syndrome, 68
Meckel-Gruber syndrome, 52
Meckel syndrome, 55, 206
Medullary cystic kidney disease (MCKD), 196
type 2, 70, 194
Medullary sponge kidneys (MSK)
distal RTA in, 152
history of, 151
laboratory investigations in, 151–152
medullary nephrocalcinosis in, 153
physical examination, 151
transtubular potassium gradient, 151–153
Membranoproliferative glomerulonephritis (MPGN)
proteinuria and, 228
treatment of, 228
Membranous glomerulonephritis, 247
Membranous nephropathy, 247
Metabolic acidosis, 165
H^+ value, 138
pCO_2 in, 138
Metabolic alkalosis, 137, 139, 313
urine chloride concentration in, 316
Metabolic diseases, 220
Methyldopa, 306
Methylprednisolone, 112
Microscopic hematuria, 226
renal biopsy and, 227
Microscopic urine evaluation, 385
Midodrine, 15
Minimal change disease (MCD), 221
Minoxidil, 306
Mixed connective tissue disease (MCTD), 268
Multicystic nephroma, 62, 159
Multilocular cystic nephroma, 159
MURCS association, 54
Mushroom poisoning, 32
Myalgias, 230
Mycobacterium tuberculosis, 346
Mycophenolate mofetil (MMF), 98
association with leukopenia and anemia, 100
side effects of, 100
Myoglobinuric ARF, 3

N

Nail-patella-like glomerulopathy, 252
Nail-patella syndrome, 188
Nance-Horan syndrome, 78
Neonatal jaundice, 397
Neonates with bilateral renal agenesis, 49–50
Nephrogenic diabetes insipidus (NDI), 82–83, 167
complication of, 82
diagnostic tests for, 82
ectopic ACTH syndrome, resulting from, 150
Nephropathic cystinosis, treatment of, 141
Nephrotic syndrome, 227
Neurogenic bladder, 157, 248–249
Newborn with unilateral renal agenesis
kidney development in, 49
symptoms, 50
Nitrite, 380
Non-parathyroid-related hypercalcemia, 31
Nonsteroidal antiinflammatory drugs (NSAIDs), 328
NPHS2 mutation, 198
NSAIDs
analgesic nephropathy, risk of, 97
for chronic kidney disease, 97
Nutcracker syndrome, 69, 246

O

Obstructive uropathy, 162, 377
Octreotide, 15
Oculoauriculo-vertebral syndrome, 54
Oligohydramnios, 68
Oncogenic osteomalacia, 130–131, 183
Oral candidiasis, 329–330
Orellanus syndrome, 32

P

PAC/PRA ratio, 295
Pallister-Hall syndrome, 54
Pamidronate, 114
Pancreatic neuroendocrine tumor, 171–173
Paragangliomas, 315–316
Parathyroidectomy, 115, 118, 231–232, 235
Paroxysmal cold hemoglobinuria (PCH), 23–24
laboratory testing, 23
Paroxysmal HTN, 291
Partial hypoxanthine-guanine phosphoribosyltransferase deficiency, 70
Parvovirus B19 infection, 23
Pauci-immune CrGN, 268
Percutaneous endoscopic gastrostomy tube placement, 388–389
Percutaneous radiofrequency ablation, 296
Percutaneous transluminal renal angioplasty (PTRA), 301–302

Persistent hypercalciuria, 329
PHA type I and II, 162–163
Pheochromocytomas, 291–292, 315–316
Phosphatonin, 236
Pierre Robin syndrome, 47
PKHD1 gene mutations, 189
Plasma aldosterone to renin ratio, 307
Plasma cortisol measurement, 148
Platelet-derived growth factor receptor alpha (PDGFRA), 338
Pneumocystis pneumonia, 100
Polycystic kidney disease (PKD), 106
Polydactyly, 55
Polymerase chain reaction (PCR), 346
Polyuria, 149–150, 172
Positive end-expiratory pressure (PEEP), 11–12
Postinfectious glomerulonephritis, 261, 274–275
Posttransplant lymphoproliferative disease (PTLD), 100–101
  Epstein Barr virus associated, 101
Potassium chloride, 170
Prednisone, 222
Prenatal ultrasonography, 377
Primary aldosteronism, 295
Primary focal and segmental glomerulosclerosis, 223
Primary hyperaldosteronism, 147, 294–295
Primary hyperoxaluria, 214
  type 2, 191–192
Probiotics, 377
Procalcitonin, 334
Procollagen-carboxy-terminal propeptide, 118, 231
Progressive kidney failure, 105–106
Prophylactic antibiotics, 387
Propofol infusion syndrome, 17
Propranolol, 145, 301–302
Protein electrophoresis, 347
Proteinuria, 204, 224
Proteus mirabilis, 357–358, 393
Proton pump inhibitors, 347
Proximal renal collecting system, 375
Proximal RTA, 155
Prune belly syndrome, 47
  cause of, 48
  mortality rate, 48
  organs affected in, 47
  prognosis of, 47–48
Pulmonary hypoplasia, 52
Pyelonephritis, 378, 381, 388, 391
Pyuria, 380

Q

QT dispersion, 95

R

Radionuclide scintigraphy with iodocholesterol, 296
Rapidly progressive glomerulonephritis (RPGN), 112
  associated with postinfectious glomerulonephritis, 112
Reinfections, 384
Relapse, 395
Renal
  abscesses, 381
  artery stenosis, 291
  biopsy, 222
  cell carcinoma, 76
  Fanconi syndrome, 78
  function, 376
  parenchymal defects, 387
Renal cysts and diabetes (RCAD) syndrome, 74
Renal lymphangiectasia, 317–318
Renal lymphangiomatosis, 80
  diagnosis of, 80
  treatment of, 80
Renal phosphate wasting, 119, 236
Renal replacement therapy (RRT), 3
  chronic, 3, 9, 12, 16
  CVVH method, 15–16
  modalities of, 3, 12
  timing of, 4
Renal transplantation from adopted sibling, 59–60
  genetic risks, 60
  IgA nephropathy after, 60
Renal tubular acidosis, type 1, 154
  acute onset of, 155–156
  associated acid-base disturbance, 155
  blood pressure in, 155
  urine ammonium in, 155
Renal vein thrombosis, 239
Renin, 319
Renin-angiotensin-aldosterone (RAA) axis, 294–295
Reninomas, 319
Renin-secreting tumor, 141–142
  captopril test for, 142
Renovascular HTN, 291
Repeat culture, 388
Reset hypernatremia, 127
Reset hyponatremia renal salt wasting, 136
Residual urine volume, 387
Respiratory alkalosis, 137
Retinal hemangioblastomas, 191
Rhabdoid tumors, 76
Rhabdomyolysis, 2, 33, 229
  CPT II deficiency-related. *See* CPT II deficiency-related rhabdomyolysis
  creatine kinase level, 18–19
  induced AKI, 19
  laboratory investigations, 19
Rheumatoid arthritis (RA), 243
Rituximab, 224
Routine blood tests, 399

S

Sacrococcygeal teratoma, 65
Saline hyperhydration, 169
Sarcoidosis, 168, 336
SARS-CoV-2 infection, 352
Schimke immunoosseous dysplasia (SIOD), 240

Schirmer test, 244
Secondary (reactive) eosinophilia, 337–338
Secondary focal and segmental glomerulosclerosis, 223
Secukinumab, 346
Segmental multicystic dysplastic kidney disease, 62, 159
Selepressin, 8, 11
Septic shock, diagnosis of, 1
Sevelamer hydrochloride, 117, 230
Sexually transmitted pathogens, 384
Short rib syndrome, 54
Sialidosis, 257
Signet ring cell carcinoma (SRCC), 245
Simultaneous kidney-pancreas (SKP) transplantation, 98
Sirolimus-related pneumonitis, 99
Sjögren syndrome, 140, 164, 336, 341, 351
  criteria for diagnosing, 165
  primary manifestation of, 164
Skin cancers, 98
Sleep apnea, 309
Slit-lamp eye examination, 219
Smith-Lemli-Opitz syndrome, 78
Sodium-loading test, 295
Sodium nitroprusside, 306
Somatostatin receptor type 2 (SSTR2), 319
Spironolactone therapy, 143, 293, 299
Spondylometaphyseal dysplasia, 240
Spot urine protein-to-creatinine ratio, 108–109
Staphylococcus aureus, 394
Staphylococcus saprophyticus, 383
Stenting of left renal artery, 308–309
Steroid-resistant nephrotic syndrome, 221
Steroid-sensitive idiopathic nephrotic syndrome, 221
Steroid therapy, 234, 348
Streptococcus viridians endocarditis, 6
Syndrome of apparent mineralocorticoid excess (AME), 145, 147
  mechanism of, 149
Syndrome of inappropriate antidiuretic hormone secretion (SIADH), 134
  diagnosis between RSW and, 136
  diagnostic criteria for, 134–135
  etiology of, 158
  euvolemic hyponatremia and, 158
  hyponatremia in, 137
  hypo-osmolality in, 158
Syphilis, sarcoidosis, 341
Systemic lupus erythematosus, 225, 239, 336
  laboratory evaluation, 225

T

Tacrolimus, 99
  for posttransplantation anemia, 100
Tamm-Horsfall protein, 194
Tanner sexual maturity rating, 339
Tenofovir, 7
Thiazide diuretic, 303
Thiazides, 301
Thoracopelvic dysplasia, 203
Throat swabs, 360
Thyroid-stimulating hormone, 397
TINU syndrome, 353
  pathogenesis of, 343
  T-cell tolerance, 343
Tobacco smoking, 307
TORCH titers, 397
Townes-Brocks syndrome, 54
Transtubular potassium gradient, 151–153, 162, 313–314
Triamterene, 296
Trimethoprim-sulfamethoxazole, 7, 391
Trisomy 13, 213
Trisomy 18, 208, 213
Trisomy 21, 213
Tuberosclerosis, 204
Tuberous sclerosis complex (TSC), 187–188
  genetic mutations, 188
  manifestations of, 188
Tubulointerstitial disease, 102, 325, 350, 363
  biomarkers, 351
Tubulointerstitial nephritis, 39, 345, 349, 365
Tumor-induced osteomalacia (TIO), 131
  diagnosis of, 131
Tumor lysis syndrome, 229
Tumor of juxtaglomerular apparatus (TJGA), 141–142
Turner syndrome, 208

U

Ultrasonography, 338
Uncomplicated infection, 379
Unilateral multiocular dysplastic kidney, 62
Unilateral renal cystic disease, 62
Upper tract signs, 381
Ureaplasma, 381
Urea-splitting organism, 381
Uremic peripheral neuropathy, 230
Ureteropelvic junction (UPJ) obstruction, 50
  indications for surgical treatment, 52
  surgical complications of, 50–52
Urinalysis, 335, 348
Urinary albumin/creatinine ratios, 326
Urinary beta-2 excretion, validity of, 2
  fractional excretion, 2
Urinary biomarker, 1
Urinary catheters, 335–336, 379
Urinary microalbumin, 227
Urinary potassium-creatinine ratio value, 147
Urinary potassium excretion, evaluation of, 146
Urinary tract infections (UTIs), 156, 335, 375, 378–379, 399
  complications of, 381
  gold-standard diagnostic tool for, 381
  grade of, 375
  laboratory evaluation, 380
  laboratory tools, 380
  modifiable risk factors for, 382
  preventive measures, 385
  recurrence, 386

Urinary tract infections (UTIs) *(Continued)*
risk factor for recurrent, 393
uncomplicated infection, 375
Urine
culture, 381, 389
dipstick studies, 380
dipstick test, 387
dye-related urine discoloration, 335
greenish discoloration of, 335
Urolithiasis, 333, 357
US-guided kidney biopsy, 338
Uterine leiomyosarcomas, 191
Uveitis, 341–342

V
VACTER-L syndrome
anomalies, 53–54
with hydrocephalus, 54
Vaginal discharge, 378
Vaginitis, 378, 393
Vesicoureteral reflux, 50, 375–376
bilateral reflux of urine, 376
degree of, 376
diagnosis of, 376
high grades of, 377
severity of, 376
treatment of, 376
unilateral reflux of urine, 376
Vitamin D deficiency, 132–133, 183
Voiding cystourethrogram (VCUG), 51, 75
examination, 376
von Hippel-Lindau syndrome, 190–191, 292
von Willebrand factor-cleaving protease (vWF-CP) activity, 197

W
Weekly dialysis treatment, 96
Wegener's granulomatosis, 237
Wells syndrome, 337
White cell cystine, 326
Wilms tumor, 68, 76, 159, 202
signs and symptoms, 76
Wilson disease, 219, 246

X
Xanthine renal stones, 333
Xanthogranulomatous pyelonephritis (XP), 76
disease, 79
laboratory tests, 79
management of, 79
unilateral and diffuse types of, 79
X-linked
Alport syndrome, 189, 198
hypophosphatemic rickets, 130, 184
recessive hypophosphatemic rickets, 327
recessive nephrolithiasis, 327

Z
Zellweger spectrum disorders (ZSDs), 210
Zellweger syndrome (ZS), 48–49, 78
PEX gene expression, 49
symptoms of, 49
treatment of, 49
Zidovudine, 7
side effects of, 3
Ziehl-Neelsen stain, 339
Zoledronic acid, 114

Pediatric Kidney Disease

A CASE-BASED APPROACH

Farahnak Assadi, MD

More than 400 true-to-life cases studies in pediatric kidney disease offer a unique opportunity for self-assessment and review.

An ideal resource for specialists and non-specialist clinicians and trainees, *Pediatric Kidney Disease: A Case-Based Approach* contains more than 400 case reports that offer **a unique learning opportunity** in this challenging field. These **accessible and instructive case studies** help readers **recognize important clinical symptoms and signs** to develop the diagnostic and management skills needed for treating patients in a routine clinical practice. With wide-ranging coverage of the kidney-related complaints most likely to be encountered, this volume is **an excellent reference or certification review tool** for residents, fellows, and clinicians who need quick access to current scientific and clinical information on managing pediatric kidney disease.

- Provides **complete, state-of-the art reviews and assessments** of kidney disease in children in a concise, templated format.
- Presents **more than 400 cases** covering acute and chronic kidney failures, congenital and hereditary kidney diseases, glomerular and vascular diseases, hereditary kidney disorders, hypertension, tubulointerstitial diseases, and urinary tract infections.
- Each case begins with a succinct summary of patient's history, signs and symptoms, examinations, and initial investigations, followed by questions and answers.
- Provides answers and comments that offer a **detailed discussion on each topic,** with further case references where appropriate.
- **An eBook version is included with purchase.** The eBook allows you to access all of the text, figures, and references, with the ability to search, customize your content, make notes and highlights, and have content read aloud.

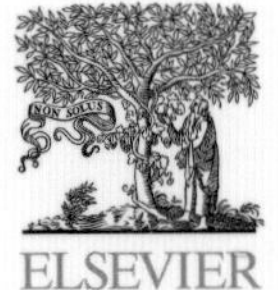

elsevierhealth.com

Take learning to the next level with access to digital content through any device.

Features include:

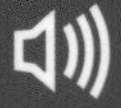

Read Aloud

Customizable Layout

Search Your Entire Library

10 Highlighter Colors

See inside front cover for access information.

Recommended Shelving Classifications
Nephrology
Pediatrics

ISBN 978-0-443-28337-6
9 780443 283376